GLOBAL CLIMATE CHANGE AND HUMAN HEALTH

GLOBAL CLIMATE CHANGE AND HUMAN HEALTH

FROM SCIENCE TO PRACTICE

George Luber

Jay Lemery

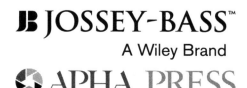

JB JOSSEY-BASS™

A Wiley Brand

APHA PRESS

AN IMPRINT OF **AMERICAN PUBLIC HEALTH ASSOCIATION**

Published by Jossey-Bass
A Wiley Brand
One Montgomery Street, Suite 1000, San Francisco, CA 94104-4594—www.josseybass.com

Jossey-Bass books and products are available through most bookstores. To contact Jossey-Bass directly call
our Customer Care Department within the U.S. at 800-956-7739, outside the U.S. at 317-572-3986, or fax
317-572-4002.

Wiley publishes in a variety of print and electronic formats and by print-on-demand. Some material included
with standard print versions of this book may not be included in e-books or in print-on-demand. If this book
refers to media such as a CD or DVD that is not included in the version you purchased, you may download this
material at http://booksupport.wiley.com. For more information about Wiley products, visit www.wiley.com.

Library of Congress Cataloging-in-Publication Data

Luber, George, editor.
  Global climate change and human health : from science to practice / George Luber, Jay Lemery.
    pages cm
  Includes index.
    ISBN 978-1-118-50557-1 (pbk.) – ISBN 978-1-118-60358-1 (epub) – ISBN 978-1-118-50557-1 (pbk.)

    1. Climatic changes—Health aspects.   2. Global warming—Health aspects.   3. Environmental
  health. I. Lemery, Jay, editor. II. Title.

  RA793.L83 2015
  615.9'02—dc23
                    2015018120

Printed in the United States of America

FIRST EDITION

PB Printing   10 9 8 7 6 5 4 3 2 1

CONTENTS

Part 1: Our Changing Planet: Emergent Risks for Human Health 1

Chapter 1 Primer on Climate Science 3

Christopher K. Uejio, James D. Tamerius, Karen Wertz, Katie M. Konchar

Chapter 2 Extreme Weather Events: The Role of Public Health in Disaster Risk Reduction as a Means for Climate Change Adaptation 35

Mark E. Keim

Chapter 3 Extreme and Changing Meteorological Conditions on the Human Health Condition 77

Daniel P. Johnson, Austin C. Stanforth, Kavya Urs Beerval

Chapter 8 Climate and Its Impacts on Vector-Borne and Zoonotic Diseases **221**

Charles B. Beard, Jada F. Garofalo, Kenneth L. Gage

Chapter 9 Addressing the Challenges of Climate Change to Food Security, Safety, and Nutrition **267**

Cristina Tirado

Chapter 10 Climate Change and Population Mental Health . . . **311**

Abdulrahman M. El-Sayed, Sandro Galea

Chapter 11 Improving the Surveillance of Climate-Sensitive Diseases **335**

*Pierre Gosselin, Diane Bélanger, Mathilde Pascal,
Philippe Pirard, Christovam Barcellos*

I have many people to thank for the privilege and opportunity to spend my days working on such an important issue. This book is dedicated to all of those who have shared their wisdom, offered mentorship, gave opportunity, and provided support, especially my mother, Maureen Ward; my mentors: Elois Ann and Brent Berlin, Carol Rubin, and Mike McGeehin; and of course, to my wife, Holly, and our sons, Lucas, Gustav, and Axel, for all of their support and love.

George Luber

*   *   *

To the educators of the Glens Falls, New York School District—may you continue to inspire; and of course, to my girls, Maeve and Zada, and my loving wife, Taryn.

Jay Lemery

Throughout history, the sky has served as a metaphor for the vast, wide open, and endless horizons. The notion that humans could in some way alter this vast expanse would have been unimaginable. It was not until our explorations into space in the 1960s that this notion began to be challenged. The first astronauts to leave the Earth reported that the atmosphere looked like a "thin blue line" in contrast to the enormous mass of the planet. Their eyes were not deceived; the atmosphere that envelops the Earth is thin—so thin that if the Earth were shrunk down to the size of a desktop globe, one would need only a sheet of plastic wrap to approximate the thickness of the atmosphere. The atmosphere is a mere sixty miles thick, compared with the eight-thousand-mile diameter of the Earth.

Following the publication of the first images from Earth's orbit, the widely held notion that the atmosphere is too vast to alter in any meaningful way was begun to be challenged by direct observational evidence. Meticulous measurements by Charles Keeling at the National Oceanic and Atmospheric Administration's (NOAA) Mauna Loa Observatory, beginning in 1956 and uninterrupted to date, have provided clear documentation of the year-on-year rise in global atmospheric carbon dioxide (CO_2) levels, providing crucial observational evidence that the chemistry of the atmosphere is changing (figure I.1).

This change is substantial. At the start of the Industrial Revolution, it has been estimated that the globally averaged concentration of CO_2 in our atmosphere was around 280 parts per million (ppm). By 1956 it was close to 320 ppm, and in the intervening fifty years, this level has risen to over 400 ppm, principally as a result of the burning of fossil fuels and land use and land cover changes.

Among its many properties, the atmosphere serves to help keep the surface of the Earth warm enough to sustain life. This is possible through the greenhouse effect in which the atmosphere allows solar radiation to pass through, generally unchanged, and trapping some of the outgoing infrared radiation that is emitted from the Earth's surface. The balance between incoming and outgoing energy is critical to maintaining some type of energy/temperature equilibrium at the Earth's surface. When this energy balance is altered, through an increase in inputs (solar energy) into the system or changes

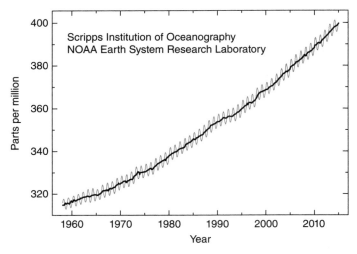

Figure I.1   Atmospheric Carbon Dioxide at Mauna Loa
Scripps Institution of Oceanography (scrippsco2.ucsd.edu/).

in Earth's atmospheric composition that alter how much of this incoming energy is captured (either naturally by volcanic emissions, or human activities such as the burning of fossil fuels or through land cover changes), changes in the Earth's surface temperature, and in turn its climate become evident.

Documenting and assessing the evidence for these potential changes in the Earth's climate system is the job of the Intergovernmental Panel on Climate Change (IPCC), a selected volunteer group of experts in the numerous disciplines and sectors with a perspective on climate change. One of the IPCC's main purpose is to undertake a periodic assessment every seven years to review and summarize the strength of the evidence around climate change, including the physical science basis and evidence, impacts in numerous sectors (e.g., agriculture, water, energy, public health), and regional impacts.

The Fourth Assessment Report of the IPCC was a landmark document and worthy of receiving the Nobel Peace Prize, not least for stating unequivocally that the Earth's climate is changing and that humans are principally responsible (IPCC 2007). This, and subsequent IPCC reports (IPCC 2012, 2013), have strengthened the evidence base on human-induced climate change. These reports have not only highlighted the complexities and magnitude of the climate change problem, but they have provided a solid evidence and rationale for action on a number of fronts. What they have concluded is that the global effects of climate change are already apparent from numerous observations of the destabilization of natural systems. These impacts include the melting and degradation of continental ice caps and glaciers, the warming and acidification of oceans, rising sea levels, an increase in frost-free days, and, not least, increases in extreme weather events such as heat waves, heavy rainfall events, drought, high storm surge, and tropical cyclones.

We can also expect substantial regional differences in the type and magnitude of these impacts. Some regions will become wetter, some dryer, and some will see no change. Consider this: the Third US National Climate Assessment reported that Grand Junction, Colorado, has warmed 3.2°F over the past century, while parts of southern Alabama actually cooled, dropping 0.6°F in the same time period (Melillo et al. 2014).

At an increasing rate, evidence is accumulating that the health threats of climate change are already affecting communities across the globe. From the direct effects of weather extremes on morbidity and mortality to the potential for profound changes in disease ecology and geography brought about by state shifts in the Earth's system, climate change will be the defining issue for public health in this century (Chan 2008).

Climate change poses to threaten health in a variety of ways. Most of the health threats of climate change that have been identified are not new ones; injury and death from heat waves and extreme weather events; reduced air quality from ozone, aeroallergens, and wildfire smoke; and from illnesses transmitted by food, water, and disease carriers such as mosquitoes and ticks. These health threats have always been with us, taking advantage of weaknesses and vulnerabilities in certain parts of our communities, particularly the young, old, the sick, economically disadvantaged, and culturally marginalized (Luber et al. 2014). For these groups, climate change represents yet another, perhaps more powerful, threat to their health and well-being.

Climate change will also threaten the critical systems and infrastructure we rely on to keep us safe and healthy: communication and transportation during emergencies, food and water systems during drought, the energy grid during prolonged heat waves. As the magnitude and frequency of extreme weather events increase, the resilience of these systems will be tested, and vulnerabilities will become more exposed. It is in this sense that climate change will serve as "risk multiplier" by amplifying both the exposures that bring about health risks and highlighting the vulnerabilities to these exposures as well.

In developing a global picture of the health impacts of climate change, it is important to acknowledge that these health impacts will differ substantially by location and pathway of exposure. These differences can be thought of as a function of the attributes of the population that confer vulnerability (the old and young, the prevalence of comorbidities, socioeconomic status), attributes of place that mediate exposure (floodplain, coastal zone, urban heat island), as well as the adaptive capacity of public health and associated infrastructure that helps maintain access to clean food and water and public health preparedness decisions that have been made in advance.

The picture is complicated, to say the least. Disentangling all of these interactions is a difficult task, requiring the expertise and perspectives of many disciplines. The purpose of this book is to bring together, in a single volume, these various perspectives—theoretical, methodological, and disciplinary—that should be brought to bear on such a critical challenge. In order to educate and empower the next generation of students and scientists to address this challenge, the four parts of this book span a science-to-practice continuum that promotes an evidence-based approach to public health practice and decision making.

Part 1, "Our Changing Planet: Emergent Risks for Human Health," begins with an overview primer on climate science, with attention to relevant concepts for public health. The next two chapters summarize the various climate-related meteorological hazards and exposures that will increasingly become emergent risks for human health.

Part 2, "The Health Consequences of Climate Change," focuses more closely on specific exposure pathways that will be altered with climate change and reviews the evidence base for the various health impacts of climate change, including waterborne disease, respiratory impacts from ozone, emissions, aeroallergens, harmful algal blooms, vector-borne and zoonotic disease, nutritional impacts, and mental health.

In Part 3, "The Public Health Approach to Climate Change," the focus turns to a discussion of the practice dimension of this book. It details the various public health strategies and approaches that are already being developed to prepare for climate change. The authors cover a wide variety of practical and methodological approaches to climate change and health assessments including public health surveillance for climate change, conducting vulnerability assessments, and modeling future health impacts. The part concludes with three chapters that describe important concepts to consider from a public health perspective: adopting a community-based approach, environmental justice as a critical dimension of risk, and the importance of communication approaches as agents of change.

Part 4, "Taking Action: Adaptation, Mitigation, and Governance," turns to an action-oriented perspective, outlining the various efforts and strategies that have been developed so far to tackle the enormous challenge of climate change. Emissions trajectories tell us that some warming is unavoidable and we must adapt. The how and why of such an endeavor is presented in the first chapter in this part before turning attention to tackling the root cause of the climate change crisis: increased emissions. This discussion focuses on a strategy to promote these mitigation efforts by seizing on the dual benefits, for both health and emissions, of certain strategies. Under-pinning both adaptation and mitigation efforts is the governance structure that allows, or prevents, this from happening, and the various institutional and governance requirements for this to indeed happen are discussed. And the last chapter explores issues of climate justice and the likelihood that the most vulnerable among us will bear the heaviest burdens of climate change.

We have included pedagogical elements to facilitate both learning and instruction. Key terms and a comprehensive glossary introduce and rein-force the lexicon of this field. Key concepts and discussion questions will keep the learner oriented to the big picture messages throughout the chap-ters. To facilitate educators, we have provided visual presentation materials (PowerPoint) to complement each lecture. And finally, because this book topic straddles both public health and clinical medicine, we have provided "Clinical Correlates" sections in each chapter to facilitate understanding and discussion of the health impacts that will face individual care providers.

We consider this last point to be a significant differentiator for our book—that this text will be relevant for both MPH and MD/DO students. So much of the intransigence of policymakers worldwide is due to a lack of clear risk assessment of the insidious and often abstract threat of climate change. And when one compounds this with the fact that cutting-edge sci-ence by its very nature is uncertain, tough decisions related to climate or energy policy are easily undercut by a fear of commitment to any particular course of action, leaving inertia as the best rational choice.

This is where you come in as a science educator. Those of us in public health and clinical medicine are ideal interlocutors, society's go-betweens in translating abstract medical science into plans for healthy living. Research in social science supports that risks identified in terms of human life, such as "your mother's risk of cancer" or "your child's risk of asthma," are much more effective fulcrums for change than abstract concepts. This is our hope for the book: to empower you with the knowledge to explain sci-ence in terms of health risks that can be readily understood and to be part of a movement to elevate public discourse to a more accurate assessment of risks and benefits. This is how meaningful change can occur and how we may have a chance to bequeath to our children a planet with a safe environ-ment and stable climate.

An instructor's supplement is available at www.wiley.com/go/luber. Additional materials such as videos, podcasts, and readings can be found at www.josseybasspublichealth.com. Comments about this book are invited and can be sent to publichealth@wiley.com.

References

Chan, M. 2008. "The Impact of Climate Change on Human Health." April 7.

IPCC. 2007. *Climate Change 2007: The Physical Science Basis. Contribution of Working Group I to the Fourth Assessment Report of the Intergovernmental Panel on Climate Change*, edited by S. Solomon,, D. Qin, M. Manning, Z. Chen, M. Marquis, K.B. Averyt, M. Tignor, and H. L. Miller. Cambridge: Cambridge University Press.

IPCC. 2012. *Managing the Risks of Extreme Events and Disasters to Advance Climate Change Adaptation. A Special Report of Working Groups I and II of the Intergovernmental Panel on Climate Change*, edited by C. B. Field, V. Barros, T. F. Stocker, D. Qin, D. J. Dokken, K. L. Ebi, M. D. Mastrandrea, et al. Cambridge: Cambridge University Press.

IPCC. 2013. *Climate Change 2013: The Physical Science Basis. Contribution of Working Group I to the Fifth Assessment Report of the Intergovernmental Panel on Climate Change*, edited by T. F. Stocker, D. Qin, G.-K. Plattner, M. Tignor, S. K. Allen, J. Boschung, A. Nauels, et al. Cambridge: Cambridge University Press.

Luber, G., K. Knowlton, J. Balbus, H. Frumkin, M. Hayden, J. Hess, M. McGeehin, et al. 2014. "Human Health." *Climate Change Impacts in the United States: The Third National Climate Assessment*, edited by J. M. Melillo, T. Richmond, and G. W. Yohe,, 220-256. Washington DC U.S. Global Change Research Program.

Melillo, J. M., T. Richmond, and G. W. Yohe, eds. 2014. *Climate Change Impacts in the United States: The Third National Climate Assessment*. Washington DC U.S. Global Change Research Program.

ACKNOWLEDGMENTS

We thank the "Clinical Correlates" editor, Cecilia Sorenson, MD; and editorial assistants Amanda Bond, Marisa Burton, Danika Evans, Sabrina Geer, DVM, Katharine Joy, and Amita Kulkarni. We also thank the Educational Materials editor, Carolyn Meyer, MD; and educational assistants Gavriel Roda and Rachel VanderWel. We are also indebted to proposal reviewers Kristie L. Ebi, Paul S. Auerbach, and Damon Chaky who provided valuable feedback on the original book proposal. Edward Avol, Qinghua Sun, Justin Remais, and Ivan Ramirez provided thoughtful and constructive comments on the complete draft manuscript.

George Luber is a Medical Anthropologist and Chief of the Climate and Health Program at the National Center for Environmental Health, Centers for Disease Control and Prevention (CDC). Since receiving his PhD in Medical Anthropology from the University of Georgia and joining CDC in 2002, he has served as an Epidemic Intelligence Service (EIS) officer and senior health scientist.

In addition to managing the Climate and Health Program at CDC, Luber is a cochair of the Climate Change and Human Health Workgroup at the US Global Change Research Program, a member of the American Anthropological Association's Presidential Task Force on Climate Change, a convening lead author for the Third US National Climate Assessment, and a lead author for the Fifth Assessment Report of the Intergovernmental Panel on Climate Change. In 2015, Luber was profiled on the Weather Channel's *Climate 25*. He is also adjunct professor in the Departments of Environmental Health, Anthropology, and Environmental Science at Emory University.

The findings and conclusions in this report are my own and do not necessarily represent the views of the Centers for Disease Control and Prevention/Agency for Toxic Substances and Disease Registry.

*　　*　　*

Jay Lemery is an Associate Professor of Emergency Medicine at the University of Colorado School of Medicine and is Chief of the Section of Wilderness and Environmental Medicine. He is the immediate past-President of the Wilderness Medical Society and is currently the EMS medical director for the US Antarctic Program. Lemery serves as a consultant for the Climate and Health Program at the Centers for Disease Control and Prevention and sits on the Institute of Medicine's Roundtable on Environmental Health Sciences, Research, and Medicine. He is a fellow of the American College of Emergency Physicians and a past term member of the Council on Foreign Relations. From 2005 to 2012, he was the director of Cornell Wilderness Medicine and a member of the Global Health Steering Committee at the Weill Cornell Medical College.

Lemery was an Echols Scholar at the University of Virginia and received his MD from the Geisel School of Medicine at Dartmouth. From 2003 to 2004, he was chief resident in emergency medicine at NYU and Bellevue Hospitals. He also holds academic appointments at the Weill Cornell Medical College and the Harvard School of Public Health (FXB Center), where he is a contributing editor for its journal *Health and Human Rights* and was guest editor for the June 2014 edition on climate justice. He is affiliate faculty of the Colorado School of Public Health.

THE CONTRIBUTORS

Lorraine C. Backer, PhD, MPH, National Center for Environmental Health, Centers for Disease Control and Prevention, Atlanta, Georgia

Christovam Barcellos, PhD, Oswaldo Cruz Foundation-Fiocruz, Rio de Janeiro, Brazil

Charles B. Beard, PhD, Division of Vector-Borne Diseases, National Center for Emerging and Zoonotic Infectious Diseases, Centers for Disease Control and Prevention, Fort Collins, Colorado

Diane Bélanger, PhD, Université Laval, Ouranos, Canada

Diarmid Campbell-Lendrum, DPhil, World Health Organization, Department of Public Health, Environmental and Social Determinants of Health, Geneva, Switzerland

Stuart Capstick, PhD, School of Psychology, Cardiff University, Cardiff, United Kingdom

Adam Corner, PhD, School of Psychology, Cardiff University, Cardiff, United Kingdom

David Driscoll, MPH, PhD, Institute for Circumpolar Health Studies, University of Alaska Anchorage, Anchorage, Alaska

Abdulrahman M. El-Sayed, MD, PhD, Mailman School of Public Health, Columbia University, New York, New York

Kristie L. Ebi, PhD, MPH, ClimAdapt, Los Altos, California

Farah Faisal, BA, International Institutions and Global Governance, Council on Foreign Relations,

Kenneth L. Gage, PhD, Division of Vector-Borne Diseases, National Center for Emerging and Zoonotic Infectious Diseases, Centers for Disease Control and Prevention, Fort Collins, Colorado

Sandro Galea, MD, MPH, DrPH, School of Public Health, Boston University, Boston, Massachusetts

Jada F. Garofalo, MS, Division of Vector-Borne Diseases, National Center for Emerging and Zoonotic Infectious Diseases, Centers for Disease Control and Prevention, Fort Collins, Colorado

Pierre Gosselin, MD, MPH, Department of Social and Preventive Medicine, Faculty of Medicine, Université Laval, Ouranos, Canada

Joy Guillemot, DrPH, World Health Organization, Department of Public Health, Environmental and Social Determinants of Health, Geneva, Switzerland

Jeremy Hess, MD, MPH, Emergency Medicine, Environmental Health, Emory University Schools of Medicine and Public Health, Atlanta, Georgia

Daniel P. Johnson, PhD, Department of Geography, Indiana University–Purdue University Indianapolis, Indianapolis, Indiana

Mark E. Keim, MD, MBA, DISASTERDOC, Lawrenceville, Georgia

Kim Knowlton, DrPH, Natural Resources Defense Council, Mailman School of Public Health, Columbia University, New York, New York

Katie M. Konchar, MS, Tallahassee, Florida

Cecilia Martinez, PhD, Center for Earth, Energy and Democracy, Minneapolis, Minnesota

Peter Montague, PhD, Environmental Research Foundation, Annapolis, Maryland

Mathilde Pascal, PhD, Institut de Veille Sanitaire, Paris, France

Nick Pidgeon, PhD, School of Psychology, Cardiff University, Cardiff, United Kingdom

Philippe Pirard, MD, Institut de Veille Sanitaire, Paris, France

Maxwell J. Richardson, MPH, MCP, Public Health Institute, Oakland, California

Linda Rudolph, MD, MPH, Center for Climate Change and Health, Public Health Institute, Oakland, California

Jan C. Semenza, PhD, MPH, MA, Office of the Chief Scientist, European Centre for Disease Prevention and Control, Stockholm, Sweden

Nicky Sheats, JD, PhD, Center for the Urban Environment, Thomas Edison State College, Trenton, New Jersey

Perry Sheffield, MD, Departments of Preventive Medicine and Pediatrics, School of Medicine, Mt. Sinai Hospital, New York, New York

Austin C. Stanforth, MS, Department of Geography, Indiana University–Purdue University Indianapolis, Indianapolis, Indiana

James D. Tamerius, PhD, Department of Geographical and Sustainability Sciences, University of Iowa, Iowa City, Iowa

Cristina Tirado, DVM, MS, PhD, University of California Los Angeles, Institute for Environment and Sustainability, Los Angeles, California

Christopher K. Uejio, PhD, Department of Geography and Program in Public Health, Florida State University, Tallahassee, Florida

Karen Wertz, MA, Department of Geography, Florida State University, Tallahassee, Florida

Carmel Williams, PhD, Fellow, School of Population Health, University of Auckland, New Zealand; Fellow, FXB Center for Health and Human Rights, Harvard TH Chan School of Public Health, Boston, Massachusetts

Lewis H. Ziska, PhD, Crop Systems and Global Change Laboratory, US Department of Agriculture, Beltsville, Maryland

GLOBAL CLIMATE CHANGE AND HUMAN HEALTH

OUR CHANGING PLANET:
EMERGENT RISKS FOR HUMAN HEALTH

CHAPTER 1

PRIMER ON CLIMATE SCIENCE

Christopher K. Uejio, James D. Tamerius, Karen Wertz, Katie M. Konchar

The notion that **carbon dioxide** (CO_2) and other greenhouse gases (GHG) emissions could accumulate in the Earth's atmosphere and increase global surface temperatures was first proposed in the nineteenth century. Indeed, in 1896, Swedish physicist and chemist Svante Arrhenius created a greenhouse law for CO_2 that is still in use today: the increase of CO_2 emissions leads to global warming (Walter 2010). However, the idea was considered unlikely at the time and was mostly forgotten until rising global temperatures in the middle of the twentieth century sparked renewed interest in the hypothesis.

In the late 1950s, Charles Keeling began measuring the atmospheric concentration of CO_2 at Mauna Loa Observatory in Hawaii, a remote observatory that is minimally affected by local CO_2 sources and thus reflects average global atmospheric CO_2 levels. Over time, repeated measurements at Mauna Loa showed a consistent upward trend in the concentration of atmospheric CO_2. Indeed, this atmospheric concentration has increased more than 42 percent since the Industrial Revolution (Siegenthaler and Oeschger 1987). This increase is consistent with the quantity of CO_2 emitted into the atmosphere by humans through the burning of fossil fuels such as oil, coal, and natural gas. As of 2008, approximately 10 billion tons of anthropogenic carbon had been released into the atmosphere, and the total mass of anthropogenic emissions was increasing annually by approximately 2 percent (Le Quéré et al. 2009).

KEY CONCEPTS

- There is a strong consensus among climate scientists that global temperatures are increasing as a result of human activities.

- Weather, natural climate variability, and long-term climate change are distinct phenomena.

- The Earth is in an energy balance, which means that the amount of energy that enters the Earth's atmosphere is equal to the amount of energy that leaves the atmosphere.

- Three primary factors affect the Earth's energy balance: variability of solar intensity, reflectivity of the Earth's surface or atmosphere, and concentration of greenhouse gases.

- Natural solar radiation cycles affect the amount of solar energy reaching the Earth's surface, but they cannot account for the average global temperature increases we are experiencing.

- The greenhouse effect is a natural process that traps energy in the Earth's system, causing average global temperatures to be warmer than they would be otherwise.

We thank the anonymous reviewers for providing critical feedback on earlier drafts of this chapter.

KEY CONCEPTS (*CONTINUED*)

- Human activities have increased the concentration of greenhouse gases in the atmosphere, which have augmented the greenhouse effect and increased average global temperatures.

- Direct and indirect observations indicate with certainty that the global climate is changing.

- Average global temperatures have increased by approximately 0.85°C since 1880.

- In addition to increasing temperatures, observations over the past century have indicated that snow and sea ice cover is decreasing, the average global sea level is rising, and precipitation patterns are changing.

- Climate models make projections of future climate change.

- Climate models strongly suggest that the increasing global temperatures and climate change in the past century are due to anthropogenic emissions of greenhouse gases.

- Average global temperatures are expected to increase between approximately 0.8°C to 4.9°C by the end of this century.

- Temperatures will increase most over land and high-latitude regions.

- There will likely be an increase in extreme heat events associated with climate change.

- Most areas will see an increase in the amount of precipitation, and rainfall events may become more intense.

Scientific Consensus

As a result of increasingly complex mathematical models of climatological processes and the development of techniques to study past climates, there is now strong agreement among climate scientists that the altered composition of the atmosphere due to emissions of CO_2 and other GHG from human activities is causing an increase in mean global temperatures. An analysis of 11,944 peer-reviewed global warming studies published between 1991 and 2011 found that 97.7 percent of the studies stated that humans are causing global warming (Oreskes 2004; Cook et al. 2013). The science that has shaped this consensus is synthesized by the Intergovernmental Panel on Climate Change (IPCC), a nonpartisan intergovernmental organization that was created in 1988 and was jointly awarded the Nobel Peace Prize in 2007. The IPCC performs periodic assessments on the status of climate change science, potential impacts, and mitigation and adaptation.

The IPCC reports reflect the evolving state of the science. The IPCC (1990) stated that "the unequivocal detection of the enhanced greenhouse effect from observations is not likely for a decade or more." In the Third Assessment (IPCC 2001), the panel concluded there was new evidence that human activities were responsible for the majority of the observed temperature increases. The Fourth Assessment Report (IPCC 2007) collectively determined with "very high confidence" (very low uncertainty) that human activities have increased global temperatures over the past fifty years. Over five hundred scientists and two thousand reviewers voluntarily contributed to the report. The recently completed Fifth Assessment (IPCC 2013) issued the strongest statement that observed warming in the past fifty years was "unequivocal." The strength of this scientific consensus is similar to the evidence linking smoking to carcinogens and cancer (Shwed and Bearman 2010).

This book looks at the climatological processes that modulate human health. This chapter, however, focuses on the physical processes associated with climate change to provide a foundation for subsequent discussions.

In particular, we discuss how greenhouse gases alter Earth's energy balance and describe recent climate trends and projections of future climate change. In addition, we present multiple converging lines of evidence that support that the climate is changing and the changes are primarily caused by human activities.

Weather, Climate Variability, Climate Change, and Scientific Theory

It is important to distinguish short-term weather changes, natural **climate variability**, and long-term climate change. People are intricately familiar with short-term weather changes in atmospheric conditions from their everyday experiences. However, it is exceedingly difficult to sense changes to climate because of its relatively slow progression and because it is masked by weather fluctuations. Confusion about these concepts can lead to incorrect interpretations and conclusions regarding climate change.

We commonly experience *weather*, the state of the atmosphere at any given moment in time, through changes in temperature, humidity, precipitation, cloudiness, and wind. Although weather changes from moment to moment, weather events such as storms may last for several hours or several days. Locations around the world tend to experience relatively unique weather patterns based on their latitude and their proximity to large water bodies and significant terrain (e.g., mountains). Collectively these features and the general circulation of the Earth's atmosphere and oceans shape a location's climate. *Climate* can be defined as the long-term average weather patterns for a specific region. More colloquially, Robert Heinlein (1973) stated, "Climate is what on an average we may expect; weather is what we actually get." J. Marshall Shepherd, former president of the American Meteorological Society, similarly stated, "Weather is your mood and climate is your personality." An operational climate definition commonly averages weather conditions over a period of thirty to fifty years.

Climate change also has a precise definition: systematic change in the long-term state of the atmosphere over multiple decades or longer. In the scientific literature, climate change may refer to a combination of human-induced and natural climatic changes or only human-induced changes. Formal statistical tests measure the probability that observed changes are outside the range of natural variability. The results are probabilistic statements about the likelihood that climate change is occurring. For example, there is at least a 99 percent chance that average global temperatures have significantly increased from 1950 to present (IPCC 2013). There is less than a 1 percent chance that we would randomly observe a similar increase in global temperatures over the same time period. Thus, scientific statements avoid using strict statements such as "I do [do not] believe" in climate change. The most robust climate changes exhibit the same trend regardless of the choice of multidecadal aggregation period (e.g., 1950–1989, 1970–2009). Due to natural climate variability, there will be periods where temperatures do not appreciably change. However, the trend over the entire period of 1950 to the present is unequivocal. Similarly, reliable studies consider globally averaged trends instead of deliberately selecting the small subset of stations where temperatures did not change.

Superimposed on long-term trends in climate is natural climate variability. Natural climate variability is often associated with oscillations in the Earth system that occur at the scale of months to decades. The El Niño Southern Oscillation (ENSO) is the best-known and important driver of year-to-year climate variability (Trenberth 1997). ENSO is associated with a two- to seven-year oscillation in sea surface temperatures (SST) in the eastern tropical Pacific, with warmer SST during El Niño. Conversely, during a La Niña event, eastern tropical Pacific SST are cooler than normal. Shifts in SST in this region have dramatic effects on the large-scale atmospheric circulation patterns around the world and can influence temperature and precipitation conditions. For example, in the eastern part of South Africa, El Niño events are frequently accompanied by drier-than-normal summers, while La Niña is associated with a slightly greater chance of above-average precipitation. However, the distribution, magnitude, and timing of the effects of ENSO vary from event to event (McPhaden, Zebiak, and Glantz 2006; Zebiak et al. 2015). Other analogous ocean-atmosphere climate variability features vary over longer periods. For example, the Pacific Decadal Oscillation alters weather throughout the Pacific Ocean and Pacific Rim, while the North Atlantic, Oscillation influences eastern North America, the Atlantic and Europe (Vuille and Garreaud 2011). The Northern and Southern annular mode, respectively, alter weather in North America/Eurasia and Antarctica.

The contention by some that climate change is "just" a theory reflects common confusion about the meaning of the term *theory*. When used colloquially, a theory is defined as an educated guess. Scientifically, however, a theory is a well-substantiated, evidence-based explanation of some aspect of the natural world. By definition, scientific theories begin as hypotheses. Over the course of repeated verification by experimental testing and observation, some hypotheses are so well supported by scientific evidence that they are accepted as theories. Climate change is one such evidence-based theory of science. Other examples are the germ theory of disease and the atomic theory of matter (American Association for the Advancement of Science 2006).

CLINICAL CORRELATES 1.1 HEAT WAVES AND THE ELDERLY

During the 2003 heat wave in Europe, a majority of the seventy thousand excess deaths were among older adults (over age sixty-five) who remained alone in their homes despite warnings to seek cooler environments (Ledrans et al. 2004; Robine et al. 2008). Older adults are particularly vulnerable to heat waves because their mobility, hearing, vision, or cognition may be compromised, making it difficult or impossible for them to process or adhere to warnings. Cardiovascular, renal, and pulmonary diseases co-morbidities, which disproportionately affect the elderly, compound cognitive and mobility issues and thus increase their vulnerability during heat waves. Primary care physicians can begin to incorporate heat vulnerability in their preventative health screening as a way to raise awareness among this population of the early warning signs of heat stress.

Elderly populations are particularly vulnerable to heat stress, a factor that should be incorporated into routine care.

Energy Balance

A basic understanding of Earth's energy balance is required to understand the theory of climate change. Our planet's temperature is dependent on how solar energy is transferred within the Earth system. The global temperature remains relatively constant because the total energy entering Earth is balanced by the energy that is released back into space. Specifically, solar energy is transmitted to Earth, and a proportion of the energy is naturally reflected back to space. However, some solar energy that enters the Earth system is absorbed by the atmosphere, oceans, and land surfaces, which causes the planet to warm. In turn, the Earth system releases (transmits) energy back into space, which precludes the accumulation of energy in the Earth system and sustains relatively constant global temperatures.

Several factors can cause the Earth's energy balance to change over time. This section discusses changes in the concentration of GHG, the greenhouse effect, GHG global warming potential, and changes in the amount of solar energy reaching Earth. Each of these factors is discussed further below.

Greenhouse Gases

We review the main GHG whose atmospheric levels have increased as a result of human activities to concentrations not seen in hundreds of thousands of years. In order of their contribution to climate change these are

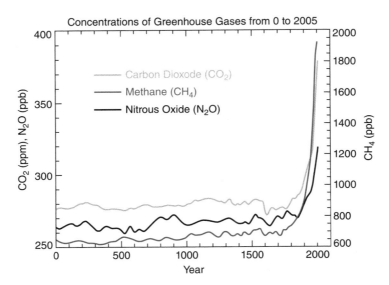

Figure 1.1 Atmospheric CO$_2$ Levels, 1958–2015

Source: NOAA (2015).

Note: Rapid increases in CO$_2$ concentrations accompanied the Industrial Revolution.

CO$_2$, methane (CH$_4$), nitrous oxide (N$_2$O), and fluorinated gases: hydrofluorocarbons, perfluorocarbons, and sulfur hexafluoride.

The most important greenhouse gas is CO$_2$ (figure 1.1). CO$_2$ is naturally emitted to and absorbed from the atmosphere through plant photosynthesis and animal respiration, volcanic eruptions, and ocean-atmospheric interactions. Although the cycle of CO$_2$ is a natural process, humans have been discharging increasing amounts of CO$_2$ through the burning of fossil fuels (oil, coal, and natural gas) for energy and transportation, solid waste, trees, and wood products. We have also been increasing atmospheric CO$_2$ through land use changes such as deforestation (Environmental Protection Agency [EPA] 2013). Human activities such as fossil fuel use and land use change have emitted so much CO$_2$ into the atmosphere that natural CO$_2$ sinks (sources of CO$_2$ absorption such as oceans and plants) and cannot absorb the excess CO$_2$ (EPA 2013). Indeed, since the eighteenth century, atmospheric CO$_2$ concentrations have increased by 40 percent from approximately 280 parts per million by volume (ppmv) to 398 ppmv in 2014. The current CO$_2$ level has not occurred for over 850,000 years (National Research Council 2010) and is not a result of natural CO$_2$ variation in the atmosphere.

Methane (CH$_4$), an important GHG, is emitted into the atmosphere through several processes. CH$_4$ is naturally emitted from wetlands and other natural areas through the decomposition of organic materials, and it is naturally removed from the atmosphere through soil and chemical reactions. Humans emit CH$_4$ through the production and use of fossil fuels and commercial livestock where it is produced from the creation and decomposition of manure in holding tanks and lagoons. The processing and decomposition of human solid waste in landfills and treatment facilities also produce CH_4. Atmospheric CH_4 levels have not been as high as they are now for 650,000 years (Environmental Protection Agency 2013).

For the 11,500 years before the Industrial Revolution, atmospheric nitrous oxide (N_2O) levels remained virtually constant. This gas is naturally released into the atmosphere through the breakdown of nitrogen by bacteria in the soil and ocean waters (denitrification). It is removed from the atmosphere through absorption by bacteria or decomposition by ultraviolet light radiation or other chemical reactions. Human causes of increased N_2O emissions stem from agriculture (e.g., synthetic fertilizers and livestock excrement), industry (e.g., nitric acid fertilizers and other synthetic products), and the combustion of solid waste and fossil fuels (Environmental Protection Agency 2013). After CO_2 and CH_4, increased atmospheric N_2O is the third largest contributor to the greenhouse effect and the largest contributor to depletion of Earth's ozone layer.

The final GHG we discuss are fluorinated gases: hydrofluorocarbons (HFCs), perfluorocarbons, and sulfur hexafluoride emitted from industrial sources. They are used as refrigerants (air conditioning for buildings and vehicles), solvents, aerosol propellants, and fire repellants. Their use as refrigerants is the primary form of their emissions. HFCs were designed to take the place of chlorofluorocarbons and hydrochlorocarbons which are being phased out internationally because they degrade the stratospheric ozone layer. However, HFCs are extremely potent GHGs. Perfluorocarbons are produced as the by-product of industrial sources such as aluminum production and the semiconductor manufacturing. Sulfur hexafluoride is produced through the transmission of electricity through electrical transmission equipment.

The Greenhouse Effect

The most discussed driver of change in Earth's energy balance is the greenhouse effect: the ability of greenhouse gases to trap heat in the atmosphere. In particular, when the planet releases or reflects energy into the atmosphere as infrared radiation (i.e., heat), GHGs absorb that radiation and prevent or slow down the loss of energy to space. GHGs essentially act like a blanket that keeps the planet warm. The natural greenhouse effect dramatically captures more of the sun's energy and raises the Earth's average temperature by 33°C. Although the natural greenhouse effect is beneficial, scientists are concerned about human actions' increasing the concentration of GHGs in the atmosphere since this will intensify the greenhouse effect.

Since the start of the Industrial Revolution in approximately 1750, human activities have added substantial quantities of GHGs to the atmosphere, thereby increasing the greenhouse effect and raising Earth's surface temperature (Environmental Protection Agency 2013). Ground-based observations observed an enhanced greenhouse effect of 2.6 Watts per meter squared (energy per area) per decade from 1986 to 2000 (Wacker et al. 2011; Wild 2012). Satellites provide a complementary record to ground-based observations of the enhanced greenhouse effect. Since 1970, less heat emitted by the Earth's surface has escaped to space, which strongly suggests more heat is being absorbed by GHGs and transferred back toward the Earth's surface (Harries et al. 2001; Feldman et al. 2015).

Greenhouse Gas Global Warming Potential

Based on its chemical structure, each GHG has a particular potential to absorb energy emitted from the Earth's surface and atmosphere, termed its global warming potential (GWP). GWPs are calculated based on the average length of time a GHG remains in the atmosphere and the amount of the heat energy it absorbs. GHGs that have a higher GWP absorb more energy and contribute more toward global warming than GHG with lower GWPs. Because changes in the atmospheric concentration of CO_2 typically occur over long periods of time (hundreds of years), the GWP of CO_2 is used as a baseline value against which other GHGs are compared. For instance, while CO_2 has a GWP of 1, CH_4 has a GWP of 21. This means that 1 pound of CH_4 is equivalent to 21 pounds of CO_2, and CH_4 has the potential to cause 21 times as much warming as CO_2 over 100 years. N_2O has a GWP of 300, HFCs 140 to 11,700, perfluorocarbons 6,500 to 9,200, and sulfur hexafluoride to 23,900 (Environmental Protection Agency 2013). Although many molecules have a greater GWP than CO_2, the abundance of CO_2 in the atmosphere and the rate that it is increasing makes it the most important GHG.

Residence Time of GHG and Climate Change Commitment

The residence time, or amount of time individual GHGs remain in the atmosphere, varies substantially. For instance, CO_2 remains in the atmosphere for 50 to 200 years, methane (CH_4) for about approximately 12 years, and nitrous oxide (N_2O) for about 120 years. For the fluorinated gases, HFCs can remain in the atmosphere in the range of 1 to 270 years, perfluorocarbons for 800 to 50,000 years, and sulfur hexafluoride for 3,200 years (Environmental Protection Agency 2013). In addition to long residence times of the GHG, it takes decades for energy in the Earth's system to equilibrate to increased GHG levels. Ocean and land temperatures will continue to increase even if all GHG emissions from human activities abruptly stopped. In other words, society is committed to additional climate changes from GHG that have already been emitted.

CLINICAL CORRELATES 1.2 INNOVATIONS IN EMERGENCY READINESS IN THE ERA OF HEAT WAVES

Epidemiological research shows that mortality in many places increases as the temperature rises (Bassil et al. 2011). Models have used temperature and humidity, as well as the time and rate of onset of these variables, to forecast when clinically significant **heat waves** may occur. These models allow for initiation of time-sensitive warnings to be released to the public. However, there is significant variability in the ways communities are affected; factors such as age, architecture, socioeconomics, prevalence of chronic disease, and relative isolation all play a part. Thus, each community has a different threshold at which heat-related illness becomes clinically apparent. Emergency medical systems (Leonardi et al. 2006), medical help lines, and emergency departments (Claessens et al. 2006) are at the forefront of detecting and treating heat-related illnesses. Research has shown that reliance on these organizations increases with rising temperatures, and the public's reliance on these institutions could therefore be an accurate indicator of the appearance of clinically relevant heat-related disease. More research is needed to determine whether real-time surveillance data generated from these clinical settings could assist public health officials in deciding when to issue heat warnings to a community. Early warnings can help to ease the toll of health-related illness, and prevention may ease the burden of such events on the health care system.

Real-time data indicate clinically significant heat waves and could be used to generate public warnings and emergency system preparedness.

Solar Radiation Cycles

Short-term solar cycles such as sunspots marginally alter the solar energy that the Earth receives. Over the past thirty years, short-term solar cycles increased the energy in the Earth system (0.017 W/m^2 per decade), but this is notably less than the greenhouse gas contribution (0.30 W/m^2 per decade) (IPCC 2013). Since 1750, there has been a slight increase in the total emitted solar energy 0.05 W/m^2 solar energy.

In addition to short-term solar cycles, gradual long-term solar cycles (10,000 to 100,000 years) also modulate the amount of solar energy reaching Earth. These cycles, referred to as Milankovitch cycles, affect the distance, orientation, and axis of the Earth relative to the sun. Indeed, the timing of the ice ages generally corresponds to periods of the Milankovitch cycles when the Earth is receiving less solar energy (Hays, Imbrie, and Shackleton 1976). Based on these predictable solar cycles, the Earth should be in the midst of a gradual cooling trend lasting 23,000 years instead of rapidly warming (Imbrie and Imbrie 1980).

Summary

In summary, there is a strong and consistent physical mechanism linking GHG to observed changes to the Earth's energy balance. GHGs absorb thermal radiation emitted by the Earth's surface and reemit this energy, further warming the Earth's surface. Human activities such as burning fossil fuels, synthesizing fertilizer and artificial coolants, and agricultural activities rapidly increased atmospheric GHG concentrations. The world is already committed to future climate changes due to the properties of GHG and the Earth's system.

Evidence of a Changing Climate

This section focuses on climatic changes that are virtually certain (99 to 100 percent probability), very likely (90 to 100 percent probability), or likely (66 to 100 percent probability) (Mastrandrea et al. 2010). There is no doubt that the climate on Earth is changing. We know this from direct observations of increasing average air and ocean temperatures, melting snow and ice, and rising average sea levels (figure 1.2). Here we examine the evidence for climate change since the first measurements were recorded in 1959 at Mauna Loa Observatory and paleoclimate records that provide physical evidence of a changing climate prior to the nineteenth century.

Temperature

Earth's surface temperatures are typically lowest near the poles and increase toward the equator. The warmer temperatures in the tropics are due to a greater amount of solar energy reaching the surface in these regions. The temperature differentials generate large-scale atmospheric circulation patterns that redistribute energy from tropical to higher-latitude regions. However, local factors such as land cover, water bodies, and terrain can modulate regional and local temperature conditions.

Global surface temperatures have been increasing since the early twentieth century. Indeed, global temperatures increased by 0.85°C (1.8°F) from 1880 to 2012 (IPCC 2013). The rate of warming since 1957 is 0.13°C (0.27°F) per decade, almost twice as fast as it had been during the previous century (Hansen et al. 2010), and all of the top ten warmest years since 1850 have occurred since 1998 (Blunden and Arndt 2013). Stated another way, no

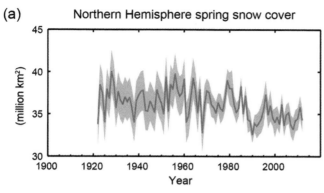

(a) Northern Hemisphere spring snow cover

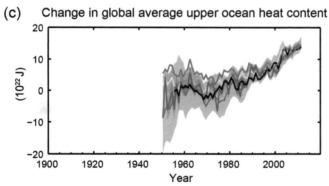

(b) Arctic summer sea ice extent

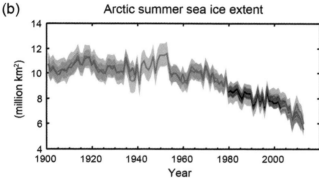

(c) Change in global average upper ocean heat content

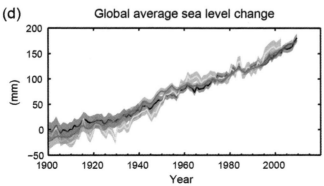

(d) Global average sea level change

Figure 1.2   Observed Changes in the Earth System Related to Climate Change

Note: Consistent with warming temperatures, the extent of Northern Hemisphere snow cover (a) from March to April and Arctic summer sea ice extent (b) from July to September are significantly decreasing. The upper ocean (0–700 meters) is also strongly warming (c), as summarized by standardized observational data sets, and (d) global average sea levels are increasing. Each line corresponds to a different data set. The lighter shading captures observational uncertainty.

Source: IPCC (2013).

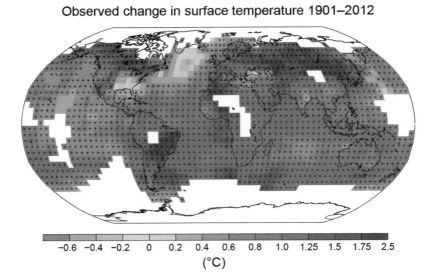

Observed change in surface temperature 1901–2012

-0.6 -0.4 -0.2 0 0.2 0.4 0.6 0.8 1.0 1.25 1.5 1.75 2.5
(°C)

Figure 1.3   Decadal Rate of Observed Temperature Changes, 1901–2012

Note: Map of the observed surface temperature change from 1901 to 2012.

Source: IPCC (2013).

person under the age of thirty has experienced a cooler-than-normal month based on global average temperatures (NOAA National Climatic Data Center 2015).

Although nearly the entire globe has experienced increasing temperatures over the past century (IPCC 2013), there is significant geographic variation with respect to the magnitude of these increases (figure 1.3). Observed temperature changes have been greatest in polar regions of the Northern Hemisphere, and air temperatures over land have increased faster than over oceans (Hansen et al. 2010). The ocean's ability to store more heat energy modulates temperature increases compared to the land surface.

Precise temperature and systematic observations did not exist prior to the late nineteenth century. Fortunately, a variety of natural records indirectly measured historic conditions. Tree rings, ocean lake microorganisms, and pollen are mechanistically linked and well associated with temperature, moisture, and other physical environmental properties of the past. Although each proxy record has its limitations, all peer-reviewed proxies exhibit the same trend.

Diurnal Temperature Cycles

Superimposed on the upward trend of global temperatures are seasonal and diurnal temperature cycles. The increase in diurnal temperatures is not straightforward. Over the past century, nighttime temperatures have increased more rapidly than daytime temperatures, resulting in a decrease in the daily temperature range (DTR; Vose, Easterling, and Gleason 2005). However, this pattern varies strongly across the world, with some regions experiencing increases in DTR and others decreases. For example, DTR has been increasing in western and eastern Europe since the 1970s (Makowski, Wild, and Ohmura 2008), whereas it significantly decreased across China from 1961 to 2008 (Zhou and Ren 2011). Local and regional trends in diurnal temperature patterns can also be modified by land surface changes due to urbanization, deforestation, and other processes. Further complicating this picture is that the global decreasing trend in DTR has flattened out since the 1990s as maximum temperatures are now increasing at rates commensurate with minimum temperatures (Vose, Easterling, and Gleason 2005).

Seasonal Temperature Cycles

In general, the timing of the warmest and the coolest times of the year have not been affected by global climate change. However, the onset of many biologically important seasonal events now occurs at a different time of the year from the past. For example, the length of the frost season is declining in many temperate regions, with later onsets and earlier cessations than was typical in the past. Remember that recent temperature increases have not been distributed evenly across the world or across seasons and geography. For instance, early summertime temperatures in the Southeast and central United States have been consistently cooler over the past fifty years (Portmann, Solomon, and Hegerl 2009).

Urban Heat Island

Warming is becoming a major problem in urban areas through a phenomenon known as the **urban heat island** (UHI) effect: a built environment that is hotter than the surrounding rural areas (Oke 1982). UHI is a result of several distinct processes. The first of these is "waste" heat released from vehicles, power plants, air-conditioning units, and other anthropogenic sources in urban regions. Second, urban areas typically absorb more radiation than rural areas. Urban streets and tall buildings composed of asphalt, concrete, and metal reflect less solar radiation than vegetated areas. Third, urban areas alter the hydrological cycle, which also changes the local temperature. Urban surfaces and storm water infrastructure move water out of the city. Thus, urban areas retain less water that can be evaporated to moderate surface temperatures. UHI effects cause increases in energy consumption (e.g., using air-conditioning units for extended periods), elevated levels of ground-level ozone, and deterioration of the living environment in urban areas.

It is important to note that while UHI effects are changing the climate at the microlevel, they are of little importance to rising temperatures at the global level with less than a 0.006°C impact on land temperatures and no impact on ocean temperatures (Solomon et al. 2007). However, UHI is a massive global problem as approximately 3 billion people live in urban areas and are directly affected by it (Rizwan, Dennis, and Liu 2008). Outdoor extreme heat increases will likely be more pronounced in large, sprawling cities with an enhanced UHI (Kalnay and Cai 2003; Stone, Hess, and Frumkin 2010). Furthermore, many of the contributors to UHI also contribute to climate change, including greenhouse gas emissions from vehicles, industrial sources, and air-conditioning units. UHI may become a more serious problem in the future as the planet continues to urbanize (Rosenzweig et al. 2011).

Hydrological Cycle

Most readers will be familiar with the hydrological cycle from their everyday experiences. Precipitation—rainfall and other solid forms of water that fall from the atmosphere to Earth's surface—occurs when the atmosphere absorbs more water vapor than it can hold. The majority of Earth's water makes its way back into the atmosphere either directly through surface evaporation or indirectly through plant transpiration. Much of the remaining liquid water runs off the land surface to a water body such as lakes, rivers, or oceans. Additional waters percolate into groundwater systems. Water may also be temporarily stored on the surface as ice or snow. Glaciers, snowpack, and groundwater are natural reservoirs that can trap water for extended periods of time.

There have been distinct geographical changes in total annual precipitation over the past century (figure 4.1). Total precipitation significantly decreased in the Mediterranean and West Africa. Drier-than-normal conditions may increase the frequency of wildfires, challenge hydropower generation, lower agriculture yields, and impair transportation on waterways. In contrast, precipitation significantly increased in the midlatitudes of both hemispheres (IPCC 2013). There is also some evidence for precipitation increases in polar areas of the Northern Hemisphere, although the strength of the conclusions is limited by patchy observations. There are inconsistent precipitation trends in the tropics and Southern Hemisphere polar regions due to uncertainties in early records.

Changes to the types and seasonal phase of precipitation may have an adverse impact on societal and ecosystem functioning. The frequency of and intensity of heavy precipitation events likely have increased over North America and Europe since 1950. This relationship is well grounded

Observed change in annual precipitation over land

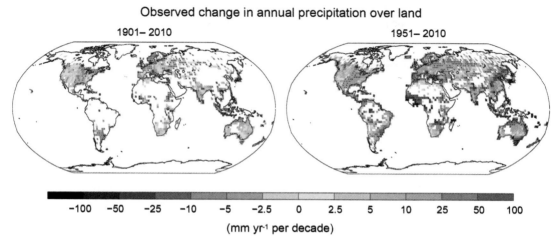

Figure 1.4   Observed Precipitation, 1901–2010 and 1951–2010 (Rates per Decade)
Source: IPCC (2013).

in physical theory since the amount of water the atmosphere can hold increases by approximately 7 percent for each additional degree Celsius of warming (Allan and Soden 2008). Furthermore, consistent with observed temperature increases, there is a trend toward fewer snowfall and more liquid rainfall events. This transition was recorded in North America, Europe, and South and East Asia (Takeuchi, Endo, and Murakami 2008; Kunkel et al. 2009). Satellite and ground-based observations support a significant decrease in snow cover extent (very high confidence) and depth (medium confidence) in spring and early summer (Brown and Mote 2009; Brown and Robinson 2011). In addition, the area, volume, and mass of almost all glaciers are decreasing across the globe (Arendt et al. 2012). Globally, 1 billion people live in watersheds with rivers fed by glacier or snowmelt. Ice loss is geographically concentrated in polar regions and high-altitude mountains such as the Andes and Himalayas.

Sea Ice Extent, Sea Level, and Ocean Acidification

Since 1978, satellite data have allowed us to observe overall Arctic sea ice shrinkage (Solomon et al. 2007). From 1979 to 2012, annual mean Arctic sea ice area had very likely decreased in the range of 3.5 to 4.1 percent per decade. On the other side of the world, Antarctic sea ice area slightly increased 1.2 to 1.8 percent. The rapid decrease of Arctic and increase of Antarctic sea ice are not contradictory findings since each pole is governed by different processes. Antarctic sea ice may be expanding due to climate change–related melting of land glaciers or increased rainfall (Zhang 2007). Strengthening wind patterns may also be responsible for observed changes

(Holland and Kwok 2012). Scientists are highly confident that there are significant regional differences in sea ice extent in Antarctica, with some regions showing increases in sea ice areas and other regions showing decreases (IPCC 2013).

For approximately the past two thousand years, average sea level changed very little. However, since the start of the twentieth century, the sea level has been rising at an accelerating pace (Environmental Protection Agency 2013). For instance, since 1961, global sea level rose at an average rate of 1.8 millimeters per year. But since 1993, that rate has accelerated to 3.1 millimeters per year (Solomon et al. 2007). Although the melting of sea ice does not directly lead to an increase in sea levels, melting glaciers, ice caps, and polar ice sheets have been contributing to **sea level rise** (Solomon et al. 2007). Equally important, the thermal expansion of ocean water is increasing the volume of water in the oceans. Specifically, as average global temperatures increase, the oceans are storing more heat. This results in increasing sea surface temperatures, which causes ocean water to thermally expand, contributing to sea level rise.

In addition to increasing sea levels, seawater chemistry has also been altered as the oceans have absorbed increasing amounts of carbon from the atmosphere. Today the oceans are about 26 percent more acidic than they were forty years ago (IPCC 2013). Tiny microscopic creatures on which the marine food chain depends are significantly affected by the calcium chemistry of ocean waters. Increased seawater acidity has also decreased the ability of these creatures to form shells (Rodolfo-Metalpa et al. 2011).

Summary

Global surface and ocean temperatures and sea levels are significantly increasing, and the rate of change continues to accelerate. Surface temperatures may be further magnified by the UHI. In turn, increased temperatures alter the timing of the seasons and length of the frost season. Increased temperatures are altering the amount, timing, and phases of precipitation and storage of liquid water. In the latter half of the twentieth century, annual precipitation increased in many midlatitude and polar regions. In North America and Europe, extreme precipitation events are becoming more intense and frequent. In North America, Europe, and South and Southeast Asia, there are fewer snowfall and more liquid precipitation events. Globally almost all glaciers are shrinking. Arctic sea ice area or extent has rapidly decreased. Thus, nonrandom climate changes are already detectable and are starting to challenge biological systems and societal well-being.

CLINICAL CORRELATES 1.3 POVERTY AND EXTREME HEAT EVENTS

Poverty is an independent risk factor for illness related to heat. It is associated with a decreased likelihood of access to medical care. It is also associated with decreased access to protective measures, such as air-conditioning (Balbus and Malina 2009), which is then compounded by the urban microclimate that escalates heat events through heat island effects (Harlan et al. 2013). The heat island effect, caused by nighttime radiation of heat from buildings, industrial heat production, and a lack of green spaces, elevates both daytime and nighttime temperatures in city neighborhoods (Smargiassi, Goldberg, and Kosatsky 2009). This effect is evident in analysis of morbidity and mortality from heat events in Phoenix, Arizona (Uejio et al. 2011; Harlan et al. 2013) and Chicago in 1995 (Semenza et al. 1996) when a disproportionate number of deaths occurred among inner-city poor. These figures highlight the need for the medical community to increase health care access and address environmental health disparities.

More resources are needed to address environmental disparities and provide protective measures against heat-related illness in urban areas.

Climate Models

How do scientists draw informed conclusions from the evidence of climatic change outlined thus far and make reasonable predictions about future change? If there were multiple Earths, a randomized trial could be conducted to determine exactly how elevated greenhouse gas levels alter the climate compared to a control Earth. Of course, we have only one planet Earth. The next-best study design is to build mathematical computer models that simulate the Earth's system and conduct trials within that model system. A climate model contains realistic representations of and interactions between the oceans, atmosphere, land surface, and cryosphere.

The backbone of climate models consists of physical equations and principles that govern the transfer of energy and mass. Climate models with increasing GHG levels over time accurately reproduce increasing temperatures, sea ice dynamics, and changing patterns of extreme weather (IPCC 2013). These models also provide additional evidence that observed climate change is caused by human activities. Detection and attribution studies attempt to determine if climate models can reproduce observed changes without elevated GHG levels (figure 1.5). Observed climate changes are outside the range of those expected by natural variability such as short-term solar radiation changes, volcanic eruptions, and other confounding processes. Only climate models with elevated greenhouse gas levels and reduced stratospheric ozone can reproduce observed climatic changes.

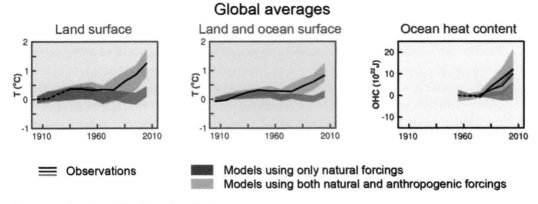

Figure 1.5   Detection and Attribution Study Results

Note: Comparison of observed and simulated climate change based on three large-scale indicators in the atmosphere, the cryosphere, and the ocean. Only climate models that account for human impacts on the atmosphere can reproduce observed temperature and heat content changes.

Source: IPCC (2013)

More than half of the observed changes in average global surface temperature from 1951 to 2010 are due to human activities based on the modeling results.

Climate Projections, Uncertainty, and Climate Feedbacks

Future climate projections are uncertain for multiple reasons. The largest contributors to uncertainty are societal choices, natural climate variability, and scientific uncertainty. The relative contribution of societal versus scientific uncertainty for climate change varies over time and region (Hawkins and Sutton 2009, 2011). *Societal choices* broadly refers to demographic, economic growth and distribution, technological, and public policy changes. Projecting future societal actions and behaviors is notoriously difficult. For instance, a high population growth rate would increase emitted carbon 12.4 gigatons per year by 2100 over a low growth rate (O'Neill et al. 2010). To put this in perspective, 31.6 gigatons of carbon were emitted in 2012. Climate change and health impact studies work with climate projections over multiple years, and ideally decades, to minimize the influence of natural climate variability.

Scientific uncertainty in climate models is introduced by the modeling techniques and incomplete knowledge of some Earth system processes. Climate modeling techniques use simplified representations of processes smaller than approximately 100 to 300 kilometers. For example, North American summer precipitation changes are more uncertain than temperature changes. Climate models have difficulty resolving clouds, water vapor, and aerosols, which are key components of convective summer precipitation. Similarly, climate projections may be more uncertain in areas with topography, near coastlines, or with large inland water bodies due to their simplified representation in global climate models (GCMs).

Scientific uncertainty also surrounds the ability of climate models to reproduce **climate feedback**. A feedback is defined as a forcing in the climate system that is both a cause and effect of itself and either acts to amplify (positive feedback) or dampen the initial forcing (negative feedback). For example, increasing surface temperatures cause highly reflective snow and ice to melt, thereby exposing dark soil and rock with lower reflectivity. This increases the solar radiation absorbed by Earth's surface, resulting in additional temperature increases and melting. Human-induced global climate change is unprecedented, so many important feedbacks have not been directly observed. Each GCM represents climate change feedbacks in subtle to moderately different ways. Climate sensitivity is defined as the average-rate global temperature increase for a doubling of CO_2 concentrations relative to preindustrial periods. The climate sensitivity depends on the representation of climate feedbacks and carbon reservoirs.

Major climate feedbacks are related to changes in the distribution of clouds, atmospheric temperature structure (changes to the relationship between temperature and altitude), vegetation type and coverage, the atmospheric concentration and distribution of water vapor, and modification of the carbon and sulfur cycles. There remains considerable uncertainty regarding feedback mechanisms, in particular those associated with clouds and the capacity of terrestrial surfaces and the ocean to absorb CO_2. (The following section provides more information on key feedbacks.)

Robustly projecting the climate change disease burden should account for societal and scientific uncertainty. Climate models provide plausible projections of future conditions based on future GHG emissions trajectories or **representative concentration pathways** (RCPs). Climate projections that use multiple RCP essentially represent some of the societal uncertainty. Using a suite of projections from ten or more climate models will capture a range of scientific uncertainty.

Rather than issue a precise forecast, scientists use scenarios to generate a plausible range of RCPs. The RCPs are bounded on the upper end by rapid GHG emission growth (RCP 8.5 Watts per meter squared, i.e., energy per area) and on the lower end by aggressive limits on GHG emissions (RCP 2.6) (Moss et al. 2010). The middle pathways suggest that GHGs stabilize at different levels (RCP 4.5, 6.0) by the end of the century.

The RCPs were recently updated in the 2013 IPCC assessment. The RCPs replace the *Special Report on Emission Scenarios* (SRES) used in the third and fourth IPCC assessments (IPCC 2001, 2007). The report describes four "scenario families" that reflect distinct and realistic demographic, technological, and economic paths, enabling projections of global GHG emissions (Nakicenovic and Swart 2000). Among the key scenarios are A1F1, A1B, and B1. A1F1 describes a world characterized by intense economic growth, a decrease in global economic disparity, low to decreasing population growth, rapid introduction of efficient technology, and a reliance on fossil energy sources. The A1B scenario is equivalent with the exception that societies use a balance of fossil and nonfossil energy resources. In scenario B1, the demographic changes are identical to those in A1F1 and A1B; however, service and information economies rapidly become predominant, clean and efficient technologies are introduced, and significant decreases in material consumption are observed.

There may be some confusion surrounding the transitions in nomenclature. To help interpret the previous literature, RCP 8.5 is analogous to the A1F1, RCP 6.0 to A1B, and RCP 4.5 to B1. The lowest RCP (2.6) is new and did not have a *Special Report on Emissions Scenarios* analogue.

Cloud Feedbacks

Feedbacks associated with clouds are still incompletely understood, and it is essential to understand their effects to improve predictions of future climatic conditions. Increasing temperatures will cause changes in the distribution and types of clouds occurring across Earth. Clouds are involved in both positive and negative feedback mechanisms by reflecting short-wave radiation back into space and by absorbing and reradiating outgoing long-wave radiation back to the surface, although different types of clouds have different radiative properties (Zelinka et al. 2013). The cumulative effect of feedback related to cloud cover is impeded by our inability to predict how the type, distribution, and characteristics of clouds will change as temperatures increase (Zelinka et al. 2013).

Carbon Reservoirs

Another source of uncertainty regarding future climate change concerns the ability of natural carbon reservoirs such as oceans and terrestrial plants to continue to uptake carbon at current rates. Slightly less than half of the total CO_2 emissions are currently absorbed by land and ocean reservoirs (Le Quéré et al. 2009). There is evidence, however, that the rate of carbon uptake by carbon reservoirs will decline as they become increasingly saturated with CO_2. Furthermore, physical characteristics of the reservoirs are modulated by increasing temperatures and anthropogenic activity (e.g., land cover change). The mechanisms underlying the uptake of carbon by land and ocean reservoirs are complex, and it remains uncertain how carbon reservoirs will absorb CO_2 in the future.

Summary

Climate models are multifaceted tools that complement observations and theory. Retrospectively, they show that natural climatic and solar variability cannot explain observed temperature increases. However, accounting for increased GHG produces similar changes to what scientists have observed. Prospectively, these models provide a range of plausible future climatic conditions. Future climate projections differ based on the magnitude and timing of climate feedbacks, natural variability, and substantial uncertainty surrounding human behavior. Nonetheless, the models continue to improve and increasingly capture the complexity of Earth's systems. The latest generation of global climate models includes the carbon cycle and dynamic vegetation.

CLINICAL CORRELATES 1.4   INTEGRATIVE APPROACHES TO HEAT RESILIENCE

Air-conditioning has become the mainstay approach to buffer the deleterious health effects of extreme heat events. Unfortunately, it places major strains on energy supplies and contributes substantially to CO_2 emissions, which in turn increase global surface temperatures. Eighty-percent of energy for air-conditioning comes from fossil fuels, and according to estimates, total world air-conditioning consumes roughly 1 trillion kilowatt hours annually, more than twice the total energy consumption of the entire continent of Africa (Dahl 2013). Given the medical necessity of cooling in the future, it is important to realize that the developing world contains thirty-eight of the largest fifty cities on the planet, the warmest of which are in the developing world (Sivak 2009). Thus, to curb the health effects of heat stress among vulnerable populations, city planners and engineers must creatively use energy-saving technologies as well as integrate traditional technologies that have a small energy footprint. These designs include passive cooling systems—evaporative cooling ("Evaporative Cooling" 2012), night flushing ("Night-Purge Ventilation" 2012), and passive downdraft evaporative cooling (Kamal 2011)—exterior heat sinks, and modification of existing structures with awnings, reflective paint, and landscaping that maximizes shade. Health care organizations should model appropriate building codes and use of indoor climate control.

Air-conditioning is both a cause of and cure for heat-related illness. Health care organizations should model green behavior in regard to indoor climate control.

Projected Future Climate Changes

Climate models are the primary tool to project long-term changes for the end of this century. Due to societal and scientific uncertainty, scientists cannot state which RCP and climate models are most likely to happen and which climate model provides the most accurate projections. This section focuses on projected temperature, hydrological cycle, and cryosphere changes. The estimates of future changes are based on the average, or an ensemble of multiple climate model projections, since the ensemble projection is typically more accurate than any individual climate model projection (Pierce et al. 2009).

Increasing Temperatures

There is significant uncertainty regarding the magnitude of future temperature increases due to our incomplete understanding of societal and physical processes. Taking this uncertainty into account, global mean surface air temperatures are expected to increase from 1986–2005 averages by approximately 0.3°C to 0.7°C by the period 2016 to 2030, and 0.8°C to 4.9°C by the period 2081 to 2100 (Kharin et al. 2013). However, mean temperature increases over land will be double the global mean increase (figure 1.6). This will be even greater in high latitudes of the Northern Hemisphere. Although mean surface temperatures over the ocean will generally not increase as rapidly as surface temperatures over land, large changes will be observed over the Arctic and the southern oceans, where the reduction of sea ice will be associated with temperature increases of approximately 2°C to 11°C by the period 2081 to 2100 (IPCC 2013). Stated another way, by the middle of this century, average annual temperatures will be higher than the hottest observed annual temperatures from 1860 to 2005 over most of the world (Mora et al. 2013).

Seasonal variation of climate will continue to evolve with anthropogenic climate change. In high and middle latitudes, the number of frost days could decrease by up to ninety days in some regions of North America and Western Europe by 2081 to 2100, and the poleward extent of permafrost areas will be reduced (Sillmann et al. 2013). The seasonal modification of temperature and precipitation will modify the seasonal and spatial range of many plants and animals, including disease vectors such as mosquitoes and allergenic plant species. The DTR will continue to decrease across much of the world, especially in high and low latitudes, due to increased cloud coverage. Many middle-latitude locations will experience increases or no change in DTR in the coming century (Kharin et al. 2013).

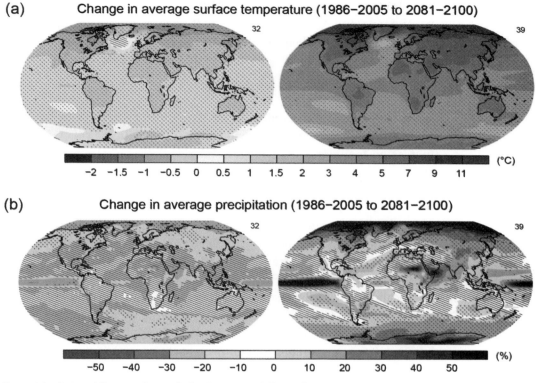

Figure 1.6   Projected Changes in Average Surface Temperature Difference for 2081–2100 versus 1986–2005 for Different RCP

Source: IPCC (2013).

Note: The average change is the mean of thirty-two climate model projections for RCP 2.6 and thirty-nine models for RCP 8.5. The figure also conveys uncertainty. In the dotted areas, the average projected changes is notably larger (two standard deviations) than natural variability. There is less confidence in the areas with hatching.

Extreme Heat Events

Extreme heat events (EHE) can be defined as periods with notably greater-than-normal surface temperatures and moisture for a specific time of year (Robinson and Dewy 1990). EHE generally occur when very hot and humid air moves into an area where people are not adapted to extreme conditions. The longer that air masses linger over a region, the greater the potential is for harm to society and the environment. Many heat metrics suggest EHE are already becoming more intense, longer lasting, frequent, and geographically widespread (IPCC 2013), a trend that is likely to continue into the future. By the end of this century, extreme heat events will be even hotter and more humid, more likely to last weeks instead of days, and more frequent.

Scientists cannot directly link individual weather events to climate change. However, they can determine the extent to which climate change is increasing the odds of an extreme event such as EHE compared to normal conditions. For example, climate change has at least doubled the probability (Stott, Stone, and Allen 2004) that an EHE event of the same magnitude of the historic European heat event of 2003 linked to seventy thousand excess deaths (Robine et al. 2008) will occur in the coming years.

Hydrological Cycle

Climate change is expected to amplify important interactions between energy in Earth's system and the intensity of the hydrological cycle. With increasing temperatures, average total global precipitation will almost certainly increase by 2050 (IPCC 2013). The rate of annual precipitation increases ranges from 1 to 3 percent per degree average annual temperature increase for all scenarios except RCP 2.5. However, there will be substantial geographical variability in projected changes. At high latitudes, precipitation is very likely to increase since warmer air holds more moisture combined with the increased transfer of tropical moisture into the region.

In the midlatitudes, there are distinct total annual precipitation trends for drylands and deserts versus relatively wet and semitropical regions. Under the high RCP 8.5 scenario, dry areas are projected to desiccate further, while precipitation is expected to increase in relatively wet midlatitude locations. Summertime monsoon precipitation will likely increase in Southeast Asia, southern India, southern regions of the West Africa, and northern Australia, whereas summertime precipitation will likely decrease in southern Africa, Mexico, and Central America (IPCC 2013). In dry regions, climate warming will accelerate land surface drying as heat goes into the evaporation of moisture and increase the frequency and severity of droughts.

The frequency and intensity of average daily precipitation events will likely increase across most midlatitude and wet tropical locations. The difference in total annual versus daily precipitation may seem incongruous for drylands and deserts; however, both trends can coexist. These regions may receive fewer precipitation events that are not compensated by the increase in relative rare extreme precipitation events. More intense precipitation will transport more pollutants, toxins, and pathogens into water bodies. Increasing atmospheric water vapor may also contribute to the greenhouse effect, further increasing the amount of energy in the system.

Sea Ice Extent, Sea Level, Ocean Acidification, Glacial Extent, and Snow Cover

The geographical extent of Arctic sea ice will continue to decrease by the end of this century under all RCP. Sea ice extent will decrease in all seasons. During the Arctic sea ice nadir in September, projected decreases range

Table 1.1   Projected Changes in Global Mean Sea Level Rise Relative to 1986–2005 for Four Representative Concentration Pathways (in meters)

Scenario	2046–2065		2081–2100	
	Mean	Likely Range	Mean	Likely Range
RCP 2.6	0.24	0.17 to 0.32	0.40	0.26 to 0.55
RCP 4.5	0.26	0.19 to 0.33	0.47	0.32 to 0.63
RCP 6.0	0.25	0.18 to 0.32	0.48	0.33 to 0.63
RCP 8.5	0.30	0.22 to 0.38	0.63	0.45 to 0.82

Note: The estimates are based on twenty-one global climate models. Rapid ice sheet changes and altered societal practices such as increasing water storage are not considered in these estimates.

from 43 to 94 percent relative to 1985 to 2006. Similarly, the apex of sea ice extent in February will also be reduced 8 to 34 percent relative to 1985 to 2006 (IPCC 2013).

Since 1870, the global sea level has risen by eight inches due to the thermal expansion of water and melting polar ice and glaciers. In the next century, future sea level rise is expected to rise at a faster rate than it has been rising for approximately the past fifty years. Various scenarios estimate different levels of sea level rise (table 1.1). Sea level rise will vary by coastal regions. Major factors that affect local and regional sea levels will be subsiding coastal land and the changing gravitational pull of large glaciers (EPA 2013; Slangen et al. 2014). With rising sea levels, we face shore erosion, loss of dry land, coastal flooding, and human population displacement. There will also be significant damage to wetlands and coastal ecosystems (EPA 2013). Logically, increased carbon emissions and subsequent absorption by the ocean will continue to increase ocean acidity. All global climate models and scenarios reflect further **ocean acidification** (IPCC 2013).

It is virtually certain that the global permafrost area will decrease in response to rising temperatures and less snow cover. Furthermore, the proportion of North America covered by snow in the spring will likely continue to decrease (Brutel-Vuilmet, Ménégoz, and Krinner 2013). Climate models do not explicitly capture local processes like glacier dynamics. Nonetheless, based on projected temperature changes, glacier area, volume, and mass are reasonably expected to continue to recede. Springtime glacier runoff is also expected to decrease.

Conclusion

We are already witnessing climate change impacts on public health, society, and ecosystems (Kovats, Campbell-Lendrum, and Matthies 2005). There is no doubt that since about 1950, the oceans and atmosphere have been warming, sea levels have been rising, and snow and ice cover have been decreasing. Observations, modeling experiments, and scientific theory implicate human activities as the largest driver of changes to the Earth's energy balance. The physical mechanism linking GHG concentrations to warming is physically sound and consistent over hundreds of thousands of years. Projecting the magnitude and geographical distribution of future climatic conditions is difficult due to uncertainty with regard to societal and physical processes. In general, there tends to be more agreement surrounding projected temperature changes and much less confidence in hydrological cycle projections.

DISCUSSION QUESTIONS

1. How have the conclusions of scientific assessments (e.g., Intergovernmental Panel on Climate Change) on whether climate change is occurring and what processes are responsible for these changes been updated over time?

2. What is the difference between natural climate variability and long-term climate change?

3. Why is it so difficult for an individual to observe long-term climate change?

4. If society somehow suddenly stopped emitting greenhouse gases, would existing greenhouse gases in the atmosphere continue to alter the climate? If so, for how long?

5. Some proposed public policies to mitigate or limit greenhouse gas emissions focus on methane, nitrous oxide, and fluorinated gases instead of carbon dioxide. What is the scientific rationale for these proposals? Discuss the relative merits and limitations of such a policy.

6. In what regions are temperatures increasing the most rapidly? Most slowly? Why?

7. What are the most important causes of sea level increases that have already happened?

8. What are the different types of evidence that support that the climate is changing?

9. What are the primary causes of uncertainty in climate model projections?

10. What are representative concentration pathways (RCPs), and why are they used?

KEY TERMS

Carbon dioxide: A colorless, odorless gas naturally occurring in our atmosphere. Over the last 150 year, global levels of this "greenhouse" gas have increased secondary to combustion of carbon-based fuels, significantly contributing to global warming. It is also a major cause of ocean acidification since it dissolves in water to form carbonic acid.

Climate feedback: Processes that change as a result of a change in forcing and cause additional climate change, for example, the "ice-albedo feedback" (as the atmosphere warms, sea ice will melt).

Climate variability: Long-term averages and variations in weather measured over a period of several decades. The Earth's climate system includes the land surface, atmosphere, oceans, and ice.

Heat wave: A prolonged period of excessively hot temperature that may be exacerbated by humidity and solar radiation. Human morbidity and mortality are known to increase during heat waves.

Ocean acidification: The ongoing decrease in the pH of the Earth's oceans, caused by the uptake of carbon dioxide from the atmosphere.

Representative concentration pathways: Four greenhouse gas concentration (not emissions) trajectories adopted by the IPCC for its fifth Assessment Report (AR5) in 2014. They represent differing predictions of future effects of climate change.

Sea level rise: A major consequence of global warming, affecting long-term coastal morphology as well as sea-level cities of the planet. Expected changes include a general shoreline retreat and increased flooding risk.

Urban heat island: A city or metropolitan area that is significantly warmer than its surrounding rural areas due to human activities.

References

Allan R. P., and B. J. Soden. 2008. "Atmospheric Warming and the Amplification of Precipitation Extremes." *Science* 321(5895):1481–84.

American Association for the Advancement of Science. 2006. "Evolution on the Front Line: An Abbreviated Guide for Teaching Evolution, from Project 2061 at AAAS." http://www.project2061.org/publications/guides/evolution.pdf

Arendt, A., T. Bolch, J. Cogley, A. Gardner, J. Hagen, R. Hock, G. Kaser, et al. 2012. "Randolph Glacier Inventory [v1. 0]: A Dataset of Global Glacier Outlines. Global land ice measurements from Space." Boulder CO: Digital Media.

Balbus, M., and C. Malina. 2009. "Identifying Vulnerable Subpopulations for Climate Change Health Effects in the United States." *Journal of Occupational and Environmental Medicine* 51:33–37.

Bassil, K., D. Col, R. Moineddin, W. Lou, A. Craig, B. Schwartz, and E. Rea. 2011. "The Relationship between Temperature and Ambulance Response Calls for Heat-Related Illness in Toronto, Ontario, 2005." *Journal of Epidemiology and Community Health* 65:829–31.

Blunden, J., and D. Arndt. 2013. "State of the Climate in 2012." *Bulletin of the American Meteorological Society* 94:S1–S258.

Brown, R., and D. Robinson. 2011. "Northern Hemisphere Spring Snow Cover Variability and Change over 1922–2010 including an Assessment of Uncertainty." *Cryosphere* 51:219–29.

Brown, R. D., and P. W. Mote. 2009. "The Response of Northern Hemisphere Snow Cover to a Changing Climate." *Journal of Climate* 22:2124–45.

Brutel-Vuilmet, C., M. Ménégoz, and G. Krinner. 2013. "An Analysis of Present and Future Seasonal Northern Hemisphere Land Snow Cover Simulated by CMIP5 Coupled Climate Models." *Cryosphere* 7:67–80.

Claessens, Y. E., P. Taupin, G. Kierzek, J. L. Pourriat, M. Baud, C. Ginsburg, J. P. Jais, E. Jougla, B. Riou, and J. F. Dhainaut. 2006. "How Emergency Departments Might Alert for Pre-Hospital Heat-Related Excess Mortality." *Critical Care* 10:R156.

Cook J., D. Nuccitelli, S. A. Green, M. Richardson, B. Winkler, R. Painting, R. Way, P. Jacobs, and A. Skuce. 2013. "Quantifying the Consensus on Anthropogenic Global Warming in the Scientific Literature." *Environmental Research Letters* 8(2):024024.

Dahl, R. 2013. "Cooling Concepts: Alternatives to Air-Conditioning for a Warm World." *Environmental Health Perspectives* 1(1):A19-A25.

Environmental Protection Agency. 2013. *Climate Change.* http://www.epa.gov/climatechange/

"Evaporative Cooling: How an Evaporative Cooler Works." 2012. Sacramento, CA: Consumer Energy Center, California Energy Commission. http://www.consumerenergycenter.org/home/heating_cooling/evaporative.html

Feldman D., W. Collins, P. Gero, M. Torn, E. Mlawer, and T. Shippert. 2015. "Observational Determination of Surface Radiative Forcing by CO_2 from 2000 to 2010." *Nature* 519(7543):339–43.

Hansen, J., R. Ruedy, M. Sato, and K. Lo. 2010. "Global Surface Temperature Change." *Reviews of Geophysics* 48:RG4004.

Harlan, S., J. Declet-Barret, W. Stefanov, and D. Petitti. 2013. "Neighborhood Effects on Heat Deaths: Social and Environmental Predictors of Vulnerability in Maricopa County, Arizona." *Environmental Health Perspectives* 121(2):197–204.

Harries, J. E., H. E. Brindley, P. J. Sagoo, and R. J. Bantges 2001. "Increases in Greenhouse Forcing Inferred from the Outgoing Longwave Radiation Spectra of the Earth in 1970 and 1997." *Nature* 410:355–57.

Hawkins, E., and R. Sutton. 2009. "The Potential to Narrow Uncertainty in Regional Climate Predictions." *Bulletin of the American Meteorological Society* 90:1095–1107.

Hawkins, E., and R. Sutton. 2011. "The Potential to Narrow Uncertainty in Projections of Regional Precipitation Change." *Climate Dynamics* 37(1–2):407–18.

Hays J. D., J. Imbrie, and N. J. Shackleton. 1976. *Variations in the Earth's Orbit: Pacemaker of the Ice Ages.* Washington, DC: American Association for the Advancement of Science.

Heinlein, R. A. 1973. *Time Enough for Love.* New York: Putnam.

Holland, P. R., and R. Kwok. 2012. "Wind-Driven Trends in Antarctic Sea-Ice Drift." *Nature Geoscience* 5(12):872–75.

Imbrie, J., and J. Z. Imbrie. 1980. "Modeling the Climatic Response to Orbital Variations." *Science* 207(4434):943–53.

Intergovernmental Panel on Climate Change. 1990. *Climate Change: The IPCC Scientific Assessment.* Cambridge: Cambridge University Press.

Intergovernmental Panel on Climate Change. 2001. *Climate Change 2001: Synthesis Report. A Contribution of Working Groups I, II, and III to the Third Assessment Report of the Intergovernmental Panel on Climate Change,* edited by R. T. Watson and the Core Writing Team. Cambridge: Cambridge University Pres.

Intergovernmental Panel on Climate Change. 2007. *Climate Change 2007: Synthesis Report. Contribution of Working Groups I, II, and III to the Fourth Assessment Report of the Intergovernmental Panel on Climate Change,* edited by R. K. Pachauri and A. Reisinger. Geneva: IPCC.

Intergovernmental Panel on Climate Change. 2013. "Summary for Policymakers." In *Climate Change 2013: The Physical Science Basis,* edited by T. F. Stocker, D. Qin, G.-K. Plattner, M. Tignor, S. K. Allen, J. Boschung, A. Nauels, et al. Cambridge: Cambridge University Press.

Kalnay, E., and M. Cai. 2003. "Impact of Urbanization and Land Use Change on Climate." *Nature* 423:528–31.

Kamal, M. A. 2011. "Reinventing Traditional Systems for Sustainable Built Environment: An Overview of Passive Downdraught Evaporative Cooling Technique for Energy Conservation." *Journal of Architectural and Planning Research* 11(2):56–62.

Kharin, V. V., F. W. Zwiers, X. Zhang, and M. Wehner. 2013. "Changes in Temperature and Precipitation Extremes in the CMIP5 Ensemble." *Climatic Change* 119:345–57.

Kovats, R. S., D. Campbell-Lendrum, and F. Matthies. 2005. "Climate Change and Human Health: Estimating Avoidable Deaths and Disease." *Risk Analysis* 25:1409–18.

Kunkel, K. E., M. Palecki, L. Ensor, K. G. Hubbard, D. Robinson, K. Redmond, and D. Easterling 2009. "Trends in Twentieth-Century US Snowfall Using a Quality-Controlled Dataset." *Journal of Atmospheric and Oceanic Technology* 26(1):33–44.

Le Quéré, C., M. R. Raupach, J. G. Canadell, G. Marland, L. Bopp, P. Ciais, T. J. Conway, S. C. Doney, R. A. Feely, and P. Foster. 2009. "Trends in the Sources and Sinks of Carbon Dioxide." *Nature Geoscience* 2:831–36.

Ledrans, M., P. Pirard, H. Tillaut, M. Pascal, S. Vandentorren, F. Suzan, G. Salines, A. Le Tertre, S. Medina, A. Maulpoix, et al. 2004. "The Heat Wave of August 2003: What Happened?" *La Revue du Praticien* 54:1289–1297.

Leonardi, G. S., S. Hajat, R. S. Kovats, G. Smith, D. Cooper, and E. Gerard. 2006. "Syndromic Surveillance Use to Detect the Early Effects of Heat-Waves: An Analysis of NHS Direct Data in England." *Sozial- und Präventivmedizin* 51:194–201.

Makowski, K., M. Wild, and A. Ohmura. 2008. "Diurnal Temperature Range over Europe between 1950 and 2005." *Atmospheric Chemistry and Physics* 8:6483–98.

Mastrandrea, M., C. Field, T. Stocker, O. Edenhofer, K. Ebi, D. Frame, H. Held, et al. 2010. *Guidance Note for Lead Authors of the IPCC Fifth Assessment Report on Consistent Treatment of Uncertainties.* Jasper Ridge, CA: Intergovernmental Panel on Climate Change.

McPhaden, M. J., S. E. Zebiak, and M. H. Glantz. 2006. "ENSO as an Integrating Concept in Earth Science." *Science* 314(5806):1740–45.

Mora, C., A. G. Frazier, R. J. Longman, R. S. Dacks, M. M. Walton, E. J. Tong, J. J. Sanchez, et al. 2013. "The Projected Timing of Climate Departure from Recent Variability." *Nature* 502(7470):183–87.

Moss, R. H., J. A. Edmonds, K. A. Hibbard, M. R. Manning, S. K. Rose, D. P. van Vuuren, T. R. Carter, et al. 2010. "The Next Generation of Scenarios for Climate Change Research and Assessment." *Nature* 463:747–56.

Nakicenovic, N., and R. Swart, eds. 2000. *Special Report on Emissions Scenarios.* Cambridge: Cambridge University Press.

National Research Council. Committee on America's Climate Choices. 2010. *Advancing the Science of Climate Change: America's Climate Choices.* Washington, DC: National Academies Press.

"Night-Purge Ventilation." 2012. San Rafael, CA: Autodesk. http://sustainability workshop.autodesk.com/fundamentals/night-purge-ventilation

"NOAA Earth System Research Laboratory: Global Greenhouse Gas Reference Network." 2015. Asheville, NC: NOAA. http://www.esrl.noaa.gov/gmd/ccgg /trends/#mlo_full

"NOAA National Climatic Data Center State of the Climate: Global Analysis for April 2015." 2015. Asheville, NC: NOAA. http://www.ncdc.noaa.gov/sotc /global/201504

Oke, T. R. 1982. "The Energetic Basis of the Urban Heat Island." *Quarterly Journal of the Royal Meteorological Society* 108(455):1–24.

O'Neill, B. C., M. Dalton, R. Fuchs, L. Jiang, S. Pachauri, and K. Zigova. 2010. "Global Demographic Trends and Future Carbon Emissions." *Proceedings of the National Academy of Sciences* 107(41):17521–26.

Oreskes N. 2004. "Beyond the Ivory Tower: The Scientific Consensus on Climate Change." *Science* 306(5702):686.

Pierce, D. W., T. P. Barnett, B. D. Santer, and P. J. Gleckler. 2009. "Selecting Global Climate Models for Regional Climate Change Studies." *Proceedings of the National Academy of Sciences* 106(21):8441.

Portmann, R. W., S. Solomon, and G. C. Hegerl. 2009. "Spatial and Seasonal Patterns in Climate Change, Temperatures, and Precipitation across the United States." *Proceedings of the National Academy of Sciences* 106:7324–29.

Rizwan, A. M., Y.C.L. Dennis, and C. Liu. 2008. "A Review on the Generation, Determination and Mitigation of Urban Heat Island." *Journal of Environmental Sciences* 20:120–28.

Robine J. M., S. L. Cheung, S. Le Roy, H. Van Oyen, C. Griffiths, J. P. Michel, and F. R. Herrmann. 2008. "Death Toll Exceeded 70,000 in Europe during the Summer of 2003." *Comptes Rendus Biologies* 331(2):171–78.

Robinson, D. A., and K. F. Dewy. 1990. "Recent Secular Variations in the Extent of Northern Hemisphere Snow Cover." *Geophysical Research Letters* 17:1557–60.

Robinson, P. J. 2001. "On the Definition of a Heat Wave." *Journal of Applied Meteorology and Climatology* 40(4):762–75.

Rodolfo-Metalpa, R., F. Houlbrèque, E. Tambutté, F. Boisson, C. Baggini, F. P. Patti, R. Jeffree, et al. 2011. "Coral and Mollusc Resistance to Ocean Acidification Adversely Affected by Warming." *Nature Climate Change* 1:308–12.

Rosenzweig, C., W. D. Solecki, S. A. Hammer, and S. Mehrotra. 2011. *Climate Change and Cities: First Assessment Report of the Urban Climate Change Research Network.* Cambridge: Cambridge University Press.

Semenza, J. C., C. H. Rubin, K. H. Falter, J. D. Selanikio, W. D. Flanders, H. L. Howe, and J. L. Wilhelm. 1996. "Heat-Related Deaths during the July 1995 Heat Wave in Chicago." *New England Journal of Medicine* 335(2):84–90.

Shwed, U., and P. S. Bearman. 2010. "The Temporal Structure of Scientific Consensus Formation." *American Sociological Review* 75:817–40.

Siegenthaler, U., and H. Oeschger. 1987. "Biospheric CO_2 Emissions during the Past 200 Years Reconstructed by Deconvolution of Ice Core Data." *Tellus B* 39:140–54.

Sillmann, J., V. V. Kharin, F. W. Zwiers, X. Zhang, and D. Bronaugh. 2013. "Climate Extremes Indices in the CMIP5 Multimodel Ensemble: Part 2. Future Climate Projections." *Journal of Geophysical Research: Atmospheres* 118:2473–93.

Sivak, M. 2009. "Potential Energy Demand for Cooling in the 50 Largest Metropolitan Areas of the World: Implications for Developing Countries." *Energy Policy* 37:1382–84.

Slangen, A., M. Carson, C. Katsman, R. van de Wal, A. Köhl, L. Vermeersen, and D. Stammer. 2014. "Projecting Twenty-First Century Regional Sea-Level Changes." *Climate Change*, 124:1–16.

Smargiassi, A., M. S. Goldberg, and T. Kosatsky. 2009. "Variation of Daily Warm Season Mortality as a Function of Micro-Urban Heat Islands." *Journal of Epidemiology and Community Health* 63:659–64.

Solomon, S., D. Qin, M. Manning, Z. Chen, M. Marquis, K. B. Avery, M. Tignor, and H. L. Miller. 2007. *Contribution of Working Group I to the Fourth Assessment Report of the Intergovernmental Panel on Climate Change, 2007.* Cambridge: Cambridge University Press.

Stone, B., J. J. Hess, and H. Frumkin. 2010. "Urban Form and Extreme Heat Events: Are Sprawling Cities More Vulnerable to Climate Change Than Compact Cities?" *Environmental Health Perspectives* 118(10):1425.

Stott P. A., D. A. Stone, and M. R. Allen. 2004. "Human Contribution to the European Heatwave of 2003." *Nature* 432:610–14.

Takeuchi, Y., Y. Endo, and S. Murakami. 2008. "High Correlation between Winter Precipitation and Air Temperature in Heavy-Snowfall Areas in Japan." *Annals of Glaciology* 49(1):7–10.

Trenberth, K. E. 1997. "The Definition of El Niño." *Bulletin of the American Meteorological Society* 78(12):2771–77.

Uejio C. K., O. V. Wilhelmi, J. S. Golden, D. M. Mills, S. P. Gulino, and J. P. Samenow. 2011. "Intra-urban Societal Vulnerability to Extreme Heat: The Role of Heat Exposure and the Built Environment, Socioeconomics, and Neighborhood Stability." *Health Place* 17(2):498–507.

Vose, R. S., D. R. Easterling, and B. Gleason. 2005. "Maximum and Minimum Temperature Trends for the Globe: An Update through 2004." *Geophysical Research Letters* 32:L23822.

Vuille, M., and R. D. Garreaud. 2011. "Ocean-Atmosphere Interactions on Interannual to Decadal Timescales." In *Handbook of Environmental Change*, edited by J. A. Matthews, P. J. Bartlein, K. R. Briffa, A. G. Dawson, A. De Vernal, T. Denham, S. C. Fritz, et al. Los Angeles: Sage.

Wacker, S., J. Gröbner, K. Hocke, N. Kämpfer, and L. Vuilleumier. 2011. "Trend Analysis of Surface Cloud-Free Downwelling Long-Wave Radiation from Four Swiss Sites." *Journal of Geophysical Research: Atmospheres* 116(D10):1–13.

Walter, M. E. 2010. "Earthquakes and Weatherquakes: Mathematics and Climate Change." *Notices of the AMS* 57(10):1278–84.

"Weather Is Your Mood and Climate Is Your Personality." 2014. Washington, DC: Office of Science and Technology Policy. https://www.whitehouse.gov /blog/2014/01/10/what-you-missed-we-geeks-weather-your-mood-and-climate-your-personality

Wild, M. 2012. "Enlightening Global Dimming and Brightening." *Bulletin of the American Meteorological Society* 93(1):27–37.

Zebiak, S. E., B. Orlove, A. G. Muñoz, C. Vaughan, J. Hansen, T. Troy, M. C. Thomson, A. Lustig, and S. Garvin. 2015. "Investigating El Niño-Southern Oscillation and Society Relationships." *Climate Change* 6(1):17–34.

Zelinka, M. D., S. A. Klein, K. E. Taylor, and T. Andrews. 2013. "Contributions of Different Cloud Types to Feedbacks and Rapid Adjustments in CMIP5." *Journal of Climate* 26:5007–27.

Zhang, J. 2007. "Increasing Antarctic Sea Ice under Warming Atmospheric and Oceanic Conditions." *Journal of Climate* 20(11):2515–29.

Zhou, Y., and G. Ren. 2011. "Change in Extreme Temperature Event Frequency over Mainland China, 1961–2008." *Climate Research* 50:125–39.

CHAPTER 2

EXTREME WEATHER EVENTS

The Role of Public Health in Disaster Risk Reduction as a Means for Climate Change Adaptation

Mark E. Keim

The incidence of natural **disasters** is increasing (Center for Research on the Epidemiology of Disasters 2009). The United States accounted for a higher proportion of global natural catastrophe losses than usual in 2012 due to a series of severe weather-related catastrophes. In 2013, natural catastrophes caused $160 billion in overall losses and $65 billion in insured losses worldwide. Some 67 percent of overall losses and 90 percent of insured losses worldwide were attributable to the United States. The year's highest insured loss was caused by Hurricane Sandy, with an estimated amount of around $25 billion (Munich Re Group 2013). Over the past century, the incidence of extreme weather (hydrometeorological) disasters has increased much more rapidly than disasters caused by geological or biological disasters (Center for Research on the Epidemiology of Disasters 2009).

In 2007, the Intergovernmental Panel on Climate Change (IPCC) concluded that changes in the climate will lead to increase in natural **hazards** into the future. More recently in 2011, the IPCC released the special report *Managing the Risks of Extreme Events and Disasters to Advance Climate Change Adaptation* (SREX), which assessed "how **exposure** and **vulnerability** to weather and climate events determine impacts and the likelihood of disasters (**disaster risk**)." Most pertinent, the SREX also examined "how disaster risk management and adaptation to climate change can reduce exposure and vulnerability to weather and climate

KEY CONCEPTS

- **Extreme weather events are a major cause contributing to the global burden of disasters.**

- **There are fifteen major public health consequences of disasters associated with extreme weather events. These consequences vary only in degree of impact among the various extreme weather disasters.**

- **Disaster risk management is a comprehensive all-hazard approach that entails developing and implementing strategies for each phase of the disaster life cycle.**

- **Disaster risk management as applied to climate change adaptation includes both preimpact disaster risk reduction (prevention, preparedness, and mitigation) as well as postimpact disaster risk transfer (risk pools and insurance policies) and disaster risk retention: (response and recovery).**

The material in this chapter reflects solely my own views. It does not necessarily reflect the policies or recommendations of the Centers for Disease Control and Prevention or the US Department of Health and Human Services.

KEY CONCEPTS (*CONTINUED*)

- **Health-related disaster risk due to extreme weather events occurs as the result of convergence of four key factors: the presence of a health *hazard* associated with an extreme weather and climate events, the degree of *exposure* to the hazard sustained by the person (or population), the degree of *vulnerability* of the person (or population) to that particular health hazard, and the degree of *resilience* of the person (or population) in order to avoid or moderate harm.**

- **Disaster risk may be reduced among populations at risk by reducing exposure to the hazard itself, decreasing the population's vulnerability, and increasing their resilience.**

events and thus reduce disaster risk, as well as increase **resilience** to the risks that cannot be eliminated."

Human vulnerability to disasters is also increasing worldwide. **Disaster risk management** is largely a task for local actors. Public health works at the local level on a daily basis and therefore is uniquely placed at the community level, where it can work in a multisectoral approach for disaster risk management to lessen human vulnerability to extreme weather events (Keim 2011).

This chapter provides an overview of the public health impacts of extreme weather events. It also examines the role of community-focused public health as a means for **disaster risk reduction** by way of lessening human vulnerability as an adaptation to extreme weather events, which are predicted to increase as a result of climate change.

Disasters Caused by Extreme Weather Events

A disaster is "a serious disruption of the functioning of a community or a society causing widespread human, material, economic or environmental losses that exceed the ability of the affected community or society to cope using its own resources" (United Nations International Strategy for Disaster Reduction 2009). Disaster consequences may include loss of life, injury, disease, and other negative effects on human physical, mental, and social well-being, together with damage to property, destruction of assets, loss of services, social and economic disruption, and environmental degradation (UNISDR 2009). The severity of these consequences is referred to as *disaster impact.* Disasters occur as a result of the combination of population exposure to a hazard, the conditions of vulnerability that are present, and insufficient **capacity** or measures to reduce or cope with the potential negative consequences.

Disasters caused by extreme weather events anticipated that may occur as a result of climate change can be categorized as associated with high precipitation (e.g., storms, floods, and landslides) or low precipitation (e.g., heat, drought, and wildfire) (Keim 2011).

Environmental disasters occur as a result of the combination of population exposure to an environmental hazard, the conditions of vulnerability that are present, and insufficient capacity or measures to reduce or cope with the potential negative consequences. Without outside assistance, these events often overwhelm the capacity of communities and societies to respond, and the resulting mismatch between needs and resources may result in a disaster declaration.

Disasters caused by extreme weather events may also be categorized as intensive **risk** and extensive risk events (UNISDR 2009). Disasters are categorized as intensive risk when intense hazards like floods and major storms strike densely populated areas with high levels of vulnerability. They are categorized as extensive risk when there is widespread risk associated with the exposure of dispersed populations to repetitive or persistent hazard conditions of low or moderate intensity. These events (e.g., the drought-flood cycle) are often of a diffusely dispersed nature yet can lead to debilitating cumulative disaster impacts.

Scope of the Problem

According to the United Nations, during the fifty-year period 1964 to 2013, disasters have affected 7 billion people with 5.2 million deaths (CRED 2009). Disasters may be caused by natural or technological hazards. Technological disasters include poisoning, chemical spills, radiation releases, structural collapses, and structural fires. Natural disasters are caused by hydrometeorological, geological, and biological hazards. Hydrometeorological disasters (including droughts, floods, storms, wildfires, and temperature extremes) are by far the most frequent disaster declarations in the world and result in the highest loss in damages (CRED 2009). Geological disasters (including earthquakes, volcanic eruptions, tsunamis, and landslides) tend to have the highest mortality rates and have resulted in the greatest loss of life worldwide (CRED 2009). Biological disasters are caused by epidemics of infectious disease (including HIV/AIDS, malaria, and tuberculosis).

Disasters caused by extreme weather events represent a significant portion of the worldwide disaster burden. As shown in figure 2.1, from 1964 to 2013, 41 percent of all disaster-related mortality were caused by hydrometeorological (climate-related) disasters. In comparison, 4 percent were caused by biological disasters and 5 percent by technological disasters (CRED 2009).

From 1980 to 2011, there were 7,009 climate-related disaster declarations worldwide, averaging 226 per year (UNISDR 2013). From 1900 to 2013, 87 percent of extreme weather disasters were associated with high precipitation events. Nearly half of these climate-related disasters worldwide were due to flooding (49 percent), and over one-third were caused by storms (38 percent) (CRED 2009). (See figure 2.2.)

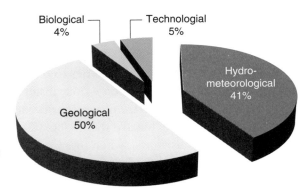

Figure 2.1   Categories of Disaster-Related Mortality
Worldwide, 1964–2013
Source: Adapted from EM-DAT (2010).

The world's poor are disproportionately affected by disasters, and the most vulnerable and marginalized people in these nations bear the brunt for a variety of reasons, including higher degree of exposure, higher degrees of vulnerability due to health disparity, and lower levels of capacity to prepare for, respond to, and recover from losses (Clack et al. 2002; National Science and Technology Council 1996; Brouewer et al. 2007; Nelson 1990; International Federation of Red Cross 2005). Table 2.1 shows the major climate-related disasters that occurred from 1900 to 2013 and the number

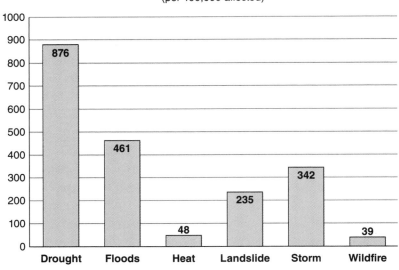

Figure 2.2   Mortality Rate among the Top Ten Disasters for Each Category of Extreme Weather Hazard, 1900–2013
Source: EM-DAT: http://www.emdat.be/database
From 1900 to 2011, extreme weather disasters caused over 19 million deaths and affected nearly 3.2 billion people worldwide (CRED 2009). In particular, meteorological hazards affect an increasing number of people and cause increasingly large economic losses likely related to climate change and increasing vulnerability of the populations affected (Thomalla 2006).

Table 2.1   World's Top Ten Extreme Weather Events Associated with Highest Mortality, 1900–2013, Ranked by Number of Deaths per Nation

Hazard	Country	Year	Number Killed (in millions)
Flood	China	1931	3.70
Drought	China	1928	3.00
Flood	China	1959	2.00
Drought	Bangladesh	1943	1.90
Drought	India	1942	1.50
Drought	India	1965	1.50
Drought	India	1900	1.25
Drought	Soviet Union	1921	1.20
Drought	China	1920	0.50
Flood	China	1939	0.50

Source: EM-DAT: http://www.emdat.be/database

Note: While there were extreme weather event disasters occurring after 1965, these events were not among the top largest in terms of number of deaths per nation.

of fatalities associated with each event. All of these disasters occurred in developing nations, and all were caused by either floods or droughts.

Public Health Impact of Extreme Weather Disasters

This chapter uses definitions of extreme weather-related disasters derived from the United Nations *Internationally Agreed Glossary of Basic Terms related to Disaster Management* (UN Department of Humanitarian Affairs 1992). This glossary is a result of a joint effort of a number of intergovernmental organizations, nongovernmental organizations, and national institutions to publish a collection of internationally agreed definitions of disaster-related basic terminology. Also for simplifying our conceptualization of the range of disaster described in this chapter, we classify extreme weather disasters into two broad categories: those associated with high levels of precipitation and those associated with low levels of precipitation.

Populations at risk for disasters face a vast range of hazards within a nearly infinite set of scenarios. This unpredictability is poorly suited to scenario-based approaches to **risk management** (Henry 2005). While the hazards that cause disasters may vary greatly, the potential public health consequences and subsequent public health and medical needs of the population do not (Keim 2006a; Federal Emergency Management Agency 1996). For example, floods, heat waves, hurricanes, and wildfires all have the potential to displace people from their homes. These hazards require the same sheltering capability with only minor adjustments based on the rapidity of onset, scale, duration, location, and intensity. Regardless of the hazard, disasters can be seen as causing fifteen public health consequences that are addressed by approximately thirty-five categories of public health and medical capabilities (Keim 2006c; Centers for Disease Control and Prevention 2011). Table 2.2 identifies the relative impact of these public health consequences.

Mortality due to Extreme Weather Disasters

Drought disasters are responsible for causing nearly 59.6 percent of these deaths. Floods were nearly 34.6 percent of these disaster-related deaths, and storms caused 4.95 percent, with the remaining less than 1 percent caused by heat waves (0.67 percent), landslides (0.14 percent), and wildfires (0.01 percent) (CRED 2009).

Mortality rates also vary according to each extreme weather hazard. The mortality rate for drought (876/100,000 affected) is the highest of all extreme weather hazards and nearly twice as high as that for floods (461/100,000). Close behind floods are the mortality rates for storms (342/100,000) and landslides (235/100,000). Heat waves and wildfires have the lowest mortality rates at 48 and 39 per 100,000, respectively (CRED 2009).

Morbidity due to Extreme Weather Disasters

Most of the morbidity related to extreme weather events occurs as injuries sustained as a result of exposure to environmental hazards such as water, wind, fire, debris, and temperature extremes.

Infectious disease epidemics following natural disasters are rare and differ according to the level of economic development of the affected nation (Keim 2010; CDC 1998, 2002; Guill and Shandera 2001; Watson, Gayer, and Connolly 2007; Ahern et al. 2005; McCarthy et al. 1994; Woodruff et al. 1990; Ivers and Ryan 2006). Although quite rare among most natural disasters, floods are associated with epidemics of communicable disease, mostly in low-income nations (Keim 2010; CDC 1998, 2002; Guill and Shandera 2001; Watson et al. 2007; Ahern et al. 2005; McCarthy et al. 1994; Woodruff et al. 1990; Ivers and Ryan 2006; Guha-Sapir and van Panhuis 2009; Floret et al. 2006) There is tremendous potential for psychosocial impacts that accompany traumatic experiences such as injury, displacement from homes, and socioeconomic disruption. Behavioral health effects are among the most debilitating long-term outcomes of environmental disasters (Krug et al. 1998; Keenan et al. 2004; Sattler et al. 2002; Goenjian et al. 2001; Caldera et al. 2001).

Extreme weather disasters can markedly affect the ability of the population to maintain and access adequate shelter, water, sanitation, hygiene,

Table 2.2 Relative Public Health Impacts of Extreme Weather Disasters

| Public Health Impact | EXTREME WEATHER DISASTERS | | | | | |
| | HIGH PRECIPITATION | | | LOW PRECIPITATION | | |
	Landslide	Storms	Flood	Drought	Wildfire	Heat
Deaths	Few to moderate	Few, but many in poor nations	Few, but many in poor nations	Few, but many in poor nations	Few	Moderate to many in rich nations
Injuries	Few to moderate	Few	Few	Unlikely	Few	Unlikely
Loss of clean water	Focal	Focal to widespread	Focal to widespread	Widespread	Focal	Unlikely
Loss of safe shelter	Focal	Focal to widespread	Focal to widespread	Focal to widespread	Focal	Focal to widespread
Loss of personal and household goods	Focal	Focal to widespread	Focal to widespread	Focal to widespread	Focal	Unlikely
Major population movements	Focal	Focal to widespread	Focal to widespread	Focal to widespread	Focal	Unlikely
Loss of routine hygiene	Focal	Focal to widespread	Focal to widespread	Widespread	Focal	Unlikely
Loss of sanitation	Focal	Focal to widespread	Focal to widespread	Focal	Focal	Unlikely
Disruption of solid waste management	Focal	Focal to widespread	Focal to widespread	Focal	Focal	Unlikely
Public concern for safety	Moderate to High	High	Moderate to High	Low to moderate	Moderate to High	Moderate to High
Increased pests	Unlikely	Focal to widespread	Focal to widespread	Focal to widespread	Unlikely	Unlikely
Loss or damage of health care system	Focal	Focal to widespread	Focal to widespread	Focal	Focal to widespread	Unlikely
Worsening of chronic illnesses	Focal	Focal to widespread	Focal to widespread	Widespread	Focal to widespread	Focal to widespread
Loss of electrical power	Focal	Focal to widespread	Focal to widespread	Focal	Unlikely	Focal
Toxic exposures	Focal	Widespread for CO poisoning	Widespread for CO poisoning	Focal	Widespread for air	Unlikely
Food scarcity	Focal	Common in low-lying coastal areas	Focal to widespread	Widespread in poor nations	Focal	Unlikely

Source: Adapted from Keim (2010).

health care, nutrition, security, public services, or utilities in order to maintain their health during a disaster event. These factors have a significant influence on morbidity following a disaster.

Low-Precipitation Events

Public Health Impact of Drought   The UN's *Internationally Agreed Glossary of Basic Terms related to Disaster Management* defines *drought* as "a period of deficiency of moisture in the soil such that there is inadequate water required for plants, animals and human beings" (UN Department of Humanitarian Affairs 1992). From 1974 to 2003, droughts occurred most frequently in Australia, Brazil, China, India, and sub-Saharan Africa (CRED 2009).

Drought-Related Mortality   Ironically, very few people die of thirst or dehydration during a drought, even in underdeveloped countries. Drought-related deaths generally occur secondary to the agricultural economic and medical side effects of drought, such as famine, malnutrition, poverty, poor public health practices, contamination of existing water supplies, infectious diseases, social strife, and heat-related illness (CRED 2009). Table 2.3 lists the world's ten droughts from 1900 to 2013 with highest mortality.

Table 2.3   Top Ten Droughts with Highest Mortality, Worldwide, 1900–2013, Ranked by Number of Deaths

Country	Year	Number of Deaths
China	1928	3,000,000
Bangladesh	1943	1,900,000
India	1942	1,500,000
India	1965	1,500,000
India	1900	1,250,000
Soviet Union	1921	1,200,000
China	1920	500,000
Ethiopia	1983	300,000
Sudan	1983	150,000
Ethiopia	1973	100,000

Source: EM-DAT: http://www.emdat.be/database

Note: While there were drought disasters occurring after 1983, these events were not among the top largest in terms of number of deaths.

Drought-Related Morbidity Most drought-related morbidity and mortality occurs in resource-poor nations. In resource-rich nations, the impact of drought is largely economic. Besides increasing the likelihood of food insecurity and famine, a drought can have catastrophic effects on the regional or national economy (Wilhite 1993). Thus, in resource-rich nations, the main health impact stems from economic stressors that result in psychosocial morbidity. Worldwide, the predominant psychosocial impacts of drought focus on the decreased quality of life, major changes in lifestyle, and increasing conflict. Disagreements are generated over water use, management of water resources, and political philosophies. The degree of social strife may be at the international, interstate, community, or individual level (Wilhite 1993).

Droughts are notable in the capacity to affect extremely large groups of people. The largest single drought during the past century is estimated to have affected 300 million people, with the top ten droughts during the past century affecting over 1 billion people (CRED 2009). Table 2.4 lists the world's ten largest droughts from 1900 to 2013. Here, the definition of *affected* includes all persons, encompassing injuries, deaths, and those displaced.

Public Health Impact of Heat Waves   The UN *Internationally Agreed Glossary of Basic Terms related to Disaster Management* defines *heat waves* as "a long lasting period with extremely high surface temperature" (UN Department of Humanitarian Affairs 1992). While there is no single

Table 2.4   World's Top Ten Largest Droughts, 1900–2013, Ranked by Number of People Affected

Country	Year	Number of People Affected
India	1987	300,000,000
India	2002	300,000,000
India	1972	200,000,000
India	1965	100,000,000
India	1982	100,000,000
China	1994	82,000,000
China	2002	60,000,000
China	2009	60,000,000
India	2000	50,000,000
China	1988	49,000,000

Source: EM-DAT: http://www.emdat.be/database

Note: While there were drought disasters occurring after 2009, these events were not among the top largest in terms of number of people affected.

agreed-on definition of an extreme heat event, most definitions refer to an extended period of time (several days or more) with unusually hot weather conditions that potentially can harm human health. Heat waves are not determined by absolute temperature alone but are dependent on other conditions specific to each location, including acclimation of the population. In addition to ambient temperatures, other environmental factors, such as humidity, air circulation, building types, and night-time temperatures, can intensify the health effects (Adrianopoli et al. 2010).

A heat emergency results when the environmental conditions of a region are such that the heat burden gained by the human body cannot be dissipated by the usual physiological mechanisms (Walker and Hogan 2003). The public health impact of heat waves may include:

- Heat illness

- Exacerbations of chronic obstructive pulmonary disease and asthma, as well as cardiovascular disease (both strokes and heart attacks)

- Short-term population displacement that results in a relatively brief need for humanitarian assistance to include safe shelter, water and food, security, sanitation, and health care among those seeking relief from the heat in their homes

Mortality   Historically heat waves had an enormous impact on human morbidity and mortality. In 1985, 800 people died as a result of heat wave affecting Milwaukee and Chicago. Additional thousands have died in subsequent urban heat waves in Cincinnati, Philadelphia, St. Louis, Kansas City, and other major US cities since the early 1990s (Adrianopoli et al. 2010). During summer 1987, a heat wave in Greece and Italy precipitated the death of approximately 3,000 people (Bailey and Walker 2007).

Table 2.5 lists the ten most extreme heat waves from 1900 to 2013 ranked according to number of deaths per nation (CRED 2009). It also reveals that all of the past century's heat waves with the highest mortality have occurred since 1980. Moreover, recently an estimated 65,000 to 70,000 people died in the 2003 heat wave that affected most of Western Europe during the hottest summer on record since 1540 (Sardon 2007; Robine et al. 2008). Stott, Stone, and Allen (2004) concluded that human activities including anthropogenic production of greenhouse gases may have contributed to the doubling of the risk of heat waves of this magnitude.

Isolated, low-income, elderly urban populations are at particular risk for mortality during heat waves. The immediate impact of the heat wave is a high incidence of heat stroke and other heat-related illnesses in the population. Over greater periods, individual physiological acclimatization to

Table 2.5 World's Top Ten Heat Waves Associated with Highest Mortality, 1900–2013, Ranked by Number of Deaths per Nation

Country	Year	Number of Deaths
Russia	2010	55,736
Italy	2003	20,089
France	2003	19,490
Spain	2003	15,090
Germany	2003	9,355
Greece and Italy	1987	3,000
Portugal	2003	2,696
India	1998	2,541
France	2006	1,388
United States	1980	1,260

Source: EM-DAT: http://www.emdat.be/database

Note: While there were heat wave disasters occurring after 2010, these events were not among the top largest in terms of number of deaths.

the heat develops, and a decrease in the direct heat injury morbidity and mortality is observed. In the long term, the most consequential impact of substantial heat waves may result from drought, wildfires, and firestorms (Bailey and Walker 2007).

Public Health Impact of Wildfires   *Wildfire* is defined as "a sweeping and destructive conflagration especially in a wilderness or a rural area" (Merriam Webster Dictionary Online n.d.). The United Nations *Internationally Agreed Glossary of Basic Terms related to Disaster Management* describes this same phenomenon as "forest/grassland fire" and defines it as "fires in forest or brush grasslands that cover extensive areas and usually do extensive damage" (UN Department of Humanitarian Affairs 1992). Wildfires have resulted in significant natural disasters all over the globe. In Australia's Ash Wednesday Fires of 1983, 75 people died, 2,539 homes were destroyed, and 300,000 domestic animals perished. In Côte d'Ivoire during forest and savanna fires in 1982 and 1983, 100 people died and 12 million hectares of land, 40,000 hectares of coffee plantations, and 60,000 hectares of cocoa plantations were destroyed. In Mongolia, steppe and forest fires in 1996 and 1997 caused 25 deaths and destroyed 10.7 million hectares of land. In Kalimantan (Borneo), during the 1982–1983 El Niño drought, fires destroyed more than 5 million hectares of forest and agricultural land, while in 1997–1998, also in Indonesia, fires on the islands of Sumatra and Borneo consumed 9 million hectares of vegetation. During the drought in the former USSR in 1987, some 14.5 million hectares of forest were destroyed by fire (World Health Organization 2009).

In 1997 and 1998, forest fires in Southeast Asia affected some 200 million people in Brunei Darussalam, Indonesia, Malaysia, the Philippines, Singapore, and Thailand. Massive movements of population fleeing the fires and smoke added to the emergency, while the increase in the number of emergency visits to hospitals during the crisis demonstrated its severity. The comparison of medical data reported during the 1997–1998 forest fire events in Southeast Asia with corresponding data in 1995 and 1996 revealed the following impact of smoke on public health, which is consistent with our knowledge of the effects of fine particles. The number of cases of pneumonia increased five to twenty-five times in southeast Borneo and one and a half to five times in South Sumatra. The number of outpatient visits with respiratory diseases in Malaysia increased two- to threefold. In September 1997 in Sumatra, the number of reported cases of upper respiratory tract infections was 50 percent higher than in the previous month (World Health Organization 1998). In fact, most of the adverse health events occur as a result of poor air quality. Deaths due to wildfires are largely due to burns and smoke asphyxiation. Table 2.6 lists the world's ten worst wildfires from 1900 to 2013, ranked according to number of deaths per nation.

Table 2.6   World's Top Ten Wildfires Associated with Highest Mortality, 1900 to 2013, Ranked by Number of Deaths per Nation

Country	Year	Number of Deaths
United States	1918	1,000
Indonesia	1997	240
People's Republic of China	1987	191
Australia	2003	180
United States	1944	121
France	1949	80
Australia	1983	75
Canada	1911	73
Australia	1939	71
Greece	1980	67

Source: EM-DAT: http://www.emdat.be/database

Note: While there were wildfire disasters occurring after 2003, these events were not among the top largest in terms of number of deaths.

The public health impact of wildfires may include burn injuries; exacerbations of chronic obstructive pulmonary disease and asthma; and population displacement that results in a need for humanitarian assistance to include safe shelter, water and food, security, sanitation, and health care. In 1991, multiple grass wildfires in the United States resulted in 226 deaths and more than 225 injuries (Bedian, Arcus, and Frankel-Cone 1994). Emergency department records showed that more than twice as many people sought treatment for smoke-related problems than did so for other traumatic injuries (Shusterman, Kaplan, and Canabarro 1993).

CLINICAL CORRELATES 2.1 FAILURE AND SUCCESS IN HOSPITALS DURING DISASTERS

During natural disasters, hospitals are considered "custodial" organizations and thus are the last to be evacuated and closed. During Hurricane Katrina, floodwaters surrounding area hospitals stranded 2,000 patients and 5,500 staff and family (Louisiana Hospital Association 2005). The hospitals had no electricity because their backup generators in basements were underwater. There was no running water, sewage treatment, refrigeration, or access to CT scanners, X-rays, laboratory information, or blood banks. Ventilators and dialysis machines could not function. Essential supplies dwindled due to transportation breakdown. Reports describe emergency surgery being done by flashlight with little or no anesthesia and family members fanning patients in sweltering rooms (Gray and Hebert 2007). Many hospitals were short-staffed and providers worked long shifts in adverse conditions while witnessing the inevitable deaths of patients who would not be sustained without life support (Davis 2005).

How should we prepare for sudden or prolonged resource shortage? Over the past fifty years, modern medical practice has become increasingly dependent on technology in diagnostics and treatment, and health care is one of the most energy-intense sectors of the economy (US Energy Information Administration 2012). Hospitals can prepare for resource shortage by adopting green energy-saving practices and identifying through institutional analysis what essential systems are necessary in emergency scenarios and how to shunt limited power to those areas. Health care providers can and must begin to train themselves to practice medicine without intensive technology or essential diagnostic testing. This approach will not only prepare us for disasters related to the environment but also abate the current financial health care crisis.

Health care is one of the most energy-intense sectors, and its systems become vulnerable during natural disasters when resources become scarce. Hospitals and providers can prepare by adopting green infrastructure and limiting unnecessary testing and interventions in the present.

High-Precipitation Events

Public Health Impact of Floods   The UN *Internationally Agreed Glossary of Basic Terms related to Disaster Management* defines *floods* as a "significant rise of water level in a stream, lake, reservoir or a coastal region" (UN Department of Humanitarian Affairs 1992). Gunn (1990) defines *flood* more specifically as "the overflow of areas that are not normally submerged with water or a stream that has broken its normal confines or has accumulated due to lack of drainage." For the purpose of this discussion, fluvial (or riverine) flooding will be characterized as either a seasonal flood or a flash flood. This is important because flash floods are often associated with a greater loss of life than seasonal riverine floods. Seasonal floods are typified by a gradual rise to flood stage that may extend across large areas over a long duration. Because seasonal floods are usually caused by a relatively gradual accumulation, warning times are usually sufficient to allow safe evacuation of nearby communities. Flash floods are characterized by a short-duration, high-volume stream flow and usually occur within six hours of a rain event, after a dam or levy fails, or after the sudden release of water from an ice or debris jam. They are accompanied by an extremely short warning and **response** time with potential for great loss of life (Centers for Disease Control and Prevention 1993a).

Coastal flooding can increase as a result of climate change–induced sea and lake level rise, coastal erosion, barrier reef loss, and storm surge associated with cyclonic tropical storms. Sea inundation of entire low-lying islands may also occur due to rogue surface waves and ocean eddies imparted by weather systems. Storm surge, produced by the high winds and vacuum effect of low-pressure cyclonic storm systems, can produce dramatically high seas that result in coastal flooding. These large storm surges, destructive and dangerous, accounted for an estimated 90 percent of deaths before a warning and evacuation system is implemented (Malilay 1997).

Mortality   Drowning is the main cause of deaths due to floods. The public health impact of floods also may include population displacement that results in a need for humanitarian assistance to include safe shelter, water and food, security, sanitation, and health care. Table 2.7 lists the world's ten floods with highest mortality from 1900 to 2013. Seven of these floods occurred in China. All ten occurred in low-resource countries.

Public health impacts of flooding include (CDC 2002):

• Damage to homes and consequent displacement of occupants, infectious disease exacerbated by crowded living conditions, and compromised personal hygiene

• Contamination of water sources

Table 2.7   World's Top Ten Floods Associated with Highest Mortality, 1900–2013, Ranked by Number of People Killed per Nation

Country	Year	Number Killed
China	1931	3,700,000
China	1959	2,000,000
China	1939	500,000
China	1935	142,000
China	1911	100,000
China	1949	57,000
Guatemala	1949	40,000
China	1954	30,000
Venezuela	1999	30,000
Bangladesh	1974	28,700

Source: EM-DAT: http://www.emdat.be/database

Note: While there were flood disasters occurring after 1999, these events were not among the top largest in terms of number of deaths.

- Disruption of sewage service and solid-waste collection
- Increased vector populations
- Injuries sustained during cleanup
- Stress-related mental health
- Substance abuse problems
- Death

Like droughts, floods are also notable in the capacity to affect extremely large groups of people. The largest single flood during the past century is estimated to have affected nearly 239 million people, with the top ten droughts during the past century affecting over 1 billion people (CRED 2009). Table 2.8 lists the world's ten largest floods, 1900 to 2013, ranked according to number of people affected.

CLINICAL CORRELATES 2.2   ARE WE READY TO ABSORB THE MENTAL HEALTH IMPACT?

According to the World Health Organization (2011), mental, neurological, and substance use disorders account for 14 percent of the global burden of disease. Current estimates place the global shortage of mental health care workers at 1.8 million, including 55,000 psychiatrists, 628,000 nurses, and 493,000 psychosocial care providers. The rippling effect of mental distress caused by natural disasters can be observed in increased rates of substance abuse (Felder et al. 2014), post-traumatic stress disorder (Chan and Rhodes 2014), child abuse (Keenan et al. 2004), and suicide (Krug et al. 1998). These conditions have the potential to undermine the social fabric of a community in which a natural disaster has occurred, impairing reconstruction efforts and economic resolution. In addition, these mental health disorders may manifest as disease through their protean interactions with physical health (Prince et al. 2007).

Although regions of the world with a disproportionate dearth of trained mental health workers are likely to experience a greater impact, industrialized nations are not immune. Currently the United States spends a relatively low percentage of total health care dollars on mental health. Studies have identified a widespread prescribing and nonprescribing provider shortage (Thomas et al. 2009), which has resulted in de facto mental health care, whereby primary care doctors or subspecialty practitioners care for roughly 50 percent of patients seeking treatment for mental health disorders. Thus, as the mental health burden from natural disasters rises, all areas of medicine are going to be called on to care for patients in need, with little funding or systems in place to do so.

Mental health care plays a crucial role in disaster recovery, and the dearth of providers domestically and globally means the care will be distributed among all specialties of medicine.

Table 2.8   World's Top Ten Largest Floods, 1900–2013, Ranked by Number of People Affected

Country	Year	Number Affected
China	1998	238,973,000
China	1991	210,232,227
China	1996	154,634,000
China	2003	150,146,000
China	2010	134,000,000
India	1993	128,000,000
China	1995	114,470,249
China	2007	105,004,000
China	1999	101,024,000
China	1989	100,010,000

Source: EM-DAT: http://www.emdat.be/database

Note: While there were flood disasters occurring after 2010, these events were not among the top largest in terms of number of people affected.

Public Health Impact of Storms   The terminology of storms is complex. A storm is any disturbed state of an astronomical body's atmosphere, especially affecting its surface, and strongly implying severe weather. It may be marked by strong wind, thunder and lightning (a thunderstorm), heavy precipitation such as ice (ice storm), or wind transporting some substance through the atmosphere (as in a dust storm, snowstorm, and hailstorm, for example).

A cyclonic storm is an area of closed, circular fluid motion rotating in the same direction as the Earth. Examples include tropical cyclones and tornadoes. A cyclone is a weather phenomenon featuring a central region of low pressure surrounded by air flowing in an inward spiral and generating maximum sustained wind speeds of 74 mph or greater. Cyclones that form over warm water between the latitudes of 30°N and 30°S are known as tropical cyclones.

A tropical cyclone is referred to as a hurricane in the Atlantic basin and the western coast of Mexico. It is called a typhoon in the western Pacific and cyclone in the Indian Ocean and Australasia (Malilay 1997). Tornadoes are different from cyclones; they generally form over land in areas of large vertical temperature gradients, and they are much smaller and briefer in duration than cyclones. When tropical cyclones make landfall, they sometimes give rise to tornadoes. Worldwide, most disaster deaths caused by storms are associated with tropical cyclones. This chapter focuses on the public health impact of tropical cyclones.

Tropical cyclones have caused an estimated 1.9 million deaths worldwide during the past two centuries (International Federation of Red Cross and Red Crescent Societies 2006). They have caused 3,322 deaths in the United States since 1940. One-third of these deaths occurred during just one storm, Hurricane Katrina in 2005 (NOAA, National Weather Service 2013). The three cyclones with highest mortality produced catastrophic loss of life: 300,000 deaths and 138,000 deaths in the Bangladesh cyclones of 1970 and 1991, respectively, and 138,000 deaths in the Myanmar cyclone of 2008 (CRED 2009). Sixteen of the world's eighteen tropical cyclones with the highest mortality occurred in the Asia-Pacific region (International Federation of Red Cross and Red Crescent Societies 2006). Table 2.9 lists the world's ten storms with the highest mortality from 1900 to 2013. All of these storms are cyclones.

Morbidity and mortality associated with cyclones differ according to the economic development of the affected population. In low-income coastal communities without early warning, evacuation, and shelter systems, drowning from storm surge accounted for an estimated 90 percent of cyclone-attributable mortality (Malilay 1997; CDC 1989). In high-income

Table 2.9 World's Top Ten Storms (Tropical Cyclones) Associated with Highest Mortality, 1900 to 2013, Ranked by Number of Deaths per Nation

Country	Year	Number of People Killed
Bangladesh	1970	300,000
Bangladesh	1991	138,866
Myanmar	2008	138,366
China	1922	100,000
Bangladesh	1942	61,000
Bangladesh	1935	60,000
China	1912	50,000
India	1942	40,000
Bangladesh	1965	36,000
Bangladesh	1963	22,000

Source: EM-DAT: http://www.emdat.be/database

Note: While there were cyclone disasters occurring after 2008, these events were not among the top largest in terms of number of deaths.

nations, most of the storm-related mortality and much of the morbidity now occurs during the postimpact cleanup period. Unfortunately, storm surge remains the primary cause of mortality following tropical cyclones in low-income nations that lack these critical **preparedness** measures (Chowdhury et al. 1992; Diacon 1992).

Injury represents the major cause of morbidity for tropical cyclones (Meredith and Bradley 2002). The top three cyclone-related injuries are lacerations, blunt trauma, and puncture wounds, with 80 percent of these injuries being confined to the feet and lower extremities (CDC 1989; Noji 1993; Philen et al. 1992). An increased incidence of animal and insect bites following tropical cyclones has also been noted (CDC 1986, 2000). Chronic diseases such as asthma and emphysema are exacerbated after cyclones and other natural disasters (Meredith and Bradley 2002; CDC 1986, 2000). There is as well a potential for exposure to hazardous materials during the impact and the cleanup phase of the disaster.

Outbreaks of infectious diseases following tropical cyclones are rare and also differ according to economic development of the affected nation (Guill and Shandera 2001; WHO 1979; Toole 1997). In high-income nations, post-hurricane infectious disease surveillance has routinely detected increases in self-limiting gastrointestinal disease and respiratory infections (CDC 2000; Lee et al. 1992), but most commonly, no increase in communicable disease is found (Toole 1997; CDC 1993b). There have been a few reports of isolated outbreaks associated with vector-borne illness in low-income nations. Interruption of health services including an antimalaria campaign may have contributed to a malaria outbreak in Haiti following Hurricane Flora in 1963 (Bissell 1983; Mason and Cavalie 1965). Following Hurricane Mitch in 1998, rates of dengue fever increased in Guatemala and Honduras, and the number of malaria cases increased in Guatemala and Nicaragua (Pan American Health Organization 1998).

Behavioral health effects are among the most debilitating long-term outcomes of tropical cyclones (WHO 1992; Ursano, Fullerton, and McCaughey 1994). Rates of suicide (Krug et al. 1998) and child abuse (Keenan et al. 2004) appear to rise. An elevated prevalence of posttraumatic stress disorder was specifically apparent in three studies of hurricane survivors in developing nations (Krug et al. 1998; Caldera et al. 2001; Goenjian et al. 2001).

CLINICAL CORRELATES 2.3   EXTREME WEATHER EVENTS AND DISRUPTIONS IN THE TREATMENT OF CHRONIC DISEASE

Extreme weather events have vast potential to displace individuals from their communities and homes. Such movement disrupts access to health care systems and severs relationships between doctors and patients. In the wake of natural disasters, care for patients is frequently interrupted. Individuals struggle to find new providers, while at the same time, doctors become overwhelmed by an influx of new patients who often arrive without medical records. Interruption of treatment may contribute to the high rates of acute exacerbations of chronic diseases such as end-stage renal disease, asthma, cardiovascular disease, and chronic obstructive pulmonary disease in the wake of natural disasters (Miller and Arquilla 2008; Chan and Sondorp 2007).

Depending on the location of the disaster and the refugee *mitigation* efforts, the responsibility for the care of displaced patients could be spread in unpredictable ways and in far-reaching locations, as was seen in the aftermath of Hurricane Katrina in 2005.

Extreme weather and resulting human movements exacerbate chronic medical problems, and the burden of treatment is spread unpredictably among health care facilities in surrounding areas.

Public Health Impact of Landslides (Debris Flows)   The term *landslide* includes all types of gravity-induced ground movements, ranging from rock falls through slides and slumps, avalanches, and flows, triggered mainly by precipitation (including snowmelt), seismic activity, and volcanic eruptions (Varnes 1978; Cruden and Varnes 1996). Landslides may also be referred to as either wet or dry mass movements. More specifically, the term *debris flow* will be used here to include wet mass movements or mudflows, and debris torrents known to be associated with high-precipitation events such as those predicted to occur more frequently as a result of climate change.

A debris flow is a rapidly moving mass of water and material that is mainly composed of sand, gravel, and cobbles, but typically includes trees, cars, small buildings, and other anthropogenic material. A debris flow typically has the consistency of wet concrete and moves at speeds in excess of 16 meters per second (Larsen et al. 2001). Many of these areas run a recurrent risk of landslides associated with the wet season. The world's largest debris flow disaster during the past century occurred in 1966 and affected 4 million people in Brazil.

The landslide associated with the highest recorded mortality in history occurred in December 1999, when several days of torrential rainfall in Vargas State, Venezuela, triggered thousands of shallow debris flows. The debris flows moved rapidly down mountainous terrain and were highly destructive as they entered densely populated areas along the Venezuelan coastline. Over eight thousand residences and seven hundred apartment buildings were destroyed, displacing up to seventy-five thousand people (Larsen et al. 2001; Wieczorek et al. 2001). The death toll is estimated to be near thirty-thousand, although exact numbers of casualties were difficult to determine due to lack of reliable census data. These debris flows also destroyed some of the port facilities in La Guaira. Warehouses at the port facility storing hazardous materials were inundated by the debris flow and came dangerously close to causing an explosion and toxic exposure with the potential to affect eighty thousand nearby residents, as well as close that nation's largest airport and second largest seaport (Keim, Humphrey, and Dreyfus 2000; "Venezuela Seeks Contractors" 2000). Table 2.10 lists the world's ten landslides associated with the highest mortality from 1900 to 2013.

Table 2.10   World's Top Ten Landslides Associated with Highest Mortality, 1900–2013, Ranked by Number of Deaths per Nation

Country	Year	Number Killed
Venezuela	1999	30,000
Soviet Union	1949	12,000
Peru	1941	5,000
Honduras	1973	2,800
Italy	1963	1,917
China	2010	1,765
Philippines	2006	1,126
India	1968	1,000
Colombia	1987	640
Peru	1971	600
China	1934	500

Source: EM-DAT: http://www.emdat.be/database

Note: While there were landslide disasters occurring after 2010, these events were not among the top largest in terms of number of deaths.

From 1990 to 1999, debris flows were second only to hurricanes as the leading cause of death due to environmental disasters in the disaster-prone Pacific basin, four times more than earthquakes and thirty times more than volcanoes (Keim 2006a).

Landslide mortality is largely related to trauma and asphyxiation. Landslide morbidity is largely associated with traumatic injuries and a disruption of water, sanitation, shelter, and the locally grown food supply of the affected population (Walker and Walter 2000).

Managing the Public Health Risk of Extreme Weather Disasters

The literature thoroughly describes how climate change affects natural disaster health risk (Van Aalst 2006; Mitchell et al. 2006; Woodruff, McMichael, and Butler 2006; Woodruff, McMichael, and Hales 2006; Huppert and Sparks 2006; Zell 2004; Parkinson and Butler 2005; Morrissey and Reser 2007; Keim 2008). Critically important are factors that directly shape the health of populations, such as education, health care, public health prevention, and infrastructure (Intergovernmental Panel on Climate Change 2007).

Disaster Risk

Risk is defined as "the probability of harmful consequences, or expected losses (deaths, injuries, property, livelihoods, economic activity disrupted or environment damaged) resulting from interactions between natural or human-induced hazards and vulnerable conditions" (UN International Strategy for Disaster Reduction 2009). **Disaster risk** is defined as "the potential disaster losses, in lives, health status, livelihoods, assets and services, which could occur to a particular community or a society over some specified future time period" (UN International Strategy for Disaster Reduction 2009). The risk equation has also been applied in various evolving derivatives to estimate disaster risk according to the following relationship (Intergovernmental Panel on Climate Change 2011; Keim 2002, 2006a, 2008, 2011; "Health Disaster Management Guidelines" 2003; British Columbia Ministry of Public Safety and Solicitor General 2003):

$$p(D) = k\,[\,p(H) \times p(V)\,] - p(R)$$

where $p(D)$ is risk of disaster impact, $p(H)$ is the probability of hazard, $p(V)$ is the probability of population vulnerability, and $p(R)$ is resilience (or **absorptive capacity**). According to this equation, disaster risk may be reduced among populations at risk by reducing exposure to the hazard itself, decreasing the vulnerability and increasing the resilience.

Disaster consequences may include loss of life, injury, disease, and other negative effects on human physical, mental, and social well-being, together with damage to property, destruction of assets, loss of services, social and economic disruption, and environmental degradation (UNISDR 2009). The severity of the consequences is referred to as disaster impact.

Principles of Disaster Risk Management

Risk Management

The overall approach to emergencies and disasters internationally has shifted from what were initially largely postimpact activities (relief and reconstruction) to a more systematic and comprehensive risk management process (Intergovernmental Panel on Climate Change 2011; Keim 2006b, 2011; Keim and Abrahams 2012; Clack et al. 2002; 17; UNISDR 2002; Schipper and Pelling 2006). The 2002 World Summit on **Sustainable Development** (WSSD) concluded, "An integrated multi-hazard, inclusive approach to address vulnerability, risk assessment, and disaster management, including **prevention**, mitigation, preparedness, response and **recovery**, is an essential part of a safer world in the twenty-first century" (UNISDR 2002).

Risk management is activity directed toward assessing, controlling, and monitoring risks. Strategies include risk assessment and control measures. These control measures in turn include transferring the risk to another party, avoiding the risk, reducing the negative effect of the risk, and accepting some or all of the consequences of a particular risk.

Disaster Risk Management

Disaster risk management is a comprehensive all-hazard approach that entails developing and implementing strategies for each phase of the disaster life cycle. As applied to climate change adaptation, it includes both preimpact disaster risk reduction (prevention, preparedness, and mitigation), as well as postimpact disaster risk transfer (risk pools and insurance policies) and disaster risk retention (response and recovery) (Schipper and Pelling 2006). The underlying drive of disaster management is to reduce risk to human life and systems important to livelihood. Climate change adaptation needs to become part and parcel of comprehensive risk management (O'Brien et al. 2006). The most notable justification is based on the proposition that if extreme weather events are expected to increase the incidence of disasters over the long term, then it is only logical for societies to reduce their own disaster risk rather than limit interventions to that of an increasingly more expense strategy of disaster response.

Disaster Risk Reduction and Climate Change Adaptation

Disaster Risk Reduction and Sustainable Development

Disaster reduction has emerged as a core element of sustainable development. According to the US National Science and Technology Council, Subcommittee on Natural Disaster Reduction (1996), "The continued upward spiral of the costs of natural disasters in the United States will be broken only by a strategy that addresses the full range of obstacles to natural disaster reduction." Reducing risk requires long-term engagement in the development process, and the actual work of disaster risk reduction is largely a task for local actors (Schipper and Pelling 2006; O'Brien et al. 2006).

Public health is uniquely placed at the community level to build human resilience to climate-related disasters (Clack et al. 2002). By focusing on vulnerability and the ability of individuals and communities to recover, vulnerability reduction places the individuals at risk at center stage and tasks the responsible authorities with enhancing social equity and promoting community cohesiveness (Werrity 2006).

Reducing the Risk of Disaster-Related Adverse Health Effects

Health-related disaster risk due to extreme weather events occurs as the result of convergence of four key factors (Intergovernmental Panel on Climate Change 2011):

1. The presence of a health **hazard** associated with an extreme weather and climate events, commonly considered as a function of frequency and impact

2. The degree of **exposure** to the hazard sustained by the person or population

3. The degree of **vulnerability** of the person or population to that particular health hazard

4. The degree of **resilience** of the person or population in order to avoid or moderate harm

In order to differentiate these key factors, it may be helpful to consider them as intrinsic or extrinsic to the individual at risk. For example, hazard frequency, impact, and degree of exposure occur as extrinsic factors. Vulnerability, however, is considered to be intrinsic to the individual person at risk and includes the major domains of demographics, education, race, language and ethnicity, and health status. Resilience is largely a measure of extrinsic response capacities and resources that include economic capacity, availability of human and material resources (e.g., food, water, shelter, sanitation, transportation, personal protective equipment, access to health care), and social capital.

Hazard Avoidance   A *disaster hazard* is defined as "a dangerous phenomenon, substance, human activity or condition that may cause loss of life, injury or other health impacts, property damage, loss of livelihoods and services, social and economic disruption, or environmental damage" (UN International Strategy for Disaster Reduction 2009).

Hazard analyses commonly begin with a comprehensive identification of all hazards that may occur within a given area or jurisdiction. Once they have been identified, they must then be assessed as to their potential severity of loss and to the probability of occurrence. In practice, for public health the process can be very difficult. The fundamental difficulty in disaster risk assessment is determining the rate of occurrence, since statistical information is not available on all kinds of past incidents (British Columbia Ministry of Public Safety and Solicitor General 2003). Furthermore, evaluating the severity of the consequences (impact) is often quite difficult for immaterial assets. Thus, best-educated opinions and available statistics are the primary sources of information (British Columbia Ministry of Public Safety and Solicitor General 2003).

Primary prevention seeks to prevent the disaster hazard exposure from ever occurring (Keim 2008). This function is consistent with the category of risk treatment known as risk avoidance; examples include land use zoning and regulations that prevent settlement in disaster-prone areas like floodplains. The risk of adverse health effects as related to specific extreme weather events varies not only according to the type, likelihood of occurrence, and impact of the hazard but also is dependent on the degree of exposure to the hazard. While people may not always have the ability to prevent disasters from occurring, the health sector can play an important role in preventing the public health impact.

Risk reduction involves methods that reduce the severity of the loss or the likelihood of the loss from occurring. Secondary prevention aims to detect the disaster hazard event early to control its advance and reduce the resulting health burden (Keim 2008). For example, secondary prevention for disasters involves accurate detection of a flash flood and early warning of the population that will allow for protective actions like evacuation. Risk-reduction activities seek to mitigate the health consequences of disasters that cannot be prevented. The risk of a public health disaster occurs when affected populations are both exposed and vulnerable to environmental hazards (Keim 2008). Exposure and vulnerability are dynamic, varying across temporal and spatial scales, and depend on economic, social, geographic, demographic, cultural, institutional, governance, and environmental factors (Intergovernmental Panel on Climate Change 2011).

Exposure Reduction   **Exposure** is defined as subjection to the influence or effects of a disaster-related health hazard. The toxicity or lethality of an environmental health hazard is often characterized by a dose-response relationship. Typically, as the degree of exposure to a health hazard increases, the human emotion of concern—itself an adverse health effect—appears in more of the population. In the case of extreme weather events, the degree of exposure of a given population to the hydrometeorological hazard (e.g., extremes of wind, temperature, and precipitation) has a direct relationship to the incidence and severity of adverse health outcomes. Persons located in close proximity to the disaster hazard have a higher risk for injury and illness as compared with those less exposed. For example, persons living in temperate climate zones may be at higher risk for exposure to hazardous extremes of temperature.

In the short term, human exposures to climate-related health hazards may be accomplished by reducing the population proximity to the hazard. This typically involves creation of a hazard map that accurately models zones where the population is at risk. In the case of landslides, tropical cyclones, floods, heat waves, and wildfires, exposure reduction is commonly achieved by temporary evacuation of the population at risk and sheltering in safe-shelter conditions. In the case of drought, reducing the impacts of exposure may also involve evacuation or migration (mainly in low-resource countries) and (in high-resource countries) also commonly involves sheltering in place with additional support being delivered to the population at risk in the way of water, food, sanitation, and health care. Long-term exposure reduction for all of these hazards most frequently involves disaster-related mitigation (UN Disaster Relief Office 1991). Mitigation may occur as both structural measures (such as wind- or flood-resistant construction, floodplain management, and planting) and nonstructural measures (such as land use regulation, water conservation, agricultural and forestry practices, and building codes) (Malilay 1997; UN Disaster Relief Office 1991). Table 2.11 lists examples of short- and long-term exposure reduction measures for extreme weather events.

Vulnerability Reduction   Human vulnerability to disasters is a complex phenomenon that includes social, economic, health, and cultural factors. Vulnerability links people with their environment and with the social forces, institutions, and cultural values that sustain them.

Human vulnerability to climate-related hazards is increasing because of rising poverty, a growing global population, and other underlying

Table 2.11   Examples of Short- and Long-Term Exposure Reduction Measures for Extreme Weather Events

Hazard	Short-Term Exposure Reduction	Long-Term Exposure Reduction
Landslides	Evacuation of hazard zones near hillsides	Land use patterns, developmental practices, natural resource conservation
Storms (tropical cyclones)	Evacuation of coastal areas and floodplains	Land use patterns, developmental practices, building construction, zoning regulation, floodplain management
Floods	Evacuation of floodplains	Land use patterns, developmental practices, building construction, zoning regulation, floodplain management
Heat waves	Evacuation of high-risk urban housing	Land use patterns, developmental practices, urban planning, building construction, zoning regulation, natural resource conservation
Wildfires	Evacuation of areas near the fire spread	Land use patterns, developmental practices, urban planning, building construction, zoning regulation
Drought	Evacuation (migration) or shelter in place with relief and public services	Land use patterns, developmental practices, urban planning, agricultural and forestry practices, zoning regulation, natural resource conservation, watershed management

development issues (O'Brien et al. 2006). Reducing human vulnerability is a key aspect of reducing climate change risk (Schipper and Pelling 2006). Given that extreme weather hazards are likely to occur, the risk of adverse health impacts is lessened by lowering human vulnerability to the hazard.

Within the context of disaster risk reduction, **vulnerability** is defined as the likelihood of suffering an adverse health effect when exposed to a given health hazard. These are characteristics and circumstances that are inherent to the specific person or population. People are not equally susceptible to the same health hazard. Differences among persons are due to such factors as demographics, socioeconomic status, social capital, and health status. The heaviest burden of every disaster most often falls disproportionately on women, children, the frail, the elderly, and those with disabilities. This degree of vulnerability has a direct relationship to the frequency and severity of adverse health outcomes. Persons more susceptible to a disaster hazard have a higher risk for injury and illness as compared with those less susceptible. For example, socially isolated elderly persons living in urban temperate climate zones are more likely to be susceptible to heat-related illness than are young adults living in the same location (Adrianopoli et al. 2010; Walker and Hogan 2003; Bailey and Walker 2007; Sardon 2007).

Healthy people are less vulnerable to the adverse effects of many disaster hazards. Health promotion programs, medical care, social support services, and social integration that result in a reduction of the existing burden of disease and injuries create greater functionality and sustained mobility in a healthier population that is less susceptible to any given extreme weather hazard. In this sense, equitable and sustainable access to public health, medical, and social services, as well as community cohesion, are essential in reducing human susceptibility to extreme weather events. Other means for vulnerability reduction include addressing its social factors by way of building social networks, public information, and education.

Building Resilience

The UN International Strategy for Disaster Reduction (2009) defines **resilience** as "the *ability* of a system, community or society exposed to hazards to resist, absorb, accommodate to and recover from the effects of a hazard in a timely and efficient manner, including through the preservation and restoration of its essential basic structures and functions [emphasis added]." More recently, the term *resilience* has been broadly used to describe actions spanning the entire disaster cycle from disaster prevention to recovery. In order to clarify this distinction, it is helpful to conceive of resilience as the ability to resile from or spring back from a stressor or shock (UN International Strategy for Disaster Reduction 2009). By definition, resilience then occurs in the postimpact phase of a disaster and is the ability to manage change in the face of shocks and stresses (UK Department for International Development 2012).

According to "Health Disaster Management Guidelines" (2003), in order to be resilient to a disaster hazard, an individual or society must be able to absorb the damage, adapt to the damage, and react in such a way so as to mitigate further damage and enable recovery.

Community Resilience   Community resilience, or the sustained ability of a community to withstand and recover from adversity (e.g., economic stress, influenza pandemic, man-made or natural disasters), has become a key policy issue in the United States, especially in recent years. While there is general consensus that *community resilience* is defined as the ability of communities to withstand and mitigate the stress of a disaster, there is less clarity on the precise resilience-building process (Chandra et al. 2011). The literature related to defining key measures and applications of building community resilience has been rather broad and lacking in the specificity required for implementation. According to one technical report published by Rand Corporation, community resilience represents a unique intersection of preparedness and emergency management, traditional public health, and community development, with its emphasis on preventative care, health promotion, and community capacity building (Chandra et al. 2011).

Health Resilience   There are also key assumptions that characterize a significant distinction between community resilience and human health resilience, especially the level of the individual person at risk for disaster-related mortality.

The resilience of a social system is determined by the degree to which the system has the necessary resources and is capable of organizing itself to develop its capacities to treat risks (e.g., implement disaster risk-reduction programs) and institute means to transfer (e.g., insurance) or manage **residual risks** (e.g., response and recovery). The thirty-five categories of public health and medical capabilities that address public health impacts of disasters (e.g., water, food, sanitation, hygiene, medical care, vector control, disease prevention) and the measure of community, societal, or organizational capacity to adapt, organize, and implement these capabilities may all be considered elements of public health resilience.

However, individuals within a population do not have the same level of resilience to the same disaster hazard. Differences among persons are typically due to social and economic factors such as health status, socioeconomic status, governmental and organizational structures (e.g., the public health and medical system), social capital, political influence, and behavioral determinants. Key to this discussion is the consideration of community infrastructure as compared to physiological constraints of the human body. Contrary to community infrastructure (neighborhoods, buildings, roadways, utilities, and commerce), the human body cannot always be expected to recover, regardless of the societal investment. In this sense, when applied to human health, it can be said that resilience is for the survivors. Once a life has been damaged by the disaster hazard beyond a certain degree, no amount of aid or assistance can enable recovery from loss of life. For this reason, disaster risk reduction that includes primary and secondary prevention measures is exceptionally pertinent to health resilience. We simply cannot expect human bodies to recover from extreme weather hazards in the same sense as we would communities.

CLINICAL CORRELATES 2.4   BUILDING COMMUNITY RESILIENCE

Community health workers have historically been integral players in disaster management (Perez and Martinez 2008). Their roles are various: providing first aid, dispensing drugs, delivering babies, giving child care advice and nutrition education, monitoring immunizations, promoting sanitation and hygiene, making health care referrals, performing school activities, making home visits, and maintaining community records. They are the sentinels and guardians of a community knowing who is sick and where to find resources. Health workers are trusted counselors because they are of the communities in which they work and may share a similar set of values (Perez and Martinez 2008). During natural disasters, they are vital players in mitigation because they understand the resources, health, and social complexities of the area affected. Research has shown that community health workers improve pregnancy and birth outcomes, health, and screening-related behaviors, as well as management of chronic disease and are vital actors in disaster situations (Richter et al. 1974).

In disaster management planning, providing education and resources to community health workers can serve twofold to mitigate negative effects of the disaster and provide feedback to higher-level systems of management.

Socioeconomic Resilience   Poverty is an important determinant of disaster risk and an important constant of resilience (Nelson 1990). Poverty is both a condition and determinant of resilience, and as such, poverty reduction is an essential component of reducing human health risk to extreme weather hazards and climate change (Thomalla 2006). Those most at risk tend to be of particular social groups, such as those with inadequate access to economic (e.g., credit, welfare) and social capital (e.g., networks, information. and relationships) (Thomalla 2006; Tapsell et al. 2002). Those populations with limited access to safe water, food security, safe housing, and public services have less absorptive capacity to the adverse effects of disaster hazards. Worldwide, loss of life from climate-related disasters is far higher among the low-resource countries. Yet within each nation, including high-resource countries, the poor are most affected (Intergovernmental Panel on Climate Change 2007, 2011; National Science and Technology Council 1996; Brouewer et al. 2007; Nelson 1990).

Building Human Resilience   Those with less resilience for responding to the disaster hazard have a higher risk for injury and illness and less likelihood for a speedy and full recovery as compared to those who are more resilient. For example, poor people living in substandard housing within temperate climate zones are more susceptible to heat-wave-related illness than are affluent, well-connected persons who prepare and otherwise ensure their own readiness for such an event. In this sense, equitable and sustainable access to education, health care, economic development, and public services is essential in building human resilience to extreme weather events.

Certain characteristics of the built environment may also affect human resilience and make individuals more prone or less prone to disaster.

Community public health and medical institutions can play an active part in lessening human vulnerability to climate-related disasters through promotion of healthy people, healthy homes, and healthy communities (Srinivasan, O'Fallon, and Dearry 2004). Healthy people are less vulnerable to disaster-related morbidity or mortality. Healthy homes are disaster resilient because they are designed and built to stay safe during extreme weather events. Healthy communities minimize exposure of people and property to natural disasters and improve social, psychological, and economic resilience of the community. Sustainable communities are disaster-resilient communities (Sidel et al. 1992).

Preparedness, response, and recovery activities all increase resilience during the postimpact phase of extreme weather events. **Preparedness** is defined as activities and measures taken in advance to ensure effective response to the impact of hazards (UN International Strategy for Disaster Reduction 2009). Preparedness also implies a certain level of resource availability and a behavioral approach focused on actions taken in advance of a disaster in order to reduce its impact. This helps to build resilience from the adverse health effects of disaster hazards.

Emergency response occurs after the impact of an event. The response phase usually begins with ad hoc local emergency response and may be followed later by a formal declaration of disaster and external assistance and emergency relief. Public health preparedness and response activities serve to build community resilience and therefore lessen human health risk. As a means of adaptation to climate change and variability, public health preparedness and response activities play a key role.

Sustainable Development and Resilience to Extreme Weather Events

The emerging vision of environmental sustainability as wedded to economic vitality and social equity is becoming important to reducing natural-hazard risk to human settlements (Olshansky and Kartez 1998). Sustainable development meets the needs of the present without compromising the ability of future generations to meet their own needs (UN Environment Programme 1972). The high property damage levels in recent disasters clearly suggest that current patterns and practices of land use and community building are not sustainable in the long run (Beatley 1998). Economic development achieved in a sustainable manner could itself be regarded as an adaptation measure for climate change (Fankhauser 1998). Climate change is the nexus where sustainable development, policy, disaster risk reduction, and communities intersect (O'Brien et al. 2006). Addressing climate change can be viewed as one component of a broad, sustainable development strategy that aims at increasing national and regional capacity to deal with climate variability as well as long-term climate change (Schipper and Pelling 2006).

Sustainable communities are where people and property are kept out of the way of natural hazards, the inherently mitigating qualities of natural environmental systems are maintained, and development is designed to be resilient in the face of natural forces (Godschalk, Kaiser, and Berke 1998). A healthy, safe community promotes the concept of resilience within the community.

Mounting evidence suggests that disaster risk may be either increased or decreased by developmental choices made associated with the built environment. Human-modified places such as homes, schools, workplaces, parks, industrial areas, farms, roads, and highways that comprise the physical and social construct (e.g., neighborhood cohesion, social patterns) of the urban environment may increase hazard exposure and also promote isolation (Bashir 2002). This isolation may result in a lack of social networks and diminished social capital that further exacerbates vulnerability to climate-related disasters (Hawe and Shiell 2000). As with all disasters in general, the impact of the built environment on the burden of illness is greater among minorities and low-income communities (Srinivasan et al. 2004). Consequently, these same populations may already experience much greater baseline burdens of disease in addition to any future increases in disaster-related morbidity and mortality associated with climate change (UN International Strategy for Disaster Reduction 2007).

Building Public Health Resilience in Sustainable Communities

The increased risk of extreme weather events brought on by climate change also presents an opportunity to build healthy and disaster-resilient homes and communities. While disasters destroy lives and property, they also create opportunities to improve safety, enhance equity, and rebuild in new or different ways. Ideally those opportunities would produce safer communities with more equitable and sustainable livelihoods for people—as the saying goes, "the opportunity to build back better" (Bolin and Stanford 1998). Community public health and medical institutions can play an active part in lessening human vulnerability to climate-related disasters through promotion of "healthy people, healthy homes and healthy communities" (Srinivasan et al. 2004). Healthy people are less likely to suffer disaster-related morbidity or mortality and are therefore more disaster resilient. Healthy homes are disaster resilient; they are designed and built to stay safe during extreme weather events. Healthy communities minimize exposure of people and property to natural disasters; in other words, sustainable communities are disaster-resilient communities (Beatley 1998). In this sense, nearly all avenues of public health promotion can act to reduce the risk of future climate-related disasters. Sustainable, cost-effective, community-based public health and medical systems strengthen population resilience to extreme weather events, and methods that reduce population vulnerability also increase resilience against natural disasters caused by climate change.

Conclusion

While humans may not always have the ability to prevent any weather-related hazards from occurring, the public health and medical sectors can play an important role in lessening or even preventing the human suffering of these disasters. Climate change adaptation, public health, and disaster risk management should all be integrated with sectoral activities and development processes (Thomalla 2006). At the community level, all three of these societal risk-reduction programs are characteristically well integrated (Allen 2006; Warner and Oré 2006). Community-based risk reduction activities that integrate public health, disaster management, and climate change adaptation lessen human vulnerability to the impacts of weather-related disasters. In this regard, public health vulnerability reduction activities that lessen disaster risk can also serve as a sustainable adaptation to extreme weather events (International Federation of Red Cross 2005).

DISCUSSION QUESTIONS

1. Identify three extreme weather hazards that could potentially occur in your home jurisdiction (city, state or province, or nation). Discuss events that may have occurred in the past.

2. Identify three major public health consequences for each of these three disaster hazards.

3. Identify ways that you may be able to reduce your risk of exposure to each of these three hazards.

4. Identify people in your home who may be highly vulnerable to each of these three disaster hazards.

5. Identify long-term strategies that may serve to reduce future population vulnerability to these three disaster hazards.

6. Identify resources and capacities within your home jurisdiction that may make population health more resilient to the impact of these three disaster hazards.

7. Identify developmental strategies by which your home jurisdiction could potentially lessen its future risk of morbidity and mortality associated with these three disaster hazards.

KEY TERMS

Absorptive capacity: A limit to the rate or quantity of impact that can be absorbed or adapted to without exceeding the threshold of loss (e.g., death, injury, or illness).

Capacity: The measure of all the strengths, attributes, and resources available to a community, society, or organization (e.g., people) that can be used to achieve agreed goals.

Disaster risk management: The systematic process of using administrative directives, organizations, and operational skills and capacities to implement strategies, policies, and improved coping capacities in order to lessen the adverse impacts of hazards and the possibility of disaster.

Disaster: A serious disruption of the functioning of a community or a society involving widespread human morbidity and mortality that exceeds the ability of the affected community or society to cope using its own resources.

Disaster risk: The potential disaster losses (e.g., loss of lives and health status) that could occur to a particular person over some specified future time period.

Disaster risk reduction: The concept and practice of reducing disaster risks through systematic efforts to analyze and manage the causal factors of disasters, including through reduced exposure to hazards, lessened vulnerability of people, wise management of land and the environment, and improved preparedness for adverse events.

Exposure: The presence of assets (e.g., people) in places that could be adversely affected by hazards.

Hazard: A dangerous phenomenon, substance, human activity, or condition that may cause loss of life, injury, or other health impacts.

Preparedness: The knowledge and capacities developed by people to effectively anticipate, respond to, and recover from the impacts of likely, imminent, or current hazard events or conditions.

Prevention: The outright avoidance of adverse impacts of hazards and related disasters.

Recovery: The restoration, and improvement where appropriate, of facilities, livelihoods, and living conditions (and health status), including efforts to reduce disaster risk factors.

Residual risk: The risk that remains in unmanaged form, even when effective disaster risk reduction measures are in place, and for which emergency response and recovery capacities must be maintained.

Resilience: The ability of a system, community, or society (and people) exposed to hazards to resist, absorb, accommodate to, and recover from the effects of a hazard in a timely and efficient manner, including through the preservation and restoration of its essential basic structures and functions (e.g., health status and essential activities of daily living).

Response: The provision of emergency services and public assistance during or immediately after a disaster in order to save lives, reduce health impacts, ensure public safety, and meet the basic subsistence needs of the people affected.

Risk: The probability of harmful consequences (e.g., morbidity and mortality) resulting from interactions between natural or human-induced hazards and vulnerable conditions.

Risk management: The systematic approach and practice of managing uncertainty to minimize potential harm and loss.

Sustainable development: Development that meets the needs of the present without compromising the ability of future generations to meet their own needs.

Vulnerability: The characteristics and circumstances of a community, system, or asset (e.g., people) that makes it (and them) susceptible to the damaging effects of a hazard.

References

Adrianopoli, C., P. Brietzke, J. Jacoby, and J. Libby. 2010. "Extreme Heat Events." In *Disaster Medicine,* edited by K. Koenig and C. Schultz, 609–31. Cambridge: Cambridge University Press.

Ahern, M., R. S. Kovats, P. Wilkinson, R. Few, and F. Matthies. 2005. "Global Health Impacts of Floods: Epidemiologic Evidence." *Epidemiological Review* 27:36–46.

Allen, K. M. 2006. "Community-Based Disaster Preparedness and Climate Change Adaptation: Local Capacity-Building in the Philippines." *Disasters* 30 (1):81–101.

Bailey, G., and J. Walker. 2007. "Heat Related Disasters." In *Disaster Medicine,* 2nd ed., edited by D. E. Hogan and J. L. Burstein, 256–88. Philadelphia: Lippincott Williams & Wilkins,

Bashir, S. A. 2002. "Home Is Where the Harm Is: Inadequate Housing as a Public Health Crisis." *American Journal of Public Health* 92:733–38.

Beatley, T. 1998. "The Vision of Sustainable Communities." In *Cooperating with Nature,* edited by R. Burby. Washington, DC: National Academies Press.

Bedian, K., A. Arcus, and C. Frankel-Cone. 1994. *Emergency Medical Response to the Oakland-Berkeley Hills Fire of October 1991.* Sacramento: California Department of Health Services.

Bissell, R. A. 1983. "Delayed-Impact Infectious Disease after a Natural Disaster." *Journal of Emergency Medicine* 1:59–66.

Bolin, R., and L. Stanford. 1998. *The Northridge Earthquake: Vulnerability and Disaster.* New York: Routledge.

British Columbia Ministry of Public Safety and Solicitor General. 2003. *Hazard, Risk and Vulnerability Analysis Toolkit.* Victoria, BC: National Library of Canada.

Brouewer, R., S. Akter, L. Brander, and E. Haque 2007. "Socioeconomic Vulnerability and Adaptation to Environmental Risk: A Case Study of Climate Change and Flooding in Bangladesh." *Risk Analysis* 27:313–26.

Caldera, T., L. Palma, U. Penayo, and G. Kullgren. 2001. "Psychological Impact of the Hurricane Mitch in Nicaragua in a One-Year Perspective." *Social Psychiatry and Psychiatric Epidemiology.* 36:108–14.

Center for Research on the Epidemiology of Disasters. 2009. "EM-DAT: The International Disaster Database." Brussels: Ecole de santé publique, Université catholique de Louvain. http://www.emdat.be/disaster-trends

Centers for Disease Control and Prevention. 1986. "Hurricanes and Hospital Emergency Room Visits—Mississippi, Rhode Island, Connecticut (Hurricanes Alicia and Gloria)." *Morbidity and Mortality Weekly Report* 34:765–70.

Centers for Disease Control and Prevention. 1989. "Deaths Associated with Hurricane Hugo—Puerto Rico." *Morbidity and Mortality Weekly Report* 38:680–82.

Centers for Disease Control and Prevention. 1993a. "Injuries and Illnesses Related to Hurricane Andrew—Louisiana." *Morbidity and Mortality Weekly Report* 42:242–43, 249–51.

Centers for Disease Control and Prevention. 1993b. "Morbidity Surveillance following the Midwest Flood—Missouri." *Morbidity and Mortality Weekly Report* 42:797–98.

Centers for Disease Control and Prevention. 1998. "Needs Assessment following Hurricane Georges—Dominican Republic." *Morbidity and Mortality Weekly Report* 1999 48:93–95.

Centers for Disease Control and Prevention. 2000. "Morbidity and Mortality Associated with Hurricane Floyd—North Carolina." *Morbidity and Mortality Weekly Report* 49:369–72.

Centers for Disease Control and Prevention. 2002. "Tropical Storm Allison Rapid Needs Assessment, Houston, Texas, June 2001." *Morbidity and Mortality Weekly Report* 51(17):365–39.

Centers for Disease Control and Prevention. 2011. *Public Health Preparedness Capabilities: National Standards for State and Local Planning.* March. http://www.cdc.gov/phpr/capabilities/Capabilities_March_2011.pdf

Chan, C. S., and J. E. Rhodes. 2014. "Measuring Exposure in Hurricane Katrina: A Meta-Analysis and an Integrative Data Analysis." *PLoS One* 9(4).

Chan, E. Y., and E. Sondorp. 2007. "Medical Interventions following Natural Disasters: Mission out on Chronic Medical Needs." *Asia-Pacific Journal of Public Health* 19:45–51.

Chandra, A., J. Acosta, S. Stern, L. Uscher-Pines, and M. V. Williams. 2011. *Building Community Resilience to Disasters: A Way Forward to Enhance National Health Security.* Santa Monica, CA: Rand.

Chowdhury, M., Y. Choudhury, A. Bhuiya, K. Islam, Z. Hussain, O. Rahman, R. Glass, and M. Bennish. 1992. "Cyclone Aftermath: Research and Directions for the Future." In *From Crisis to Development: Coping with Disasters in Bangladesh*, edited by H. Hossain, C. P. Dodge, and F. H. Abed, 101–33. Dhaka, Bangladesh: University Press.

Clack, Z., M. Keim, A. Macintyre, and K. Yeskey. 2002. "Emergency Health and Risk Management in Sub-Saharan Africa: A Lesson from the Embassy Bombings in Tanzania and Kenya." *Prehospital and Disease Medicine* 17(2):59–66.

Cruden, D. M., and D. J. Varnes. 1996. "Landslide Types and Processes." In *Landslides: Investigation and Mitigation*, edited by A. K. Turner and R. L. Schuster, 36–75. Washington, DC: National Research Council.

Davis, R. 2005. "Hope Turns to Anguish at Intensive-Care Unit." *United States Today*, September 16.

Diacon, D. 1992. "Typhoon Resistant Housing in the Philippines: The Core Shelter Project." *Disasters* 16:266–71.

EM-DAT: The International Disaster Database. Centre for Research on the Epidemiology of Disasters. Available at http://www.emdat.be/database. Accessed on August 16, 2015.

EM-DAT, C.R.E.D. 2010. "The OFDA/CRED International Disaster Database. 2001." Belgium: Université Catholique de Louvain.

Fankhauser, S. 1998. *The Costs of Adapting to Climate Change.* Washington, DC: Global Environment Facility.

Federal Emergency Management Agency. 1996. *SLG 101: Guide for All-Hazard Emergency Operations Planning.* Washington, DC: FEMA. http://www.fema.gov/pdf/plan/slg101.pdf

Felder, S. S., J. Seligman, C. K. Burrows-McElwain M. E. Robinson, and E. Hierholzer. 2014. "Disaster Trauma: Federal Resources That Help Communities on Their Road to Recovery." *Disaster Medicine and Public Health Preparedness* 8:174–78.

Floret, N., J. Viel, F. Mauny, et al. 2006. "Negligible Risk for Epidemics after Geophysical Disasters." *Emerging Infectious Diseases* 12:543–48.

Godschalk, D., E. Kaiser, and P. Berke. 1998. "Confronting Natural Hazards with Land-Use." In *Cooperating with Nature*, edited by R. Burby. Washington, DC: National Academies Press.

Goenjian, A. K., L. Molina, A. M. Steinberg, L. M. Fairbanks, M. L. Alvarez, H. A. Goenjian, and R. S. Pynoos. 2001. "Posttraumatic Stress and Depressive Reactions among Nicaraguan Adolescents after Hurricane Mitch." *American Journal of Psychiatry* 158:788–94.

Gray, B., and K. Hebert. 2007. "Hospitals in Hurricane Katrina: Challenges Facing Custodial Institutions in a Disaster." *Journal of Health Care for the Poor and Underserved* 18:283–98.

Guha-Sapir, D., and W. van Panhuis. 2009. "The Andaman Nicobar Earthquake and Tsunami 2004: Impact on Diseases in Indonesia." *Prehospital and Disaster Medicine* 24:493–99.

Guill C. K., and W. X. Shandera. 2001. "The Effects of Hurricane Mitch on a Community in Northern Honduras." *Prehospital and Disaster Medicine* 16:124–29.

Gunn, S.W.A. 1990. *Multilingual Dictionary of Disaster Medicine and International Relief.* Dordrecht, Netherlands: Kluwer Academic.

Hawe, P., and A. Shiell. 2000. "Social Capital and Health Promotion: A Review." *Social Science and Medicine* 51:871–85.

"Health Disaster Management Guidelines for Evaluation and Research in the Utstein Style. United States." 2003. *Prehospital and Disaster Medicine* 17 (Suppl. 3). http://www.wadem.org/guidelines/intro.pdf

Henry, R. 2005. "Defense Transformation and the 2005 Quadrennial Defense Review," *Parameters* (Winter):5–15.

Huppert, H., and S. Sparks. 2006. "Extreme Natural Hazards: Population Growth, Globalization and Environmental Change." *Philosophical Transactions of the Royal Society of London A: Mathematical, Physical and Engineering Sciences,* 364:1875–88.

Intergovernmental Panel on Climate Change. 2007. *Impacts, Adaptation and Vulnerability.* Geneva: United Nations Working Group II. http://www.ipcc.ch /ipccreports/ar4-wg2.htm

Intergovernmental Panel on Climate Change. 2011. *Special Report on Managing the Risks of Extreme Events and Disasters to Advance Climate Change Adaptation.* http://ipcc-wg2.gov/SREX/images/uploads/SREX-All_FINAL.pdf

International Federation of Red Cross. 2005. *World Disaster Report 2005.* Geneva: International Federation of Red Cross.

International Federation of Red Cross and Red Crescent Societies. 2006. *World Disaster Report 2006.* Bloomfield, CT: Kumarian Press.

Ivers, L. C., and E. T. Ryan. 2006. "Infectious Diseases of Severe Weather-Related and Flood-Related Natural Disasters." *Current Opinions in Infectious Diseases* 19:408–14.

Keenan, H. T., S. W. Marshall, M. A. Nocera, and D. K. Runyan. 2004. "Increased Incidence of Inflicted Traumatic Brain Injury in Children after a Natural Disaster." *American Journal of Preventive Medicine* 26:189–93.

Keim, M. 2002. "Intentional Chemical Disasters." In *Disaster Medicine*, edited by D. Hogan and J. Burstein, 340–48. Philadelphia: Lippincott Williams & Wilkins.

Keim, M. 2006a. "Pacific Health Summits for Sustainable Disaster Risk Management." *Pacific Health Dialog* 13(1):4–51.

Keim, M. 2006b. "Disaster Preparedness" In *Disaster Medicine,* edited by Greg Ciottone, 164–73. Philadelphia: Mosby-Elsevier.

Keim M. 2006c. "Landslides." In *Disaster Medicine,* edited by Greg Ciottone, 509–13. Philadelphia: Mosby-Elsevier.

Keim, M. 2008. "Building Human Resilience: The Role of Public Health Preparedness and Response as an Adaptation to Climate Change." *American Journal of Preventive Medicine* 35:508–16.

Keim, M. 2010. "Environmental Disasters." In *Environmental Health: From Global to Local*, edited by H. Frumkin, 843–75. San Francisco: Jossey-Bass.

Keim, M. 2011. " Preventing Disasters: Public Health Vulnerability Reduction as a Sustainable Adaptation to Climate Change." *Disaster Medicine and Public Health Preparedness* 5:140–48.

Keim, M., and J. Abrahams. 2012. "Health and Disaster." In *The Routledge Handbook of Hazards and Disaster Risk Reduction*, edited by B. Wisner, J. C. Gaillard, and I. Kelman. London: Routledge.

Keim, M., A. Humphrey, and A. Dreyfus. 2000. *Situation Assessment Report involving the Hazardous Material Disaster Site at LaGuaira Port, Venezuela. CDC Report to Office of Foreign Disaster Assistance.* Washington, DC: US Agency for International Development, January 10.

Krug, E. G., M. Kresnow, J. P. Peddicord, L. L. Dahlberg, K. E. Powell, A. E. Crosby, and J. L. Annest. 1998. "Suicide after Natural Disasters." *New England Journal of Medicine* 338:373–78.

Larsen, M., G. Wieczorek, L. Eaton, B. A. Morgan, and H. Torres-Sierra. 2001. "Natural Hazards on Alluvial Fans: The Venezuela Debris Flow and Flash Flood Disaster." US Geological Survey Fact Sheet 103–01.

Lee, L. E., V. Fonseca, K. M. Brett, J. Sanchez, R. C. Mullen, L. E. Quenemoen, S. L. Groseclose, and R. S. Hopkins. 1992. "Active Morbidity Surveillance after Hurricane Andrew—Florida." *Journal of the American Medical Association* 270:591–94.

Louisiana Hospital Association. 2005. "Hurricane Katrina Evacuation Report." Unpublished worksheet. Baton Rouge: LHA.

Malilay, J. 1997. "Floods." In *The Public Health Consequences of Disasters*, edited by E. R. Noji, 287–300. New York: Oxford University Press.

Mason, J., and P. Cavalie. 1965. "Malaria Epidemic in Haiti following a Hurricane." *American Journal of Tropical and Medical Hygiene* 14:533–39.

McCarthy, M. C., J. He, K. C. Hyams, A. El-Tigani, and I. O. Khalid. 1994. "Acute Hepatitis E Infection during the 1988 Floods in Khartoum, Sudan." *Transactions of the Royal Society of Tropical and Medical Hygiene* 88:177.

Meredith, J. T., and S. Bradley. 2002. "Hurricanes." In *Disaster Medicine*, edited by D. E. Hogan and J. L. Burstein, 179–86. Philadelphia: Lippincott Williams & Wilkins.

Miller, A. C., and B. Arquilla. 2008. "Chronic Diseases and Natural Hazards: Impact of Disasters on Diabetic, Renal and Cardiac Patients." *Prehospital and Disaster Medicine* 23(2):185–94.

Mitchell, J., J. Lowe, R. Wood, and M. Vellinga. 2006. "Extreme Events due to Human-Induced Climate Change." *Philosophical Transactions of the Royal Society of London A: Mathematical, Physical and Engineering Sciences* 364:2117–33.

Morrissey, S., and J. Reser. 2007. "Natural Disasters, Climate Change and Mental Health Considerations for Rural Australia." *Australian Journal of Rural Health* 15:120–25.

Munich Re Group. 2013. "Natural Catastrophe Statistics for 2012 Dominated by Weather Extremes." Press release. January 3, http://www.munichre.com/en/media_relations/press_releases/2013/2013_01_03_press_release.aspx

National Science and Technology Council. 1996. *Natural Disaster Reduction: A Plan for the Nation.* Washington, DC: Committee on the Environment and Natural Resources, Subcommittee on Natural Disaster Reduction.

Nelson, D. 1990. "Mitigating Disasters: Power to the Community." *International Nursing Review* 37:371.

NOAA. National Weather Service. 2013. *Natural Hazard Statistics.* http://www.nws.noaa.gov/om/hazstats.shtml

Noji, E. K. 1993. "Analysis of Medical Needs during Disasters Caused by Tropical Cyclones: Anticipated Injury Patterns." *Journal of Tropical and Medical Hygiene* 96:370–76.

O'Brien, G., P. O'Keefe, J. Rose, and B. Wisner. 2006. "Climate Change and Disaster Management." *Disasters* 30(1):64–80.

Olshansky, R., and J. Kartez. 1998. *Cooperating with Nature*, edited by R. Burby. Washington, DC: National Academies Press.

Pan American Health Organization. 1998. "Impact of Hurricane Mitch on Central America." *Epidemiology Bulletin* 19:1–14.

Parkinson, A., and J. Butler. 2005. "Potential Impacts of Climate Change on Infectious Diseases in the Arctic." *Journal of Circumpolar Health* 64:478–86.

Perez, L., and J. Martinez. 2008. "Community Health Workers: Social Justice and Policy Advocates for Community Health and Well-Being." *American Journal of Public Health* 98:11.

Philen, R., D. Combs, L. Miller, L. M. Sanderson, R. G. Parrish, and R. Ing. 1992. "Hurricane Hugo-Related Deaths: South Carolina and Puerto Rico, 1989." *Disasters* 16:53–59.

Prince, M., V. Patel, S. Saxena, M. Maj, J. Maselko, M. Phillips, and A. Rahman. 2007. "No Health without Mental Health." *Lancet* 370:859–77.

Richter, R. W., B. Bengen, P. A. Alsup, B. Bruun, M. M. Kilcoyne, and B. D. Challenor. 1974. "The Community Health Worker: A Resource for Improved Health Care Delivery." *American Journal of Public Health* 63:1056–61.

Robine, J. M., S.L.K. Cheung, S. Le Roy, H. Van Oyen, C. Griffiths, J. P. Michel, and F. R. Herrmann. 2008. "Death Toll Exceeded 70,000 in Europe during the Summer of 2003." *Comptes Rendus Biologies* 331:171–78.

Sardon, J. P. 2007. "The 2003 Heat Wave." *European Communicable Disease Bulletin* 12(3):226.

Sattler, D. N., A. J. Preston, C. F. Kaiser, V. E. Olivera, J. Valdez, and S. Schlueter. 2002. "Hurricane Georges: A Cross-National Study Examining Preparedness, Resource Loss, and Psychological Distress in the US Virgin Islands, Puerto Rico, Dominican Republic, and the United States." *Journal of Traumatic Stress* 15:339–50.

Schipper, L., and M. Pelling. 2006. "Disaster Risk, Climate Change and International Development: Scope for, and Challenges to, Integration." *Disasters* 30(1):19–38.

Shusterman, D., J. Kaplan, and C. Canabarro. 1993. "Immediate Health Effects of an Urban Wildfire." *Western Journal of Medicine* 158:133–38

Sidel, V., E. Onel, H. Geiger, J. Leaning, and W. H. Foege. 1992. "Public Health Responses to Natural and Human-Made Disasters." In *Public Health and Preventive Medicine*, 13th ed., 1173–86. Norwalk, CT: Appleton and Lange.

Srinivasan, L. R., M. A. O'Fallon, and A. Dearry. 2004. "Creating Healthy Communities, Healthy Homes, Healthy People: Initiating a Research Agenda on the Built Environment and Public Health." *American Journal of Public Health* 9:1446–50.

Stott, P. A., D. A. Stone, and M. R. Allen. 2004. "Human Contribution to the European Heatwave of 2003." *Nature* 432:610–14.

Tapsell, S., E. Penning-Rowsell, S. Tunstall, and T. L. Wilson. 2002. "Vulnerability to Flooding: Health and Social Dimensions." *Philosophical Transactions of the Royal Society of London A: Mathematical, Physical and Engineering Sciences* 360:1511–25.

Thomalla, F. 2006. "Reducing Hazard Vulnerability: Towards a Common Approach between Disaster Risk Reduction and Climate Adaptation." *Disasters* 30(1):39–48.

Thomas, K., A. Ellis, T. Konrad, C. Holzer, and J. Morrissey. 2009. "County-Level Estimates of Mental Health Professional Shortage in the United States." *Psychiatric Services* 60:1323–28.

Toole, M. J. 1997. "Communicable Disease and Disease Control." In *The Public Health Consequences of Disasters*, edited by E. K. Noji, 79–100. New York: Oxford University Press.

UK Department for International Development. 2012. *Defining Disaster Resilience*. http://www.fsnnetwork.org/sites/default/files/dfid_defining_disaster_resilience.pdf

UN Department of Humanitarian Affairs. 1992. *Internationally Agreed Glossary of Basic Terms related to Disaster Management*. DHA 93/36. Geneva. http://reliefweb.int/sites/reliefweb.int/files/resources/004DFD3E15B69A67C1256C4C006225C2-dha-glossary-1992.pdf

UN Disaster Relief Office. 1991. "Risk Reduction Measures." In *Mitigating Natural Disasters: Phenomena, Effects and Options*. New York: United Nations.

UN Environment Programme. 1972. *Declaration of the United Nations Conference on the Human Environment*. http://www.unep.org/Documents.Multilingual/Default.asp?DocumentID=97&ArticleID=1503

UN International Strategy for Disaster Reduction. 2002. *World Summit on Sustainable Development*. Geneva. http://www.un.org/esa/sustdev/documents/WSSD_POI_PD/English/WSSD_PlanImpl.pdf

UN International Strategy for Disaster Reduction. 2007. *Building Disaster Resilient Communities: Good Practices and Lessons Learned*. Geneva. http://www.unisdr.org/we/inform/publications/596

UN International Strategy for Disaster Reduction. 2009. *Terminology on Disaster Risk Reduction*. http://www.unisdr.org/eng/library/UNISDR-terminology-2009-eng.pdf

UN International Strategy for Disaster Reduction. 2013. *Disaster Statistics*. 2013. http://www.unisdr.org/we/inform/disaster-statistics

US Energy Information Administration. 2012. *Commercial Buildings Energy Consumption Survey.* http://www.eia.gov/consumption/commercial

Ursano, R. J., C. S. Fullerton, and B. G. McCaughey 1994. "Trauma and Disaster." In *Individual and Community Responses to Trauma and Disaster: The Structure of Human Chaos,* edited by R. J. Ursano, B. G. McCaughey, and C. S. Fullerton, 3–27. Cambridge: Cambridge University Press.

Van Aalst, M. 2006. "The Impacts of Climate Change on the Risk of Natural Disasters." *Disasters* 30(1):5–18.

Varnes, D. J. 1978. "Slope Movement Types and Processes." In *Landslides: Analysis and Control,* edited by R. L. Schuster and R. J. Krizek, 11–33. Washington, DC: National Research Council.

"Venezuela Seeks Contractors for Hazardous Cleanup." 2000. *Hazardous Substances Spill Report* 3(2).

Walker, J. S., and D. E. Hogan. 2003. "Heat Emergencies." In *Emergency Medicine: A Comprehensive Study Guide,* 6th ed., edited by J. E. Tintinalli, G. D. Kelen, and J. S. Stapcyzynski, 1183–90. New York: McGraw-Hill.

Walker, P., and J. Walter 2000. *World Disasters Report.* Geneva: International Federation of Red Cross and Red Crescent Societies.

Warner, J., and M. T. Oré. 2006. "El Niño Platforms: Participatory Disaster Response in Peru." *Disasters* 30:102–17.

Watson, J. T., M. Gayer, and M. A. Connolly. 2007. "Epidemics after Natural Disasters." *Emerging Infectious Diseases* 13(1):1. http://www.cdc.gov/ncidod/EID/13/1/1.htm

Werrity, A. 2006. "Sustainable Flood Management: Oxymoron or New Paradigm?" *Area* 38(1):16–23.

Wieczorek, G. F., M. C. Larson, L. S. Eaton, B. A. Morgan, and J. L. Blair. 2001. "Debris-Flow and Flooding Hazards Associated with the December 1999 Storm in Coastal Venezuela and Strategies for Mitigation." US Geological Survey. http://pubs.usgs.gov/of/2001/ofr-01–0144/

Wilhite, D. A. 1993. "Drought Mitigation Technologies in the United States: With Future Policy Recommendations." International Drought Information Center technical report series 93–1.

Woodruff, B. A., J. M. Toole, D. C. Rodriguez, E. W. Brink, E. S. Mahgoub, M. M. Ahmed, and A. Babikar. 1990. "Disease Surveillance and Control after a Flood in Khartoum, Sudan." *Disasters* 14:151–63.

Woodruff, R., T. McMichael, and C. Butler. 2006. "Action on Climate Change: The Health Risks of Procrastinating." *Australian and New Zealand Journal of Public Health* 30:567–71.

Woodruff, R., T. McMichael, and S. Hales. 2006. "Climate Change and Human Health: Review of the Evidence." *Lancet* 367(9513):59–69.

World Health Organization. 1979. "The Risk of Disease Outbreaks after Natural Disasters." *WHO Chronicle* 33:214–16.

World Health Organization. 1992. *Psychosocial Consequences of Disasters: Prevention and Management.* Geneva: World Health Organization.

World Health Organization. 1998. *Health Sector Emergency Preparedness Guide. Tazmania.* Geneva: World Health Organization.

World Health Organization. 2009. *Vegetation Fires.* https://apps.who.int/inf-fs/en/fact254.html.

World Health Organization. 2011. "Human Resources for Mental Health: Workforce Shortages in Low and Middle-Income Countries." *Human Resources for Health Observer* 8.

Zell, R. 2004. "Global Climate Change and the Emergence/Re-Emergence of Infectious Diseases." *International Journal of Medical Microbiology* 293(suppl.):16–26.

CHAPTER 3

EXTREME AND CHANGING METEOROLOGICAL CONDITIONS ON THE HUMAN HEALTH CONDITION

Daniel P. Johnson, Austin C. Stanforth

Investigating the impact of weather or climate variability on human health requires a substantial multidisciplinary foundation (Huang et al. 2011). Understanding the spectrum of disorders, climate-induced triggers, social and environmental vulnerability to local-scale changes in climate, and sustainability mitigation practices requires involvement from a broad scientific community. These processes are only a sampling of the many environmental concerns that the scientific community, and indeed the overall population of Earth, is concerned with regarding changes to climate and health. Each one of these has plagued humankind throughout its history to some degree. We note that our use of *climate* and *climate change* refers specifically to regional and meteorological variability within this chapter. Although we do not take a stance on the current climate change discussion, current climate and ecological models tend to predict an increased frequency and, in many cases, intensity of extreme weather conditions (Patz et al. 2000). With these concerns, it is vitally important for the scientific community to respond in a robust and meaningful way to promote the integration of research findings across disciplines.

In the United States, many people feel they are not as vulnerable to meteorological or longer-term climatic change as those within developing countries due to their health infrastructure and the political arguments downplaying climate change research. Arguably these

KEY CONCEPTS

- Investigating weather or climate variability's impact on human health requires a substantial multidisciplinary foundation. It is vitally important for the scientific community to respond in robust and meaningful ways to promote the integration of research findings across disciplines.

- This chapter portrays findings related to social, environmental, and individual risk factors to weather and climate-related health hazards. It demonstrates developing approaches using geospatial technologies and how they can be used to pinpoint areas of concern, a data set that is usually not available to the public health community, first responders, and to clinicians on the frontlines in any situation.

- It is vital for health professionals, from first responders to clinicians, to understand the basic fundamentals of modeling the effects of weather and climate variability and change on human health. An understanding of their limitations is also warranted so improvements can continue to be made in the future.

beliefs potentially make the United State more vulnerable. The increased number of heat waves during the past few years (many of which have been predicted by climate modeling), drought events across the nation, vector-borne disease prevalence, extreme precipitation events (which lead to flooding and a concern about the quality of water), and other assorted weather-related disasters (tornados, hurricanes, thunderstorm events) tend to confirm many concerns about the increasing risk of human health to weather events in the United States. These issues alone should be cause for alarm to the general population of the United States, but they also bring a plethora of additional health constraints. Therefore, it is vital that a new generation of clinicians be trained to be aware of the potential dangers that climate change poses to human health. These clinicians and other health scientists need to be aware of surveillance techniques that can be used to predict areas of concern. This work can prove important both for first responders (emergency management personnel and medical clinicians) and the broad range of social and environmental scientists engaged in such techniques.

This chapter portrays findings related to the social, environmental, and individual risk factors to meteorological-related health hazards. It demonstrates developing approaches using geospatial technologies and how they can be used to pinpoint areas of concern. A data set of this resolution is usually not known to the public health community, first responders, and clinicians on the frontlines in any situation. We discuss current and potential surveillance techniques for extreme heat, extreme precipitation and flooding, water quality, and vector-borne disease as well as how they could potentially be blended within a clinical framework. We conclude with a discussion of future work on vulnerability, its modeling, and the potential impacts these newer systems may have on the health of individuals and first aid responses. Finally, we present a discussion on our research into creating a process of developing a model for pinpointing extreme heat health risk using geospatial technologies that lends itself well to the interdisciplinary foundation.

Social, Environmental, and Individual Factors within Well-Known Climate-Related Health Risks

Two of the most discussed and well-known climate-related concerns within the scientific literature are extreme heat and extreme precipitation events, the latter of which lead to flooding, water quality, and vector-borne disease concerns. These climate health concerns have some similarities regarding the social dimensions of vulnerability. Differences arise in the types of hazards socially vulnerable groups are exposed to. Individual risk factors are, in many cases, different for each climate-related phenomenon. However, they share some similarities, as will be evident in the following discussions of who is commonly most affected. As our case study will explain in more detail, there have often been two types of vulnerability studies: physical, which identifies potential victims based on their physical location, and social, where victims are identified by their ability to adapt to or endure an event. Combining the aspects of physical and social identification of risk factors lead to the foundation of improved modeling, as will be evident in our case study example.

Extreme Heat

Extreme heat is a leading cause of weather-related fatality in the United States. In any given year, more people die from extreme heat than any other weather-related cause of mortality (McGeehin and Mirabelli 2001; Luber and McGeehin 2008). In fact, during a typical summer in the United States, more people die from excessive temperatures than from flooding, lightning, tornados, and hurricanes combined. This is a little-known fact, as the general public perception considers heat to be of no particular concern (Akerlof et al. 2010). This perception of heat is dangerous and could contribute to the increase in mortality witnessed across the United States. In addition to this lack of perception is an inclination to not modify behavior during episodes of extremely hot weather (Bassil and Cole 2010). These issues likely lead to an increase in heat health complications; however, heat-related mortality is often underreported within the United States since many causes of death are linked to cardiac or respiratory problems that were exasperated or exaggerated due to the extreme heat, but weather is often not listed as a contributing cause. Therefore, extreme heat could be exponentially more dangerous to public health than current figures show (Johnson et al. 2011).

The earliest widely discussed extreme heat event (EHE) in the United States was the 1995 Chicago episode. This EHE led to over 750 deaths in approximately five days (Dematte et al. 1998). Many of those who died were socially isolated, a common individualized risk factor (Browning et al. 2006; Duneier 2006). In addition, their social situation required these people, mostly aged individuals, to reside in subsidized housing in multistory buildings, and many of them were in fact afraid to venture out due to high crime rates in the neighborhood (Browning et al. 2006; Duneier 2006). These characteristics created a perfect storm of environmental, individual, and social factors that contributed to a disaster of significant dimensions.

Fortunately, the United States has not witnessed a heat-related disaster in any one city of this magnitude since. It has been argued that we might not witness another because that event was possibly the result of a variety of situations that came about in Chicago that are now included in forecasting. However, this does not alleviate the concern regarding extreme heat. A primary environmental stressor that is associated with mortality to extreme heat is the urban heat island (UHI) effect (Johnson and Wilson 2009; Harlan et al. 2006). This urban health threat is perhaps the second greatest health concern discovered in cities after the witnessed decreases in air quality during the nineteenth century. The UHI is simply described as the notable air temperature differences between the rural and urban contiguous zone. The city is much warmer (by many degrees Celsius) due to a decrease in vegetation and a significant increase in the **built environment**, or building materials, which tend to absorb heat during the day and emit it into the surrounding environment, adding to the sensible heat individuals are exposed to during the day and evening. However, the UHI effect is not spatially homogeneous across the entire extent of urbanized development. There are pockets of extreme heat locations in different areas of the city next to areas of cooler temperature. These are termed more **microurban heat islands (micro UHIs)**. Unfortunately, many of the locations within cities that contain the socially disadvantaged are spatially congruent with areas of these micro UHIs (Johnson et al. 2012; Johnson and Wilson 2009). This suggests that the socially vulnerable within many different cities are located in areas where there is a significant heat-related environmental stressor.

Not surprisingly there are numerous social indicators of vulnerability to extreme heat that may tend to alter in levels of importance from one city to the next (Johnson et al. 2009, 2013). Some of these specific population characteristics will be discussed in more depth within the case study at the end of the chapter.

Flooding and Extreme Precipitation Events

Current theories of the changing climate include the expectation of a warming atmosphere, which will result in more frequent flooding and extreme precipitation events (EPEs) (Whitfield 2012). A warmer atmosphere can retain more water vapor than a cooler one. This aspect of water vapor maintains a positive feedback mechanism in the atmosphere. The warmer the atmosphere becomes, the more water vapor it can maintain, and because it is a greenhouse gas, it can lead to increased warming. Provided with this well-known meteorological fact of increased atmospheric moisture, it is probable that flooding and extreme precipitation events will occur (Whitfield 2012). However, many of the impacts that will be experienced will occur at a local scale rather than the global one typically assumed

(Shaw and Riha 2011). In a warmer climate there would tend to be more evaporation of liquid water, and it is uncertain how this would affect the overall hydrological cycle.

The greatest concern with EPEs and their associated flood events is the land cover change occurring at drastic rates throughout the world. Considering current population patterns, the projected increases in human population undoubtedly will cause urbanized and built environment land forms to continue to be the largest growing land cover type. The built environment is defined as areas that are built up or modified in such a way by human activity. Impervious roads, buildings, sidewalks, and even some city parks could be included under the heading of built environment. The predominant land cover type being replaced is dependent on the area of the world being investigating, but is typically vegetated. For example, in Indianapolis, the predominant land cover type being replaced by urban and suburbanization is agricultural land. In Rio de Janeiro, the principal type of land cover being changed is tropical rain forest. The alteration of the original type of land cover can have a significant impact on the effect that EPEs will have on the local hydrological system (Tang et al. 2011; Thompson 2012). For example, if a forested area in a hilly location is deforested and is then exposed to an EPE, it is highly probable that the soil will be heavily eroded and transported. This sediment is then integrated into runoff, which eventually leads into streams and similar systems. This moving sediment can increase stream bed height, clog dam or sewer systems, and lead in increased flood potential.

EPEs will likely have their impact felt more significantly in urbanized areas. This is due to the fact that within urban areas, the predominant land cover types are impervious to liquid water, so any rainfall flows toward the lowest location. For example, in an EPE that produces locally five inches of rainfall in the urbanized area, most of this liquid water will not disperse into the ground but rather flow into constructed drainage systems, and it will fall too quickly for sewer systems to handle and cause an urban flooding event. The flooding event itself is not of particular concern to the public health community, but the implications, especially in cities where there is a **combined sewer overflow system**, are considerably troubling (Nilsen et al. 2011; Patz et al. 2008). Combined sewer overflow systems are drainage systems established in many major cities that are designed to divert both storm water and the sanitation to the sewer system. When this system becomes taxed beyond its intended capabilities, it can essentially fail. A direct result of a system failure could lead to increased likelihoods of effluent, or sewage, from the sanitation or sewer system becoming present on the surface—in many cases an impermeable surface. The potential health effects of such an event are understandably significant.

Modeling the vulnerability to EPE effects potentially requires more spatially discrete modeling techniques than what is outlined in the EHEs previously. Such an undertaking would require significant amounts of data. A system would require data on elevation, impervious surface, soil type (for percolation), buildings and other built environment variables, and drainage capacity. Currently, many cities are beginning to place more advanced monitors in their combined sewer overflow systems to measure their efficiency. Data from these monitors could be used as ancillary data within any surveillance system. Conjoined with these types of data and considering the magnitude of an EPE covering a city, it is possible to determine which areas within a city are more likely to have more significant issues handling rainfall accumulation. Areas with increased amounts of impervious surface are likely to be more vulnerable to high precipitation events just as they had increased vulnerability to higher temperature risk during EHEs (Boegh et al. 2009; Zhang, Zhong et al. 2009; Zhang, Odeh et al. 2009).

CLINICAL CORRELATES 3.1 EXTREME PRECIPITATION EVENTS, WATER TREATMENT, AND HUMAN HEALTH

Expanding areas of urbanization across the United States coupled with increasing extreme precipitation events pose significant threats to human health. During times of low precipitation, urban environments collect substances such as heavy metals, chemical pollutants, and pathogens on their impervious surfaces. When extreme precipitation occurs, treatment capacities of water facilities are overwhelmed, and these chemicals and pathogens are released into surface, drinking, and recreational waters. It is estimated that 6 to 40 percent of the 99 million cases of acute gastroenteritis that occur annually in the United States can be attributed to contaminated drinking water. We know that more than half of contaminated drinking water outbreaks in the past sixty years have followed extreme rainfall (Curriero et al. 2001). In addition to bacterial exposures, toxic substances such as copper, zinc, and lead, as well as pesticides and hormonally active compounds, accumulate on roads, roofs, and parking lots and are released into the drinking and surface waters during extreme precipitation events, never even seeing a treatment facility. These substances have the propensity to create neurotoxicity and act as carcinogens when ingested (Gaffield et al. 2003). The individuals most at risk from these types of environmental contamination are children, the elderly, pregnant women, and the immunocompromised. Physical factors that put communities at risk can be measured through indexes such as the normalized built-up difference index (NDBI) and thus be used to target improvements in domestic water management.

Extreme precipitation events unleash toxic man-made compounds as well as infectious pathogens into drinking and recreational waters, posing significant risks to human health.

Water Quality

The debate regarding water quality is highly related to the previous discussion of flooding and EPEs. Sediment or chemicals (e.g., petroleum products, acids, alkalines) can accumulate on impervious surfaces and can be carried into local streams, lakes, reservoirs, and ultimately the oceans during a pulse of precipitation (Miles 2009). This could be problematic at the conclusion of a drought when the precipitation event causes a pulse of chemical activity that had been accumulating during the dry period, and may cause an acidification pulse into the local freshwater system (Whitehead, Wade et al. 2009). Surprisingly, the larger concern with climate change and its impact on water has been with supply (Whitehead, Wade et al. 2009; Whitehead, Wilby et al. 2009).

Relatively minor evidence has been presented within the scientific literature on the impact to quality until relatively recently (clearly quality would affect supply, but most studies until recently have focused on the lack of water quantity regardless of its quality). Not surprisingly, many research scenarios do not project an increase in the quality of water due to climate changes. Quite to the contrary, research suggests water quality will significantly decrease due to a variety of chemical and physical imbalances produced by disruptions in the hydrological cycle and the natural land cover replacement witnessed through urban- and suburbanization. The major concern to date is the impact on drinking water. Disruptions in the physiochemical processes could reduce the natural filtration process of freshwater sources, both groundwater and surface water, and could make it undrinkable (Delpla et al. 2009). Additional concerns are now being brought up about the numerous waterborne diseases that are likely to increase due to these same physiochemical filtration disruptions.

Many of these waterborne diseases are a by-product of the combined sewer overflow system being overwhelmed and sewer effluent making its way into freshwater systems used for harvesting drinking water and recreational areas such as reservoirs and beaches (Patz et al. 2008). Such effluent, including phosphorus and nitrogen concentrations from fertilizers, can lead to cyanobacterial blooms in waterborne habitats, a leading concern for potable water supplies and recreational water contact (Hunter 2003).

Another waterborne issue that is strongly related to water quality is cholera. Prevalence of this bacterial illness has been found to be affected by river nutrient discharge, possibly a result of fertilizer concentrations and upstream precipitation (Jutla et al. 2011). Apart from its relationship to water quality, a study in Tanzania demonstrated that a 1°C increase in temperature raised the relative risk of cholera by 15 to 29 percent (Traerup, Ortiz, and Markandya 2011). Cholera is perhaps one of the more well-known waterborne diseases due to the advances made by John Snow in London during the nineteenth century. The prevalence of this disease has recently been on the rise and is thought to correlate strongly to climate change, potentially through **teleconnections** via oceanic-atmospheric oscillations such as the El Niño Southern Oscillation (Rodo et al. 2002). Teleconnections refer to climate anomalies that are related but separated by great distances; a change in climate can therefore reach geographically diverse regions across the globe. Researchers have been able to produce predictive systems to forecast the likelihood of encountering jellyfish swarms, harmful algal blooms, and even cholera-carrying phytoplankton (Constantin de Magny and Colwell 2009). These types of resources can help predict outbreaks across the world, as well as in our own yards.

During the summer 2012, the hottest on record for the United States, many people used the beaches and water from Lake Michigan in Chicago to cool themselves during heat events and other abnormally hot days. However, numerous beaches were closed to the public because of many of the disease issues we have noted. For example, the water was considered to be beyond safe levels for *Escherichia coli*, most likely a result of sewer effluent. Anyone visiting the water for recreational purposes was at increased risk for waterborne disease. Modeling risk for contaminated water is difficult because it is typically considered a problem not only for people considered to be socially vulnerable but for the broader community. Certainly individuals without economic and social means might delay a visit to a physician or other medical personnel due to financial concerns, putting them at a higher risk, but trying to identify who is at the highest risk at a very local scale would prove extremely difficult without knowledge of the contamination concentration and dispersion.

Vector-Borne Disease

Some of the initial concerns regarding climate change and human health, especially as they relate to a warming climate, is the likely and evolving threat that vector-borne disease could become more widespread due to the migration of vectors. Vectors could spread out of their endemic zones, creating new areas of epidemic due to reduced climatic stress placed on them outside their indigenous environment or due to the expansion of suitable habitat. This expansion can be both altitudinal and longitudinal (Ceccato et al. 2012; Freed and Cann 2013; Medlock et al. 2013). As an environment transforms due to climate stresses, it could become more suitable for harmful vectors. In many cases, these could be predicted in a longitudinal pattern; however, since there is an expectation of altitudinal expansion of vector habitat, one could expect the expansion to be less predictable in areas of high topographic change. Therefore, altitudinal habitat change needs to be modeled and accounted for accurately. The implications for such spread are evident, as clinicians have begun to see signs of vector-borne infectious disease in areas congruent to endemic zones, such as dengue fever in the southern United States and meningitis in sub-Saharan Africa (Eisen and Moore 2013; Erickson et al. 2010; Ceccato et al. 2014).

Since vectors lend themselves well to habitat suitability modeling, they have been researched in the context of climate change since initial indications of greenhouse warming. **Remote-sensing** techniques are capable of examining both the global and local scale for certain disease vectors by identifying suitable habitats for vectors. However, some species can escape the resolution of such sensors. For example, the *Culex pipiens pipiens* species prefers small areas in which to breed (tree holes, cups, cow footprints full of water, underground storm tunnels) that are far too small or inaccessible for satellite-based remote sensing instruments to detect (Poncon et al. 2007). However, other species habitats are more observable and can be readily detected, or contributing data (such as remotely sensed precipitation and temperature measurements) can identify areas of concern for vectors such as malaria (Lawless et al. 1988; Cleckner, Allen, and Bellows 2011; Ceccato et al. 2012, 2014). In this context of remotely sensed synoptic habitat, the spatial resolution of the sensor plays an important role in the range and effectiveness of modeling. The spatial resolution is effectively the pixel size of the image; the area on the ground that is covered by a pixel is the image. Usually designated in meters, a sensor with a 30-meter spatial resolution would contain pixels covering a 30-by-30 meter area on the ground. Usually the higher the spatial resolution of the sensor (and the smaller the pixel size), the smaller the overall area that can be covered by the sensor, otherwise known as the instantaneous field of view.

The challenge to modeling vector-borne disease within the framework established throughout this discussion is the temporal nature of the phenomenon. With EHE, EPE, flooding, and water quality, the distribution does not spatially change as rapidly as a disease vector. When dealing with vector-borne disease, one is not actually able to model the behavior and movement of the individual vector. The synoptic habitat is the base layer, and the biophysical environment is modeled in relation to suitability. These variables can change but do not fluctuate significantly when compared to an individual vector's movement. This is an area of inefficiency in remote sensing as these different times could have drastically different meteorological conditions and lead to a poor synoptic representation of the habitat due to the limited instantaneous view or temporal resolution of the sensor.

Case Study

Historically, vulnerability studies have been conducted through social or **physical vulnerability** study methods. Studies focusing on the vulnerability of social characteristics use socioeconomic data to identify individuals who have an increased level of difficulty adapting to any oppressive event, which is understood to be an external negative force that tests an individual's resilience or adaptive capabilities. The method is not focused on a particular type of event; rather **social vulnerability** studies identify any person or group who would experience trouble during any oppressive event (Cutter and Finch 2008). This demonstrates how social vulnerability studies have been able to identify who, within a population, will be at a greater risk, but cannot definitively identify where those populations are located or the likelihood that an event will affect them.

Physical vulnerability is the study of specific events or oppressive systems, each focusing on a particular physical component. Each event type, whether a flood or hurricane, is considered independently. **Physical studies** specifically identify the location of the population that will experience the hardest impact within an environment, such as those living in flood zones, but they cannot identify which of those people are less able to adapt to or survive the specific oppressive event (Wisner 2004). Recently work has been done to combine the social and physical study designs to create a more precise vulnerability analysis to consider both the physical location of vulnerable studies and also identify who is more vulnerable within the affected areas (Johnson et al. 2009, 2012).

The following sections describe the individual components and steps that go into such an analysis conducted during a heat wave.

CLINICAL CORRELATES 3.2 EXTREME HEAT EVENTS, AGING POPULATIONS, AND HEALTH CARE SPENDING

In 2009, the number of persons over sixty-five years of age in the United States numbered 39.6 million, representing 12.9 percent of the total population. This demographic is expected to rise to 72.1 million by 2030. Older populations have unique health needs that are likely to be exacerbated with rising ambient temperature and therefore must be considered as we make projections of future health care costs.

Human mortality has been shown to increase on hot days, often attributed to cardiovascular and respiratory collapse, and the elderly are disproportionately affected for medical as well as social reasons (Davis et al. 2003). Aging is associated with a decreased physiological ability to adjust to heat, especially when concurrent chronic and degenerative disease exists. Cognitive disability compounds these factors by altering risk perception and protective behaviors (Astrom, Forsberg, and Rocklov 2011). The trend in increasing mortality among the elderly exists worldwide (Astrom et al. 2011).

The financial cost of caring for an aging population is daunting: Medicare spending currently represents 14 percent of the federal budget ($492 billion; Henry Kaiser Family Foundation 2014) and is expected to increase by two-thirds in the next ten years. With projected increases in extreme heat events and other natural disasters, the needs of the elderly are likely to be more than are projected by current estimates that do not account for climate change. Hospital administrations and clinicians must prepare for this increased demand in services and curtail their systems-based practices to be able to meet the rising need with a limited financial budget.

Climate change poses unique risks to elderly patients, a rising demographic in the United States. Clinicians, hospitals, policymakers, and financial planners must prepare for these unique needs.

Social Vulnerability

The socioeconomic variables used in vulnerability studies have been well established within the background literature (Cutter, Boruff, and Shirley 2003; O'Neill et al. 2005; McMichael et al. 2008; Harlan et al. 2006). These variables are consistent with attributes of a population that is less able to adapt to oppressive forces and events due to either a corporeal or financial inability to deal with adverse conditions. Age, for example, is a common vulnerability variable because it represents a demographic that is less capable of physically dealing with hazardous events such as heat waves. This variable considers both the elderly (age sixty-five and older) and young (below age five) populations, who are less capable of taking care of themselves. Both age demographics represent individuals who have decreased mobility and independence and often require the assistance of a caregiver to relocate them to cooler environments or assist with rehydration (Ebi et al. 2004). Those who are elderly also commonly have chronic illnesses that exacerbate their risk of heat morbidity. Many cardiovascular, neurological, respiratory, or other chronic illnesses have a strong correlation to adverse health outcomes during heat waves, such as hospitalization or death. This is because the chronic illnesses exacerbate the impact that heat has on the individual's body (Semenza et al. 1996; Shen et al. 1998).

Finances have also been found to be representative of vulnerability status in many studies (McMichael et al. 2008; Naughton et al. 2002). This is commonly attributed to its influence on a variety of other variables. Those with better wages often have higher educational attainment and a more stable job. People living below the poverty line typically take up residence in lower-rent neighborhoods, consisting of older buildings with less insulation and built-in dense groups. Older buildings have been known to be more difficult to keep at an appropriate temperature and, depending on the location, rarely have air-conditioning (Davis 1997; O'Neill et al. 2005). Financial situations can also demonstrate whether the household has the monetary ability to afford pool memberships or other activities that could provide relief during a heat wave or other oppressive event (Changnon, Kunkel, and Reinke 1996). A list of common input variables, both social and physical, for social vulnerability studies can be found in table 3.1.

Table 3.1 Vulnerability Variables

Socioeconomic	Total	Total population: Total
	White	Total population: White alone
	Black	Total population: Black or African American alone
	AIAN	Total population: American Indian and Alaska Native alone
	Asian	Total population: Asian alone
	NHPI	Total population: Native Hawaian and Other Pacific Islander alone
	Other_race	Total population: Some other race alone
	total_under5	Total population: 5 years and younger
	total_65up	Population 65 years and over: Total
	M65up_alone	Population 65 years and over: In households; In nonfamily households; Male householder; Living alone
	F65up_alone	Population 65 years and over: In households; In nonfamily households; Female householder; Living alone
	Grouplive_65up	Population 65 years and over: In group quarters; comunal living
	M_NS	Population 25 yeares and over: Male; No schooling completed
	M_NHS	Population 25 yeares and over: Male; Educational attainemnt; below high school
	M_HSG	Population 25 yeares and over: Male; High school graduate (Include equivalency)
	F_NS	Population 25 yeares and over: Female; Educational attainemnt; No schooling completed
	F_NHS	Population 25 yeares and over: Female; Educational attainemnt; below high school
	F_HSG	Population 25 yeares and over: Female; High school graduate (Include equivalency)
	households	Households: Total
	MHI	Households: Median hosuehold income
	Poverty total	Population for whom poverty status is determined: Income below poverty level
	Poverty5under	Population for whom poverty status is determined: Income below poverty level; 5 years and under
	Poverty65up	Population for whom poverty status is determined: Income below poverty level; 65 years and over
Environmental	Mean_temp	approximate surface temperature of residential spaces from Satellite Thermal band
	NDBI	Normalized Difference Build-up Index estimate of built environment within residential space
	NDVI	Normalized Difference Vegetation Index estimate of built environment within residential space

Note: These input variables, social and physical, for vulnerability assessment were tested against a dependent outcome, mortalities during the heat wave, to designate which variables were the best predictors of risk.

Physical Vulnerability

Studies that focus on physical attributes and locations that impart an oppressive force on a population are considered a hazard first analysis. This type of study is most commonly used in flood analysis, because there are specific physical characteristics or boundaries where the oppressive influence is more common. The methodology can also be used in heat vulnerability studies by quantifying the thermal impact on neighborhoods through the land surface temperature (LST) and other physical attributes. These variables can explain the impact of the UHI, a phenomenon that describes the process of concrete and other built materials absorbing solar energy and reemitting it into the local environment (Zha, Gao, and Ni 2003; Johnson et al. 2012). This causes the urban environment to be significantly warmer than the surrounding rural areas (Chen et al. 2006). Advances in remote-sensing technologies have discovered that the UHI is not a singular or continuous event, but rather affects sections of a city disproportionately based on the density of constructed materials. Areas of higher density, with more concrete, have a larger storage capacity for the solar energy and can therefore store and reemit more energy that less dense areas (Zha et al. 2003; Zhang and Wang 2008).

Other common environmental variables that can quantify negative impacts within the urban environment are the normalized built-up difference index (NDBI) and the normalized difference vegetation index (NDVI). The NDBI identifies cement and other constructed or impervious surfaces and offers supportive information to the LST data (Jensen 2007). Higher NDBI values are normally associated with increased urban construction, which is linked to increased temperature, air pollutants, and precipitation runoff, all of which have a negative impact on vulnerable populations.

The NDVI identifies areas of increased vegetation, which is considered to be a protective variable. Vegetation absorbs heat and other solar energy during photosynthesis, which can reduce the thermal impact on local populations (Quattrochi and Luvall 1997; Chen et al. 2006; Jensen 2007). Healthy vegetation also purifies the air we breathe and provides protection during precipitation events. Plants absorb water for growth and storage during high rain events; the roots also stabilize the soil to reduce erosion, causing a decrease in damage during large precipitation events.

The cumulative impact of these environmental variables can assist in identifying areas of a city at increased risk. Therefore, satellite imagery can be used to identify and quantify the influence an environment has on local populations for vulnerability studies. The LST and NDBI can be used to document the discontinuous thermal impact between urban areas, and NDVI can document areas of relief from the negative meteorological influences (Johnson et al. 2012). Figure 3.1 demonstrates the relationship between the environmental variables. The figure demonstrates how LST and NDBI identify similar regions of the city, while high NDVI values are in opposing areas.

CLINICAL CORRELATES 3.3 VULNERABLE POPULATIONS AND "NO REGRETS" SOLUTIONS

Extreme climate events have wide-reaching consequences to the mental and physical health and the long-term prosperity of socially and economically disadvantaged populations. Traditionally, demographic factors such as age, ethnicity, employment status, education, and household size have been used to create risk maps in order to direct resources to vulnerable communities. However, these traditional assessments often overlook hidden populations in communities that on average appear resilient: illegal immigrants, victims of domestic abuse, child runaways, the homeless, persons with substance abuse problems, the mentally ill, and people with AIDS or other stigmatized diseases (Enarson 2007). What puts these populations at special risk during an emergency situation is their fear of trusting conventional help and a lack of social connections to rely on. One way to connect with these populations is to increase the availability of trained psychologists and social workers in emergency departments, which become last-resort places for help. Staff with dedicated time to speak with these special populations would allow for individual risk mapping and resource problem solving. This is an example of a "no-regrets" solution that would increase resilience and decrease vulnerability for this hidden population in the present and the future.

Health care systems must invest in safety nets for populations at risk for adverse outcomes during natural disasters and extreme climate events.

Identifying Risk

Statistical methods can be used to identify which variables, social and physical, are the best predictors of vulnerability across a study area. Principal component analysis (PCA) can be used to identify discontinuities in vulnerability because it uses data reduction techniques to simplify the data relationships. This allows the PCA to identify trends, or underlying patterns, in the data by identifying features that are more significant to the understanding of a dependent variable (DeCoster 2004). These trends identify which input variables are more important to the understanding of the dependent's variability and allows for a reduction in the quantity of input variables needed to explain the variance, similar to the reduction techniques done in previous studies (Cutter et al. 2003; Harlan et al. 2006). This allows a user to include only those that explain the greatest amount of the dependent variable's variation; this can simplify the input variables' relationship, reduce confounding errors, and allow for the mapping of high-risk potential (StatSoft 2011). The dependent

Physical Variables

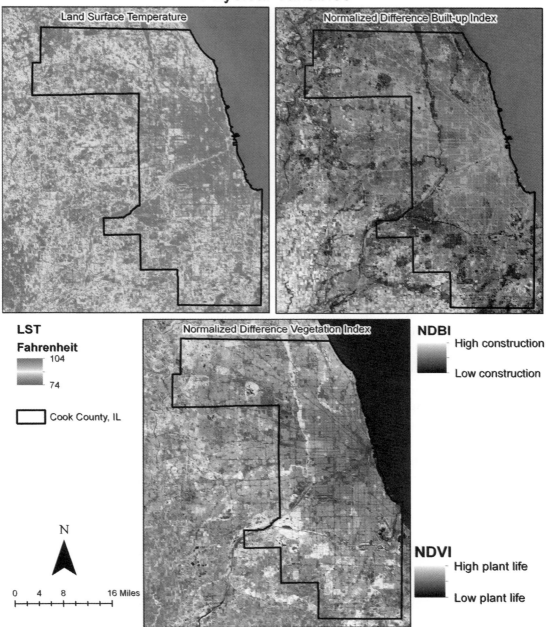

Figure 3.1 Similarities of the Remotely Captured Physical Variables

Note: The LST and NDBI demonstrate higher values for the densely built environment areas, while the NDVI highlights opposing areas where vegetation is more prevalent.

variable is an incidence of the event being studied. For vulnerability studies, negative health outcomes or mortalities caused by the event are often used (Semenza et al. 1996). Therefore, mortalities during heat waves, which list heat as a main or contributing cause of death, can be used as the dependent variable. PCA can identify how well each of the input variables is able to explain the variation in mortality occurrences within an environment. Those variables, which explain a larger percent of the mortality variation, represent a higher risk to the population. The PCA output will consist of a list of components that identify the variables that best explain the variance among the dependent variables. Once the relationship between an input variable and the dependent is determined, it can be related back to the original input variable data set. This will allow for a vulnerability weight to be created for each variable type within a boundary; the summation of each boundary's risk weight can create a risk map that represents a real-world hierarchy of vulnerability.

To better explain these methods, we offer an example of our study of the Chicago 1995 heat wave. Social vulnerability input variables were collected through the use of US Census data from 1990. The census has population data collected at various boundary resolutions (census tracts versus block groups); a previous study found the census tract to perform the best under these circumstances (Stanforth 2011). Vulnerability variables (financial, age, education) identified from the literature can be extrapolated from the census at this boundary. The physical variables (LST, NDVI, NBDI) were downloaded from a US Geological Survey (USGS) online database, and consisted of a Landsat 5 TM satellite image acquired on July 1, 1995. Satellite environmental data can be joined to the census boundary through the use of geographic information science (GIS) methodologies and computer software designed for geospatial analysis. These steps convert all the data into comparable quantitative variables for statistical analysis and merged the data sets into the census tract boundaries, which became distinct neighborhoods for vulnerability assessment and comparison (Johnson et al. 2009).

The results from the study of the 1995 heat wave in Chicago demonstrated how age, financial situation, education, and LST were all strong predictors of the variability found within the mortality data (Johnson et al. 2012; Stanforth 2011). This demonstrates that the results from this study identified important variables that can indicate the vulnerability of local populations, many of which were similarly found in previous vulnerability studies (Cutter et al. 2003; Harlan et al. 2006, 2013). Understanding the relationship between the individual variables and the vulnerable ranking, the results can be used to map areas of higher risk by merging the PCA outputs to their original boundary features (Johnson et al. 2009). Identifying areas at higher risk can allow for preventative mitigation practices to be established in an attempt to reduce the local population's risk or protect individuals who live in those areas. Should a high-risk area have a high LST, tree planting programs could serve as a proactive mitigation project. Additional attempts to address high-risk areas could be as simple as identifying which hospitals or cooling centers are located within high-risk areas; those establishments should see an increase in visitors during a heat wave so extra staff should be scheduled. Figure 3.2 demonstrates a heat vulnerability map created for

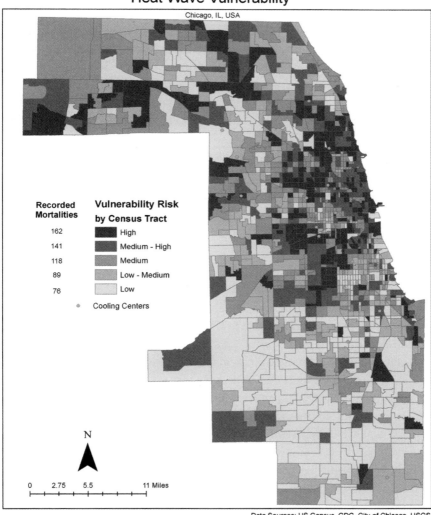

Figure 3.2   A Heat Risk Vulnerability Map for Chicago, 1990s

Note: City-sponsored cooling centers are also identified on the map. Centers that are in higher-risk areas should be considered priority locations for activation during oppressively hot weather.

Chicago circa 1995, with city-sponsored cooling centers located. The centers located in higher-risk areas should be the priority centers to open during a heat wave.

Physical vulnerability studies are applicable only to specific locations and time because physical features are constantly changing due to erosion or development (Johnson et al. 2013). It is understandable then that this analysis, which has a physical vulnerability component, is also limited by the constraints of the boundaries and time when the data were collected. The results are therefore directly applicable only to the Chicago area around the time of the 1990s (Johnson et al. 2012, 2013). The city is a dynamic system, always changing; construction is occurring within it, and population demographics change as neighborhood property values shift. In contrast, the general relationship between vulnerability prediction and the social variables should be relatable to other studies (e.g., age and poverty will normally be predictive of vulnerability), but the actual weight each variable holds will not be consistent between geographical areas or time periods (Johnson et al. 2013). Due to the distinct nature of both the social and physical variables at each study location and period, the identification of vulnerable locations within a city will need periodic updating to remain current, and individual cities will require their own analysis.

Conclusion

Modeling the health effects of climate change is a vital part of our preparation for its effects. Health impacts are both environmental and societal and will undoubtedly be felt as the climate and cities change. The effects of climate change on human health is often overlooked by the popular media; press releases seem more concerned with monetary and insurance costs associated with large meteorological events, as well as glacial retreat, Antarctic ice loss, or general denial of scientific research for more long-term climate change claims. It is vital for health professionals, from first responders to clinicians, to understand the basic fundamentals of modeling such scenarios as we demonstrated in this case study. This could lead to a better understanding of model effectiveness and procedures within the general population. This is important in order to properly prepare decision makers and the most vulnerable populations for the effects of our changing climate; this includes helping to prepare for extreme events and improve policy in anticipation of such events. Moreover, as such models become more commonplace in the decision support environment, an understanding of their limitations is also warranted so improvements can continue to be made in the future.

DISCUSSION QUESTIONS

1. List some of the situations in which modeling of environmental risks would be beneficial, and enumerate some of the benefits.

2. The authors note that the results from a study of the 1995 heat wave in Chicago demonstrated how age, financial situation, education, and land surface temperature were all strong predictors of the variability found within the mortality data. List and briefly discuss several ways in which such a study could be used in real time to direct preparation or recovery efforts.

3. Discuss the limitations of modeling vector-borne disease as reviewed in this chapter. Can you think of ways in which these limitations could be overcome?

4. What other events have a physical or environmental component (consider other disease vectors or even volcanic eruptions), and how could advanced warning methods be used to improve resilience?

5. If you were a public health official, how could you use advanced warnings to prepare? What services or procedures would you enact to reduce vulnerability during a projected extreme heat event? Vector disease outbreak? Other oppressive event?

KEY TERMS

Built environment: Areas that are built up or modified by human activity—for example, impervious roads, buildings, sidewalks, and even some city parks.

Combined sewer outflow system: Drainage systems established in many major cities that are designed to divert both storm water and the sanitation/sewer system. When this system becomes taxed beyond its intended capabilities, it can fail.

Microurban heat island: Pockets of extreme heat locations in different areas of the city next to areas of cooler temperature.

Physical studies: Studies that identify the location of the population that will experience the hardest impact within an environment but cannot identify which of those affected people are less able to adapt to or survive the specific oppressive event (Wisner 2004).

Physical vulnerability: Physical characteristics or boundaries that are susceptible to hazard and may become a source of harm themselves.

Remote sensing: The use of aerial sensors technologies to detect and classify objects on Earth.

Social vulnerability: The variables consistent with attributes of a population able to adapt to oppressive forces and events due to a corporeal or financial inability to deal with adverse conditions.

Teleconnections: Climate anomalies that are related but separated by great distances; a change in climate can therefore affect geographically diverse regions across the globe.

References

Akerlof, K., R. DeBono, P. Berry, A. Leiserowitz, C. Roser-Renouf, K. L. Clarke, A. Rogaeva, M. C. Nisbet, M. R. Weathers, and E. W. Maibach. 2010. "Public Perceptions of Climate Change as a Human Health Risk: Surveys of the United States, Canada and Malta." *International Journal of Environmental Research and Public Health* 7:2559–2606.

Astrom, D., B. Forsberg, and J. Rocklov. 2011. "Heat Wave Impact on Morbidity and Mortality in the Elderly Population: A Review of Recent Studies." *Maturitas* 69:99–105.

Bassil, K. L., and D. C. Cole. 2010. "Effectiveness of Public Health Interventions in Reducing Morbidity and Mortality during Heat Episodes: A Structured Review." *International Journal of Environmental Research and Public Health* 7:991–1001.

Boegh, E., R. N. Poulsen, M. Butts, P. Abrahamsen, E. Dellwik, S. Hansen, C. B. Hasager, et al. 2009. "Remote Sensing Based Evapotranspiration and Runoff Modeling of Agricultural, Forest and Urban Flux Sites in Denmark: From Field to Macro-Scale." *Journal of Hydrology* 377:300–16.

Browning, C. R., D. Wallace, S. L. Feinberg, and K. A. Cagney. 2006. "Neighborhood Social Processes, Physical Conditions, and Disaster-Related Mortality: The Case of the 1995 Chicago Heat Wave." *American Sociological Review* 71:661–78.

Ceccato, P., C. Vancutsem, R. Klaver, J. Rowland, and S. J. Connor. 2012. "A Vectorial Capacity Product to Monitor Changing Malaria Transmission Potential in Epidemic Regions of Africa." *Journal of Tropical Medicine*, 1–6. doi:10.1155/2012/595948

Ceccato, P. S., C. P. Trzaska, O. Garcia-Pando, J. del Corral Kalashnikova, R. Cousin, M. B. Blumenthal, M. Bell, S. J. Connor, and M. C. Thomson. 2014. "Improving Decision-Making Activities for Meningitis and Malaria." *Geocarto International* 29:19–38.

Changnon, S. A., K. E. Kunkel, and B. C. Reinke. 1996. "Impacts and Responses to the 1995 Heat Wave: A Call to Action." *Bulletin of the American Meteorological Society* 77:1497–1506.

Chen, X.-L., H.-M. Zhao, P.-X. Li, and Z.-Y. Yin. 2006. "Remote Sensing Image-Based Analysis of the Relationship between Urban Heat Island and Land Use/Cover Changes." *Remote Sensing of Environment* 104:133–46.

Cleckner, H. L., T. R. Allen, and A. S. Bellows. 2011. "Remote Sensing and Modeling of Mosquito Abundance and Habitats in Coastal Virginia, USA." *Remote Sensing*, 3:2663–81.

Constantin de Magny, G., and R. R. Colwell. 2009. "Cholera and Climate: A Demonstrated Relationship." *Transactions of the American Clinical and Climatological Association* 120:119–28.

Curriero, F. C., J. A. Patz, J. B. Rose, and S. D. Lele. 2001. "The Association between Extreme Precipitation and Waterborne Disease Outbreaks in the United States, 1948–1994." *American Journal of Public Health* 91:1194–99.

Cutter, S. L., B. J. Boruff, and W. Shirley. 2003. "Social Vulnerability to Environmental Hazards." *Social Science Quarterly* 84:242–61.

Cutter, S. L., and C. Finch. 2008. "Temporal and Spatial Changes in Social Vulnerability to Natural Hazards." *Proceedings of the National Academy of Sciences of the United States of America* 105:2301–2306.

Davis, M. 1997. "The Radical Politics of Shade." *Capitalism, Nature, Socialism* 8:35–39.

Davis, R., P. Knappenberger, P. Michaels, and W. Novicoff. 2003. "Changing Heat-Related Mortality in the United States." *Environmental Health Perspectives* 111:1712–18.

DeCoster, J. 2004. "Data Analysis in SPSS." http://www.stat-help.com/notes.html

Delpla, I., A. V. Jung, E. Baures, M. Clement, and O. Thomas. 2009. "Impacts of Climate Change on Surface Water Quality in Relation to Drinking Water Production." *Environment International* 35:1225–33.

Dematte, J. E., K. O'Mara, J. Buescher, C. G. Whitney, S. Forsythe, T. McNamee, R. B. Adiga, and I. M. Ndukwu. 1998. "Near-Fatal Heat Stroke during the 1995 Heat Wave in Chicago." *Annals of Internal Medicine* 129:173–81.

Duneier, M. 2006. "Ethnography, the Ecological Fallacy, and the 1995 Chicago Heat Wave." *American Sociological Review* 71:679–88.

Ebi, K. L., K. A. Exuzides, E. Lau, M. Kelsh, and A. Barnston. 2004. "Weather Changes Associated with Hospitalizations for Cardiovascular Diseases and Stroke in California, 1983–1998." *International Journal of Biometeorology* 49(1):48–58.

Eisen, L., and C. G. Moore 2013. "*Aedes (Stegomyia) aegypti* in the Continental United States: A Vector at the Cool Margin of Its Geographic Range." *Journal of Medical Entomology* 50:467–78.

Enarson, E. 2007. "Identifying and Addressing Social Vulnerabilities." In *Emergency Management: Principles and Practice for Local Government,* 2nd ed., edited by W. Waugh and K. Tierney, 257–78. Washington, DC: IMCA Press.

Erickson, R. A., S. M. Presley, L.J.S. Allen, K. R. Long, and S. B. Cox. 2010. "A Dengue Model with a Dynamic *Aedes albopictus* Vector Population." *Ecological Modelling* 221:2899–2908.

Freed, L. A., and R. L. Cann. 2013. "Vector Movement Underlies Avian Malaria at Upper Elevation in Hawaii: Implications for Transmission of Human Malaria." *Parasitology Research* 112:3887–95.

Gaffield, S., R. Goo, L. Richards, and R. Jackson. 2003. "Public Health Effects of Inadequately Managed Stormwater Runoff." *American Journal of Public Health* 39:1527–33.

Harlan, S. L., A. J. Brazel, L. Prashad, W. L. Stefanov, and L. Larsen. 2006. "Neighborhood Microclimates and Vulnerability to Heat Stress." *Social Science and Medicine* 63:2847–63.

Harlan, S. L., J. H. Declet-Barreto, W. L. Stefanov, and D. B. Petitti. 2013. "Neighborhood Effects on Heat Deaths: Social and Environmental Predictors of Vulnerability in Maricopa County, Arizona." *Environmental Health Perspectives* 121:197–201.

Henry Kaiser Family Foundation. 2014. "The Facts on Medicare Spending and Financing." http://kff.org/medicare/fact-sheet/medicare-spending-and-financing-fact-sheet/.

Huang, C. R., P. Vaneckova, X. M. Wang, G. FitzGerald, Y. M. Guo, and S. L. Tong. 2011. "Constraints and Barriers to Public Health Adaptation to Climate Change: A Review of the Literature." *American Journal of Preventive Medicine* 40:183–90.

Hunter, P. R. 2003. "Climate Change and Waterborne and Vector-Borne Disease." *Journal of Applied Microbiology* 94:37S-46S.

Jensen, J. R. 2007. *Remote Sensing of the Environment: An Earth Resource Perspective.* Upper Saddle River, NJ: Pearson Prentice Hall.

Johnson, D. P., V. Lulla, A. C. Stanforth, and J. Webber. 2011. "Remote Sensing of Heat-Related Risks: The Trend towards Coupling Socioeconomic and Remotely Sensed Data." *Geography Compass* 5:767–80. doi:10.1111/j.1749–8198.201.00442.x

Johnson, D. P., A. Stanforth, V. Lulla, and G. Luber. 2012. "Developing an Applied Extreme Heat Vulnerability Index Utilizing Socioeconomic and Environmental Data." *Applied Geography* 35(1):23–31.

Johnson, D. P., J. J. Webber, K.U.B. Ravichandra, V. Lulla, and A. C. Stanforth. 2013. "Spatiotemporal Variations in Heat-Related Health Risk in Three Midwestern US Cities between 1990 and 2010." *Geocarto International*, January 20, 1–20.

Johnson, D. P., and J. S. Wilson. 2009. "The Socio-Spatial Dynamics of Extreme Urban Heat Events: The Case of Heat-Related Deaths in Philadelphia." *Applied Geography* 29:419–34.

Johnson, D., J. Wilson, and G. Luber. 2009. "Socioeconomic Indicators of Heat-Related Health Risk Supplemented with Remotely Sensed Data." *International Journal of Health Geographics* 8:57.

Jutla, A. S., A. S. Akanda, J. K. Griffiths, R. Colwell, and S. Islam. 2011. "Warming Oceans, Phytoplankton, and River Discharge: Implications for Cholera Outbreaks." *American Journal of Tropical Medicine and Hygiene* 85:303–308. doi:10.4269/ajtmh.2011.11–0181

Lawless, J. G., J. F. Paris, P. D. Sebesta, R. K. Washino, and B. L. Wood. 1988. "Identification and Monitoring of Vector-Borne Disease Environments Utilizing Remote-Sensing Imagery." *Aviation Space and Environmental Medicine* 59:482–82.

Luber, G., and M. McGeehin. 2008. "Climate Change and Extreme Heat Events." *American Journal of Preventive Medicine* 35:429–35.

McGeehin, M. A., and M. Mirabelli. 2001. "The Potential Impacts of Climate Variability and Change on Temperature-Related Morbidity and Mortality in the United States." *Environmental Health Perspectives*, 109:185–89.

McMichael, A. J., P. Wilkinson, R. S. Kovats, S. Pattenden, S. Hajat, B. Armstrong, N. Vayanapoom, et al. 2008. "International Study of Temperature, Heat and Urban Mortality: The 'ISOTHURM' Project." *International Journal of Epidemiology* 1, 1121–31.

Medlock, J. M., K. M. Hansford, A. Bormane, M. Derdakova, A. Estrada-Pena, J. C. George, I. Golovljova, et al. 2013. "Driving Forces for Changes in Geographical Distribution of *Ixodes ricinus* Ticks in Europe." *Parasites and Vectors* 6:1.

Miles, E. L. 2009. "On the Increasing Vulnerability of the World Ocean to Multiple Stresses." *Annual Review of Environment and Resources* 34:17–41.

Naughton, M. P., A. Henderson, M. C. Mirabelli, R. Kaiser, J. L. Wilhelm, S. M. Kieszak, C. H. Rubin, and M. A. McGeehin. 2002. "Heat-Related Mortality during a 1999 Heat Wave in Chicago." *American Journal of Preventive Medicine* 221–27.

Nilsen, V., J. A. Lier, J. T. Bjerkholt, and O. G. Lindholm. 2011. "Analysing Urban Floods and Combined Sewer Overflows in a Changing Climate." *Journal of Water and Climate Change*, 2:260–71.

O'Neill, M. S., A. Zanobetti, and J. Schwartz. 2005. "Disparities by Race in Heat-Related Mortality in Four US Cities: The Role of Air Conditioning Prevalence." *Journal of Urban Health*, 82:191–97.

Patz, J. A., M. A. McGeehin, S. M. Bernard, K. L. Ebi, P. R. Epstein, A. Grambsch, D. J. Gubler, et al. 2000. "The Potential Health Impacts of Climate Variability and Change for the United States: Executive Summary of the Report of the Health Sector of the US National Assessment." *Environmental Health Perspectives* 108:367–76.

Patz, J. A., S. J. Vavrus, C. K. Uejio, and S. L. McLellan. 2008. "Climate Change and Waterborne Disease Risk in the Great Lakes Region of the US." *American Journal of Preventive Medicine* 35:451–58.

Poncon, N., C. Toty, G. L. Ambert, G. Le Goff, C. Brengues, F. Schaffner, and D. Fontenille. 2007. "Population Dynamics of Pest Mosquitoes and Potential Malaria and West Nile Virus Vectors in Relation to Climatic Factors and Human Activities in Camargue, France." *Medical and Veterinary Entomology* 21:350–57.

Quattrochi, D. A., and J. C. Luvall. 1997. "High Spatial Resolution Airborne Multispectral Thermal Infrared Data to Support Analysis and Modeling Tasks in EOS IDS Project ATLANTA." Huntsville, AL: Global Hydrology and Climate Center.

Rodo, X., M. Pascual, G. Fuchs, and A.S.G. Faruque. 2002. "ENSO and Cholera: A Nonstationary Link Related to Climate Change?" *Proceedings of the National Academy of Sciences of the United States of America* 99:12901–12906.

Semenza, J. C., C. H. Rubin, K. H. Falter, J. D. Selanikio, W. D. Flanders, H. L. Howe, and J. L. Wilhelm. 1996. "Heat-Related Deaths during the July 1995 Heat Wave in Chicago." *New England Journal of Medicine* 335:84–90.

Shaw, S. B., and S. J. Riha. 2011. "Assessing Possible Changes in Flood Frequency due to Climate Change in Mid-Sized Watersheds in New York State, USA." *Hydrological Processes* 25:2542–50.

Shen, T. F., H. L. Howe, C. Alo, and R. L. Moolenaar. 1998. "Toward a Broader Definition of Heat-Related Death: Comparison of Mortality Estimates from Medical Examiners' Classification with Those from Total Death Differentials during the July 1995 Heat Wave in Chicago, Illinois." *American Journal of Forensic Medicine and Pathology* 19:113–18.

Stanforth, A. 2011. "Identifying Variations of Socio-Spatial Vulnerability to Heat-Related Mortality During the 1995 Extreme Heat Event in Chicago, IL, USA." Master's thesis, IUPUI, Indianapolis.

StatSoft. 2011. *Electronic Statistics Textbook.* Tulsa, OK: StatSoft. http://www.statsoft.com/textbook/

Tang, L. H., D. W. Yang, H. P. Hu, and B. Gao. 2011. "Detecting the Effect of Land-Use Change on Streamflow, Sediment and Nutrient Losses by Distributed Hydrological Simulation." *Journal of Hydrology* 409:172–82.

Thompson, J. R. 2012. "Modelling the Impacts of Climate Change on Upland Catchments in Southwest Scotland Using MIKE SHE and the UKCP09 Probabilistic Projections." *Hydrology Research* 43:507–30.

Traerup, S.L.M., R. A. Ortiz, and A. Markandya. 2011. "The Costs of Climate Change: A Study of Cholera in Tanzania." *International Journal of Environmental Research and Public Health* 8:4386–4405.

Whitehead, P. G., A. J. Wade, and D. Butterfield. 2009. "Potential Impacts of Climate Change on Water Quality and Ecology in Six UK Rivers." *Hydrology Research* 40:113–22.

Whitehead, P. G., R. L. Wilby, R. W. Battarbee, M. Kernan, and A. J. Wade. 2009. "A Review of the Potential Impacts of Climate Change on Surface Water Quality." *Hydrological Sciences Journal/Journal des sciences hydrologiques* 54:101–23.

Whitfield, P. H. 2012. "Floods in Future Climates: A Review." *Journal of Flood Risk Management* 5:336–65.

Wisner, B. 2004. *At Risk: Natural Hazards, People's Vulnerability, and Disasters.* London: Routledge.

Zha, Y., J. Gao, and S. Ni. 2003. "Use of Normalized Difference Built-Up Index in Automatically Mapping Urban Areas from TM Imagery." *International Journal of Remote Sensing* 24:583–94.

Zhang, J., and Y. Wang. 2008. "Study of the Relationships between the Spatial Extent of Surface Urban Heat Islands and Urban Characteristic Factors based on Landsat ETM+ Data." *Sensors* 8:7453–68.

Zhang, X., T. Zhong, K. Wang, and Z. Cheng. 2009. "Scaling of Impervious Surface Area and Vegetation as Indicators to Urban Land Surface Temperature Using Satellite Data." *International Journal of Remote Sensing* 30:841–59.

Zhang, Y. S., I.O.A. Odeh, and C. F. Han. 2009. Bi-Temporal Characterization of Land Surface Temperature in Relation to Impervious Surface Area, NDVI and NDBI, Using a Sub-Pixel Image Analysis." *International Journal of Applied Earth Observation and Geoinformation* 11:256–64.

PART 2

THE HEALTH CONSEQUENCES OF CLIMATE CHANGE

CHAPTER 4

CHANGES IN HYDROLOGY AND ITS IMPACTS ON WATERBORNE DISEASE

Jan C. Semenza

Adjustment of existing surveillance practices for infectious diseases is necessary for monitoring climate change–related threats to public health. This chapter discusses the climate change impacts on the **hydrological cycle** and waterborne diseases. It touches on elevated water temperature and precipitation extremes and discusses specific waterborne diseases in detail.

Rising global temperatures increase the rate of evaporation of the Earth's surface water, which in turn causes an increase in water vapor in the **atmosphere**. Water vapor is itself a greenhouse gas and therefore perpetuates the warming cycle. As the planet warms, changes in both the frequency and intensity of precipitation are expected to occur, with a variety of results. Heavy rainfall may flush pathogens into waterways, contaminating water catchment areas, treatment plants, beaches, and coastal waterways. Floods may result in an increased number of waterborne epidemics, and droughts may necessitate the use of poor-quality water sources, increasing the risk of microbiological threats. Increased temperatures will allow certain pathogens, such as *Salmonella* and *Vibrio* (non-*cholerae*), to thrive. The incidence of vector-borne diseases, such as West Nile virus and malaria, may also increase as the result of floods or heavy rainfall events, which provide vector breeding grounds.

Vulnerability, impact, and adaptation assessment can help prepare society for changes in the hydrological cycle. Prediction of meteorological events should

KEY CONCEPTS

- **Vulnerability, impact, and adaptation assessment can improve risk management of water resources and prepare society for changes in the hydrological cycle such as failures of the water supply.**

- **Monitoring and reporting of contaminated beaches and enforcing beach closures can reduce illnesses from bathing in recreational waters.**

- **Upgrading aging water treatment and distribution systems, including improved water filter operations, is warranted to cope with extremes of the hydrological cycle and prevent breakthrough of filters.**

- **Risk assessments are needed by municipal water providers to help manage heavy precipitation discharge by augmenting sewer system storage capacity or droughts through increasing drinking water supplies.**

be incorporated into public health practice and combined with concurrent epidemiological monitoring. Steps should also be taken to manage water quality, such as increasing the capacity of water treatment and sewage management systems.

Changes in Hydrology due to Climate Change

The climate system comprises several interconnected subsystems: the **atmosphere**, the **hydrosphere** (rivers, lakes, and oceans), the **cryosphere** (ice and snow), the **lithosphere** (soils), and the **biosphere** (ecosystems) (figure 4.1). Historically, many factors have influenced the climate, such as volcanic activity, atmospheric composition, the Earth's orbit around the sun, and solar activity. At least since the eighteenth century, human activity has also contributed to changes in the climate, particularly to the warming of the global climate; in fact, it is estimated that the total warming effect of human activities is responsible for a least ten times that of what can be attributed to natural factors such as solar activity (Intergovernmental Panel on Climate Change 2007). However, increasing temperatures due to **anthropogenic activity** are only one manifestation of global climate change; another manifestation is change to the hydrological cycle, which describes the continuous movement of water on Earth (figure 4.1). The water-holding capacity of the atmosphere is a function of temperature and increases by about 8 percent per degree Celsius (Trenberth 1999). The most important greenhouse gas (GHG) in the atmosphere is water vapor, which lets visible light pass through but absorbs part of the infrared radiation from the Earth, and thus retains the heat in the system. This cycle not only increases temperatures but also increases evaporation, which adds to the atmospheric moisture content; changes in both frequency and intensity of extreme (high and low) precipitation are expected to occur (Semenza 2012).

Another manifestation of global climate change is the increasing trend in the heat content of the oceans. The capacity of water to absorb heat is approximately twenty times greater than that of the atmosphere (Levitus et al. 2012). Over 90 percent of the warming of the Earth can be attributed to the warming of the world's ocean. Particularly the top layers of the ocean (the uppermost 700 meters depth) have shown an increasing warming trend but also the deeper ocean (between 700 and 2,000 meters depth) has warmed (Levitus et al. 2012). The rate of increase in sea surface temperature over the last twenty-five years is the largest ever measured in any previous twenty-five-year period (Frankignoul and Kestenare 2005). The hydrology of freshwater quantity and quality is also affected by global climate change. Changes in river flow are difficult to detect due to substantial natural variability, but increased river flow during the winter months in more northern

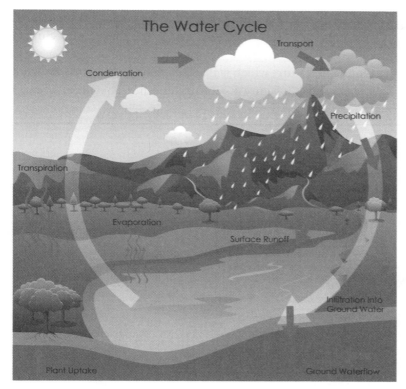

Figure 4.1   The Hydrological Cycle

Note: This illustration was produced under ECDC framework contract: Tender 0J/2008/04/11—PROC/2008/005 Lot 2 by RIVM.

latitudes and lower river flows during the summer in southern latitudes have been observed (Stahl et al. 2010). Increases in river floods might be due to improved reporting, but river flow droughts seem to be on the rise and associated with the increase in hot spells and heat waves.

These changes to the hydrology can affect waterborne diseases because their **environmental exposure pathways** are intricately linked to local climate and weather conditions (figure 4.1) (Boxall et al. 2009). Certain waterborne pathogens cannot multiply outside the human or animal host (e.g., *Norovirus, Cryptosporidium, Camplylobacter*) while others can multiply in the environment (e.g. *Vibrio, Salmonella*) (Semenza, Herbst, et al. 2012).

This chapter discusses the climate change impacts on the hydrological cycle and waterborne diseases; it touches on elevated water temperature, precipitation extremes, and flooding and discusses specific waterborne disease in more detail. The discussion is based on a systematic literature review of peer-reviewed articles on climate change and food- and waterborne pathogens (Semenza, Herbst, et al. 2012; Semenza, Höser, et al. 2012). Detailed information was extracted from these articles and entered into an electronic database. The information was then tagged with terms from a predefined climate change ontology (library of terms or a line listing of technical expressions). The web of connections emerged for all the different aspects documented in the literature, which is illustrated in the semantic network maps in figures 4.2 and 4.3. Figure 4.2 illustrates different sources of water

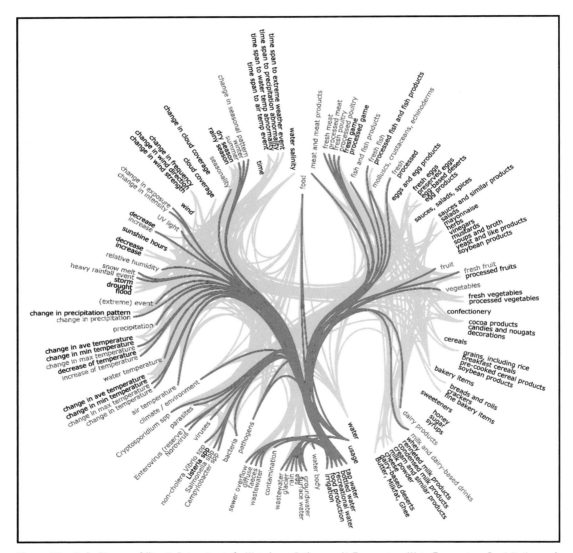

Figure 4.2   Radar Diagram of Climatic Determinants for Waterborne Pathogens: Air Temperature, Water Temperature, Precipitation, and Heavy Rainfall Event, by Pathogen from the Climate Change Knowledgebase for Food- and Waterborne Diseases, 1998–2009

Source: Semenza, Herbst et al. (2012).

Note: The terms *air temperature, water temperature, precipitation,* and *heavy rainfall event* have been extracted from the peer-reviewed literature for the individual pathogens listed. The terms from peer-reviewed articles were quantified by pathogen and mapped on a radar diagram, a graphical method of plotting multivariate data on a two-dimensional chart, on multiple axes originating from the same pole.

Axes (spokes) with different scales.

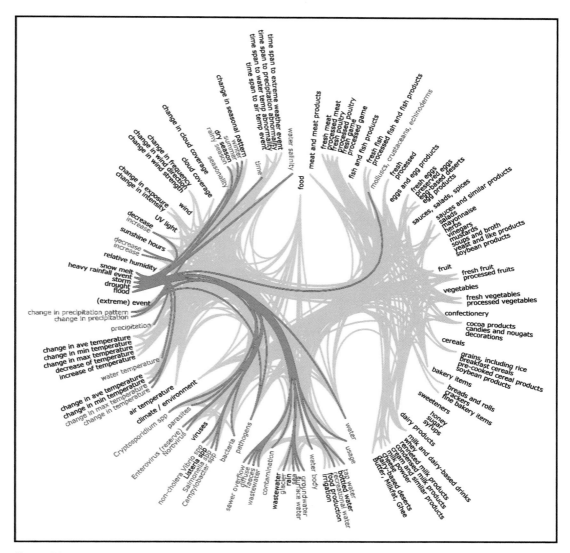

Figures 4.3

(irrigation water, water for food production, recreational water, bottled water, and tapwater) that have been linked to food- and waterborne pathogens, and figure 4.3 maps extreme events (floods, droughts, storms, heavy rainfall events, and snow melt) that have been linked to these pathogens. This database lends itself for data-mining and analysis, and is presented below.

Water Temperature

The link between water temperature and *Vibrio* and *Campylobacter* has been extensively investigated in the peer-reviewed literature, but much

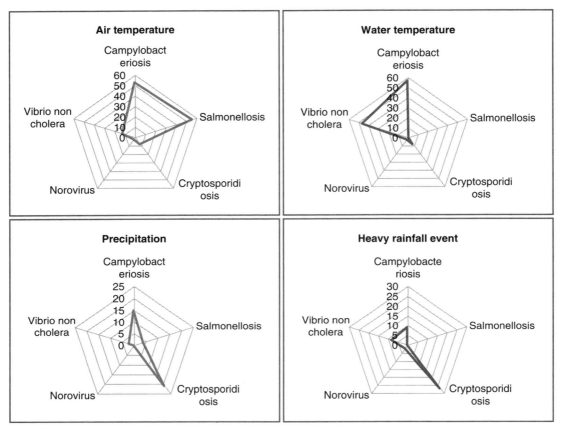

Figure 4.4   Radar Diagram of Climatic Determinants for Waterborne Pathogens: Air Temperature, Water Temperature, Precipitation, and Heavy Rainfall Event, by Pathogen from the Climate Change Knowledgebase for Food- and Waterborne Diseases, 1998–2009

Source: Semenza, Herbst et al. (2012).

Note: The terms *air temperature, water temperature, precipitation,* and *heavy rainfall event* have been extracted from the peer-reviewed literature for the individual pathogens listed. The terms from peer-reviewed articles were quantified by pathogen and mapped on a radar diagram, a graphical method of plotting multivariate data on a two-dimensional chart, on multiple axes originating from the same pole.

Axes (spokes) with different scales.

less so for other waterborne pathogens such as *Cryptosporidium, Salmonella,* or *Norovirus* (figure 4.4) (Semenza, Herbst, et al. 2012). Elevated river water temperature and lower flow rates during the warmer summer months result in inactivation of certain waterborne pathogens such as *Norovirus* and *Campylobacter* (table 4.1) (Schijven and de Roda Husman 2005). Conversely, these pathogens can survive longer during the colder winter months, which explains in part the higher concentrations in river water. However, *Listeria, Vibrio,* and *Salmonella* concentrations can increase at elevated temperatures, of particular concern in marine environments where indigenous *Vibrio* can readily replicate above temperatures of 19°C (table 4.1) (Baker-Austin et al. 2012).

Table 4.1   Climate Change and Waterborne Diseases: Environmental Effects, Pathogen Fate, and Microbial Risk

Climate Change	Effects	Consequences	Microbial Risk
Water temperature increase	Replication of marine bacteria (*Vibrio*)	Bacterial blooms in marine environments	Increased risk
	Die-off of enteric pathogens (e.g., *Norovirus, Campylobacter*)	Lower concentrations of pathogens in surface water	Decreased risk
	Water purification at the treatment plant more efficient	Elimination of pathogens from drinking water	Decreased risk
	Organic matter and nutrients dissolve better	Challenges for water treatment: less efficient	Increased risk
Extended seasons for agriculture and leisure activities	Altered demand on water treatment plant	Opportunities for exposures (e.g., contamination of irrigation water)	Increased or decreased risk
	Shortened winter season with lower snow cover and reduced flooding due to snow melt	Reduced stress on water treatment plants	Decreased risk
Precipitation increase	Runoff, sediments, organic matter, nutrients	Challenges for water treatment: less efficient	Increased risk
	Peak concentrations of pathogens in surface water	Challenges for water treatment: less efficient	Increased risk
	Flooding of wells or water treatment plants	Water treatment at risk	Increased risk
	Storm water runoff and combined sewage overflow	Water treatment at risk Recreational water contamination	Increased risk
	Groundwater contamination with fecal pathogens	Water treatment insufficient	Increased risk
Drought	Changes in water sources	Insufficient treatment options	Increased risk
	Concentration of pathogens	Challenges for water treatment: less efficient	Increased risk

For example, environmental monitoring of *Campylobacter* from ponds, rivers, and recreational water bodies showed that recovery rates are higher in winter and fall but lower in summer and spring (Carter et al. 1987; Obiri-Danso and Jones 1999). However, other reports do not confirm these findings; no significant relationship between *Campylobacter* concentrations and surface water temperatures was found in Greece and Poland (Abulreesh,

Paget, and Goulder 2006). Although *Campylobacter* does not readily die off at 4°C in water, it is nonetheless vulnerable to environmental stresses such as freezing, desiccation, elevated temperatures, or ultraviolet exposure (Blaser 2000; Jones 2001). Concentration of *Vibrio* bacteria increases during times of elevated surface water temperatures and zooplankton blooms (Lipp, Huq, and Colwell 2002). Peak concentrations are found primarily in the later parts of the summer and early autumn and reveal a direct association with salinity and water temperatures. *Vibrio* propagates with mounting surface water temperatures during continued periods of advantageous environmental conditions. The seasonal window was related to water temperatures from 12°C to 15°C, up to an optimum of 26°C (Randa, Polz, and Lim 2004). In Israel, infections were significantly associated with elevated temperatures during the preceding month; indeed in hot climates, the minimum temperature is the determining factor contributing to the growth of *Vibrio* (Paz et al. 2007). Not surprisingly, 78 percent of all infections occur between May and October (Daniels et al. 2000). In immunocompromised individuals bathing in contaminated waters with open wounds, infection can lead to severe necrotic ulcers, septicemia, and death (Lindgren et al. 2012).

Precipitation

In the scientific literature, the effect of precipitation has been studied extensively for *Campylobacter* and *Cryptosporidium* but less so for other waterborne pathogens such as *Vibrio, Norovirus, Salmonella,* or *Listeria* (figure 4.4) (Semenza, Herbst et al. 2012). Rain events can flush pathogens from surrounding areas into streams or lakes and contaminate the water source of water treatment plants (table 4.1). The intensity of such rain events can exceed or simply overwhelm the capacity of the treatment plant and result in water treatment failure. Infiltration of pathogenic *Cryptosporidium* oocysts into drinking water reservoirs poses a technical challenge since the oocysts are resistant to chlorination. Heavy rain events (figures 4.3 and 4.4) have been associated with a number of waterborne outbreaks in many countries (Curriero et al. 2001; Jean et al. 2006; Singh et al. 2001; Semenza and Nichols 2007).

In developing countries, the pathogens involved and the exposure pathways might differ. For example, cholera outbreaks have been associated with heavy rain in developing countries (Griffith, Kelly-Hope, and Miller 2006); a hepatitis A outbreak has been associated with the contamination of a water source due to heavy rain in Korea (Lee, Lee, and Kwon 2008); and outbreaks of enterovirus infections have been linked to extreme precipitation in Taiwan (Jean et al. 2006).

The presence of fecal coliform in drinking water is an indication of water treatment failure and has been linearly associated with rainfall that occurred the preceding day (Richardson et al. 2009). Elevated concentrations of enteric pathogens due to runoff is a problem particularly during the first heavy rain event of the season. It can flush organic matter and microbial nutrients into water distribution system and foster coliform regrowth in treated water (LeChevallier, Schulz, and Lee 1991). Open water reservoirs are at risk for posttreatment contamination with fecal matter from domestic or wild animals that shed *Giardia* and *Cryptosporidium.*

Precipitation events have also been associated with coastal water contamination from surface runoff (Heijs, Wilkinson, and Couriel 2002; Hsu and Huang 2008; Haramoto et al. 2006; Crowther, Kay, and Wyer 2001). Seawater contamination is of particular concern during heavy precipitation events when outfalls from urban storm water contaminate the beaches (Brownell et al. 2007; McCarthy et al. 2007; Soyeux, Blanchet, and Tisserand 2007). These storm events can result in runoff and loading of coastal waters with pathogens, nutrients, and toxic chemicals that may adversely affect aquatic life and public health. This is particularly concerning in coastal watersheds, where human development and population increases have led to urbanization of coastal areas (Mallin et al. 2000; Gaffield et al. 2003). In southern California, urban runoff affects coastal water quality most significantly during the storm season (Dwight et al. 2002; Noble et al. 2003; He and He 2008). The intensity of storms, a manifestation of global climate change, is related to greater bacterial concentrations in ocean water at Santa Monica beaches (Ackerman and Weisberg 2003; Schiff, Morton, and Weisberg 2003). **Storm runoff** also carries other pathogens, including viruses and parasites, into coastal waters (Schiff, Morton, and Weisberg 2003; Griffin et al. 2003). For example, a positive link has been established between measured precipitation and observed coastal water contamination with *Enterococcus* bacteria in southern California (Semenza, Caplan, et al. 2012). Exposure to elevated concentrations of bacteria in bathing waters at southern California beaches has been associated with an increased health risk (Haile et al. 1999; Dwight et al. 2004). An estimated 1.4 million enteric and respiratory illnesses occur at these beaches each year as a result of exposure to contaminated water, but surveillance data for this region do not exist (Brinks et al. 2008).

Mathematical climate change models of future precipitation project a decrease in predicted *Enterococcus* levels through the majority of this century (Semenza, Caplan, et al. 2012). These findings hold potentially beneficial implications for public health, although the variability of storminess might actually increase in southern California in this century ("California

Climate Adaptation Strategy" 2009), which calls for innovative adaptation and surveillance strategies (Lindgren et al. 2012).

Droughts

Precipitation extremes include both high and low extremes (figure 4.3). Interestingly, one study found that in the twentieth century, 10 percent of waterborne disease outbreaks from Wales and England was indeed associated with heavy precipitation, but 20 percent of waterborne outbreaks was associated with prolonged periods of low rainfall (Senhorst and Zwolsman 2005). Low extremes in prolonged dry periods or droughts can significantly diminish river discharge and thus augment the concentration of effluent pathogens. River discharge was significantly reduced during the dry summer of 2003, which affected water quality (Senhorst and Zwolsman 2005). Reductions in the rate of water flow can pose problems for the clearance capacity of water treatment plants (table 4.1) (Senhorst and Zwolsman 2005). Water quality can also be affected by the fact that residues and minerals are more concentrated in dwindling water supplies. Less mobile, disabled, or elderly people might be particularly at risk due to lack of access to safe water. The use of poor-quality water sources due to increased demand can create microbiological threats, such as the use of contaminated irrigation water on crops in the field.

However, water availability may or may not be associated with the microbiological water quality. For example, extended periods of low precipitation levels in more southern latitude countries might also result in reductions in the pathogen load of river water due to longer residence time and higher inactivation of these pathogens. For example, *Norovirus* is inactivated through ultraviolet light, drought, or reductions in relative humidity.

Flooding

Heavy precipitation can generate excessive runoff and cause natural disasters such as flooding (figure 4.3). However, flooding can also occur due to river overflow, rapid snow melt, tidal or storm surge, flash flood, tsunami, and so on. Injuries are the major public health concern, but microbiological risk has also been documented. Flooding of agricultural land contaminated with waterborne pathogens, poor drainage, and backed-up sewage systems can quickly become a public health emergency. The contaminated floodwaters can transport the pathogens to drinking water wells and infiltrate the water distribution system (table 4.1). Standing water can also become a breeding ground for vector-borne diseases. Floods and increased water flows can lead to contamination of drinking, recreational, irrigation, or water drinking water supplies and thus increase the risk of waterborne epidemics (World Health Organization [WHO] 2011). A number of microbial agents have been associated with floods; these include cholera (Sur et al. 2000), cryptosporidiosis (Katsumata et al. 1998), leptospirosis (Sarkar et al. 2002), unspecified diarrhea (Kunii et al. 2002; Mondal, Biswas, and Manna 2001; Heller, Colosimo, and Antunes 2003), poliomyelitis (van Middelkoop et al. 1992), rotavirus (Fun et al. 1991), and typhoid and paratyphoid (Vollaard et al. 2004).

The majority of these outbreaks due to flooding have occurred in developing countries, whereas in developed countries, there is much less evidence of epidemics following such natural disasters (Semenza and Menne 2009). In Europe, for example, flooding has seldom been linked to an increased risk of epidemics of waterborne diseases, but a few exceptions exist and have been documented for the United Kingdom (Reacher et al. 2004), Finland (Miettinen et al. 2001), Czech Republic (Kriz et al. 1998), and Sweden (Ebi 2006).

CLINICAL CORRELATES 4.1 FIFTY YEARS OF CHOLERA

We are in the midst of the seventh global cholera pandemic, which began in Indonesia in 1961. Unlike the prior six pandemics that burned out after five to twenty years, the current strain of *Vibrio cholerae* O1 has undergone two serotype changes (Ryan 2011) and has persisted (See figure 4.5). It remains endemic in fifty countries and reemerges catastrophically during natural disasters, civil unrest, and the breakdown of public health measures. Examples are evident in the Rwandan refugee camps in 1994 and in 2010 following the earthquakes in Haiti (Orata, Keimv, and Boucher 2014).

Recently the current pandemic strain of *V. cholerae,* El Tor, has undergone a hybridization with the classic serotype and become significantly more virulent, killing 1 to 5 percent of its hosts as compared to traditional rates of less than 1 percent (Ryan 2011). There are currently two killed oral vaccines approved for use, Dukoral and Shanchol. Both require multiple doses and provide a limited time frame of immunity. The World Health Organization does not currently recommend routine use of the vaccines in the immediate outbreak of an epidemic, as data are insufficient to predict whether immunity is conferred fast enough to curb the spread of disease and the cost of administration is high. It instead recommends focusing efforts on providing clean drinking water and rehydration as primary management strategies.

Global climate change is likely to intensify preexisting public health emergencies such as cholera. Health care providers must stay informed on these issues to maximize appropriate patient care and curb the further spread of communicable diseases.

Waterborne Pathogens

Campylobacter

Campylobacteriosis is caused by thermophilic *Campylobacter,* with *C. jejuni* being the most common species in humans (Blaser 2000). Symptoms include watery, sometimes bloody diarrhea, abdominal pain, fever, headache, and nausea (Young, Davis, and Dirita 2007). *Campylobacter* are incapable of reproducing outside animal hosts, such as poultry or pigs, and cannot grow in the presence of air. These bacteria are extremely susceptible to a number of environmental stressors, including heat and cold stress, ultraviolet light, and acidic conditions. *C. jejuni* tends to survive in various biological environments better at 4°C than at 25°C. Lakes, rivers, streams, and other surface water sources can become polluted with *Campylobacter* by defecating wild birds or domestic animals that harbor the bacteria. Humans can get exposed through contaminated food or water but also through exposure to sewage effluent during combined sewer overflows (Murphy, Carroll, and Jordan 2006). Risk factors for campylobacteriosis are a function of age, season, and degree of urbanization (Doorduyn et al. 2010).

Ambient temperature has been associated with the incidence campylobacteriosis although not consistently (Bi et al. 2008; Fleury et al. 2006; Kovats et al. 2005; Patrick et al. 2004). As noted, *Campylobacter* is not capable of reproducing outside its animal host, and the seasonal incidence peak does not occur during the hottest time of the year, which might explain in part the inconsistent findings in the literature. Rain in early spring can also trigger campylobacteriosis outbreaks. Households supplied by private water sources tend to be more susceptible to contamination during extreme weather events; indeed, outbreaks tend to occur more often in rural areas than in metropolitan areas with a municipal water source (Hearnden et al. 2003; Pebody, Ryan, and Wall 1997). Extreme rainfall events as a result of climate change might therefore augment the risk of surface and groundwater contamination. Conversely, in more southern latitude countries, climate change might increase the reliance on rainwater during dry spells or droughts. If the harvesting of rainwater increases, *Campylobacter* in untreated roof runoff water might contribute to an increased risk of both animal and human disease (Palmer et al. 1983; Savill et al. 2001).

Salmonella

Among all the *Salmonella* species, *S. enterica* is the species that mostly affects humans and causes gastroenteritis, with nausea, vomiting, and diarrhea six to forty-eight hours after ingestion. While the disease tends to be self-limited, the elderly and immunocompromised can suffer from bacteremia or endovascular complications (Crum-Cianflone 2008). Food is a major source of exposure for humans because *Salmonella* has the ability to persist and reproduce outside the host (European Food Safety Authority 2010; Gantois et al. 2009). Contaminated drinking or irrigation water is also a source of exposure that has resulted in outbreaks (Angulo et al. 1997). The water can become contaminated through fecal pollution by infected individuals but also by other vertebrates, such as birds and reptiles, poultry, cattle, and sheep. Environmental sampling has documented that the bacteria can persist in a dry environment over extended periods of time; it has been recovered from two-and-a-half-year-old dried excrement (Stine et al. 2005). In wet environments, soil, and sediment, *Salmonella* can also survive relatively long and even multiply for up to a year (Winfield and Groisman 2003).

Salmonella usually grow within a temperature range of between 10°C to 47°C, where temperature accelerates the growth rate, but growth at 6°C to 8°C is still possible. This biological determinant manifests itself in the incidence of *Salmonella,* which is highly seasonal. An increase in weekly temperatures has been linked with elevated incidence in different countries (Fleury et al. 2006; Kovats et al. 2004; Naumova et al. 2007; Nichols 2010; Zhang, Bi, and Hiller 2008; D'Souza et al. 2004). Under climate change scenarios, a warmer world should experience a mounting disease burden. However, *Salmonella* incidence has decreased in many countries over the past few years. This decrease is in part due to effective public health interventions such as vaccination of animal hosts or culling of infected poultry flocks. It is also possible that the influence of temperature on *Salmonella* incidence has been attenuated by other measures, such as health education and health promotion, which has resulted in a decline of salmonellosis over the years (Lake et al. 2009). Seasonal *Salmonella* concentrations in water environments are related to monthly maximum precipitation in summer and fall following fecal contamination events (Craig, Fallowfield, and Cromar 2003; Martinez-Urtaza et al. 2004). Floods caused by heavy rainfall events may disrupt water treatment and sewage systems and contribute to increased exposure to *Salmonella* and other pathogens (table 4.1). Thus, effective public health interventions should be able to mitigate adverse impacts of climate change.

Cryptosporidium

Cryptosporidium is an intestinal parasite that causes watery diarrhea that spontaneously resolves over a couple of weeks in otherwise healthy patients but can be severe and even life threatening in immunocompromised individuals. The disease in humans is predominantly caused by the two species *C. parvum* and *C. hominis*, although a number of other species are pathogenic for humans (Slifko et al. 1997). *Cryptosporidium* generates sturdy oocysts that can sustain significant environmental impacts such as chlorine. Once released, the oocysts can survive in moist soil or water for months and remain infectious even under varying temperatures (Kovats et al. 2000). *Cryptosporidium* oocysts appear to be widespread in drinking water resources, including rivers, streams, lakes, and reservoirs; it is found in over half of the samples tested in the United Kingdom and in 97 percent of surface waters in the United States (Gray 1994). The effect of predators (e.g., rotifer) on the survival of the oocysts in water is not yet fully understood; therefore die-off rates cannot be given (Stott et al. 2003). The small size of *Cryptosporidium* makes their removal by filtration during water and wastewater treatment a difficult task (Rose, Huffman, and Gennaccaro 2002). Die-off can be achieved using ultraviolet light (Rose, Huffman, and Gennaccaro 2002) and dry heat (King and Monis 2007). Chlorine is not an appropriate disinfectant (Rose, Huffman, and Gennaccaro 2002). Ozone is more effective in inactivating *Cryptosporidium* oocysts than chlorine (Rose, Huffman, and Gennaccaro 2002; King and Monis 2007).

Contamination of water supplies and subsequent outbreaks of cryptosporidiosis have been linked to heavy rainfall events (Semenza and Nichols 2007; Aksoy et al. 2007; Hoek et al. 2008; Smith et al. 2006), as the concentration of *Cryptosporidium* oocysts in river water increases significantly during rainfall events. Thus, heavy precipitation can result in the persistence of oocysts in the water distribution system and the contamination of drinking water reservoirs from springs and lakes. A rise in precipitation is predicted to lead to an increase in cryptosporidiosis, although the strength of the relationship varies with the kind of climate category (Jagai et al. 2009). As noted, dry weather conditions preceding a heavy rain event have also been associated with drinking water outbreaks (Nichols et al. 2009).

CLINICAL CORRELATES 4.2 *CRYPTOSPORIDIUM*

Cryptosporidium is a ubiquitous and tenacious organism that is highly resistant to conventional means of disinfection (chlorination and filtration) owing to its small size (4–6 micrometers) and cystic structure (Rose, Huffman, and Gennaccaro 2002). Despite even stringent standards for water turbidity in wastewater treatment facilities, outbreaks still frequently occur (Goldstein et al. 1996).

In developing countries *Cryptosporidium* accounts for 6.1 percent of cases of diarrhea in HIV-negative patients and 24 percent of cases in HIV-positive patients, while in developed countries, it causes 2.1 percent and 13.8 percent of illnesses, respectively (Adal, Sterling, and Guerrant 1995).

In the immunocompromised population, it can often be a fatal disease (Dillingham, Lima, and Guerrant 2002). Even when not fatal, infection may cause dire yet subtle complications. Among children living in impoverished areas, infection has been shown to lead to impaired weight gain in the month following symptomatic and even asymptomatic infection, which occurs without a subsequent catch-up growth period (Checkley et al. 1997). Among patients with chronic diseases, infection has been observed to interfere with the absorption and therapeutic levels of antiretroviral and antituberculous drugs (Dillingham, Lima, and Guerrant 2002), which can affect the transmission of these highly communicable diseases.

Cryptosporidium **is a common climate-sensitive disease that health care providers must be aware of in order to prevent complications among vulnerable patients.**

Norovirus

Noroviruses cause acute gastroenteritis in humans. Symptoms include projectile vomiting, watery nonbloody diarrhea with abdominal cramps, nausea, myalgia, malaise, and headaches, occasionally also with low-grade fever. Noroviruses are ubiquitous and highly resistant in the environment. They can survive for long periods on different surfaces, at temperatures below 0°C and up to 60°C and in fluids with up to 10 parts per million (ppm) chlorine. In surface waters, an average *Norovirus* genome load of 10^4 to 10^6 genomic equivalents per liter can be found (Pusch et al. 2005). In many surface waters, *Norovirus* can be detected during all seasons (Pusch et al. 2005; Hörman et al. 2004; Gerba and Albert 2007). In Finland, *Norovirus* survived for four months during a period of low temperatures and ice-covered surface waters. In this case, an originally foodborne *Norovirus* strain caused a second waterborne outbreak 70 kilometers downstream (Kukkula et al. 1999). Transmission during outbreaks is complex. Often an initial food-borne or waterborne transmission is followed by secondary person-to-person transmission. Waterborne *Norovirus* outbreaks are less common, but well investigated and are often caused by sewage contamination of wells and groundwater or recreational water (Carrique-Mas et al. 2003; Nygard et al. 2003). Cross-contamination during the repair of public water pipelines (Merbecks et al. 2004) or back-siphonage within household installations also occurs. Outbreaks linked to private water suppliers occur more often and have a much higher overall incidence rate than outbreaks linked to public water supplies (Smith et al. 2006; Blackburn et al. 2004). If public water supplies are contaminated, they cause higher infection rates because higher numbers of people use these supplies (Hui 2006). Food-borne norovirus outbreaks have been linked to climate and weather events;

for example, heavy rainfall and floods may lead to wastewater overflow, which can contaminate shellfish farming sites. Floodwater has been associated with a *Norovirus* outbreak in Austria (Schmid et al. 2005). The magnitude of rainfall has also been related to viral contamination of the marine environment with peaks in diarrhea incidence (Miossec et al. 2000). The predicted increase of heavy rainfall events under climate change scenarios could lead to an increase in *norovirus* infections because floods are known to be linked to *norovirus* outbreaks.

Vibrio (Noncholera)

Bacteria of the genus *Vibrio* include several species, the most important being *V. cholerae*, which causes cholera. *V. vulnificus* and *V. parahaemolyticus* are other clinically important species that, unlike *V. cholerae*, are endemic in Europe and the United States and can infect open wounds that can necrotise and cause septicemia in individuals bathing in marine waters. Vibrios are halophytic organisms known to have their natural habitat in the warm waters of coastal areas (Lipp, Huq, and Colwell 2002); their growth is mainly dependent on temperature and salinity (Morris and Kris 2008). Due to higher temperatures, the bacteria reach their highest concentrations in summer and early autumn (Lipp, Huq, and Colwell 2002); if the environmental conditions are unfavorable for growth and multiplication, *Vibrio* enter a dormant phase.

The occurrence of *V. vulnificus* and *V. parahaemolyticus* in the marine environment is clearly associated with the growth of zooplankton, shellfish, and fish. Relatively higher *Vibrio* concentrations are observed in zooplankton than in the surrounding water column (Lipp, Huq, and Colwell 2002). In Spain, *Vibrio* is frequently isolated during red tides (Lipp, Huq, and Colwell 2002). An increase in water temperature promotes the growth of *Vibrio*, which become particularly concentrated in shellfish. The largest known outbreak of illness caused by *V. parahaemolyticus* occurred in Alaska in 2004 (McLaughlin et al. 2005). Passengers on a cruise ship ate raw local Alaskan oysters and developed diarrhea. This outbreak demonstrated a change in the spatial distribution of *Vibrios* and the correlation between *Vibrio* growth and high temperatures. Rising ocean water temperatures allowed the spread of subtropical *Vibrio* to the north. The northernmost documented oyster source contaminated with *V. parahaemolyticus* was immediately extended by 1,000 kilometers (McLaughlin et al. 2005).

In Israel, a high number of *V. vulnificus* wound infections and bacteremia were noted during the summer months of 1996, which were the hottest ever recorded in Israel in the previous forty years (Paz et al. 2007). Infections were significantly correlated with high temperatures during the preceding weeks. Paz et al. (2007) noted that in hot climates, the minimum temperature is the most important factor contributing to the growth of *Vibrio*. During daytime, temperature is always higher than 15°C, so the growth of *Vibrios* is unlimited. Minimum temperatures occur at night, and if they drop below 15°C, the growth of *Vibrios* will be interrupted.

In the Baltic Sea, *V. vulnificus* infections occur during hot summer months and augment with water temperatures above 20°C (Baker-Austin et al. 2012). The Baltic Sea has experienced an unprecedented rate of warming over the past three decades with recent peak temperatures never before documented since the inception of instrumental measurements in this region. Simultaneously, northern Europe witnessed an unexpected emergence of *Vibrio* infections with a clear link between elevated sea surface temperatures during extended summer seasons (Dalsgaard et al. 1996; Ruppert et al. 2004; Lukinmaa et al. 2006; Andersson and Ekdahl 2006; Frank et al. 2006). These open wound infections from recreational water use can necrotize and cause septicemia; in immunocompromised individuals, these infections can be fatal (Lukinmaa et al. 2006; Andersson and Ekdahl 2006; Frank et al. 2006). There is strong empirical evidence that anthropogenic climate change drives the emergence of *Vibrio* infections in this region of the world (Baker-Austin et al. 2012).

Other Infectious Diseases

Listeriosis is a serious infection caused by food or drinking water contaminated with the bacterium *Listeria*. About three to seventy days (average three weeks) after ingestion, the infected person suffers from fever, muscle aches, and sometimes gastrointestinal symptoms such as nausea or diarrhea. The only relevant human pathogenic species is *L. monocytogenes,* which is found in soil, surface water, plants, animals, and food. Under optimal conditions, the bacteria multiply at temperatures ranging from −0.4°C to +45°C and are considered a psychrophilic bacterium capable of multiplying in a refrigerator at +4°C (Greifenhagen and Noland 2003). However, growth rates increase at elevated temperatures. During heat waves, a breakdown of the cold chain for (processed) food could not only propagate the (re-) growth of *Listeria* but also of other pathogens such as *C. perfringens* and *S. aureus.*

Another health concern is the free-living amoeba *Naegleria fowleri* that can cause primary amebic meningoencephalitis and death. It is often found in warm freshwater environments such as pools, hot springs, lakes, natural mineral water, and resort spas (Heggie 2010). During an unusually hot summer month in 2010, an individual was infected by this amoeba and subsequently died after local freshwater exposures at much higher latitude than previously described (Kemble et al. 2012). It is possible that hot weather conditions due to climate variability and long-term climate change could affect the distribution and frequency of primary amebic meningoencephalitis. Algal blooms might become more prevalent in recreational waters under climate change scenarios. Yet there is not much evidence that organisms that bloom in coastal waters such as *Aeromonas hydrophila* have been associated with human disease.

Community-acquired pneumonia caused by *Legionella pneumophila* has been associated with air conditioners and water systems in buildings, such as water taps, showerheads, and other sources of aerosol. Wet periods of elevated humidity and temperature have been linked to Legionnaires' disease in several locations (Fisman et al. 2005; Ricketts et al. 2009). Climate change projects a higher frequency, intensity, and duration of heat waves. During periods of excessive heat, the temperature of water in buildings might increase as well as air-conditioner use. Whether this will lead to growth of *L. pneumophila* and pose a threat to the health of the public has not been ruled out yet.

Vector-borne diseases that are transmitted by insect vectors are also water-related diseases, since the insects complete part of their life cycle in water. These insects include mosquitoes, black flies, and a number of biting midget species that transmit diseases such as dengue, West Nile fever, malaria, Rift Valley fever, or river blindness. The arthropod vectors are subjected to abiotic conditions such as increased temperature, which influences vector competence, boosts mosquito reproduction rates, prolongs their breeding season, and accelerates virus replication within vectors. Moreover, precipitation patterns, floods, and droughts are also important determinants of these diseases. The association of these diseases with climate change is covered in chapter 2 and has been discussed extensively elsewhere (Semenza and Menne 2009).

CLINICAL CORRELATES 4.3 HOW SAFE IS OUR WATER SUPPLY?

In 2012, the World Health Organization announced attainment of the Millennium Development Goal (MDG) of reducing the number of individuals without "sustainable access to safe drinking water" by half. One major information gap that remains is the quality of the water. Even in the best of public water treatment scenarios, outbreaks of water-related disease still occur (MacKenzie et al. 1994). In a recent study conducted by UNICEF and USAID, households were questioned about their drinking water access. As a proxy for "sustainable access to safe drinking water," individuals were asked if they had "use of an improved water source," where "improved" was generalized to imply only a mechanism of handling water that aimed to decrease the likelihood that it would cause disease or infection (UNICEF and World Health Organization 2012). Since there is no agreed definition of *safe* and no widely used and inexpensive means of testing drinking water for pathogens, it is difficult to predict if attainment of this MDG will result in a decrease in the global burden of gastrointestinal disease. In addition, we are at this point unable to predict with regional certainty the effects of climate change on local water access. Medical personnel will likely be at the forefront of monitoring this impact.

Access to safe water is a difficult milestone to define, achieve, and assess. It is requisite to achieve modern health standards and may be threatened by changing climates.

Adaptation Strategies

Even in the absence of conclusive evidence, public health practitioners are obliged to address credible risks from climate change through adaptation strategies (Semenza 2013). Vulnerability, impact, and adaptation assessment can help prepare society for changes in the hydrological cycle (European Centre for Disease Prevention and Control 2010; Semenza, Suk, et al. 2012). The European Centre for Disease Prevention and Control (2012) has developed a decision-making tool for public health practitioners to help assess threats of climate change-associated waterborne diseases (figures 4.5 and 4.6) (European Centre for Disease Prevention and Control 2012). It is a software tool for quantitative microbial risk assessments under different climate change scenarios (Schijven et al. 2013). It is designed to assist decision makers in risk analysis in order to prioritize different intervention options and allocate funds accordingly. Twenty-two modules break down each step of the fate and behavior of selected microorganism during their transmission from environmental sources to humans. The exposure pathways include drinking water, bathing water, oysters, egg (products) or chicken filets (figure 4.5). The tool is built for use by default values from the literature or under user settings with local data. Based on these computations, a specific risk can be quantified, and mitigating steps can be taken. For example, drinking water quality can be improved by upgrading the water treatment and distribution systems (Semenza et al. 1998). In England and Wales, *Cryptosporidium* contamination was addressed by improvements in the treatment plants such as filtration of previously unfiltered water and by adoption of drinking water regulations (Semenza and Nichols 2007). These measures had a profound impact on spring peaks of *Cryptosporidium*, traditionally associated with heavy rain events (figure 4.7).

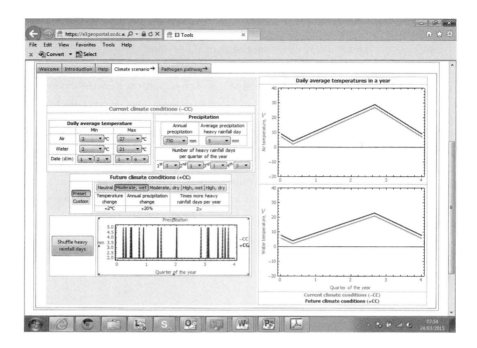

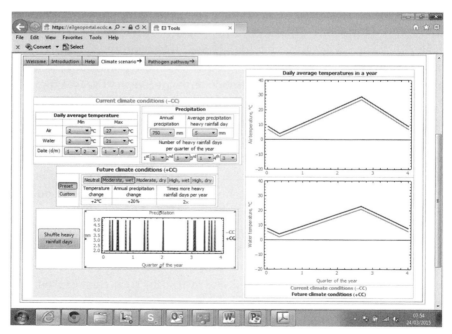

Figure 4.5   Screenshots of the Pages of the Climate Scenarios of the Climate Change Modules for Quantitative Microbial Risk Assessment Tool

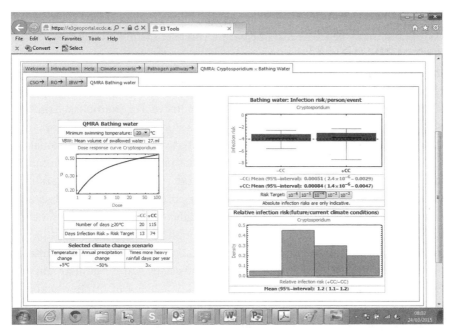

Figure 4.6 Screenshots of the Pages of the Infection Risk from *Cryptosporidium* Exposure from Bathing Water from the Climate Change Modules for Quantitative Microbial Risk Assessment Tool

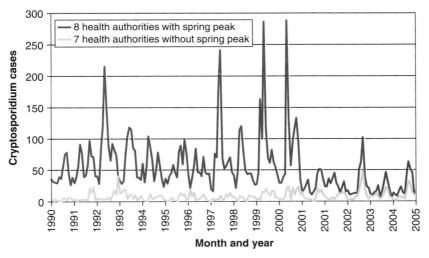

Figure 4.7 *Cryptosporidium* Cases in Two Groups of Health Authorities in Northwest England, 1990–2005
Source: Adapted from Semenza and Nichols (2007).

Other adaptation strategies include augmenting sewer system storage capacity to minimize wet weather discharges (David and Matos 2005). Storage and advanced physical chemical treatment of stormwater could significantly reduce overflow volumes. Even though settling in sedimentation tanks would reduce the overflow, microorganism concentrations could nevertheless remain high, which could potentially be treated online with ultraviolet disinfection (Soyeux et al. 2007). Holding tanks for storm water, water diversion, levees, reservoirs, dikes, or mechanical barriers are all measures that need to be reconsidered under the changing circumstances of climate change. They need to be judiciously applied since many of these measures are mutually exclusive. For example, a drinking water reservoir cannot simultaneously act as a storm water holding tank; they are supposed to be either full or empty, respectively, in order to be functional.

The challenges outlined in this chapter call for a number of adaptation interventions such as higher water quality standards, prudent use of desalination, gray water reclamation, but also greater public outreach and education campaigns. Moreover, monitoring metrological conditions and epidemiological intelligence will increasingly be part of public health practice aiming to protect the health of the public (Semenza 2013). Climate change has impacts on the hydrological cycle, and waterborne diseases call for adjustments to existing surveillance practices (Lindgren et al. 2012). For example, enhanced collaboration between surveillance for human cases of *Vibrio* and laboratory monitoring of bivalve shellfish could prevent *Vibrio* outbreaks due to seafood consumption. Climate change adaptation strategies should be designed to improve public health preparedness and facilitate the response to emerging threats from waterborne diseases and thereby help contain human and economic costs. Society will have to accept these adaptive strategies to mitigate the negative consequences of the anticipated extremes of the hydrological cycle.

Conclusion

The effects of climate change on the hydrosphere have important implications for water availability, quality, and supply. Waterborne and vector-borne pathogens are also closely correlated to the changing dynamics of water. Public health interventions are essential for both mitigation and monitoring of the effects of climate change and should guide intervention in these areas.

DISCUSSION QUESTIONS

1. Describe the differential impact of climatic events on waterborne pathogens, including bacteria, parasites, and viruses.

2. Discuss public health interventions to address the threats of climate change from waterborne pathogens.

3. Describe extremes of the hydrologic cycle and associated disease outbreaks.

KEY TERMS

Anthropogenic activity: Any human activity, commonly used to refer to activities that result in the production of greenhouse gases.

Atmosphere: The gaseous envelope surrounding the Earth.

Biosphere: The aggregate of the Earth's ecosystems.

Cryosphere: The part of the Earth's surface where water exists as ice.

Environmental exposure pathways: The physical means by which pathogens gain access to susceptible hosts.

Hydrological cycle: Describes the continuous movement of water on, above, and below the surface of the Earth.

Hydrosphere: The waters of the Earth's surface, referred to collectively.

Lithosphere: The crust and upper mantle of the Earth.

Storm runoff: Precipitation that results from a storm or from snow and/or ice melt and overwhelms both natural and man-made absorptive capacities. Storm runoff often carries debris and pollutants and results in contamination of waterways, and any physical space it contacts.

References

Abulreesh, H. H., T. A. Paget, and R. Goulder. 2006. "Campylobacter in Waterfowl and Aquatic Environments: Incidence and Methods of Detection." *Environmental Science and Technology* 40:7122–31.

Ackerman, D., and S. Weisberg. 2003. "Relationship between Rainfall and Beach Bacterial Concentrations on Santa Monica Bay Beaches." *Journal of Water and Health* 1(2):85–89.

Aksoy, U., C. Akisu, S. Sahin, S. Usluca, G. Yalcin, F. Kuralay, et al. 2007. "First Reported Waterborne Outbreak of Cryptosporidiosis with Cyclospora Co-Infection in Turkey." *Eurosurveillance* 12(7).

Andersson, Y., and K. Ekdahl. 2006. "Wound Infections due to *Vibrio cholerae* in Sweden after Swimming in the Baltic Sea." *Eurosurveillance* 8:E060803.2.

Angulo, F. J., S. Tippen, D. J. Sharp, B. J. Payne, C. Collier, J. E. Hill, T. J. Barrett, et al. 1997. "A Community Waterborne Outbreak of Salmonellosis and the Effectiveness of a Boil Water Order." *American Journal of Public Health* 87:580–84.

Baker-Austin, C., J. Trinanes, N. Taylor, R. Hartnell, A. Siitonen, and J. Martinez-Urtaza. 2012. "Emerging Vibrio Risk at High Latitudes in Response to Ocean Warming." *Nature Climate Change* 13:73–77.

Bi, P., A. Cameron, Y. Zhang, and K. Parton. 2008. "Weather and Notified Campylobacter Infections in Temperate and Sub-Tropical Regions of Australia: An Ecological Study." *Journal of Infection* 57:317–23.

Blackburn, B. G., G. F. Craun, J. S. Yoder, V. Hill, R. L. Calderon, N. Chen, et al. 2004. "Surveillance for Waterborne-Disease Outbreaks Associated with Drinking Water—United States, 2001–2002." *MMWR Surveillance Summary* 53(8):23–45.

Blaser, M. J. 2000. "*Campylobacter jejuni* and Related Species." In *Principles and Practices of Infectious Diseases*, 5th ed., edited by G. L. Mandell, J. E. Bennett, and R. Dolin, 2276–85. Philadelphia: Churchill Livingston.

Boxall, A. B., A. Hardy, S. Beulke, T. Boucard, L. Burgin, P. D. Falloon, P. M. Haygarth et al. 2009. "Impacts of Climate Change on Indirect Human Exposure to Pathogens and Chemicals from Agriculture." *Environmental Health Perspectives* 117:508–14.

Brinks, M., R. Dwight, N. Osgood, G. Sharavanakumar, D. Turbow, M. El-Gohary, J. S. Caplan, and J. C. Semenza. 2008. "Health Risk of Bathing in Southern California Coastal Waters." *Archives of Environmental and Occupational Health* 63:123–35.

Brownell, M., V. Harwood, R. Kurz, S. McQuaig, J. Lukasik, and T. Scott. 2007. "Confirmation of Putative Stormwater Impact on Water Quality at a Florida Beach by Microbial Source Tracking Methods and Structure of Indicator Organism Populations." *Water Research* 41:3747–57.

California Climate Adaptation Strategy. 2009. "A Report to the Governor of the State of California in Response to Executive Order S-13–2008."

Carrique-Mas, J., Y. Andersson, B. Petersen, K. O. Hedlund, N. Sjogren, and J. Giesecke. 2003. "A Norwalk-Like Virus Waterborne Community Outbreak in a Swedish Village during Peak Holiday Season." *Epidemiology and Infection* 131:737–44.

Carter, A. M., R. E. Pacha, G. W. Clark, and E. A. Williams. 1987. "Seasonal Occurrence of Campylobacter spp. in Surface Waters and Their Correlation with Standard Indicator Bacteria." *Applied Environmental Microbiology* 53:523–26.

Checkley, W., R. H. Gilman, L. D. Epstein, M. Suarez, J. F. Diaz, L. Cabrera, R. E. Black, and C. R. Sterling. 1997. "Asymptomatic and Symptomatic Cryptosporidiosis: Their Acute Effect on Weight Gain in Peruvian Children." *American Journal of Epidemiology* 145:156–63.

Craig, D., H. Fallowfield, and N. Cromar. 2003. "Effectiveness of Guideline Faecal Indicator Organism Values in Estimation of Exposure Risk at Recreational Coastal Sites." *Water Science and Technology* 47:191–98.

Crowther, J., D. Kay, and M. Wyer. 2001. "Relationships between Microbial Water Quality and Environmental Conditions in Coastal Recreational Waters: The Fylde Coast, UK." *Water Research* 35:4029–38.

Crum-Cianflone, N. F. 2008. "Salmonellosis and the GI Tract: More Than Just Peanut Butter." *Current Gastroenterology Reports* 10:424–31.

Curriero, F., J. Patz, J. Rose, and S. Lele. 2001. "The Association between Extreme Precipitation and Waterborne Disease Outbreaks in the United States, 1948–1994." *American Journal of Public Health* 91:1194–99.

D'Souza, R., N. Becker, G. Hall, and K. Moodie. 2004. "Does Ambient Temperature Affect Foodborne Disease?" *Epidemiology* 151:86–92.

Dalsgaard, A., N. Frimodt-Møller, B. Bruun, L. Høi, and J. L. Larsen. 1996. "Clinical Manifestations and Molecular Epidemiology of *Vibrio vulnificus* Infections in Denmark." *European Journal of Clinical Microbiology and Infectious Diseases* 15:227–32.

Daniels, N. A., B. Ray, A. Easton, N. Marano, E. Kahn, A.L.I. McShan, L. Del Rosario, et al. 2000. "Emergence of a New *Vibrio parahaemolyticus* Serotype in Raw Oysters: A Prevention Quandary." *Journal of the American Medical Association* 284:1541–45.

David, L. M., and J. S. Matos. 2005. "Combined Sewer Overflow Emissions to Bathing Waters in Portugal: How to Reduce in Densely Urbanised Areas?" *Water Science and Technology* 52:183–90.

Dillingham, R. A., A. A. Lima, and R. L. Guerrant. 2002. "Cryptosporidiosis: Epidemiology and Impact." *Microbes and Infection* 4:1059–66.

Doorduyn, Y., W. E. Van Den Brandhof, Y. T. Van Duynhoven, B. J. Breukink, J. A. Wagenaar, and W. Van Pelt. 2010. "Risk Factors for Indigenous *Campylobacter jejuni* and *Campylobacter coli* Infections in the Netherlands: A Case-Control Study." *Epidemiology and Infection* 138(10):1391–1404.

Dwight, R. H., D. B. Baker, J. C. Semenza, and B. H. Olson. 2004. "Health Effects Associated with Recreational Coastal Water Use in Urban vs. Rural California." *American Journal of Public Health* 94:565–67.

Dwight, R., J. Semenza, D. Baker, and B. Olson. 2002. "Association of Urban Runoff with Coastal Water Quality in Orange County, California." *Water and Environmental Research* 74:82–99.

Ebi, K. 2006. "Floods and Human Health." In *Climate Change and Adaptation Strategies for Human Health*, edited by B. Menne and K. Ebi, 99–127. Darmstadt: Steinkopff.

European Centre for Disease Prevention and Control. 2010. *Climate Change and Communicable Diseases in the EU Member Countries: Handbook for National Vulnerability, Impact and Adaptation Assessments.* Stockholm: ECDC.

European Centre for Disease Prevention and Control. 2012. *Climate Change and Food and Water-Borne Diseases: A Tool for Quantitative Microbial Risk Assessment.* Stockholm: ECDC.

European Food Safety Authority. 2010. *The Community Summary Report on Trends and Sources of Zoonoses, Zoonotic Agents and Food-Borne Outbreaks in the European Union in 2008.* Parma, Italy: European Food Safety Authority.

Fisman, D. N., S. Lim, G. A. Wellenius, C. Johnson, P. Britz, M. Gaskins, J. Maher, et al. 2005. "It's Not the Heat, It's the Humidity: Wet Weather Increases Legionellosis Risk in the Greater Philadelphia Metropolitan Area." *Journal of Infectious Diseases* 192:2066–73.

Fleury, M., D. F. Charron, J. D. Holt, O. B. Allen, and A. R. Maarouf. 2006. "A Time Series Analysis of the Relationship of Ambient Temperature and Common

Bacterial Enteric Infections in Two Canadian Provinces." *International Journal of Biometeorology* 50:385–91.

Frank, C., M. Littman, K. Alpers, and J. Hallauer. 2006. "*Vibrio vulnificus* Wound Infections after Contact with the Baltic Sea, Germany." *Eurosurveillance* 11(8):E060817.1.

Frankignoul, C., and E. Kestenare. 2005. "Observed Atlantic SST Anomaly Impact on the NAO: An Update." *Journal of Climate* 18(19):4089–94.

Fun, B., L. Unicomb, Z. Rahim, N. Banu, G. Podder, J. Clemens, F. P. Van Loon, et al. 1991. "Rotavirus-Associated Diarrhea in Rural Bangladesh: Two-Year Study of Incidence and Serotype Distribution." *Journal of Clinical Microbiology* 29:1359–63.

Gaffield, S., R. Goo, L. Richards, and R. Jackson. 2003. "Public Health Effects of Inadequately Managed Stormwater Runoff." *American Journal of Public Health* 93:1527–33.

Gantois, I., R. Ducatelle, F. Pasmans, F. Haesebrouck, R. Gast, T. J. Humphrey, and F. Van Immerseel. 2009. "Mechanisms of Egg Contamination by *Salmonella enteritidis*." *FEMS Microbiology Reviews* 33:718–38.

Gerba, C. P., and B. Albert. 2007. "Virus Occurrence and Survival in the Environmental Waters." In *Perspectives in Medical Virology*, edited by A. Bosch, 91–108. Dordrecht: Elsevier.

Goldstein, S. T., D. D. Juranek, O. Ravenholt, A. W. Hightower, D. G. Martin, J. L. Mesnik, S. D. Griffiths, A. J. Bryant, R. R. Reich, and B. L. Herwaldt. 1996. "Cryptosporidiosis: An Outbreak Associated with Drinking Water Despite State-of-the-Art Water Treatment." *Annals of Internal Medicine* 124:459–68.

Gray, N. F. 1994. *Drinking Water Quality: Problems and Solutions.* Chichester, UK: Wiley.

Greifenhagen, S., and T. L. Noland. 2003. *Forest Research Information Paper: A Synopsis of Known and Potential Diseases and Parasites Associated with Climate Change.* Sault Ste. Marie: Ontario Ministry of Natural Resources, Ontario Forest Research Institute.

Griffith, D. C., L. A. Kelly-Hope, and M. A. Miller. 2006. "Review of Reported Cholera Outbreaks Worldwide, 1995–2005." *American Journal of Tropical Medicine and Hygiene* 75:973–77.

Haile, R., J. Witte, M. Gold, R. Cressey, C. McGee, R. Millikan, A. Glasser, et al. 1999. "The Health Effects of Swimming in Ocean Water Contaminated by Storm Drain Runoff." *Epidemiology* 10:355–63.

Haramoto, E., H. Katayama, K. Oguma, Y. Koibuchi, H. Furumai, and S. Ohgaki. 2006. "Effects of Rainfall on the Occurrence of Human Adenoviruses, Total Coliforms, and *Escherichia coli* in Seawater." *Water and Science Technology* 54:225–30.

He, L., and Z. He. 2008. "Water Quality Prediction of Marine Recreational Beaches Receiving Watershed Baseflow and Stormwater Runoff in Southern California, USA." *Water Research* 42:2563–73.

Hearnden, M., C. Skelly, R. Eyles, and P. Weinstein. 2003. "The Regionality of Campylobacteriosis Seasonality in New Zealand." *International Journal of Environmental Health Research* 13:337–48.

Heggie, T. 2010. "Swimming with Death: *Naegleria fowleri* Infections in Recreational Waters." *Travel Medicine and Infectious Disease* 8:201–206.

Heijs, J., D. Wilkinson, and E. Couriel. 2002. "Project CARE: Reducing Wet Weather Overflows to Improve Beach Water Quality: Council Action in Respect of the Environment." *Water and Science Technology* 46(6–7):35–46.

Heller, L., E. Colosimo, and C. Antunes. 2003. "Environmental Sanitation Conditions and Health Impact: A Case-Control Study." *Revista da Sociedade Brasileira de Medicina Tropical* 36(1):41–50.

Hoek M. R., I. Oliver, M. Barlow, L. Heard, R. Chalmers, and S. Paynter. 2008. "Outbreak of *Cryptosporidium parvum* among Children after a School Excursion to an Adventure Farm, South West England." *Journal of Water and Health* 6:333–38.

Hörman, A., R. Rimhanen-Finne, L. Maunula, C. H. von Bonsdorff, N. Torvela, A. Heikinheimo, and M. L. Hänninen. 2004. "Campylobacter spp., *Giardia* spp., *Cryptosporidium* spp., Noroviruses, and Indicator Organisms in Surface Water in Southwestern Finland, 2000–2001." *Applied and Environmental Microbiology* 70(1):87–95.

Hsu, B., and Y. Huang. 2008. "Intensive Water Quality Monitoring in a Taiwan Bathing Beach." *Environmental Monitoring and Assessment* 144:463–68.

Hui, K. E. 2006. "Reasons for the Increase in Emerging and Re-Emerging Viral Infectious Diseases." *Microbes and Infection* 8:905–16.

Intergovernmental Panel on Climate Change. 2007. *Climate Change 2007: The Physical Science Basis. Contribution of Working Group I to the Fourth Assessment Report of the Intergovernmental Panel on Climate Change.* Cambridge: Cambridge University Press.

Jagai, J. S., D. A. Castronovo, J. Monchak, and E. N. Naumova. 2009. "Seasonality of Cryptosporidiosis: A Meta-Analysis Approach." *Environmental Research* 109:465–78.

Jean, J., H. Guo, S. Chen, C. Liu, W. Chang, Y. Yang, and M. C. Huang. 2006. "The Association between Rainfall Rate and Occurrence of an Enterovirus Epidemic due to a Contaminated Well." *Journal of Applied Microbiology* 101:1224–31.

Jones, K. 2001. "Campylobacters in Water, Sewage and the Environment." *Symp Ser Soc Appl Microbiol* 30:68S–79S.

Katsumata, T., D. Hosea, E. B. Wasito, S. Kohno, K. Hara, P. Soeparto, and I. G. Ranuh. 1998. "Cryptosporidiosis in Indonesia: A Hospital-Based Study and a Community-Based Survey." *American Journal of Tropical Medicine and Hygiene* 59:628–32.

Kemble, S., R. Lynfield, A. DeVries, D. Drehner, W. Pomputius, M. Beach, G. S. Visvesvara, A. J. da Silva, et al. 2012. "Fatal *Naegleria fowleri* Infection Acquired in Minnesota: Possible Expanded Range of a Deadly Thermophilic Organism." *Clinical Infectious Diseases* 54:805–809.

King, B. J., and P. T. Monis. 2007. "Critical Processes Affecting Cryptosporidium Oocyst Survival in the Environment." *Parasitology* 134:309–23.

Kovats, R., S. Edwards, D. Charron, J. Cowden, R. D'Souza, K. L. Ebi, C. Gauci, et al. 2005. "Climate Variability and Campylobacter Infection: An International Study." *International Journal of Biometeorology* 49:207–14.

Kovats, R., S. Edwards, S. Hajat, B. Armstrong, K. Ebi, and B. Menne. 2004. "The Effect of Temperature on Food Poisoning: A Time-Series Analysis of Salmonellosis in Ten European Countries." *Epidemiology and Infection* 132:443–53.

Kovats, S., B. Menne, A. J. McMichael, R. Bertollini, and C. Soskolne. 2000. *Climate Change and Stratospheric Ozone Depletion: Early Effects on Our Health in Europe.* Geneva: World Health Organization.

Kriz, B., C. Benes, J. Castkova, and J. Held, eds. 1998. *Monitoring of the Epidemiological Situation in Flooded Areas of the Czech Republic in Year 1997.* Prodebrady, Czech Republic: National Institute of Public Health.

Kukkula, M., L. Maunula, E. Silvennoinen, and C. H. von Bonsdorff. 1999. "Outbreak of Viral Gastroenteritis due to Drinking Water Contaminated by Norwalk-Like Viruses." *Journal of Infectious Diseases* 180:1771–76.

Kunii, O., S. Nakamura, R. Abdur, and S. Waka. 2002. "The Impact on Health and Risk Factors of the Diarrhoea Epidemics in the 1998 Bangladesh Floods." *Public Health* 116(2):68–74.

Lake, I. R., I. A. Gillespie, G. Bentham, G. L. Nichols, C. Lane, G. K. Adak, and E. J. Threlfall. 2009. "A Reevaluation of the Impact of Temperature and Climate Change on Foodborne Illness." *Epidemiology and Infection* 137:1538–47.

LeChevallier, M., W. Schulz, and R. Lee. 1991. "Bacterial Nutrients in Drinking Water." *Applied and Environmental Microbiology* 57:857–62.

Lee, C. S., J. H. Lee, and K. S. Kwon. 2008. "Outbreak of Hepatitis A in Korean military Personnel." *Japanese Journal of Infectious Diseases* 61:239–41.

Levitus, S., J. I. Antonov, T. P. Boyer, O. K. Baranova, H. E. Garcia, R. A. Locarnini, A. V. Mishonov, et al. 2012. "World Ocean Heat Content and Thermosteric Sea Level Change (0–2000 m), 1955–2010." *Geophysical Research Letters* 39(10). doi:10.1029/2012GL051106

Lindgren, E., Y. Andersson, J. E. Suk, B. Sudre, and J. C. Semenza. 2012. "Monitoring EU Emerging Infectious Disease Risk due to Climate Change." *Science* 336:418–19.

Lipp, E. K., A. Huq, and R. R. Colwell. 2002. "Effects of Global Climate on Infectious Disease: The Cholera Model." Clin Microbiol Rev. 15:757–70.

Lukinmaa, S., K. Mattila, V. Lehtinen, M. Hakkinen, M. Koskela, and A. Siitonen. 2006. "Territorial Waters of the Baltic Sea as a Source of Infections Caused by *Vibrio cholerae* Non-O1, Non-O139: Report of 3 Hospitalized Cases." *Diagnostic Microbiology and Infectious Disease* 54(1):1–6.

MacKenzie, W. R., N. J. Hoxie, M. E. Proctor, S. Gradus, K. A. Blair, D. E. Peterson, J. J. Kazmierczak, et al. 1994. "A Massive Outbreak in Milwaukee of Cryptosporidium Infection Transmitted through the Public Water Supply." *New England Journal of Medicine* 331:161–67.

Mallin, M., K. Williams, E. Esham, and R. Lowe. 2000. "Effect of Human Development on Bacteriological Water Quality in Coastal Watersheds." *Ecological Applications* 10:1047.

Martinez-Urtaza, J., M. Saco, J. de Novoa, P. Perez-Pineiro, J. Peiteado, A. Lozano-Leon, and O. Garcio-Martin. 2004. "Influence of Environmental Factors and Human Activity on the Presence of Salmonella Serovars in a Marine Environment." *Applied and Environmental Microbiology* 70:2089–97.

McCarthy, D., V. Mitchell, A. Deletic, and C. Diaper. 2007. "*Escherichia coli* in Urban Stormwater: Explaining Their Variability." *Water and Science Technology* 56(11):27–34.

McLaughlin, J., A. DePaola, C. Bopp, K. Martinek, N. Napolilli, C. Allison, S. L. Murray, E. C. Thompson, M. M. Bird, and J. P. Middaugh. 2005. "Outbreak of *Vibrio parahaemolyticus* Gastroenteritis Associated with Alaskan Oysters." *New England Journal of Medicine* 353:1463–70.

Merbecks, S-S., D. Beier, A. Gruschwitz, L. Müller, and M. Partisch. 2004. "An Accumulation of Norovirus Illnesses as a Result of Contaminated Drinking Water" *RKI Epidemiologisches Bulletin* 36:301–302.

Miettinen, I., O. Zacheus, C. von Bonsdorff, and T. Vartiainen. 2001. Waterborne Epidemics in Finland in 1998–1999." *Water and Science Technology* 43(12):67–71.

Miossec, L., F. Le Guyader, L. Haugarreau, and M. Pommepuy. 2000. "Magnitude of Rainfall on Viral Contamination of the Marine Environment during Gastroenteritis Epidemics in Human Coastal Population." *Revue d'épidémiologie et de santé publique* 48(2):S62–S71.

Mondal, N., R., Biswas, and A. Manna. 2001. "Risk Factors of Diarrhoea among Flood Victims: A Controlled Epidemiological Study." *Indian Journal of Public Health* 45:122–27.

Morris, J., and H. Kris. 2008. *Cholera and Other Vibrios.* Orlando, FL: Academic Press.

Murphy, C., C. Carroll, and K. N. Jordan. 2006. "Environmental Survival Mechanisms of the Foodborne Pathogen *Campylobacter jejuni.*" *Journal of Applied Microbiology* 100(4):623–32.

Naumova, E. N., J. S., Jagai B., Matyas A. DeMaria Jr., I. B. MacNeill, and J. K. Griffiths. 2007. "Seasonality in Six Enterically Transmitted Diseases and Ambient Temperature." *Epidemiology and Infection* 135:281–92.

Nichols, G. 2010. "Mapping out the Causes of Infectious Diseases: A Case Study on the Multiple Factors Involved in *Salmonella enteritidis* Infections." In *Environmental Medicine,* edited by R. L. Maynard, J. G. Ayres, G. L. Nichols, and R. M. Harrison, 102–105. London: Hodder.

Nichols, G., C. Lane, N. Asgari, N. Q. Verlander, and A. Charlett. 2009. "Rainfall and Outbreaks of Drinking Water Related Disease in England and Wales." *Journal of Water and Health* 7(1):1–8.

Noble, R., S. Weisberg, M. Leecaster, C. McGee, J. Dorsey, P. Vainik, and V. Orozco-Borbón. 2003. "Storm Effects on Regional Beach Water Quality along the Southern California Shoreline." *Journal of Water and Health* 1(1):23–31.

Nygard, K., M. Torven, C. Ancker, S. B. Knauth, K. O. Hedlund, J. Giesecke, Y. Andersson, and L. Svensson. 2003. "Emerging Genotype (GGIIb) of Norovirus in Drinking Water, Sweden." *Emerging Infectious Diseases* 9:1548–52.

Obiri-Danso, K., and K. Jones. 1999. "The Effect of a New Sewage Treatment Plant on Faecal Indicator Numbers, Campylobacters and Bathing Water Compliance in Morecambe Bay." *Journal of Applied Microbiology* 86(4): 603–14.

Orata, F. D., P. S. Keimv, and Y. Boucher. 2014. "The 2010 Cholera Outbreak in Haiti: How Science Solved a Controversy." *PLoS Pathogens* 10(4).

Palmer, S., P. Gully, J. White, A. Pearson, W. Suckling, D. Jones, J. C. Rawes, and J. L. Penner. 1983. "Waterborne Outbreak of Campylobacter Gastroenteritis." *Lancet* 1(8319):287–90.

Patrick, M., L. Christiansen, M. Waino, S. Ethelberg, H. Madsen, and H. Wegener. 2004. "Seven Effects of Climate on Incidence of *Campylobacter* spp. in Humans and Prevalence in Broiler Flocks in Denmark." *Applied and Environmental Microbiology* 0(12):7474–80.

Paz, S., N. Bisharat, E. Paz, O. Kidar, and D. Cohen. 2007. "Climate Change and the Emergence of *Vibrio vulnificus* Disease in Israel." *Environmental Research* 103:390–96.

Pebody, R., M. Ryan, and P. Wall. 1997. "Outbreaks of Campylobacter Infection: Rare Events for a Common Pathogen." *Communicable Disease Report* 7(3):R33–37.

Pusch, D., D. Y. Oh, S. Wolf, R. Dumke, U. Schroter-Bobsin, M. Höhne, I. Röske, and E. Schreier. 2005. "Detection of Enteric Viruses and Bacterial Indicators in German Environmental Waters." *Archives of Virology* 150:929–47.

Randa, M. A., M. F. Polz, and E. Lim. 2004. "Effects of Temperature and Salinity on Vibrio vulnificus Population Dynamics as Assessed by Quantitative PCR." *Applied and Environmental Microbiology* 70:5469–76.

Reacher, M., K. McKenzie, C. Lane, T. Nichols, I. Kedge, A. Iversen, P. Hepple, et al. 2004. "Health Impacts of Flooding in Lewes: A Comparison of Reported Gastrointestinal and Other Illness and Mental Health in Flooded and Non-Flooded Households." *Communicable Disease and Public Health* 7(7):39–46.

Richardson, H., G. Nichols, C. Lane, I. Lake, and P. Hunter. 2009. "Microbiological Surveillance of Private Water Supplies in England: The Impact of Environmental and Climate Factors on Water Quality." *Water Research* 43:2159–68.

Ricketts, K. D., A. Charlett, D. Gelb, C. Lane, J. V. Lee, and C. A. Joseph. 2009. "Weather Patterns and Legionnaires' Disease: A Meteorological Study." *Epidemiology and Infection* 137:1003–1012.

Rose, J. B., D. E. Huffman, and A. Gennaccaro. 2002. "Risk and Control of Waterborne Cryptosporidiosis." *FEMS Microbiology Reviews* 26(2):113–23.

Ruppert, J., B. Panzig, L. Guertler, P. Hinz, G. Schwesinger, S. Felix, and W. Friesecke. 2004. "Two Cases of Severe Sepsis due to *Vibrio vulnificus* Wound Infection Acquired in the Baltic Sea." *European Journal of Clinical Microbiology and Infectious Diseases* 23:912–95.

Ryan, E. T. 2011. "The Cholera Pandemic, Still with Us after Half a Century: Time to Rethink." *PLoS Neglected Tropical Diseases* 5(1).

Sarkar, U., S. Nascimento, R. Barbosa, R. Martins, H. Nuevo, I. Kalofonos, I. Grunstein, et al. 2002. "Population-Based Case-Control Investigation of Risk Factors for Leptospirosis during an Urban Epidemic." *American Journal of Tropical Medicine and Hygiene* 66:605–10.

Savill, M., J. Hudson, A. Ball, J. Klena, P. Scholes, R. Whyte, et al. 2001. "Enumeration of Campylobacter in New Zealand Recreational and Drinking Waters." *Journal of Applied Microbiology* 91(1):38–46.

Schiff, K., J. Morton, and S. Weisberg. 2003. "Retrospective Evaluation of Shoreline Water Quality along Santa Monica Bay Beaches." *Marine Environmental Research* 56:245–53.

Schijven J., and A. de Roda Husman. 2005. "Effect of Climate Changes on Waterborne Diseases in the Netherlands." *Water and Science Technology* 51(5):79–87.

Schijven, J., A. M. de Roda Husman, M. Bouwknegt, J. E. Suk, S. Rutjes, and J. C. Semenza. 2013. "Estimating Climate Change Vulnerabilities from Food and Waterborne Diseases." *Risk Analysis* 33:2154–67.

Schmid, D., I. Lederer, P. Much, and A.-M. Pichler. 2005. "Allerberger Outbreak of Norovirus Infection Associated with Contaminated Flood Water, Salzburg." *Eurosurveillance* 10(24):E050616.3.

Semenza, J. C. "Human Health Effects of Extreme Weather Events." In *The Praeger Handbook of Environmental Health*, edited by R. H. Friis, Volume 3, Chapter 20, 419–36.

Semenza, J. C. 2013. "Climate Change Adaptation to Infectious Diseases in Europe." In *Climate Change and Global Health*, edited by C. D. Butler, Chapter 23, 193–205. Wallingford, Oxfordshire: UK CABI.

Semenza, J. C., and B. Menne. 2009. "Climate Change and Infectious Diseases in Europe." *Lancet Infectious Diseases* 9:365–75.

Semenza J. C., C. Höser, S. Herbst, A. Rechenburg, J. Suk, T. Frechen, and T. Kistemann. 2012. "Knowledge Mapping for Climate Change and Food and Waterborne Diseases." *Critical Reviews in Environmental and Science Technology* 42:378–411.

Semenza, J. C., and G. Nichols. 2007. "Cryptosporidiosis Surveillance and Water-Borne Outbreaks in Europe." *Eurosurveillance* 12(5):E13–4.

Semenza, J. C., J. E. Suk, V. Estevez, K. L. Ebi, and E. Lindgren. 2012. "Mapping Climate Change Vulnerabilities to Infectious Diseases in Europe." *Environmental Health Perspectives* 120:385–92.

Semenza, J. C., J. S. Caplan, G. Buescher, T. Das, M. V. Brinks, and A. Gershunov. 2012. "Climate Change and Microbiological Water Quality at California Beaches." *Ecohealth* 9(3):293–97.

Semenza, J. C., L. Roberts, A. Henderson, J. Bogan, and C. H. Rubin. 1998. "Water Distribution System and Diarrheal Disease Transmission: A Case Study in Uzbekistan." *American Journal of Tropical Medicine and Hygiene* 59:941–46.

Semenza, J. C., S. Herbst, A. Rechenburg, J. E. Suk, C. Höser, C. Schreiber, and T. Kistemann. 2012. "Climate Change Impact Assessment of Food- and Waterborne Diseases." *Critical Reviews in Environmental and Science Technology* 42:857–90.

Senhorst, H., and J. Zwolsman. 2005. "Climate Change and Effects on Water Quality: A First Impression." *Water and Science Technology* 51(5):53–59.

Singh, R., S. Hales, N. de Wet, R. Raj, M. Hearnden, and P. Weinstein. 2001. "The Influence of Climate Variation and Change on Diarrheal Disease in the Pacific Islands." *Environmental Health Perspectives* 109:155–59.

Slifko, T. R., D. Friedman, J. B. Rose, and W. Jakubowski. 1997. "An In Vitro Method for detecting Infections Cryptosporidium Oocysts with Cell Culture." *Applied Environmental Microbiology* 63(9): 3669–75.

Smith, A., M. Reacher, W. Smerdon, G. K. Adak, G. Nichols, and R. M. Chalmers. 2006. "Outbreaks of Waterborne Infectious Intestinal Disease in England and Wales, 1992–2003." *Epidemiology and Infection* 11:1–9.

Soyeux, E., F. Blanchet, and B. Tisserand. 2007. "Stormwater Overflow Impacts on the Sanitary Quality of Bathing Waters." *Water and Science Technology* 56(11):43–50.

Stahl, K., H. Hisdal, J. Hannaford, L. M. Tallaksen, H.A.J. van Lanen, E. Sauquet, S. Demuth, M. Fendekova, and J. Jodár. 2010. "Streamflow Trends in Europe: Evidence from a Dataset of Near-Natural Catchments." *Hydrology and Earth System Sciences* 14(12):2367–82.

Stine, S. W., I. Song, C. Y. Choi, and C. P. Gerba. 2005. "Effect of Relative Humidity on Preharvest Survival of Bacterial and Viral Pathogens on the Surface of Cantaloupe, Lettuce, and Bell Peppers." *Journal of Food Protection* J68(7):1352–58.

Stott, R., E. May, E. Ramirez, and A. Warren. 2003. "Predation of Cryptosporidium Oocysts by Protozoa and Rotifers: Implications for Water Quality and Public Health." *Water and Science Technology* 47(3):77–83.

Sur, D., P. Dutta, G. Nair, and S. Bhattacharya. 2000. "Severe Cholera Outbreak following Floods in a Northern District of West Bengal." *Indian Journal of Medical Reseach* 112:178–82.

Trenberth, K. 1999. "Conceptual Framework for Changes of Extremes of the Hydrological Cycle with Climate Change." *Climate Change* 42:327–39.

UNICEF and World Health Organization. 2012. "Progress on Drinking Water and Sanitation: UNICEF/WHO Joint Monitoring Programme Update." UNICEF and World Health Organization.

van Middelkoop, A., J. van Wyk, H. Küstner, I. Windsor, C. Vinsen, B. Schoub, S. Johnson, and J. M. McAnerey. 1992. "Poliomyelitis Outbreak in Natal/KwaZulu, South Africa, 1987–1988. 1. Epidemiology." *Transactions of the Royal Society of Tropical Medicine and Hygiene* 86(1):80–82.

Vollaard, A., S. Ali, H. van Asten, S. Widjaja, L. Visser, C. Surjadi, and J. T. van Vissel. 2004. "Risk Factors for Typhoid and Paratyphoid Fever in Jakarta, Indonesia." *JAMA* 291(21):2607–15.

WHO, ed. 2011. Guidance on Water Supply and Sanitation in Extreme Weather Events. Copenhagen, Denmark: WHO.

Winfield, M. D., and E. A. Groisman. 2003. "Role of Nonhost Environments in the Lifestyles of Salmonella and *Escherichia coli*." *Applied and Environmental Microbiology* 69:3687–94.

Young, K. T., L. M. Davis, and V. J. Dirita. 2007. "Campylobacter jejuni: Molecular Biology and Pathogenesis." *Nature Reviews Microbiology* 5:665–79.

Zhang, Y., P. Bi, and J. Hiller. 2008. "Climate Variations and Salmonellosis Transmission in Adelaide South Australia: A Comparison between Regression Models." *International Journal of Biometeorology* 52:179–87.

CHAPTER 5

OZONE, OPPRESSIVE AIR MASSES, AND DEGRADED AIR QUALITY

Kim Knowlton

Despite general improvements in air quality over the past forty years in the United States, there remain sources of pollutants that can aggravate heart and respiratory conditions like asthma and lead to millions of lost workdays and missed school days. Furthermore, climate change is having effects on the environment in several ways that can exacerbate oppressive air masses, degrade air quality, and harm human health. Several specific pollutants are affected by climate change and degraded air quality, including ground-level ozone smog; particulate matter (especially fine particulates); cookstove, wildfire, and landscape smoke that can travel hundreds of kilometers downwind; dusts and airborne pathogens associated with drought and dust storms; and allergenic mold or moisture in indoor air when poststorm flood damage affects residences, schools, health institutions, and businesses. Climate change is already fueling environmental shifts that can increase exposure to air pollutants in many regions. Unfortunately, there is also a parallel rise in some factors that make people more vulnerable to air pollution exposures: a US population in which young children and the elderly are increasing in proportion, rising asthma and obesity rates, more and more households living in economic disadvantage, and communities of color faced with multiple exposures to air pollutants that have long-term, cumulative health effects.

Exposures to climate-sensitive air pollution are increasing in many regions, and at the same time underlying population vulnerabilities are also increasing: the high proportion of aging baby boomers; increasing rates of asthma, diabetes, and obesity; and the highest rates of economic disadvantage in decades. With these two

KEY CONCEPTS

- **Climate change affects weather patterns in ways that can reduce atmospheric mixing and make oppressive, health-harming air masses occur more frequently in many regions, often in combination with local topography and population growth.**

- **Ground-level ozone smog is a widespread threat to respiratory health because of rising temperatures that enhance the formation chemistry of ground-level ozone in the atmosphere.**

- **Heat-trapping carbon pollution from burning fossil fuels is the source of climate change; that combustion is also the source for numerous other health-harming air pollutants, notably a variety of air toxics and particulates. Particles are also formed from a variety of other climate-sensitive sources, including wildfires, drought, and dust storms.**

KEY CONCEPTS (*CONTINUED*)

- Climate change fuels extreme rainfall events and increases sea levels, which worsen coastal storm surge damage. Mold and moisture from storm-related flooding can compromise indoor air quality and harm respiratory health and have been linked to longer-term psychosocial impacts.

- Strategies to control oppressive air masses and improve degraded air quality include identifying local vulnerabilities to air pollution, tracking air pollution–related health threats, designing communities and transportation systems to be more resilient to climate change, and public health practitioners' and clinicians' involvement in outreach toward developing strategies to limit carbon and associated air pollutants and prepare for those health-harming effects that cannot be avoided.

coincident trends in exposure and vulnerability, several strategies can be employed to prepare for climate change: identifying local vulnerabilities to air pollution, tracking air pollution–related health threats and accessing publicly available monitoring resources, designing communities and transportation systems to be more resilient to climate change, and promoting the active engagement of health care providers, vulnerable communities, and policymakers in discussing and developing strategies to limit carbon pollution and associated air pollutants and adapt to those health-harming effects that are unavoidable. It is critical to remember that reducing fossil fuel combustion limits heat-trapping carbon pollution and can thus help limit some of the worse air pollution effects of climate change while simultaneously reducing other health-harming air pollutants like fine particles and air toxics also generated by fossil fuel combustion. These air quality improvements benefit everyone and go hand in hand with the longer-term benefits of healthier, more climate-secure communities for generations to come.

Climate Change and Air Quality

Climate change is caused largely by human-made heat-trapping pollution emitted by burning fossil fuels in the two hundred years since the Industrial Revolution. In the last fifty years, atmospheric temperatures have risen at an accelerating pace in most quarters of the globe, and in particular across the Northern Hemisphere. Rising atmospheric (and ocean) temperatures in turn influence global and regional precipitation, humidity, wind patterns, and pressure systems in ways that affect local meteorology and air quality (Kinney 2008; Jacob and Winner 2009). Climate change will likely offset some of the expected improvements in air quality that would be otherwise enjoyed from reductions in primary pollution sources and precursor emissions (Hogrefe 2012).

Effects of Rising Temperatures

Rising temperatures can substantially increase summer energy use, especially in areas not already adapted

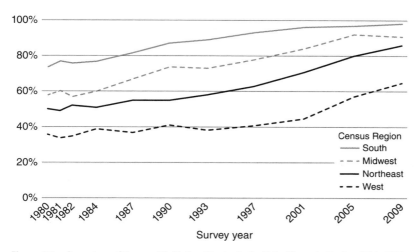

Figure 5.1   Percentage of Homes with Air-Conditioning in the United States by Region, 1980–2009

Source: Energy Information Administration, http://www.realclearenergy.org/charticles/2011/08/29/air_conditioning
_trends_in_the_us_106266.html

to warm weather, where homes and businesses may rely on window air-conditioning (A/C) units rather than central air. Nationally, A/C use is increasing, and an estimated 87 percent of US homes have some type of A/C. There are regional differences in air-conditioner use and type used (see figure 5.1). The South had close to 100 percent use by 2009, and the highest percentage (85 percent) of central air A/C systems (figure 5.1). The least air-conditioned region is the West, with 62 percent of homes using A/C in 2009, but central air comprising 75 percent of installations. And in the Northeast, 85 percent of homes have A/C but a mere 44 percent of those are central air.

No matter the region, providing peak summer electrical demand is a major draw on electrical power grids. "Peaker plants" are electrical power plants that run only during times of peak demand for electricity, which usually occurs during hot summer afternoons and evenings when workplaces and homes demand power to run electronics and appliances, including A/C. Possible electrical power failures (blackouts) remain a concern because periods of weather-driven peak demand can be expected to worsen with climate change and coincide with periods of greatest reliance on A/C (Anderson and Bell 2012). Air-conditioning units generate waste heat into the surrounding urban environment, and power plants that provide electricity to run A/C units are powered mostly by fossil fuels including coal, which emit both greenhouse gases and health-harming co-pollutants such as fine particles, polycyclic aromatic hydrocarbons (PAHs), sulfur and **nitrogen oxides**, benzene, and mercury (Perera 2008).

Meteorological Variables

Climate change can affect air pollutant concentrations through its effects on several meteorological variables, including temperature, humidity, wind speed and direction, and mixing height. Many chemical reactions are temperature dependent, notably ozone formation chemistry, so rising temperatures tend to increase ozone concentrations, absent other change in its precursor emissions (Kinney 2008). For example, there has been a long-term decrease in ozone attributable to reductions in the anthropogenic (human-produced) emissions that combine to form ozone, including **nitrogen oxides** (NO_x) and **volatile organic compounds** (VOCs) in recent decades. Both NO_x and VOCs come from mobile sources (cars, trucks, other on-road and off-road vehicles, and internal combustion engines), industrial sources (fuel burning, solvent use, other industrial processes), and natural sources like biological growth and decay, lightning, and forest and grassland fires. There have also been large interannual variations in average concentrations of these ozone precursors because of weather and temperatures. The summer of 1988 was among the hottest on record in the Northeast United States, which experienced a record high number of exceedances up to that time (Jacob and Winner 2009). However, the summer of 1992 was among the coolest due to the longer-term cooling effects of the 1991 eruption of Mt. Pinatubo and the sulfur particles it emitted into the atmosphere that blocked incoming solar radiation (Harries and Futyan 2006). As a result, 1992 was cool, and it had a low number of exceedances: ten times fewer high-ozone episodes than in 1988 (Jacob and Winner 2009).

A warming atmosphere can hold more moisture. With the contribution of human-caused recent warming, water vapor content since 1988 has been increasing roughly 6 to 7.5 percent per degree Celsius warming of the lower atmosphere (Santer et al. 2007). Periods of increased humidity can affect local air quality and health on an individual scale in many ways: high humidity can diminish ambient aeroallergen concentrations as pollen grains and spores tend to clump together and become less inhalable; conversely, higher humidity makes perspiration and associated body cooling less successful during extreme heat.

Wind speed and direction shift in ways that are fairly complex and sensitive to local topography and microclimates, as well as changes in larger ocean and regional atmospheric air transport patterns. Winds greatly affect which upwind source areas will affect local background air pollution and locations that will be affected by transport of local pollutants downwind, but it is not yet entirely clear how a warmer climate affects patterns of wind speed and direction overall (Fiore et al. 2012). Other climate-sensitive meteorological characteristics that also affect local and regional air quality include stagnant air conditions, changes in vertical mixing depth in the lower atmosphere that affect mixing height, and the degree of dilution of atmospheric pollutants. Global climates are projected to become more stagnant in the future, with weaker global circulation and a decreasing frequency of midlatitude cyclones (Jacob and Winner 2009). With more atmospheric stagnation and the continued correlation between ground-level ozone and rising temperatures in polluted regions, there is likely to be a net detrimental effect of warming on human health (Bell et al. 2007; Jacob and Winner 2009).

In a recent finding related to convection and vertical atmospheric mixing, one provocative study (Anderson et al. 2012) found that violent weather with large convective storms injects water vapor high into the stratosphere over the United States. They suggest that theoretically, this could shift stratospheric ozone chemistry and dramatically increase ozone loss there. By extension, there would be increased risk of increased human cancer rates if more incident ultraviolet light were allowed to reach the ground surface as a result of more stratospheric ozone destruction.

Local meteorology and regional weather patterns affect not only the formation chemistry but also the dilution, transport, and distribution of air pollutants locally and across regions. Rising temperatures make chemical reactions progress more rapidly in general. Ambient ozone concentrations are indeed strongly correlated with temperature (Hogrefe 2012). In a warming world, secondary chemical reactions like those that form ozone smog at ground level in the atmosphere proceed more rapidly, leading to higher ozone concentrations. Ozone precursor emissions (VOCs and NO_x) are emitted from vehicles, power plants, or other industrial sources and combine into ozone more rapidly in warmer temperatures. Temperature-sensitive changes in the production rate of **biogenic emissions**, chemical compounds that are emitted naturally from vegetation sources, are also climate-sensitive factors (Ebi and McGregor 2008; Fiore et al. 2005; Jacob and Winner 2009; Jacobson 2008; Tagaris et al. 2010).

This effect is projected to continue into the future as well. A modeling study of fifty large cities east of the Mississippi projected a 68 percent increase in unhealthy summer ozone days by the 2050s due to the effect of rising temperatures under a high carbon-emissions climate change scenario (Bell et al. 2007). Biogenic precursor emissions of ozone also tend to increase in warmer temperatures, adding even more source input to the ozone formation reactions (Fiore et al. 2005).

Transport of Air Pollution

Wildfire smoke can be transported long distances downwind hundreds, even thousands, of kilometers to affect intercontinental background levels of particulates. National Aeronautics and Space Administration (NASA) satellite imagery shows the long-distance transport of wildfire smoke from Canada in June 2015, across the continental United States and throughout the Midwest, reminding us that what appear to be local effects of climate change all too often reach far beyond country or state boundaries.

CLINICAL CORRELATES 5.1   HUMAN HEALTH EFFECTS OF OZONE

Acute and chronic ozone exposure has been associated with significant adverse health effects in humans, including cardiopulmonary and respiratory morbidity and premature mortality (Berman et al. 2012). Abrupt daily increases in ozone concentrations have been shown to decrease pulmonary function (Mudway and Kelly 2000), increase asthma exacerbation rates, and increase emergency department visits (Choi et al. 2011). Ozone has also been associated with an increased relative risk of death from all cardiopulmonary causes (Jerrett et al. 2009). A recent assessment (Berman et al. 2012) found that as many as twenty-five hundred ozone-related premature deaths, 3 million cases of acute respiratory symptoms, and 1 million school days could have been avoided annually could the nation attain the 75 parts per billion (ppb) standard goal.

Ozone not only contributes to global warming but also causes measurable negative health effects during periods of acute exposure.

Chemical Transformation

The warming effects of climate change alone, absent precursor emissions change, will increase summertime surface ozone in polluted regions by an estimated 1 to 10 ppb in coming decades, with the largest effects in urban areas during pollution episodes (Jacob and Winner 2009). This "climate penalty" means that stronger emission controls will be needed to meet a given air quality standard, even with expected overall reductions in pollution emissions from ongoing regulatory efforts (Jacob and Winner 2009; Hogrefe 2012).

The effect of climate change and rising temperatures on particulate matter (PM) is more complicated than for ozone (Kinney 2008; Jacob and Winner 2009). The effects of rising temperatures tends to vary by PM species, with sulfates and primary PM (formed directly by mechanical rather than chemical processes) also increasing, versus nitrated and organic components decreasing in concentration as they move from particulate to gaseous phase (Kinney 2008). Aerosols and PM can also reduce solar radiation at the surface by reflecting sunlight upward or by absorbing sunlight before it reaches the ground (Wang, Dickinson, and Liang 2009), having a further feedback effect on temperatures.

Cloud Formation and Deposition of Air Pollutants

Climate change can affect cloudiness in several ways that affect air pollution concentrations. Natural biogenic emissions from plants contribute to haze and decreased visibility and are important ozone precursors. This is one reason that the southeastern United States, with its abundance of coniferous and hardwood forests, has persistent ground-level ozone compliance issues. Questions still remain about the net global effect that biogenics, soot, and other aerosols could have in the future on cloud formation under a changing climate, since they can have either cooling or warming effects. Different types of aerosols can affect cloud formation differently. They can act as seeds for cloud formation, reflect incoming radiation away from the surface, and have a cooling effect. Conversely they can reduce cloudiness, as often happens in northern China, with a warming effect. And aerosols or soot from burning biofuels absorb sunlight in the troposphere rather than scattering it back to space, with a warming effect (Wang et al. 2009). Aerosols also affect clouds' areal extent and other characteristics. More work is needed to determine the local, regional, and global net dynamics and trade-offs between cloud formation, air pollution, and climate.

Climate change is likely to affect the ways in which pollutants are deposited out of the atmosphere, either during precipitation events or by dry deposition onto surfaces of vegetation, buildings, and other objects (Hogrefe 2012). Excessive nitrogen deposition, a by-product of fossil fuel combustion, animal husbandry, and intensive use of fertilizers, can tilt ecosystem processes toward deterioration of downstream water quality (Grulke and Schilling 2008). These processes, coupled with rising temperatures and changing precipitation patterns, could destabilize ecosystems further and exacerbate fire risks.

Air Pollutants Affected by Climate Change

Several major air pollutants, notably ground-level ozone and particulates, are sensitive to climate conditions and are affected by climate change. These pollutants increase air pollution days that can be hazardous to health and exacerbate underlying respiratory and cardiovascular disease, causing increases in emergency room visits, hospitalizations, and premature mortality.

Ground-Level Ozone

Ozone (O_3) is probably the most frequently cited climate-sensitive air pollutant. It is not emitted directly but instead is a secondary pollutant formed in the atmosphere from photochemical reactions between ozone precursor compounds that include NO_x and VOCs, themselves health-harming pollutants. The current global tropospheric O_3 concentration is double that of preindustrial times and is expected to increase by 50 percent by 2020 (Grulke and Schilling 2008).

In urban settings, power plants, industrial and vehicle-based fossil fuel emissions, and chemical solvents provide ample sources for the NO_x and VOCs that are the precursors of O_3. In the presence of sunlight, these precursor compounds undergo temperature-dependent photochemical reactions that form O_3, the major component of the ground-level air pollution commonly known as smog. The formation chemistry is a complex, multistep process, with some of the intermediate constituents also capable of destroying ozone in a process called titration.

The most abundant atmospheric VOC, methane (CH_4), a potent greenhouse gas, is typically outpaced by anthropogenic nonmethane VOCs (NMVOCs) in urban and suburban ozone formation chemistry (Shea et al. 2008). Globally, methane has a key role in determining atmospheric concentrations of ozone because it reacts slowly and affects global background concentrations of O_3. Thus, reducing CH_4 reduces O_3 concentrations in both polluted urban regions and rural areas (West et al. 2006). Strategies to reduce methane could provide cost-effective ways to reduce O_3 internationally and yield air quality, public health, and climate benefits. One study suggests that by reducing about 20 percent of global anthropogenic methane, an estimated 30,000 premature deaths could be prevented globally in 2030 or an estimated 370,000 deaths between 2010 and 2030 (West et al. 2006).

Health Effects of Ozone

Acute and chronic exposures to ground-level ozone have been associated with a wide range of morbidities, as well as premature mortality (Bell et al. 2004; Bell, Dominici, and Samet 2005; Ito, De Leon, and Lippmann 2005; Levy, Chermerynski, and Sarnat 2005) in toxicological studies, clinical trials, longitudinal epidemiological studies, and cohort epidemiological studies (Berman et al. 2012). Decreased lung function, increases in school absenteeism and lost workdays, exacerbations of asthma symptoms, and increased hospital admissions and emergency room visits have been linked to acute ground-level ozone exposures (Bell et al. 2004; Kinney 2008; Sheffield et al. 2011; Choi et al 2011; Berman et al. 2012). For example, when the Atlanta, Georgia, Olympics in 1996 limited automobile traffic and associated VOC emissions, peak daily O_3 declined 28 percent, pediatric emergency room asthma visits declined by 11 percent, and acute care asthma events fell by more than 40 percent (Friedman et al. 2001). Beyond these acute effects, longer-term ozone exposures lead to loss of years of productive life (Jerrett et al. 2009). An estimated 160 million people in the United States live in areas with unhealthy levels of summertime ozone. A health impact assessment found that annually, around fourteen hundred to twenty-five hundred ozone-related premature deaths, 3 million cases of acute respiratory symptoms, and 1 million school loss days could have been avoided nationally by full attainment of the current 75 ppb standard (Berman 2012). Even greater health benefits could be achieved with a more stringent primary standard.

Particulates: Sources and Health Effects

While both coarse and fine particulates come from natural and anthropogenic sources, diesel and fossil-fuel burning vehicles and industries are the major sources in cities and suburban areas (Shea et al. 2008). Particulate matter is also generated by several climate-sensitive environmental changes, including forest fires, drought, and desertification. Airborne particulates come from many sources: secondary pollutants formed by chemical reactions of pollutant gases, dust particles raised from road surfaces by traffic, and particles emitted by industrial and agricultural activities. Fine particulates (2.5 micrometers in diameter or smaller) are known to harm human health (Shea et al. 2008). Recently fine particulates have been shown to decrease precipitation in areas downwind of their production and reduce photosynthetic activity and growth of plants on chalky soils, that is, those rich in calcium carbonate (Grulke and Schilling 2008).

The combustion of charcoal, animal dung, and plant matter in indoor cooking and heating by an estimated 4 billion people is having a dramatic impact on climate change and dramatically increasing mortality from children's respiratory infections and chronic obstructive pulmonary disease worldwide (Pinkerton et al. 2012). It is estimated that 1.9 million people annually die from exposures to cookstove and cooking fire smoke, mostly children and women, because of indoor use patterns and cultural traditions that place these family members in close contact with smoke, often in relatively unvented conditions. Many more—an estimated 3 billion people—develop respiratory illnesses such as pneumonia, emphysema, lung cancer, and heart disease (UN Foundation 2012).

The warming effect of soot, whether from cookstoves, industrial boilers, power plants, or ship boilers, is twice as great as previously estimated by the 2007 Intergovernmental Panel on Climate Change (IPCC) report, according to a 2013 study (Bond et al. 2013). Roughly 8 million tons of soot are produced annually worldwide, and they can have various warming effects. They can absorb solar energy, pass it on to the atmosphere, and add to global warming caused by anthropogenic greenhouse gases; they can shrink cloud droplet size and brighten clouds; they can land on ice and snow and darken it sufficiently to absorb more sunlight and melt; but now it is understood that soot's net warming effect is second only to carbon dioxide (CO_2) (Bond et al. 2013). Next, understanding the inventories of soot being produced by developing regions and these particles' interactions with clouds will help fill important research gaps.

Wildfires

Wildfire smoke is a complex and toxic brew of hundreds of different chemical compounds, from fine particles to ozone precursors to mercury, many of them potentially health harming (Delfino et al. 2009; Dennekamp and Abramson 2011; Johnston et al. 2012; Johnston et al. 2002; Marlier et al. 2013; Shea et al. 2008). (See chapter 2 for more information on ways that heat and drought can affect wildfire risks and associated health impacts.) Premature death from injuries, burns, smoke inhalation and cardiovascular and respiratory illness, increased hospital and emergency room visits, exacerbation of asthma, allergies, chronic obstructive pulmonary disease, displacement, and loss of homes with associated mental stress are among the adverse health impacts of wildfires (Dennekamp and Abramson 2011; Kinney et al. 2008; Shea et al. 2008).

The observed increase in western US wildfire activity since the 1980s has caused atmospheric organic carbon concentrations to increase 30 percent relative to 1970 to 1984, and in future decades, climate change is likely to exacerbate wildfires further (Spracklen et al. 2007; Westerling and Bryant 2008). Research suggests that some western forests will become more susceptible to wildfire as high concentrations of O_3 air pollution increase plant transpiration and exacerbate tree drought stress (Grulke and Schilling 2008). This could increase their vulnerability to both insect pest attacks and wildfire. The particulate and carbonaceous aerosol components of wildfire smoke could increase as air pollutants of concern in the future, with projected climate change (Marlier et al. 2013; Spracklen et al. 2009). By the 2050s, climate change could increase the summer organic carbon aerosols over the western United States by an estimated 40 percent and elemental carbon by 20 percent, with important consequences for air quality (Spracklen et al. 2009).

CLINICAL CORRELATES 5.2   HEALTH EFFECTS OF FINE PARTICULATE MATTER

Fine particulate matter, generated through diesel and fossil-fuel burning vehicles, industrial processes, and climate-sensitive environmental changes, have been shown to cause negative acute and chronic health problems. Studies show that elevations in ambient particulate matter are associated with increases in myocardial infarction and accelerated atherosclerosis (Zhang et al. 2009). Other studies show that each 10 micrograms per cubic meter elevation in fine particulate air pollution is associated with approximately a 4 percent, 6 percent, and 8 percent increased risk of all-cause, cardiopulmonary, and lung cancer mortality, respectively (Pope et al. 2002).

In addition to accelerating global climate change, ambient fine particulate matter has a significant negative impact on human health.

Wildfires and Health   The range of air toxics included in wildfire smoke surprises most people, even clinicians: wildfire smoke produces large amounts of carbon monoxide, carbon dioxide, NO_x, ozone precursors and O_3, particulate matter or PM (both coarse PM_{10} and finer $PM_{2.5}$), VOCs, metals including mercury, organic acids, and other air toxics (Dennekamp and Abramson 2011; Shea et al. 2008). Associations between bushfire smoke PM_{10} and respiratory hospitalizations and emergency room visits in Australian studies are consistent with those found in urban air pollution exposure studies (Dennekamp and Abramson 2011). Worldwide, an estimated 339,000 people annually perish from the combined effects of wildfire and landscape fire smoke (Johnston et al. 2012).

People exposed to smoke from wildfires or landscape fires may not realize the health risks to which they are being exposed. The Children's Health Study found that after the 2003 California wildfires, even the smell of fire smoke, having penetrated indoors, could persist for more than six days and has been associated with continued respiratory symptoms: sore throat, cough, bronchitis, wheezing, and asthma attacks (Kunzli et al. 2006). Clinicians should take care to both diagnose and counsel carefully, even at locations far distant and downwind of fire source areas, since fire smoke can travel hundreds of miles downwind and still affect air quality measurably. One study found that $PM_{2.5}$ from 2002 wildfires in northern Quebec, Canada, traveled over one thousand kilometers southward to affect air quality in Baltimore, Maryland (Kinney 2008).

Drought

A devastating drought struck much of the United States in 2011 and 2012, the most widespread in fifty years. (See chapter 9 on food and nutrition security for more information on ways that climate change affects drought, crops, and nutritional aspects of human health.) Over thirteen hundred counties across twenty-nine states were declared by the US Department of

Agriculture as drought disaster areas in 2012 (Natural Resources Defense Council 2012). Billion-dollar disasters in 2011 and 2012 affected 67 percent of US counties in forty-three states, and the combined heat and drought damage estimates were among the highest (Center for American Progress 2012). Drought affects not only the farm households that are directly involved in production and agriculturally based communities in the Midwest and Great Plains states. Rising food prices affect families across the country and globally (Redman 2012). Drought has a wide range of respiratory effects on health that, until now, have not often been seen as a whole spectrum. Climate change may exacerbate these health impacts in future across many regions.

Drought Effects on Respiratory Health   Periods of drought have long affected North America, and the memory of the 1930s Dust Bowl is vivid still for many. Since then, periods of drought hit the Great Plains in the 1950s and 1980s, with "significant negative economic and societal consequences" (Centers for Disease Control/US Environmental Protection Agency 2010). However, the ongoing effects of climate change are likely to increase the severity of future droughts into this century (Dai 2011; Schwalm et al. 2012). Increasing air temperature (even in nondrought periods) can lead to excessive soil and vegetation drying and loss of ground cover (National Weather Service 2013), poor soil quality, diminishing soil and surface water, and reduced crop yields. The interspersed extreme rainfall events that can punctuate drought periods increase runoff and erosion, compounding the effects of enhancing drought. This cycle can lead to soils, dusts, and soil-borne pathogens that can become airborne and have far-reaching health impacts (CDC/US EPA 2010).

The potentially health-harming respiratory effects of droughts include increased mobilization of dusts from dry soils. These dusts can irritate bronchial passages and lungs, exacerbating asthma symptoms and increasing risks of acute respiratory infection, bronchitis, and bacterial pneumonia. Because associated dry soils and hot temperatures also increase wildfire risks, risk of smoke inhalation means potentially increased exposures to $PM_{2.5}$, ozone, and a host of air toxics that can harm respiratory health. During drought periods, harmful algal blooms in freshwater bodies can increase, and some species generate aerosolized toxins. Transmission patterns of vector-borne illnesses like West Nile virus, hantavirus, coccidiomycosis, and dengue fever can be affected by drought, since these periods can put animal and insect vectors into closer contact with human hosts as both species vie for shrinking water resources. Recreational water use becomes riskier as water body levels decline, injuries increase, water temperatures rise, and risk of contact with thermophilic waterborne pathogens like *Naegleria folweri* ("the brain-eating amoeba") increase. Mental and behavioral health suffers during drought, in part from the economic and cultural stress it puts on communities. As drought places human communities in competition with one another for water resources, basic sanitation and hygiene can suffer, which can increase local transmission of illnesses. And in a bigger frame, large health care institutions rely on large-scale water supplies not only for drinking but also for energy, patient care, sterilization, refrigeration, and other services, so drought in many ways compromises critical aspect of health care delivery as well as public health (CDC /US EPA 2010).

CLINICAL CORRELATES 5.3   WILDFIRES, DROUGHT, AND HUMAN HEALTH

Although direct impacts of wildfires tend to occur in restricted geographical regions, they have potential to affect the health of populations hundreds of miles away (Kinney 2008). Smoke from the combustion of biomass contains myriad chemicals known to be detrimental to human health (Naeher et al. 2007). Examples include carbon monoxide, organic acids, mercury, and fine particulate matter. Some experts compare the impact of particulate matter produced by wildfires to that of industrial urban environments where fine particulate matter is associated with a wide range of adverse health effects, including neonatal and cardiorespiratory mortality, exacerbations of respiratory and cardiovascular conditions, and pathophysiological changes such as inflammation, oxidative stress, and coagulation (Pope and Dockery 2006). Carbon monoxide poisoning can manifest as headache, confusion, and coma in severe cases. Mercury can cause neurological toxicity, and a study from the National Center for Atmospheric Research found that 48 tons of mercury are redistributed by wildfires annually in the United States (Lipsher 2007). It is unclear how the metal is affecting human health, although experts suspect it is entering waterways and drinking water.

Clinicians should take care to both diagnose and counsel carefully, even at locations far distant and downwind of fire source areas, since fire smoke can travel hundreds of miles downwind and still affect air quality measurably.

Coccidiomycosis and Respiratory Health   A recently reemergent fungal infectious illness, coccidiodomycosis or "valley fever," is on the rise, with rapidly increasing numbers in the US southwestern border region (Centers for Disease Control 2013a). Coccidiomycosis was first recognized and reported over one hundred years ago, but since the early 1990s, its incidence has increased dramatically. Valley fever is caused by inhalation of fungal spores that reside in desert soils, which can become airborne during periods of drought, when soils are more easily crumbled or pulverized, and can sub-sequently become airborne and be dispersed by high winds. Between these dry periods that contribute to airborne pathogen transport, the spores reside and thrive in relatively moist soils, leading to the phrase "grow and blow" to describe the life cycle of Coccidiomycoses. It is estimated that in endemic regions, 30 to 60 percent of residents are exposed to the fungus at some time in their lives (Centers for Disease Control 2013b).

For most people, the infection clears on its own, but for those few who develop severe infections with its flulike symptoms that can last for weeks or turn into chronic pneumonia, medical treatment is needed. The infec-tion can spread from the lungs throughout the body, causing meningitis or even death. Fever, chest pain, coughing, rash, and muscle aches are among its range of symptoms. Groups most at risk for the more severe dissemi-nated infection form of valley fever are women in their third trimester of pregnancy, people with weakened immune systems, or who are of African American, Asian, Hispanic, or Filipino descent (CDC/US EPA 2010). Cali-fornia State prisons have seen high incidence rates as the construction of new prison facilities in endemic areas disturbed spores and then put large numbers of inmates in potential contact with dusty, fungus-laden soil (Pap-pagianis 2007). Approximately 20,000 new cases are reported nationally each year in the United States, but an estimated 150,000 may be infected. Far fewer cases are diagnosed across the Arizona-Mexico border, although the pathogen's progress obviously does not stop at the border (Centers for Disease Control 2013a).

All of this highlights the need for more health care providers and labo-ratories to be trained to recognize and diagnose valley fever and prevent its spread beyond the areas in which it is now endemic in the United States (see Clinical Correlates 5.4). Expanding awareness of valley fever among clini-cians and the public can help minimize delays in diagnosis and treatment (Centers for Disease Control 2013b).

Summers in and around Phoenix, Arizona, have taken a new twist in recent years. Besides the searing temperatures that summer brings to the region, residents turn to the horizon with an eye to the towering dust storms, or haboobs, which have appeared out of the desert landscape in summer to darken the air with massive columns of particulates and dusts. Named for the Arabic term for "blasting," these large-scale haboobs, intense dust storms with sometimes blasting winds, have become a more regular feature of sum-mers in the desert Southwest (Wikipedia 2015). While dust storms have long been part of desert life, more of these dust storms seem to be occurring recently. Some of the meteorological conditions that can contribute to the formation of major dust storms and haboobs include drought, which can diminish the amount of ground-covering vegetation, leaving more open fields that can serve as sources of dust. The widespread drought and heat of recent summers, notably 2011 and 2012, contributed to some ideal local conditions in parts of the desert Southwest. Eye and respiratory protection and taking shelter is advisable in the face of these approaching clouds.

Health Effects of Particulate Matter

Particle pollution contains solids and liquid droplets so small that they can penetrate deeply into lungs and cause serious health problems. The health effects of particle pollution or particulates, especially fine particles with average aerodynamic diameters of 2.5 microns or less ($PM_{2.5}$), include premature death in people with preexisting heart or lung disease; nonfatal heart attacks; irregular heartbeat; aggravated asthma; decreased lung function in children and adults; and increased respiratory symptoms, such as irritation of the airways, coughing, or difficulty breathing (Shea et al. 2008; US Environmental Protection Agency 2013). People vulnerable to particulates include those with heart or lung diseases, children, and older adults. Exposures to $PM_{2.5}$ differ by race/ethnicity, age, and socioeconomic status (SES) in the United States: Hispanics generally have the highest exposures, as do young persons up to nineteen years of age and persons with lower SES (Bell and Ebisu 2012). However, even healthy people can be negatively affected by high levels of particle pollution.

Mold and Fungi

Extreme rainfall events, along with sea level rise that can worsen storm surge and coastal flooding, are being fueled by climate change (Intergovernmental Panel on Climate Change 2012). Together they can cause moisture damage in residences, businesses, schools, and other institutions. The associated growth of indoor molds can have health-harming respiratory effects (Fisk, Lei-Gomez, and Mendell 2007; Institute of Medicine 2004, 2011; Mudarri and Fisk 2007; Reid and Gamble 2009; Sheffield et al. 2011), and exposure to dampness and mold in homes has also been linked to depression (Shenassa et al. 2007). Exposure to *Alternaria alternata* in US homes is associated with higher prevalence of current asthma symptoms. In a survey of 831 US housing units, higher levels of *A. alternata* antigens measured in indoor dust increased the odds of having asthma symptoms in the past year, relative to the lowest tertile (adjusted odds ratio was 1.84, 95 percent confidence interval [CI], 1.18 to 2.85 for the third tertile) (Salo et al. 2006). Besides prevalence, asthma's persistence and severity of symptoms have been strongly associated with sensitization and exposure to the widespread fungus *A. alternata*, though few studies have done indoor exposure assessment.

Increasing carbon dioxide levels in the atmosphere can also exacerbate spore production and total antigen production in molds like *Alternaria*, an allergenic fungus so ubiquitous that this response may contribute to the increasing prevalence of allergies and asthma (Wolf et al. 2010). Furthermore, mold and moisture are exacerbated by flooding associated with tropical storms and intense rainfall events that are fueled by climate change.

Challenges exist in characterizing mold exposures in indoor environments. These allergens have not been characterized as well as other indoor allergens such as dust mite, cockroach, and pet (Salo et al. 2006). Measuring moisture conditions indoors, evaluating damage to home building materials, and surveying for mold growth visually are the current means of establishing potential mold health issues when respiratory symptoms are reported. Human exposures to fungal allergens have been estimated by indirect methods using spore or fungal colony counts in air or dust samples as a proxy of exposure. Thus the absence of standardized measurement techniques for evaluation of fungal allergen exposures has been a major constraint in risk assessment. Because interpretation of fungal exposure data is both complex and contentious, no universally recognized exposure thresholds exist, but these would be tremendously helpful in guiding remediation efforts to reestablish healthy indoor environments after flooding (Salo et al. 2006).

Implementing best practices in mold remediation remains challenging nationwide. Licensing for mold remediation does not exist in all states. This can leave homeowners with moisture and mold damage wondering where to turn for top-notch cleanup assistance. It remains to be seen whether a unified set of mold remediation guidelines can be developed that could serve as a best-practices guide for contractors, cleanup specialists, and homeowners nationwide and if one consistent framework for national certification of mold remediation can be established.

Air Pollution–Vulnerable Populations

Some of the groups most susceptible to air pollution are children, people with preexisting heart or lung disease, people with diabetes, athletes, and outdoor workers (Balbus and Malina 2009; Makri and Stilianakis 2008; Pinkerton et al. 2012; Sheffield and Landrigan 2011). Socioeconomic factors and economic disadvantage increase people's susceptibility to air pollution health effects in terms of both increased, disproportionate exposures and reduced coping capacities and access to health care (Makri and Stilianakis

2008). The homeless are especially vulnerable to air pollution, with high rates of respiratory infections and self-reported lung diseases including asthma, chronic bronchitis, and emphysema that are double the rates in the general population; asthma rates in homeless children have been reported as six times the national rate (Ramin and Svoboda 2009). However, the homeless may be a challenging population to locate, protect, and serve, and comorbidities including depression and schizophrenia are also common. Developing strategies to communicate climate health risks widely and in ways that speak to local community needs will be essential in the years ahead. The active engagement of leaders from all highly vulnerable communities in developing effective outreach will be critical.

Double-Whammy for People with Asthma

Climate change is projected to worsen many of the existing health issues that face Americans, and the clinicians who serve them. One season that is already challenging is the dog days of summer, which include the hottest, most sultry months—typically July and August in the Northern Hemisphere. Heat can compound respiratory and cardiovascular illnesses, increasing rates of emergency room visits and hospitalizations. Late summer sees rampant seasonal allergy symptoms from ragweed pollen beginning in August and lasting into October. An estimated 36 million people in the United States have seasonal allergies (Natural Resources Defense Council 2007), and ragweed causes more allergies than any other plant pollen. And among people with asthma, approximately 70 percent also have allergies (American Academy of Allergy, Asthma and Immunology/National Allergy Bureau 2013), making the possibility of both allergy and asthma symptoms far more than an inconvenience for some patients.

Ground-level ozone concentrations tend to be higher in the hotter temperatures of late summer, since ozone's formation chemistry is temperature dependent. So the health "double-whammy" of higher exposures to ozone smog plus ragweed pollen can be a challenge to children and adults trying to enjoy sports, back-to-school activities, or just a day in the late-summer sun.

Clinicians should take note that in future decades, climate change could make those hot, cloudless days even tougher. Rising CO_2 concentrations make ragweed grow larger and produce more pollen per plant. In the years ahead, especially in and around cities where vehicle and industrial sources are concentrated, with ragweed pollen seasons increasing in length (Ziska et al. 2011), there could be more people sensitized to ragweed, more severe symptoms if peak pollen concentrations increases, or the need to counsel patients to sustain allergy medication over a longer time period, beginning earlier and lasting later into the season.

CLINICAL CORRELATES 5.4   DROUGHT AND REEMERGENCE OF DISEASE: COCCIDIOMYOCISIS

According to the Centers for Disease Control (2013a), Coccidiomyocisis, a fungal pathogen capable of causing respiratory as well as disseminated disease, is on the rise in the southwestern United States and Mexico. Exposure occurs from inhalation of the fungal spores that reside in desert soils. Periods of drought cause the spores to become airborne and dispersed by winds. Although 30 to 60 percent of residents living in endemic regions may be exposed, certain populations (including women in third trimester of pregnancy and immunocompromised individuals) are susceptible to significant disease. Symptoms include a flulike illness and pneumonia followed by the possibility of spread throughout the body and central nervous system. Clinicians in endemic and even nearby drought-affected areas need to be aware of the potential for this disease, as its distribution is subject to change with the climate.

Drought and changing climate in the desert southwestern regions of the United States mean that local clinicians must be attuned to symptoms of reemergent disease such as Coccidiomyocisis to avoid missed and delayed diagnosis.

Future Projections of Climate Change's Effects on Air Pollution

Studies have modeled temperature-dependent ozone air pollution into future decades with climate change's influence. These forward-looking ozone modeling efforts suggest that climate change alone will increase summertime surface ozone in polluted regions of the United States by 1 to 10 ppb this century, with the largest effects in urban areas during pollution episodes (Fiore et al. 2012; Jacob and Winner 2009). Changes in extreme climate conditions may intensify the extreme meteorological conditions that encourage high-ozone episodes in many parts of the world. Changes in regional high-ozone episodes by the 2050s appear to depend mainly on assumptions about precursor inventories: three major pollutant regions—North America, Europe, and East Asia—would see increases in the number of days with hazardous eight-hour ozone concentrations (thirty-nine to seventy-nine days per summer by the 2050s) under a fossil fuel-intensive, high greenhouse gas-emissions A1F1 scenario (Lei, Wuebbles, and Liang 2012). The A1 storyline and scenario family describes a future world of very rapid economic growth, global population that peaks in midcentury and declines thereafter, and the rapid introduction of new and more efficient technologies. Major underlying themes are convergence among regions, capacity building, and increased cultural and social interactions, with a substantial reduction in regional differences in per capita income. A1F1 is fossil fuel intensive (http://www.ipcc.ch/ipccreports/tar/wg1/029.htm).

Several studies have used a combination of the output from current-day epidemiological studies' air pollution exposure-response coefficients and future climate-health risk assessments to estimate health impacts from future climate-sensitive air pollution model projections. Bell et al. (2007) modeled temperature-dependent ozone by the 2050s in fifty large eastern cities, assuming constant precursor emissions, and found a 68 percent increase in unhealthy summertime ozone days by the 2050s relative to the 1990s and a 2.1 percent increase in asthma hospitalizations across all the cities, ranging as high as 4.7 percent from O_3 exposures. Sheffield et al. (2011) considered potential effects of climate change on ozone-related emergency room visits for asthma in the 2020s, driven by climate-sensitive temperature changes, and found a median 7.3 percent increase occurring in fourteen metropolitan New York City counties by the 2020s (Sheffield et al. 2011).

A study that looked at the metropolitan New York City region and the effects of climate change on human health found that by the 2050s, projected ozone-related premature mortality increases by 4.5 percent across the region, compared to the 1990s (Knowlton et al. 2004). Other studies have estimated that globally by 2050, there could be four thousand additional premature deaths each year attributable to climate change-connected PM increases, and 300 due to O_3 increases (Russell et al. 2010; Tagaris et al. 2010).

Mitigation: Health Benefits of Reducing Carbon Pollution and Associated Co-Pollutant Air Pollution

It is important to remember that many of the fossil fuel combustion sources of heat-trapping carbon pollution are also sources of local-scale co-pollutants like PM, ozone precursors, air toxics, and metals that can have health-harming effects on local air quality. By reducing carbon pollution and moving toward less fossil fuel use, those co-pollutants can simultaneously be reduced in ways that can provide substantial current health benefits in terms of immediate air quality improvements and through initiatives that provide more access to walkable, bikable local transportation networks, enhanced exercise and fitness opportunities, and increased social contacts in the community.

Nationally, the 1970 Clean Air Act (CAA) is the foundational statute that protects human health and welfare from air pollution, via the National Ambient Air Quality Standards. The CAA limits major climate-sensitive air pollutants or precursors in the United States. Since being enacted in 1970, the CAA plus its 1990 amendments prevented more than 160,000 premature deaths in 2010 and will prevent a projected 230,000 deaths in 2020 (US EPA 2011).

Local initiatives to reduce health-harming air pollution exposures include strategies to improve local air quality and reduce emissions of heat-trapping carbon pollution. For example, the New York City West Harlem Environmental Action, along with the Natural Resources Defense Council and Environmental Defense Fund, were instrumental in developing initiatives to take diesel buses off the streets and reduce the high concentrations of bus depots in residential neighborhoods among communities of color.

New York City is also among the communities that passed prohibiting trucks and buses from idling their engines when they stop for more than a few minutes. Passage of these local laws and making enforcement a neighborhood priority can lead to appreciable differences to health. New York City, for example, not only allows agents of the Department of Parks and Recreation and the Department of Sanitation to issue idling summonses, appearance tickets, and violation notices but gives citizens the ability to report truck violations. Switching to cleaner fuels in transportation and energy sourcing and instituting regulations that require the latest emission controls can make a big difference in air quality. For example, efforts in New York City to take diesel buses off the streets and retrofit oil furnaces so they burn cleaner fuel have improved air quality there.

Triple Wins: Cutting Carbon Pollution and Air Pollution, and Improving Community Health

The transportation systems that communities put in place, as well as overall community form and proximities of living, working, recreational and community spaces, have enormous impacts on transportation energy demand, associated air pollution emissions, overall air quality, and community health. For example, one study of ninety-eight US communities suggests that for every 10 percent of the population that takes public transportation to work, long-term ozone levels decrease by 9 percent (Bell and Dominici 2008).

Eliminating short automobile trips (eight or fewer kilometers or about five miles round-trip) and substituting bicycle trips instead can help limit average urban $PM_{2.5}$ and O_3 concentrations. In a study that considered this switch for eleven Upper Midwest cities, $PM_{2.5}$ would decline by 0.1 micrograms per cubic meter; and summer O_3 would increase slightly in cities but decline regionally, resulting in net annual health benefits of $4.9 billion. About 25 percent of $PM_{2.5}$ and most of the O_3 benefits would occur in rural areas downwind of cities. Across the study region of approximately 31 million people, mortality would decline annually by almost thirteen hundred deaths because of improved air quality and increased exercise. Making 50 percent of short trips by bicycle would save approximately $3.8 billion annually from avoided mortality and reduced health care costs. The combined benefits of improved air quality and physical fitness were estimated at over $8 billion annually (Grabow et al. 2012).

Cutting Pollution with Walkable, Bikable, Active Transit in New York City

Even in New York City, where residents have long prided themselves on getting a bit more exercise than their fellow Americans might expect—sprints to catch the bus, walking blocks from apartment to subway station—obesity and type 2 diabetes are epidemic, with 40 percent of elementary and middle school children overweight or obese. This exceeds the 30 percent rate nationwide (Lee 2012). Moreover, obesity is the second leading cause of deaths in the United States behind tobacco. Physical inactivity not only contributes to the second through fourth leading causes—obesity, high blood pressure, and high blood glucose—it is the fifth leading cause itself. The built environment—the streets, buildings, and neighborhoods where we work and live—can play a vital role in encouraging healthy physical activities (Patz et al. 2007). When cities are redesigned to promote fitness and discourage fossil fuel–based transit, the triple win of personal fitness, better air quality today, and reductions in heat-trapping carbon pollution combines to limit the worst of climate change's effects (Patz et al. 2007).

Nationwide, 40 percent of car trips are less than two miles (Patz et al. 2007), and 62 percent of all trips are less than six miles (US Department of Energy 2013); these could easily be translated into a bike trip. In 2009, 5 percent of walk trips and 11 percent of bike trips were to or from work (US Department of Energy 2013). Active transport has the potential to move past recreation and become a way of life for many Americans.

In May 2013, New York City began its first public subscription bike-share program, CitiBike, with sponsorship from Citibank to place six thousand bikes at 330 stations in Manhattan and parts of Brooklyn. Within less than a month, over 1 million rider-miles had been logged by CitiBike participants (Donohue 2013). Bike share kiosk programs in other locations have found that well-planned, ongoing community engagement is needed to reach a wide variety of residents and make these programs a long-term success accessible to a wide cross-section of city residents (Stewart et al. 2013). New York City has a large population of willing riders, and Hudson River public greenways. While CitiBike represents an innovative effort to reduce emissions and promote physical activity in New York City, it is not yet accessible in many poorer neighborhoods to members of the subpopulations who are most vulnerable to asthma. The fate of active transport in the Big Apple may depend on the support of people whose lives and health it's changing for the better.

Adaptation: Climate Health Preparedness and Reducing Air Pollution Vulnerability

Despite increasing exposures to climate-sensitive air pollution in many regions and the rise in underlying population vulnerability to that pollution, several strategies are available to prepare for climate change (Natural Resources Defense Council 2011):

- Identifying local vulnerabilities to air pollution at an individual, neighborhood, and community level by conducting air pollution vulnerability assessments

- Tracking air pollution–related health threats and establishing publicly available resources that allow the public to easily access daily monitoring data and forecasts

- Designing buildings, communities, and transportation systems to be more resilient to climate change

- Promoting outreach, communication, and the active engagement of health care providers, vulnerable communities, and policymakers in discussing and developing strategies to limit carbon pollution and associated air pollutants and adapt to the health-harming effects that cannot be avoided

Communication and outreach to share knowledge about air pollution vulnerabilities under a changing climate are critical for health care providers and administrators. As highly trusted messengers, clinicians and public health professionals as well as hospitals can become beacons of learning about climate preparedness, healthy eating, healthy energy sourcing, creating sustainable climate-smart communities, and much more—before people become ill or come with questions about healing.

There is no legislation or federal mandate that requires states to have a climate health adaptation plan or make climate action plans that target the most vulnerable communities to prepare. In fact, only about one-third of US states currently have a state climate preparedness plan with public health considerations in them. More states need to become prepared to meet changing health concerns, identify and prioritize planning to reduce climate health impacts or prepare for extreme weather events fueled by climate change, and learn from the experiences of people in the local neighborhoods who are most affected. In recent years, online interactive mapping tools and maps of climate health vulnerabilities including air pollution have been developed, which can be applied as a screening tool for discussing local vulnerability assessment needs (Natural Resources Defense Council 2011, 2012).

Creating healthier, more vibrant communities reflects the triple wins of reducing air pollution now; living healthier, more active lifestyles; and simultaneously reducing community carbon footprints with cleaner, more sustainable transportation and energy system choices. It is critical to remember that some of the worst air pollution effects of climate change remain preventable by significantly reducing fossil fuel combustion and thereby limiting heat-trapping carbon pollution. Reductions in fossil fuel combustion have the additional benefit of simultaneously reducing other health-harming air pollutants like $PM_{2.5}$ and air toxics. These health benefits for everyone go hand in hand with the longer-term benefits of healthier, more climate-secure communities for generations to come.

Conclusion

Research is needed to better assess the links between climate change, meteorology, air pollution, and health outcomes and to perform future modeling simulations to estimate the respiratory health effects of a changing climate, via air pollution changes (Grulke and Schilling 2008; Pinkerton et al. 2012; Reid and Gamble 2009). To accomplish this, some knowledge gaps and research needs demand further investigation:

- Gaps in environmental data, such as updating future projections of global ozone precursor emissions inventories and transboundary transport, especially for lower- and middle-income countries

- Studying how climate change and its effects on meteorology will affect PM concentrations locally in co-pollutant hot spots near fossil fuel emissions sources

- Looking at the combined effects of CO_2 and temperature on mold and interactions between these and other variables

- Experimental and field studies to examine how allergen content, distribution, growth, and genetic variation of pollens and of molds (indoor and outdoor) may be altered in response to changing CO_2 concentration, bioavailability, and temperature

- Ways that climate change (mediated by changes in precipitation, air humidity, and wind patterns) modifies pollutant deposition to landscapes and vegetation

- Evaluating how the impacts of urban warming or land use changes may exacerbate climate change's effects on desertification and loss of vegetation, which increase the likelihood and extent of dust storms; establishing better-bounded inventories of soot being produced by developing regions

- More investigation of soot particles' interactions with clouds

Other knowledge gaps pertain to the current understanding of human health impacts from air pollution exposures and local variations in both exposures and underlying vulnerabilities. For example, studies needed include:

- Health impact assessments for air pollution exposures that account for cumulative, long-term exposures to multiple air pollutants species

- Downscaling models of climate change effects on local air quality and its synergistic, cumulative effects on human health, especially in the most climate-vulnerable communities with different adaptive capacity

- Studies of how changes in humidity, precipitation, and extreme weather events affect respiratory exposures to mold, especially those brought on by flooding

- How underlying population vulnerability factors may change in the future, especially given a combination of vulnerability factors in some locations or among certain communities

- Considering how climate-forced drought and desertification and the long-term transport of mineral dusts will affect respiratory health

- Investigating how prescribed fires and wildfires contribute to regional air quality

- How climate change affects the frequency and intensity of forest fires regionally and, in turn, their likely impact on local and downwind human exposures to respiratory irritants

- Analyses of how drought conditions enhance wildfire risks and affect transport and subsequent case incidence of Coccidiomycoses or other infectious illnesses

- Investigation of source areas of haboob events across a wider area of the desert Southwest to help determine if they bear any relationship to changing incidence patterns of infectious disease or respiratory illnesses

- Evaluation of the extent to which climate change could alter time spent indoors versus outside, and time-behavior patterns for air pollution exposure assessments

- Local evaluations into how climate change could affect the frequency, intensity, and extent of forest fires and smoke production; associated smoke impact on human respiratory exposures; and possible interventions to limit harmful effects

A third type of knowledge gap comes from the need for monitoring data and ensuring better compatibility and consistency of meteorological, air quality/environmental, and health impact data sets across timescales. These might include:

- Linking existing long-term data sets on molds, fungi, and valley fever occurrence to those on respiratory illness and diseases that are available through the Environmental Public Health Tracking Network

- Creating a network of monitoring sites capable of detecting wildfire smoke downwind of source areas and estimating the contributing of wildfire smoke emissions to local air pollution as a way of better estimating smoke's effects on public health and of developing early warning systems to give advance warning of potentially harmful smoke conditions approaching far downwind

- Quantifying wildfire smoke exposures and health outcomes, as well as for other air pollutants with more centralized, real-time environmental monitoring linked with health tracking data at similar spatial and timescales nationwide

- Establishing a larger network of continuous or daily monitoring sites in air pollution–vulnerable communities across the United States

Despite advances in improving air quality overall in recent decades, climate change is making it more challenging to meet the goal of providing increasingly healthy air to breathe for communities everywhere. The effects of heat-trapping carbon pollution not only increase atmospheric temperatures but also alter key meteorological characteristics and flow patterns, and they affect the degree to which local pollutants are dispersed and how widely they may affect human health. To come to grips with this climate penalty with rising temperatures that make it tougher to achieve air quality compliance goals and the combined health impacts that increasingly include frequent extreme rainfalls, flood damage, drought, heat waves, and windstorms can have on respiratory health, adaptation and health preparedness strategies must be developed. This has become an urgent priority, because while these climate-sensitive effects on air quality and related exposures are increasing, many of the population's underlying health vulnerabilities are also on the rise: asthma prevalence increasing in all age categories, a rapidly aging American population, many families suffering from economic disadvantage, and communities faced with the health effects of long-term exposure to multiple air pollutants, whose effects are cumulative. In the face of these challenges, strong coordination and continuing active engagement among communities, clinicians, policymakers, and researchers is vital to move us toward healthier, more secure communities. Prevention of even more negative respiratory health effects today means limiting carbon pollution and harmful co-pollutants at their source. Better preparedness to face tomorrow's climate changes can be achieved by making climate health preparedness a national priority that also becomes a part of everyday conversation.

DISCUSSION QUESTIONS

1. America is in the midst of a national obesity health crisis. An estimated 17 percent of children aged two to nineteen years are obese, or 12.5 million kids. Since 1980, prevalence has almost tripled (Ogden and Carroll 2010). No matter what a person's age, getting daily physical exercise is important, and for many people making exercise a priority remains challenging. With climate change, are the messages becoming mixed? For example, encouraging children to go outdoors and get more exercise and play to stay physically fit flies in the face of concerns that in warmer summer months, ground-level ozone can threaten respiratory health, even for healthy athletes, especially in late afternoon hours after school in many parts of the country. And early-morning hours can be high-pollen hours during certain seasons of the year. How might clinicians, public health professionals, teachers, and parents work with available knowledge sources to best counsel their patients or their children to make the most health-enhancing choices about outdoor activities?

2. In trying to make decisions about how to project the future effects of climate change on air quality and the associated human health effects, how would you decide what combination of assumptions to use about, for example, precursor emissions inventories, population projections, changing prevalence over time of the health outcome being studied, and land use and land cover changes that can affect air quality? If incorporating each of these future projections introduces some level of uncertainty into modeling, should you include any at all?

3. China is in the midst of an air pollution crisis and in recent years, stories in the international press have shown compelling images of the visibly high concentrations of particulate and other air pollution in China's booming cities. Yet some have argued that the visible need

for improved regulation to improve air quality and reduce "traditional" air pollutants also affords a golden opportunity to make advances in limiting heat-trapping carbon pollution (see Buckley's *New York Times* article "Silver Lining in China's Smog As It Puts Focus on Emissions"). Do you think that an air quality or health crisis is what it takes to act as a policy lever to enact more long-lasting, health-protective policies? Why or why not? Can you name any parallels in domestic pollution-regulation policies? What do you think it would take to go beyond crises and move toward more health protective air pollution policies before public health is endangered?

4. One argument forwarded to avoid deeper regulation of air pollution is that society cannot afford to cut air pollution more significantly, not more than the gains already accomplished in the forty-plus years since the Clean Air Act was first passed, because stricter regulation of air pollution from industry or vehicles will cost jobs. This argument has been forwarded from business and industrial interests regarding regulation of toxic air pollutants; today, it is also applied in continuing efforts to limit carbon pollution from power plants. Others (often those in the public health and environmental justice community) counter that society cannot afford not to limit air pollutants and/or carbon pollution, since the associated health effect costs run into the billions in health effects and lives lost. Play devil's advocate and write a paragraph defending each side of the issue of figuring costs into air pollution regulation issues.

5. Go to the US Environmental Protection Agency website or other sources to gather some supporting information on costs related to air pollution regulation. Develop one to three points with supporting evidence on each side of the argument about why we should or should not limit either air toxics or carbon pollution. On the basis of your own evidence, select which you think is the more convincing argument and state why you were convinced of its merits.

KEY TERMS

Biogenic emissions: Chemical compounds that are emitted by natural sources. These include some volatile organic compounds emitted from trees and vegetation, such as monoterpenes and isoprenes, as well as emissions of nitrogen compounds from soil.

Nitrogen oxides (NO_x): A class of precursor compounds that, when combined in the atmosphere in the presence of sunlight along with VOCs, can form ground-level ozone, a major component of smog.

Volatile organic compounds (VOCs): Along with nitrogen oxides, precursor compounds of ozone, a major component of smog.

References

American Academy of Allergy, Asthma and Immunology/National Allergy Bureau. 2013. *Allergy Statistics.* http://www.aaaai.org/about-the-aaaai/newsroom /allergy-statistics.aspx

Anderson, G. B., and M. L. Bell. 2012. "Lights Out: Impact of the August 2003 Power Outage on Mortality in New York." *Toxicology* 3(2):1–5.

Anderson, J. G., D. M. Wilmouth, J. B. Smith, and D. S. Sayres. 2012. "UV Dosage Levels in Summer: Increased Risk of Ozone Loss from Convectively Injected Water Vapor." *Science Express,* July 27. doi.10.1126/science.1222978

Balbus, J. M., and C. Malina. 2009. "Identifying Vulnerable Subpopulations for Climate Change Health Effects in the United States." *Journal of Occupational and Environmental Medicine* 51:33–37.

Bell, M. L., and F. Dominici. 2008. "Effect Modification by Community Characteristics on the Short-Term Effects of Ozone Exposure and Mortality in 98 US Communities." *American Journal of Epidemiology* 167:986–97.

Bell, M. L., F. Dominici, and J. M. Samet. 2005. "Meta-Analysis of Ozone and Mortality and Comparison to a Multi-City Study." *Epidemiology* 16:436–45.

Bell, M. L., and K. Ebisu. 2012. "Environmental Inequality in Exposure to Airborne Particulate Matter Components in the United States." *Environmental Health Perspectives* 120:1699–1704.

Bell, M. L., R. G. Goldberg, C. Hogrefe, P. L. Kinney, K. Knowlton, B. Lynn, J. Rosenthal, C. Rosenzweig, and J. A. Patz. 2007. "Climate Change, Ambient Ozone, and Health in 50 US Cities." *Climatic Change* 82: 61–76. doi:10.1007 /s10584–006–9166–7

Bell, M. L., A. McDermott, S. L. Samet, J. M. Zeger, and F. Dominici. 2004. "Ozone and Mortality in 95 U.S. Urban Communities, 1987 to 2000." *Journal of the American Medical Association* 292:2372–78.

Berman, J. D., N. Fann, J. W. Hollingsworth, K. E. Pinkerton, W. N. Rom, A. M. Szema, P. N. Breysse, R. H. White, and F. C. Curriero. 2012. "Health Benefits from Large-Scale Ozone Reduction in the United States." *Environmental Health Perspectives* 120:1404–10. http://dx.doi.org/10.1289/ehp.1104851

Bond, T. C., S. J. Doherty, D. W. Fahey, P. M. Forster, T. Berntsen, B. J. DeAngelo, M. G. Flanner, et al. 2013. "Bounding the Role of Black Carbon in the Climate System: A Scientific Assessment." *Journal of Geophysical Research: Atmospheres* 118:5380–5552. doi:10.1002/jgrd.50171

Buckley, C. 2013. "Silver Lining in China's Smog as It Puts Focus on Emissions." *New York Times,* September 1, 6–8. http://www.nytimes.com/2013/09/01/world/asia /silver-lining-in-chinas-smog-as-it-puts-focus-on-emissions.html?hpw&_r=0

Center for American Progress. 2012. *Heavy Weather: How Climate Destruction Harms Middle- and Low-Income Americans.* http://www.americanprogress .org/wp-content/uploads/2012/11/ExtremeWeather.pdf

Centers for Disease Control and Prevention. 2011. "Borders, Budgets, and the Rising Risk of Disease." *Public Health blog entry* by Ali S. Khan, July 6. http://blogs .cdc.gov/publichealthmatters/2011/07/borders-budgets-disease/

Centers for Disease Control and Prevention. 2013a. *Valley Fever: Awareness Is Key.* http://www.cdc.gov/Features/ValleyFever/index.html

Centers for Disease Control and Prevention. 2013b. Coccidiomycosis ("Valley Fever"). http://www.cdc.gov/fungal/diseases/coccidioidomycosis

Centers for Disease Control and Prevention and U.S. Environmental Protection Agency, National Oceanic and Atmospheric Agency, and American Water Works Association. 2010. *When Every Drop Counts: Protecting Public Health during Drought Conditions—A Guide for Public Health Professionals.* Atlanta: US Department of Health and Human Services. http://www.cdc.gov/nceh/ehs /Publications/Drought.htm

Choi, M., F. C. Curriero, M. Johantgen, M.E.C. Mills, B. Sattler, and J. Lipscomb. 2011. "Association between Ozone and Emergency Department Visits: An Ecological Study." *International Journal of Environmental Health Research* 21:201–21. doi:10.1080/096–3123.2010.533366

Dai, A. 2011. "Drought under Global Warming: A Review." *WIREs Climate Change* 2:45–65. doi:10.1002/wcc81

Delfino R. J., S. Brummel, J. Wu, H. Stern, B. Ostro, M. Lispett, A. Winer, et al. 2009. "The Relationship of Respiratory and Cardiovascular Hospital Admissions to the Southern California Wildfires of 2003." *Occupational and Environmental Medicine* 66(3):189–97.

Dennekamp, M., and M. J. Abramson. 2011. "The Effects of Bushfire Smoke on Respiratory Health." *Respirology* 16:198–209.

Donohue, P. 2013. "Citi Bike Program Will Soon Top Mark of 1 Million Miles Traveled." *New York Daily News*, June 20. http://www.nydailynews.com/new-york /citi-bike-program-speeding-1st-milestone-article-1.1378709

Ebi, K. L., and G. McGregor. 2008. "Climate Change, Tropospheric Ozone and Particulate Matter, and Health Impacts." *Environmental Health Perspectives* 116(11):1449–55.

Fiore, A. M., L. W. Horowitz, D. W. Purves, H. Levy, M. J. Evan, Y. Wang, Q. Li, et al. 2005. "Evaluating the Contribution of Changes in Isoprene Emissions to Surface Ozone Trends over the Eastern United States." *Journal of Geophysical Research—Atmospheres* 110:12303.

Fiore, A. M., V. Naik, D. V. Spracklen, A. Steiner, N. Unger, M. Prather, D. Bergmann, et al. 2012. "Global Air Quality and Climate." *Chemical Society Reviews* 41:6663–83.

Fisk, W. J., Q. Lei-Gomez, and M. J. Mendell. 2007. "Meta-Analyses of the Associations of Respiratory Health Effects with Dampness and Mold in Homes." *Indoor Air* 17:284–96.

Friedman, M. S., K. E. Powell, L. Hutwanger, L. M. Graham, and W. G. Teague. 2001. "Impact of Changes in Transportation and Commuting Behaviors during the 1996 Summer Olympic Games in Atlanta on Air Quality and Childhood Asthma." *JAMA* 285:897–905.

Grabow, M. L., S. N. Spak, T. Holloway, B. Stone Jr., A. C. Mednick, and J. A. Patz. 2012. "Air Quality and Exercise-Related Health Benefits from Reduced Car Travel in the Midwestern United States." *Environmental Health Perspectives* 120(1):68–76.

Grulke, N., and S. Schilling. 2008. *Air Pollution and Climate Change*. Washington, DC: US Department of Agriculture, Forest Service, Climate Change Resource Center. http://www.fs.fed.us/ccrc/topics/air-pollution.shtml

Harries, J. E., and J. M. Futyan. 2006. "On the Stability of the Earth's Radiative Energy Balance: Response to the Mt. Pinatubo Eruption." *Geophysical Research Letters* 33:L23814. doi:10.1029/2006GL027457

Hogrefe, C. 2012. "Emissions versus Climate Change." *Nature Geoscience* 5(10):685–86.

Institute of Medicine. 2004. *Damp Indoor Spaces and Health*. Washington, DC: Committee on Damp Indoor Spaces and Health, Institute of Medicine, National Academies of Sciences.

Institute of Medicine. 2011. *Climate Change, the Indoor Environment, and Health*. Washington, DC: Committee on the Effect of Climate Change on Indoor Air Quality and Public Health. Institute of Medicine, National Academies of Sciences.

Intergovernmental Panel on Climate Change. 2012. *Managing the Risks of Extreme Weather Events and Disasters to Advance Climate Change Adaptation (SREX): A Special Report of Working Groups I and II of the IPCC*, edited by C. Field and coauthors. Cambridge: Cambridge University Press.

Ito, K., S. F. De Leon, and M. Lippmann. 2005. "Associations between Ozone and Daily Mortality." *Epidemiology* 16:446–57. doi:10.1097/01.ede.0000165821.90114.7f

Jacob, D. J., and D. A. Winner. 2009. "Effect of Climate Change on Air Quality." *Atmospheric Environment* 43(1):51–63.

Jacobson, M. Z. 2008. "On the Causal Link between Carbon Dioxide and Air Pollution Mortality." *Geophysical Research Letters* 35(3):L03809. doi:10.1029/2007GL031101

Jerrett, M., R. T. Burnett, C. A. Pope III, K. Ito, G. Thurston, D. Krewski, Y. Shi, et al. 2009. "Long-Term Ozone Exposure and Mortality." *New England Journal of Medicine* 360:1085–95. doi:10.1056/NEJMoa0803894

Johnston, F. H., S. B. Henderson, Y. Chen, J. T. Randerson, M. Marlier, R. DeFries, P. Kinney, et al. 2012. "Estimated Global Mortality Attributable to Smoke from Landscape Fires." *Environmental Health Perspectives* 120:695–701. http://dx.doi.org/10.1289/ehp.1104422

Johnston, F. H., A. M. Kavanagh, D. M. Bowman, and R. K. Scott. 2002. "Exposure to Bushfire Smoke and Asthma: An Ecological Study." *Medical Journal of Australia* 176:535–38.

Kinney, P. L. 2008. "Climate Change, Air Quality, and Human Health." *American Journal of Preventive Medicine* 35:450–67.

Knowlton, K., J. E. Rosenthal, C. Hogrefe, B. Lynn, S. Gaffin, R. Goldberg, C. Rosenzweig, et al. 2004. "Assessing Ozone-Related Health Impacts under a Changing Climate." *Environmental Health Perspectives* 112:1557–63.

Kunzli, N., E. Avol, J. Wu, W. J. Gauderman, E. Rappaport, J. Millstein, J. Bennion, et al. 2006. "Health Effects of the 2003 Southern California Wildfires on Children." *American Journal of Respiratory and Critical Care Medicine* 174:1221–28.

Lee, K. K. 2012. "Developing and Implementing the Active Design Guidelines in New York City." *Health and Place* 18:5–7.

Lei, H., D. J. Wuebbles, and X.-Z. Liang. 2012. "Projected Risk of High-Ozone Episodes in 2050." *Atmospheric Environment* 59:567–77.

Levy, J., S. Chermerynski, and J. Sarnat. 2005. "Ozone Exposure and Mortality." *Epidemiology* 16:458–68. doi:10.1097/01.ede.0000165820.08301.b3

Lipsher, S. 2007. "Wildfire Smoke a Culprit in Mercury's Spread." *Denver Post*, October 19.

Makri, A., and N. I. Stilianakis. 2008. "Vulnerability to Air Pollution Health Effects." *International Journal of Hygiene and Environmental Health* 211:326–36.

Marlier, M. E., R. S. DeFries, A. Voulgarakis, P. L. Kinney, J. T. Randerson, D. T. Shindell, Y. Chen, et al. 2013. "El Niño and Health Risks from Landscape Fire Emissions in Southeast Asia." *Nature Climate Change* 3:131–36.

Mudarri, D., and W. J. Fisk. 2007. "Public Health and Economic Impact of Dampness and Mold." *Indoor Air* 17:226–35.

Mudway I. S., and F. J. Kelly. 2000. "Ozone and the Lung: A Sensitive Issue." *Molecular Aspects of Medicine*, 21:1–48.

Naeher, L. P., M. Brauer, M. Lipsett, J. T. Zelikoff, C. D. Simpson, J. Q. Koenig, and K. R. Smith. 2007. "Woodsmoke Health Effects: A Review." *Inhalation Toxicology*, 19(1):67–106.

Natural Resources Defense Council. 2007. *Sneezing and Wheezing: How Global Warming Could Increase Ragweed Allergies, Air Pollution, and Asthma*, by K. Knowlton, M. Rotkin-Ellman, and G. Solomon. http://www.nrdc.org/globalwarming/sneezing/sneezing.pdf

Natural Resources Defense Council. 2011. *Climate Change Threatens Health*. www.nrdc.org/climatemaps

Natural Resources Defense Council. 2012. *Extreme Weather 2012*. www.nrdc.org/extremeweather

National Weather Service, Lubbock, Texas. 2013. "Intense Cold Front Produces Severe Winds and Blowing Dust—17 October 2011." http://www.srh.noaa.gov/lub/?n=events-2011–20111017-haboob

Ogden, C., and M. Carroll M. 2010. "Prevalence of Obesity among Children and Adolescents: United States, Trends 1963–1965 through 2007–2008." Division of Health and Nutrition Examination Surveys. http://www.cdc.gov/nchs/data/hestat/obesity_child_07_08/obesity_child_07_08.pdf

Pappagianis, D. 2007. "Coccidiomycosis in California State Correctional Institutions." *Annals of the New York Academy of Sciences* 1111:103–11.

Patz, J. A., H. K. Gibbs, J. A. Foley, J. A. Rogers, and K. R. Smith. 2007. "Climate Change and Global Health: Quantifying a Growing Ethical Crisis." *EcoHealth* 4:397–405. doi:10.1007/s10393–007–0141–1

Perera, F. P. 2008. "Children Are Likely to Suffer Most from Our Fossil Fuel Addiction." *Environmental Health Perspectives* 116:987–90.

Pinkerton, K. E., W. N. Rom, M. Akpinar-Elci, J. R. Balmes, H. Bayram, O. Brandli, J. W. Hollingsworth, et al. 2012. "An Official American Thoracic Society Workshop Report: Climate Change and Human Health." *Proceedings of the American Thoracic Society* 9(1):3–8.

Pope, C. A. III, R. T. Burnett, M. J. Thun, E. E. Calle, and G. D. Thurston. 2002. "Lung Cancer, Cardiopulmonary Mortality and Long Term Exposure to Fine Particulate Air Pollution." *Journal of the American Medical Association* 287:1132–41.

Pope, C. A. III, and D. W. Dockery. 2006. "Health Effects of Fine Particulate Air Pollution: Lines That Connect." *Journal of the Air and Waste Management Association* 56:709–42.

Ramin, B., and T. Svoboda. 2009. "Health of the Homeless and Climate Change." *Journal of Urban Health* 86:654–64.

Redman, J. 2012. "Connecting the Dots of Extreme Weather." *Albert Lea Tribune*, July 20. http://www.albertleatribune.com/2011/07/20/connecting-the-dots-of-extreme-weather/

Reid, C. E., and J. L. Gamble. 2009. "Aeroallergens, Allergic Disease, and Climate Change: Impacts and Adaptation." *EcoHealth* 6:458–70;. doi:10.1007/s10393–009–0261-x

Russell, A. G., E. Tagaris, K. Liao, and P. Amar. 2010. "Climate Impacts on Air Pollution and the Related Health Impacts and Increased Control Costs." Paper presented at the American Meteorological Association's 12th Conference on Atmospheric Chemistry and the 2nd Symposium on Aerosol-Cloud-Climate Interactions as part of the 90th American Meteorological Society Annual Meeting, January 16–21, Atlanta, GA.

Salo, P. M., S. J. Arbes Jr., M. Sever, R. Jaramillo, R. D. Cohn, S. J. London, and D. C. Zeldin. 2006. "Exposure to *Alternaria alternata* in US Homes Is Associated with Asthma Symptoms." *Journal of Allergy and Clinical Immunology* 118:892–98.

Santer, B. D., C. Mears, F. J. Wentz, K. E. Taylor, P. J. Glecker, T.M.L. Wigley, T. P. Barnett, et al. 2007. "Identification of Human-Induced Changes in Atmospheric Moisture Content." *Proceedings of the National Academies of Sciences of the United States of America* 104:15248–53.

Schwalm, C. R., C. A. Williams, K. Schaefer, D. Baldocchi, T. A. Black, A. H. Goldstein, B. E. Law, et al. 2012. "Reduction in Carbon Uptake during Turn of the Century Drought in Western North America." *Nature Climate Change* 5:551–56.

Shea, K. M., R. T. Truckner, R. W. Weber, and D. B. Peden. 2008. "Climate Change and Allergic Disease." *Journal of Allergy and Clinical Immunology* 122:443–53.

Sheffield, P. E., K. Knowlton, J. L. Carr, and P. L. Kinney 2011. "Modeling of Regional Climate Change Effects on Ground-Level Ozone and Childhood Asthma." *American Journal of Preventive Medicine* 41:251–57.

Sheffield, P. E., and P. J. Landrigan. 2011. "Global Climate Change and Children's Health: Threats and Strategies for Prevention. *Environmental Health Perspectives* 119:291–98. doi:10.1289/ehp.1002233

Shenassa, E. D., C. Daskalakis, A. Liebhaber, M. Braubach, and M. J. Brown. 2007. "Dampness and Mold in the Home and Depression: An Examination of Mold-Related Illness and Perceived Control of One's Home as Possible Depression Pathways." *American Journal of Public Health* 97:1893–99.

Spracklen, D. V., J. A. Logan, L. J. Mickley, R. J. Park, R. Yevich, A. L. Westerling, and D. A. Jaffe. 2007. "Wildfires Drive Interannual Variability of Organic Carbon Aerosol in the Western US in Summer." *Geophysical Research Letters* 34(16). L16816. doi:1029/2007GL030037

Spracklen, D. V., L. J. Mickely, J. A. Logan, R. C. Judman, R. Yevich, M. D. Flannigan, and A. J. Westerling. 2009. "Impacts of Climate Change from 2000 to 2050 on Wildfire Activity and Carbonaceous Aerosol Concentrations in the Western United States." *Journal of Geophysical Research* 114:D20301. doi:10.1029/2008JD010966

Stewart, S. K., D. C. Johnson, and W. P. Smith. 2013. "Bringing Bike Share to a Low-Income Community: Lessons Learned Through Community Engagement, Minneapolis, Minnesota; 2011." *Preventing Chronic Disease* 10:120274. doi: http://dx.doi.org/10.5888/pcd10.120274

Tagaris, E., K.-J. Liao, A. J. DeLucia, L. Deck, P. Amar, and A. G. Russell. 2010. "Sensitivity of Air Pollution–Induced Premature Mortality to Precursor Emissions under the Influence of Climate Change." *International Journal of Environmental Research and Public Health* 7:2222–37.

United Nation (UN) Foundation. 2012. *Global Alliance for Clean Cookstoves.* http://www.unfoundation.org/assets/pdf/global-alliance-for-clean-cookstoves-factsheet.pdf

US Department of Energy. 2013. *Transportation Energy Data Book: Edition 32,* edited by S. C. Davis and S. W. Diegel. Oak Ridge, TN: Oak Ridge National Laboratory.

US Environmental Protection Agency. 2013. *Particulate Matter—Health.* http://www.epa.gov/pm/health.html

US EPA. 2011. *The Benefits and Costs of the Clean Air Act from 1990 to 2010: Final Report—Rev. A.* Washington, DC: Office of Air and Radiation, April. http://www.epa.gov/cleanairactbenefits/prospective2.html

Wang, K., R. E. Dickinson, and S. Liang 2009. "Clear Sky Visibility Has Decreased over Land Globally from 1973 to 2007." *Science* 323:1468–70.

West, J. J., A. M. Fiore, L. W. Horowitz, and D. L. Mauzerall. 2006. "Global Health Benefits of Mitigating Ozone Pollution with Methane Emission Controls." *Proceedings of the National Academies of Sciences of the United States of America* 103:3988–93.

Westerling, A. L., and B. P. Bryant. 2008. Climate Change and Wildfire in California." *Climatic Change* 87(Suppl. 1):S231–49. doi:10.1007/s10584–007–9363-z

Wikipedia. 2015. "Haboobs." http://en.wikipedia.org/wiki/Haboob

Wolf, J., N. R. O'Neill, C. A. Rogers, M. L. Muilenberg, and L. H. Ziska. 2010. "Elevated Atmospheric Carbon Dioxide Concentrations Amplify *Alternaria alternata* Sporulation and Total Antigen Production." *Environmental Health Perspectives* 118:1223.

Zhang, Z., E. Whitsel, P. M. Quibrera, R. Smith, D. Liao, G. L. Anderson, and R. J. Prineas. 2009. "Ambient Fine Particulate Matter Exposure and Myocardial Ischemia in the Environmental Epidemiology of Arrhythmogenesis in the Women's Health Initiative (EEAWHI) Study." *Environmental Health Perspectives* 117:751–56.

Ziska, L. H., K. Knowlton, C. A. Rogers, D. Dalan, N. Tierney, M. A. Elder, W. Filley, et al. 2011. "Recent Warming by Latitude Associated with Increased Length of Ragweed Pollen Season in Central North America." *Proceedings of the National Academies of Sciences of the United States of America* 108:4248–51.

CHAPTER 6

EFFECTS OF CLIMATE CHANGE ON NONINFECTIOUS WATERBORNE THREATS

Lorraine C. Backer

The Earth's climate has warmed over the last 150 years, increasing the global average surface temperature about 1°C, increasing sea level about 20 centimeters, and decreasing snow cover in the Northern Hemisphere about 5 percent (Bindoff et al. 2007). The associated potential **public health** consequences include changes in **disease risk** and distribution subsequent to changes in disease ecology. Other consequences include premature deaths from extreme heat and cold, increased frequencies of extreme weather events, as well as morbidity and mortality from deteriorating air, food, and water quality (Confalonieri et al. 2007). Climate change will also directly affect the Earth's freshwater systems and the ocean. The resources provided by fresh and marine waters include clean water for drinking, agriculture, and industrial uses; seafood; recreation opportunities; transportation; and energy. As climate changes, these resources may be placed at risk. For example, changes in precipitation patterns, particularly an increased frequency of extreme precipitation events, will wash nutrients and other land-based pollutants into local waterways and eventually the ocean, where they will be incorporated into the food web. This chapter focuses on threats from cyanobacteria and algae blooms.

KEY CONCEPTS

- **Human activities and climate change interact to increase public health risks from exposure to cyanobacteria and algal toxins in drinking and recreational waters and in seafood.**

- **Climate change–induced changes to freshwaters and the ocean may favor proliferation of harmful cyanobacteria and algae.**

The findings and conclusions in this report are my own and do not necessarily represent the views of the Centers for Disease Control and Prevention/Agency for Toxic Substances and Disease Registry.

Harmful Algal Blooms

The term **harmful algal bloom** (HAB) refers to the proliferation of cyanobacteria or algae to concentrations that can threaten human, animal, and environmental health (Erdner et al. 2008). Direct effects of HABs include terrestrial and aquatic animal illnesses and deaths from exposure to toxins accumulated in seafood or entrained in aerosols. Specific routes of human exposure to HABs and related toxins include eating contaminated seafood, inhaling contaminated aerosols during water-related recreational or occupational activities, and drinking contaminated water (Backer et al. 2003, 2010; Backer, Kirkpatrick et al. 2005a; Backer, Rogers et al. 2005b; Fleming et al. 2005; Kirkpatrick et al. 2006). HABs can also cause environmental degradation by increasing **biological oxygen demand**, creating dense noxious algal mats, and preventing sunlight from reaching lower levels of the water column. These effects in turn have negative effects on fisheries, local economies, and coastal communities (World Health Organization 2009).

Freshwater cyanobacteria

Cyanobacteria (sometimes referred to as blue-green algae) are ubiquitous in freshwater ecosystems and may form **harmful cyanobacteria blooms,** dense blooms that are a threat to people, animals, and ecosystems. Cyanobacteria are capable of producing **cyanotoxins**, a group of structurally diverse compounds that include highly potent neurologic, liver, and kidney toxins, including anatoxin, cylindrospermopsin, **microcystins**, nodularins, and saxitoxons (Falconer 1993, 1998).

People can be exposed acutely or chronically to cyanotoxins in drinking and recreational waters. For example, in the past, occasional drinking water treatment system failures allowed cyanotoxins to enter community water supplies and caused outbreaks of gastrointestinal illness in the United States and Australia (see reviews by Falconer 1998; Carmichael 2001). A more serious event occurred in Brazil, where patients received fatal doses of microcystins when kidney dialysis water became contaminated (Carmichael 2001). Chronic exposure to low doses of microcysins, toxins produced by *Microcystis aeruginosa*, has been associated with high frequencies of liver cancer in people who drank ditch water in China (Yu 1989; Yu et al. 1989; Nishiwaki-Matsushima et al. 1992; Yu 1995).

In developed countries, sophisticated drinking water treatment and distribution systems make it less likely that people will be exposed to cyanotoxins through their drinking water. In these countries, the most common exposure to cyanotoxins occurs during recreational activities on water bodies with ongoing blooms. Initial studies did not find an association between individuals sailing or fishing in water with cyanobacterial blooms and self-reported symptoms, such as eye irritation or sore throat (Philipp, Brown, and Francis 1992). However, later studies found that those who were exposed to waters with concentrations of cyanobacteria more than 5,000 cells per milliliter during recreational activities were more likely to report at least one symptom during the week following exposure than were those exposed to waters that did not contain cyanobacteria (Pilotto et al. 1977). Reported symptoms included itchy skin rashes, hay-fever-like symptoms, gastrointestinal distress, and allergic reactions, as well as more severe symptoms such as headaches, fever, and blistering in the mouth.

A more recent study found that people who used personal watercraft on lakes with high cyanobacteria concentrations were twice as likely to report symptoms, particularly respiratory symptoms, than those who used their personal watercraft on lakes with low cyanobacteria concentrations (Stewart et al. 2006). Studies by Backer et al. (2008, 2010) examined exposures to aerosols generated by recreational activities on small lakes with ongoing *M. aeruginosa* blooms. Water, aerosol, personal breathing zone samples collected while people were engaged in recreational activities, and nasal swabs collected after exposure all contained low but measurable concentrations of microcystins. However, study participants did not report increases in symptoms following exposures.

The effects of harmful cyanobacteria blooms are not limited to people. Animals may also be exposed to and subsequently become ill from toxin-producing cyanobacteria blooms. During hot, dry summer months, algae flourish in small ponds where domestic animals (e.g., horses and cattle) drink and may result in fatal exposures to cyanotoxins (see Senior 1960 and Stewart et al. 2008 for review). Pets, particularly dogs, are at risk for acute fatal poisonings when they swim in or drink from ponds with dense toxin-producing blooms. In fact, an animal poisoning is often the first indication that a bloom has formed in a lake or pond. During the 2012 summer months, warmer-than-average temperatures and drought combined to support cyanobacteria blooms in many Georgia farm ponds. At least four dairy cows from one small ranch died from acute cyanobacteria toxin poisoning after drinking water from one of these ponds (University of Georgia 2012).

In addition to producing toxins that may become aerosolized during active blooms, intense cyanobacteria blooms generate foul odors and hydrogen sulfide when they senesce, or die off. Homeowners living near small lakes with ongoing blooms reported severe upper respiratory symptoms and irritating odors late in the bloom season (typically August and September).

During the late summer and early fall of 2009, people living near Lake Menomin and Tainter Lake in Wisconsin complained of unpleasant odors and respiratory symptoms they believed were associated with dying cyanobacteria blooms. On two separate occasions, representatives from the Bureau of Environmental and Occupational Health, Division of Public Health, State of Wisconsin, conducted air monitoring near the lakes for ammonia, hydrogen sulfide, and volatile organic compounds (VOCs), and collected air samples for laboratory analysis of various mercaptans and other sulfur-containing compounds. On September 17, 2009, air monitoring detected ammonia near both lakes (0.2 to 0.5 parts per million [ppm]) and hydrogen sulfide at Lake Menomin (0.2 to 0.8 ppm). In addition, air samples collected on September 29, 2009, found detectable amounts of diethyl disulfide and diethyl trisulfide in the air (290 parts per billion [ppb] and 500 ppb, respectively) around Tainter Lake (personal communication, Mark Werner, November 23, 2009). Although there are no national ambient air quality standards for ammonia or the sulfides detected near the lakes, Wisconsin does have ambient air standards for ammonia (0.60 ppm) and hydrogen sulfide (0.24 ppm), based on a 24-hour average (http://docs.legis.wisconsin.gov/code/admin_code/nr/445.pdf). For comparison, the National Institute for Occupational Safety and Health (NIOSH) recommends a maximum ten-hour time-weighted-average (TWA) occupational exposure of 25 ppm (fifteen-minute TWA of 35 ppm) for ammonia and a ten-minute TWA of 10 ppm of hydrogen sulfide (http://www.cdc.gov/niosh/npg/default.html). Currently, there are no recommended exposure limits for diethyl disulfide or diethyl trisulfide. Thus, although the odors generated by the dying bloom were noxious, there was little assumed acute risk for healthy people. However, many of the people who reported adverse effects had underlying chronic diseases, such as asthma or allergies, which could be exacerbated by these exposures (personal communication, Mark Werner and Ryan Wosniak).

Another example of the effects of cyanobacteria blooms on animals is the 2012 bird die-off at the Paul S. Sarbanes Ecosystem Restoration Project at Poplar Island, Chesapeake Bay, Maryland, associated with an outbreak of avian botulism compounded by a cyanobacteria bloom that produced microcystins (personal communication, Peter McGowan, January 23, 2013) (http://www.fws.gov/fieldnotes/regmap.cfm?framesFlag=0&arskey=33275&callingKey=executive_summary&callingValue=Poplar Island). A total of 769 birds and 8 mammals were collected, and 564 birds and all of the mammals died. Avian botulism was detected in 6 of 17 (35 percent) birds examined, and microcystins were detected in 16 of 25 (64 percent) birds tested. The birds were negative for common outbreak-associated infections, including avian influenza. The intoxicated birds were weak, dehydrated, and had paralysis of the wings and legs and drooping head symptoms that suggested neurotoxin poisoning such as that associated with avian botulism. However, these same symptoms were found in several birds negative for avian botulism but positive for microcytsin poisoning. No other cyanotoxins were found in water samples where blooms were present.

The effects from cyanobacteria blooms are not limited to direct exposure to such freshwater bodies with ongoing blooms. For example, sea otters living off the California coast became intoxicated by microcystins entrained in freshwater flows (Miller et al. 2010). Extensive blooms of cyanobacteria occurred in three nutrient-impaired rivers that flow into the Monterey Bay National Marine Sanctuary. Microcystin concentrations up to 2,900 ppm were detected in upstream waters within a kilometer of the ocean, and the deaths of twenty-one southern sea otters, a federally listed threatened species, were attributed to microcystin poisoning. In addition, farmed and free-living shellfish consumed by both people and the otters biomagnified microcystins to as much as 107 times the concentrations found in ambient waters. This event confirmed that both animals and people are at risk for microcystin poisoning when eating shellfish harvested at the land-sea interface (Miller et al. 2010).

Some nations have developed guidelines or regulations defining acceptable levels of cyanotoxins and cyanobacteria cells in drinking or recreational waters, and a newly published compendium of this guidance (Chorus 2012) is available online (http://www.uba.de/uba-info-medien-e/4390.html). The report demonstrates that the regulatory approach to protect people and the environment from cyanobacteria blooms varies by country. For example, in the United States, the states are largely responsible, and they primarily rely on guidelines published by the World Health Organization (WHO) or on risk assessments based on the WHO data (WHO 2003) to manage drinking water sources and recreational water bodies. It is notable that the WHO guidelines were based on cell concentrations rather than on cyanotoxin concentrations and that not all cyanobacteria blooms produce toxins. Resource managers and public health officials face competing priorities of protecting public health by closing a water body with a significant but possibly not toxic algal bloom and protecting the local tourism economy by keeping a water body with a visible, aesthetically unappealing bloom open for use.

In addition to using the WHO guidance, some states have done their own risk assessments to develop guidelines to support public health decision making, such as posting advisories or closing water bodies (Graham, Loftin, and Kamman 2009). For example, the Office of Environmental Health Hazard Assessment of the California Environmental Protection

Agency issued guidance on six cyanotoxins in 2012 (Butler, Carlisle, and Linville 2012). That guidance provides recommended action levels that may be applied by local, regional, state, or tribal entities to reduce or eliminate human and animal exposures to cyanobacteria toxins.

Other states have taken steps to protect their populations from cyanobacteria blooms. One example is Oklahoma, which was the first US state to pass legislation limiting exposure to freshwater algae (the bill can be viewed at http://legiscan.com/gaits/view/366438). The law requires the Oklahoma Tourism and Recreation Department to maintain a public website with freshwater cyanobacteria bloom information (www.checkmyoklake.com). The legislation defines the health-related warning thresholds: tourism officials will warn lake users if algae cell counts exceed 100,000 cells per milliliter and microcystin concentrations exceed 20 micrograms per liter. These levels conflict with WHO guidelines, which consider cell concentrations of 100,000 cells per milliliter indicative of a high probability of health effects (Chorus and Bartram 1999).

Another example is Kansas, which has taken a multifaceted approach to protecting its citizens that includes a website where people can get information and report potential blooms (http://www.kdheks.gov/algae-illness/index.htm) and an extensive outreach and education campaign that includes social media communication. Each Monday during the bloom season of 2012 and 2013, Odin, the Old English Bulldog, had a new message on the Kansas Department of Environmental Health (KDEH) Facebook page. Since Odin began starring in these messages, the number of KDEH Facebook friends has increased from 29 to nearly 400 (personal communication, Janet Neff, June 27, 2012).

Marine Algae

Seafood constitutes a significant proportion of the world's food supply, and more than 70 million tons are harvested each year. Per capita global annual seafood consumption averaged about 17 kilograms in 2008 (FAO Fisheries and Agricultural Department 2010), and estimated seafood consumption was 9 kilograms per person per year in the United States in 2000 (Spalding 1995). Although it is an important and popular food source, seafood is associated with a number of public health risks. In fact, seafood ranked third on the list of products most frequently associated with foodborne disease (Lipp and Rose 1997). One type of seafood-related disease, ciguatera fish poisoning, is the most commonly reported food poisoning caused by a chemical toxin (Centers for Disease Control and Prevention 1996).

Ciguatera fish poisoning (CFP) results from eating large reef fish contaminated with ciguatera toxins or ciguatoxins. Ciguatoxins, or their precursors, are produced by *Gambierdiscus toxicus* algae, are modified through metabolic pathways in the food web, and accumulate in fish, particularly larger carnivorous species such as barracuda (Heymann 2004).

From 2003 to 2012, 282 ciguatera fish poisoning cases were reported in Florida (data from Lazensky 2008). Four of Florida's sixty-seven counties contributed 71 percent of cases: Miami-Dade (43 percent), Palm Beach (15 percent), Broward (8 percent), and Monroe counties (5 percent). These southern coastal counties are located in close proximity to the Caribbean and the Bahamas. For many CFP cases, exposure occurred when they ate toxic fish, primarily barracuda and grouper, they caught themselves. Other species associated with Florida CFP cases are amberjack, snapper, tuna, kingfish, eel, trevally, sea bass, mackerel, hogfish, mahi-mahi, and mixed species in a ceviche dish.

In all, 243 (86 percent) cases were classified as outbreak associated (i.e., there were several people sick), 37 (13 percent) were single cases, and 2 (0.7 percent) were unknown (see table 6.1). To confirm exposure to ciguatoxins, leftover fish samples were tested for the presence of ciguatoxins at the FDA Laboratory on Dauphin Island.

CFP was acquired in Florida in 241 (86 percent) cases, in another state in 2 (0.7 percent) cases, and outside the United States in 39 (14 percent) cases. In case reports where the origin of the fish was captured in the

Table 6.1   Ciguatera Fish Poisoning, Frequency by Year, in Florida, 2003–2012

Year	Number of Cases
2003	7
2004	4
2005	10
2006	32
2007	29
2008	53
2009	49
2010	20
2011	48
2012	30

Source: Lazensky (2008).

Note: Florida's broad public health surveillance case definition for CFP includes clinically compatible illness and a history of fish consumption within twenty-four hours before onset of symptoms (Florida Department of Health 2014). Symptoms associated with CFP include abdominal cramps; nausea; vomiting; diarrhea; numbness and prickling sensation on lips and tongue, fingers and toes; metallic taste; muscle aches; rash; blurred vision; and sensitivity to hot and cold temperatures. To be considered a case of CFP, the victim must have eaten a species of fish that could be contaminated with ciguatoxins. CFP is not nationally notifiable, but many states choose to report cases.

electronic record (n = 33), the origin was most often the Bahamas (30, or 91 percent of cases), followed by Cuba (2, or 6 percent of cases), and St. Thomas (U.S. Virgin Islands) (1, or 3 percent of cases).

The year with the highest number of CFP cases (53) was 2009. Since then, at least 20 cases have been reported each year. The number of cases of CFP remains consistent even though the US annual consumption of fish and shellfish gradually decreased from 16.6 pounds in 2004 to 15.8 pounds per person in 2010 (Gall and Kern 2012). In addition, significant underreporting is suspected, as not all cases present to a physician. Finally, only a subset of cases that do seek medical attention will be accurately diagnosed with CFP and then reported to public health officials.

CLINICAL CORRELATES 6.1 THE HUMAN HEALTH RISKS OF CIGUATOXINS

Ciguatera toxin is one of the most common nonbacterial causes of fish-related food poisoning in the United States ("Marine Toxins" 2013). The disease is caused by consumption of certain tropical reef fish that bioaccumulate toxins from the algae *Gambierdiscus toxicus*. Although most cases are limited to the algae's geographical range of Florida and Hawaii, changing marine climates could have unpredictable effects on algae populations and cases of disease could rise. In addition, specialty fish are often shipped around the country, causing the disease to manifest outside its endemic range. Therefore, it is important for health care providers to be able to recognize the symptoms of poisoning.

Ciguatoxin is a heat and acid stable, odorless, tasteless (Lehane and Lewis 2000) compound that causes hyperpolarization of sodium channels in an array of tissues (Lewis et al. 1991), leading to a broad array of neurological symptoms. Common manifestations include paresthesias, numbness, headache, ataxia, vertigo, weakness, paralysis, and cranial nerve dysfunction (Tunik 2011). Gastrointestinal symptoms and hemodynamic instability also occur. Treatment is supportive, yet effects may last weeks. The differential diagnosis for ciguatoxin poisoning includes paralytic shellfish poisoning, stroke, eosinophilic meningitis, organophosphate poisoning, tetrodotoxin poisoning, and more. Clinicians must take a careful history to uncover this rare yet important cause of climate sensitive biopoisoning.

Ciguatera poisoning is a climate-sensitive cause of biopoisoning that clinicians must be aware of.

In cases where symptom data were entered into Florida's electronic database for reportable diseases (MERLIN), the following symptoms were reported by cases: nausea (185), joint pain (183), blurred vision (23), diarrhea (223), metallic taste (42), muscle pain (208), numbness (187), enhanced sensitivity to hot and cold temperatures (196), prickling sensation (179), and vomiting (138).

While most cases develop ciguatera fish poisoning after eating ciguatoxic fish, rare cases of sexual transmission and mother-to-child transmission have been reported. One case of mother-to-child transmission was reported by a mother who noticed a change in behavior in her three-year-old child following breast-feeding. She reported that the child experienced unusual sensitivity to hot and cold temperatures (Lazensky 2008).

Educational campaigns and outreach efforts targeted to medical providers may have contributed to enhanced awareness in recent years. While progress has been made, ongoing environmental changes that support the growth of *G. toxicus* and its expansion into the marine food web suggest that the incidence of CFP may increase over time (Gingold, Strickland, and Hess 2014).

The vast majority of food poisoning cases associated with seafood ingestion are caused by postharvest contamination with infectious organisms (e.g., *Salmonella* spp., *Campylobacter* spp., *Clostridium botulinum*, *Shigella* spp., *or Listeria* spp.), with toxins of bacterial origin (e.g., scombroid poisoning from high levels of histamine produced by *Vibrio* spp.), or are the result of allergies to shellfish (Lipp and Rose 1997). Other adverse health effects are associated with eating seafood contaminated with chemicals such as mercury. Another group of diseases is characterized by both acute and chronic neurological symptoms of varying intensity and duration associated with eating shellfish and reef fish. These diseases are caused when people eat seafood contaminated with potent neurotoxins naturally produced by marine algae.

Certain species of marine microalgae, such as dinoflagellates and diatoms, produce some of the most powerful known natural toxins. These toxins, called **phycotoxins**, may accumulate in a variety of marine organisms. These toxins are not destroyed by cooking or food preservation (e.g., heating, boiling, freezing, drying, or salting) and there are no antidotes against their biological activity (Schantz 1973). People who eat phycotoxin-contaminated seafood are at risk for a number of diseases, including neurotoxic shellfish poisoning (NSP), paralytic shellfish poisoning (PSP), amnesic shellfish poisoning (ASP), diarrhetic shellfish poisoning (DSP), and azaspiracid shellfish poisoning (AZP), as well as ciguatera fish poisoning (CFP). The brevetoxins associated with NSP may also be incorporated into sea spray during blooms, causing respiratory irritation in beach visitors. Detailed reviews of these syndromes have been published (Anderson 1994; Backer et al. 2003, 2008; Baden et al. 1995; Baden and Trainer 1993;

Clark et al. 1999; Falconer 1993; Fleming, Backer, and Rowan 2002; Halstead and Schantz 1984; Kirkpatrick et al. 2006; Tester 1994; Van Dolah 2000). A brief summary of the organisms, toxins, and clinical characteristics of these syndromes is in table 6.2.

CLINICAL CORRELATES 6.2 MONITORING PARALYTIC SHELLFISH TOXINS

The Washington State Department hosts one of the longest-running biotoxin monitoring programs. Since 1957, it has studied fluctuations in the concentrations of toxins in shellfish and has found a positive correlation between ocean temperature and the prevalence of the toxin-producing algae that are bio accumulated by shellfish (Moore et al. 2009). Many of these toxins cause significant human disease. For example, Saxitoxin, produced by the algae *Alexandrium catenella,* is covered by the UK Chemical Weapons convention because of its deadly potential (Moira 2003). When consumed in oysters, scallops, clams, and other shellfish, it interacts with sodium channels in nerve and muscle tissue, causing progressive numbness, headache, fever, nausea, vomiting, and diarrhea. In a dose-dependent relationship, these neurological complications can progress to respiratory arrest and death (Scoging 1998). Local health departments need to remain vigilant about predicting potential for toxic exposures from these algae and shellfish and make necessary closures. Underestimations of harm could lead to unnecessary illness, whereas overestimations could affect the local fishing economy.

Paralytic shellfish poisoning is a climate-sensitive environmental risk that needs ongoing monitoring and awareness on behalf of public health officials and clinicians in order to appropriately mitigate risks.

Table 6.2   Characteristics of Human Diseases and Conditions Caused by Eating Seafood Contaminated with Phycotoxins

	Diseases and Conditions					
Characteristic	Paralytic Shellfish Poisoning (PSP) and Puffer Fish Poisoning	Neurotoxic Shellfish Poisoning (NSP)	Diarrhetic Shellfish Poisoning (DSP)	Amnesic Shellfish Poisoning (ASP)	Azaspiracid Shellfish Poisoning (AZP)	Ciguatera Fish Poisoning (CFP)
Main area with endemic disease	Temperate areas worldwide	Gulf of Mexico, southern US coast, New Zealand	Europe, Japan	East and West Coasts of North America	Europe	Tropical coral reefs
Associated foods	Bivalve shellfish, some herbivorous fish and crabs	Bivalve shellfish	Bivalve shellfish	Bivalve shellfish, possibly some fin fish species	Bivalve shellfish	Large reef fish

(Continued)

	Diseases and Conditions					
Characteristic	Paralytic Shellfish Poisoning (PSP) and Puffer Fish Poisoning	Neurotoxic Shellfish Poisoning (NSP)	Diarrhetic Shellfish Poisoning (DSP)	Amnesic Shellfish Poisoning (ASP)	Azaspiracid Shellfish Poisoning (AZP)	Ciguatera Fish Poisoning (CFP)
Acute symptoms	Gastrointestinal Respiratory Cardiovascular Neurological, progressing to paralysis	Gastrointestinal Respiratory Cardiovascular Neurological Muscular aches	Gastrointestinal Other: chills, headache, and fever	Gastrointestinal Respiratory Cardiovascular Neurological	Gastrointestinal	Gastronintestinal Neurological Cardiovascular
Chronic symptoms	Unknown	Unknown	Unknown Possible carcinogen	Amnesia	Unknown	Paresthesias
Treatment	Supportive care Possibly respiratory support	Supportive care	Supportive care	Supportive care	Supportive care	Intravenous mannitol Supportive care Tricyclic antidepressants
Incubation time	5–30 minutes	30 minutes-24 hours	Less than 24 hours	Less than 24 hours	Less than 24 hours	Less than 24 hours
Duration	Days	Days	Days	Years	Days	Months
Death rate	1–14 percent	0 percent	0 percent	3 percent	Unknown	0.1–12 percent
Toxin (number)	Saxitoxin (20 or more)	Brevetoxin (10 or more)	Okadaic acid and dinophysistoxins (6 or more)	Domoic acid	Azaspiracid	Ciguatoxin (10 or more) Maitotoxin Scaritoxin
Toxin-producing organism	Dinoflagellates: *Gymnodinium catenatum, Pyrodinium bahamense* var. *compressum, Alexandrium* spp.	Dinoflagellate: *Karenia brevis* (formerly *Gymnodinium breve*)	Dinoflagellates: *Dinophysis* spp., *Prorocentrum lima*	Diatoms: *Pseudo-nitzschia* spp.	Dinoflagellate: *Protoperidinium* spp.	Epibenthic dinoflagellates: *Gambierdiscus toxicus*, possibly *Ostreopsis* spp.; *Coolia* spp.; or *Prorocentrum* spp.

Sources: Backer et al. (2003); Baden, Fleming, and Bean (1995); Baden and Trainer (1993); Fleming et al. (2001).

Climate Change and Harmful Algal Blooms

There is mounting evidence that potentially harmful algal blooms (HABs) and cyanobacteria blooms are occurring more frequently and across a wider geographic area than in the past (Viviani 1992; Epstein, Ford, and Colwell 1994; Halstead and Schantz 1984; Tester 1994;

Todd 1994; Glibert, Anderson, and Gentien 2005; Moore et al. 2008). Scientists disagree about whether this increase is associated with man-made influences (e.g., Hallegraeff et al. 1992) or natural processes (e.g., Sellner et al. 2003). However, the ultimate threat posed by a bloom likely derives from a combination of the overall increases in nutrients and other inputs associated with human activities into aquatic environments worldwide, and shifts in ocean conditions, large-scale climate oscillations, and changes in local weather patterns associated with climate change (Moore et al. 2008; Backer and Moore 2010).

CLINICAL CORRELATES 6.3 POLYBROMINATED DIPHENYL ETHERS

One of the most ubiquitous man-made persistent organic pollutants, the polybrominated diphenyl ethers (PBDEs), have been steadily accumulating in the environment since the late 1970s (Alaee and Weening 2002). They are found throughout the world, from core samples collected from the Bornholm deep in the Baltic Sea (Nylund et al. 1998), to human breast milk (Meironyte, Noren, and Bergman 1999). These chemicals enter drinking water sources and the food chain when sewers, landfills, and industrial sites overflow and chemicals are leached into soils. Leaching events may be accelerated by extreme weather, flooding, and other forms of climate change. Limited data are available about the human-toxic potential of PBDEs. Observational studies of factory workers exposed to PBDEs have shown sensory and motor abnormalities, as well as thyroid abnormalities (Darnerud et al. 2001). In rodent models, they appear fetotoxic, reducing fetal weights, causing severe generalized edema, and reducing ossification of the skull and long bones. Several studies have also shown complex malfunction of the thyroid gland and the immune system. More research is needed to understand the potentially vast effects of these chemicals in order to mediate effects and inform regulatory boards.

PBDEs are a climate-sensitive environmental pollutant that has wide-reaching and relatively unknown human health implications.

The ongoing and predicted changes to the ocean associated with climate change and increases in atmospheric carbon dioxide concentrations include increasing water temperatures; changes to upper ocean density, which will alter vertical water mixing; changes to nutrient supplies from the intensification or weakening of **upwelling**; ocean acidification; and changes to the timing and amount of freshwater inflows (Moore et al. 2008). The effects of these changes on marine HABs and HAB-related public health issues are not well understood, partly because there have been few ecologically relevant laboratory experiments and there are no long-term data sets for HAB events and HAB-related diseases (see Moore et al. 2008 for review). However, since climate change is expected to affect the factors that limit the growth of all algae (temperature, light, and nutrient availability), the responses of various HAB species will vary with their ecological and physiological diversity (Finkel et al. 2010). For example, as global temperatures increase, both ocean temperatures and freshwater runoff to the coast will increase stratification of the water column. Highly stratified water (e.g., warm freshwater overlaying cooler saltwater) undergoes less vertical mixing, thus decreasing the available supply of nutrients in surface waters normally contributed by deeper waters (Tozzi, Schofield, and Falkowski 2004). The conditions of increased temperatures and nutrient depletion favor organisms with lower nutrient requirements and those, such as **dinoflagellates** (the group of phytoplankton to which most harmful marine microalgae belong), with the ability to vertically migrate to nutrient-rich regions in the water column (Tozzi et al. 2004).

CLINICAL CORRELATES 6.4 HEALTH IMPLICATIONS OF HARMFUL ALGAE BLOOMS

Climate change is leading to more frequent and widespread HABs, thus increasing the incidence of human exposures. The impacts of HABs are diverse and may affect both coastal and inland communities. For example, *Kareina brevis,* the dinoflagellate responsible for Florida's red tide (Hoagland et al. 2009), blooms on an annual basis with varying degrees of intensity (Heil and Steidinger 2009). The cells of these organisms contain potent neurotoxins, which when lysed by wind and waves become aerosolized and can travel up to a mile inland (Fleming et al. 2005). Studies have linked the blooming of these algae with upper and lower respiratory symptoms including rhinorrhea, cough, and bronchoconstriction, especially in those with asthma and elderly people. High-intensity blooming events have been shown to correlate with increased emergency department use in nearby coastal areas (Kirkpatrick et al. 2006). Climate change and resulting changes to oceans may increase the intensity and occurrence of HABs, the costs of which include exacerbation of chronic illness and increased volumes of patients in emergency departments.

Increased incidence of HABs leads to exacerbation of chronic respiratory illness and increases patient volumes in nearby emergency departments.

In addition to nutrients, pH is an important contributor to the success or failure of specific species of ocean phytoplankton. Since the beginning of the Industrial Revolution, the atmospheric concentration of carbon dioxide increased from about 280 ppm to 380 ppm (Bindoff et al. 2007). The ocean readily absorbs atmospheric carbon dioxin to increase the concentrations of carbon dioxide and bicarbonate in seawater, making it more acidic (Bindoff et al. 2007). Since the Industrial Revolution, the pH of seawater has dropped from 8.2 pH units to 8.1 pH units. pH is measured on a logarithmic scale; thus a 0.1 decrease represents a 30 percent increase in the concentration of free hydrogen ions (Caldiera and Wickett 2003; Riebesell 2004; Orr et al. 2005; Bindoff et al. 2007). If carbon dioxide emissions continue at current levels, seawater pH could drop an additional 0.6 pH units (Moore et al. 2008). The additional free hydrogen ions compete with calcium ions for carbonate ions, which are used by calcifying organisms to produce calcium carbonate (e.g., for shells). Corals are the best known of the calcifying organisms; however, about 70 percent of global calcium carbonate is accounted for by planktonic organisms, including some phytoplankton. Thus, a more acidic ocean environment would likely favor noncalcifying organisms, such as the dinoflagellates (again, the phytoplankton group comprising most harmful algae).

Changes in the timing and amount of stream flow and snowmelt may also affect the distribution of bloom events, possibly putting new populations of people and animals at risk. For example, in coastal regions experiencing increased freshwater flows, new areas may be exposed to freshwater cyanobacteria toxins present in stream plumes that extend farther offshore (see the earlier sea otter example), whereas regions experiencing decreased freshwater flows might see marine HAB events farther upstream (GEOHAB 2006).

Even given the uncertainty in predicting how climate change will affect phytoplankton, some changes have been observed already. For example, *Gambierdiscus toxicus* and other dinoflagellate microalgae responsible for ciguatera fish poisoning are generally either epiphytic (they grow on another plant for support but derives its own nutrients) or benthic (they grow on or within the bottom surfaces, such as sediments) and are typically not affected by the oceanographic processes experienced by planktonic (i.e., drifting) algae. However, their growth is dependent on the temperature and salinity of surrounding waters. Hales, Weinstein, and Woodward (1999) found strong positive correlations between the annual incidence of CFP and warming of the sea surface near a group of Pacific islands during El Niño Southern Oscillation events. The investigators observed the opposite effect in a group of islands where the sea surface cooled during El Niño events. *G. toxicus* may also expand its range into higher latitudes as water temperatures rise more generally due to climate change, thus expanding the number of people potentially at risk (Tester 1994).

Climate-change-induced damage to corals may also increase the risk for CFP. Dead corals form a hospitable surface for colonization by filamentous and calcareous macroalgae, a substrate preferred by the CFP-associated dinoflagellates (Hallegraeff, Anderson, and Cembella 1995). Physical damage to coral reefs has been associated with both increased abundance of *G. toxicus* (Lewis 1986) and CFP outbreaks (Ruff and Lewis 1994; de Sylva 1994). Degradation of the reef environment may also be caused by other man-made forces, including tourism, the aquarium trade, ship groundings, and natural forces possibly associated with climate change, including eutrophication, freshwater runoff, and sedimentation (Lehane and Lewis 2000).

Warming ocean temperatures may also exacerbate public health risks from *Alexandrium catenella*, which produces the saxitoxins associated with PSP. *A. catenella* shows accelerated growth and causes shellfish to become toxic in the Puget Sound, Washington, when temperatures are greater than 13°C, which typically occurs between July and November (Nishitani and Chew 1984; Moore et al. 2009). As the ocean warms, the number of days this temperature is exceeded will likely increase, possibly promoting more prolonged blooms and increased public health risks and costs (Moore et al. 2008).

Climate-induced changes in ocean currents may also affect local or regional risks from HAB toxins. For example, ASP outbreaks along the northern Pacific coast of the United States are apparently modulated by an eddy that resides offshore of the Straits of Juan de Fuca. There is a fairly steady supply of nutrients to support growth of *Pseudo-nitzschia multiseries*, the organism associated with ASP. Surface currents transport materials from the eddy to adjacent shelf waters (MacFadyen, Hickey, and Foremann 2005), providing a direct link between the toxin-producing algae and coastal razor clams and creating a periodic public health hazard for people harvesting the clams (Backer and McGillicuddy 2006). Currently NOAA researchers are able to predict which beaches will harbor toxin-contaminated clams, and they produce a bulletin with information about areas that are safe for harvesting (Trainer and Suddleson 2005). However, climate-induced changes in the supply of nutrients, such as changes in upwelling or in coastal freshwater inflows (MacFadyen et al. 2005) or the specific movements of this eddy may modulate this public health risk or make the risk less easy to predict.

Increased surface temperatures from global climate change are also affecting cyanobacteria bloom distribution and temporal extent (Paerl and Huisman 2009). Extraordinary blooms of *Microcystis aeroginosa* have occurred in Lake Erie. For example, in August 2003, a massive bloom that produced high concentrations of microcystins formed in western Lake Erie. The bloom produced foul-smelling algal mats that washed ashore, making beaches and boating areas unusable and affecting local sport fishing

(Backer and McGillicuddy 2006). This bloom was only the latest in a trend over the last decade (Bridgeman 2005), and blooms have lasted well into the fall, when the lake should have been too cold to support substantial algae growth.

Conclusion

As the Earth's climate changes, there will likely be increases in health threats associated with changes in the Earth's freshwater systems and the oceans that support rapid growth of cyanobacteria and algae. Increased contamination of drinking water sources, recreational waters, and aquatic food resources pose challenges for water resource managers and those responsible for ensuring seafood quality and has important implications for public health.

DISCUSSION QUESTIONS

1. Researchers have suggested that we seed the ocean with iron to support extensive algal blooms that will sequester CO_2. What might be the unintended consequences of this action?

2. How might climate change affect risks from eating seafood?

3. Besides threats to human health, what other long-term effects might occur as the result of increased freshwater cyanobacteria blooms?

KEY TERMS

Biological oxygen demand: The amount of dissolved oxygen needed by aerobic biological organisms in a body of water to break down the organic material present in water sample at a certain temperature over a specific time period.

Cyanobacteria: Class of organisms (sometimes referred to as blue-green algae) that contain photosynthetic pigments and can perform oxygenic photosynthesis (Skulbert et al. 1993). Their algae-like morphology and photosynthetic capabilities have historically made them difficult to classify. Cyanobacteria represent the oldest living organisms on Earth, and produce most of the Earth's oxygen.

Cyanotoxins: A group of chemically diverse compounds produced as secondary metabolites by cyanobacteria. These include anatoxin-a, anatoxin-a(s), cylindropsermopsin, microcystins, nodularins, and saxitoxins (Carmichael and Falconer 1993).

Dinoflagellates: Microalgae that are ubiquitous in liquid habitats, including terrestrial snow, Antarctic ice slush, and seawater in the spaces between sand grains. Their life cycles and the fossil record reflect years of successful adaptations to environmental changes (Steidinger 1993).

Disease risk: The chance of getting a certain disease in a certain amount of time. The risk depends on all the factors (genetic makeup, environmental factors, lifestyle choices) that would affect whether one gets the disease.

Harmful algal bloom: The proliferation of algae to concentrations that can threaten human, animal, and environmental health. Harmful algal blooms may become dense enough to deplete the amount of oxygen in the water and prevent light from reaching the lower depths of the water column. These blooms may also produce toxins that can accumulate in the algae, ambient waters, and the food web.

Harmful cyanobacteria blooms: Extensive or dense blooms of cyanobacteria that cause harm to the local ecology, animals, or people.

Microcystins: A group of structurally similar cyanotoxins that induce liver damage.

Phycotoxins: A group of chemically diverse compounds produced as secondary metabolites by marine microalgae. These compounds include numerous derivatives of saxitoxin, okadaic acid, brevetoxin, ciguatoxin, and domoic acid polyethers (e.g., brevetoxins), saxitoxins.

Public health: The science and art of protecting and improving the health of communities through research and education.

Upwelling: Wind-driven motion of dense, cool, and typically nutrient-rich water toward the ocean surface, replacing the warmer, usually nutrient-depleted surface waters. The nutrient-rich upwelled water stimulates the growth and reproduction of primary producers, such as phytoplankton.

References

Alaee, M., and R. Weening. 2002. "The Significance of Brominated Flame Retardants in the Environment: Current Understanding, Issues and Challenges." *Chemosphere* 46:579–82.

Anderson, D. 1994. "Red Tides." *Scientific American* 271(2):62.

Backer, L. C., W. Carmichael, B. Kirkpatrick, C. Williams, M. Irvin, Y. Zhou, T. B. Johnson, et al. 2008. "Recreational Exposure to Microcystins during a *Microcystis aeruginosa* bloom in a Small Lake." *Marine Drugs* 6(2):389–406.

Backer, L. C., L. E. Fleming, A. Rowan, Y.-S. Cheng, J. Benson, R. H. Pierce, J. Zaias, et al. 2003. "Recreational Exposure to Aerosolized Brevetoxins during Florida Red Tide Events." *Harmful Algae* 2:19–28.

Backer, L. C., B. Kirkpatrick, L. Fleming, Y.-S. Cheng, R. Pierce, J. Bean, R. Clark, et al. 2005a. "Occupational Exposure to Aerosolized Brevetoxins during Florida

Red Tide Events: Impacts on a Healthy Worker Population." *Environmental Health Perspectives* 113:644–49.

Backer, L., and D. J. McGillicuddy Jr. 2006. "Harmful Algal Blooms: At the Interface between Coastal Oceanography and Human Health." *Oceanography* 19(2):94–106.

Backer, L. C., S. V. McNeel, T. Barber, B. Kirkpatrick, C. Williams, M. Irvin, Y. Zhou, et al. 2010. "Recreational Exposure to Microcystins during Algal Blooms in Two California Lakes." *Toxicon* 55:909–21.

Backer, L. C., and S. K. Moore. 2010. "Harmful Algal Blooms: Future Threats in a Warmer World." In *Environmental Pollution and Its Relation to Climate Change*, edited by A. E. Nemr, 485–512. New York: Nova Science.

Backer, L. C., H. Rogers, L. Fleming, B. Kirkpatrick, and J. Benson. 2005b. "Phyco-toxins in Marine Seafood." In *Toxins in Food*, edited by W. M. Dabrowski and Z. E. Sikorski, 155–89. Boca Raton, FL: CRC Press.

Baden, D., L. Fleming, and J. Bean. 1995. "Marine Toxins." In *Handbook of Clinical Neurology: Intoxications of the Nervous System Part II. Natural Toxins and Drugs*, edited by F. A. deWolff, 141–75. Amsterdam: Elsevier Press.

Baden, D., and V. L. Trainer 1993. "Mode of Action of Toxins of Seafood Poisoning." In *Algal Toxins in Seafood and Drinking Water*, edited by I. R. Falconer, 49–74. San Diego: Academic Press.

Bindoff, N. L., J. Willebrand, V. Artale, A. Cazenave, J. Gregory, S. Gulev, K. Hanawa, et al. 2007. "Observations: Oceanic Climate Change and Sea Level." In *Climate Change 2007: The Physical Science Basis. Contribution of Working Group I to the Fourth Assessment Report of the Intergovernmental Panel on Climate Change*, edited by S. Solomon, D. Qin, M. Manning, Z. Chen, M. Marquis, K. B. Avery, M. Tignor, et al. Cambridge: Cambridge University Press.

Bridgeman, T. B. 2005. "The Microcystis Blooms of Western Lake Erie (2003–2004)." Paper presented at the 48th Annual Meeting of the International Association for Great Lakes Research, Ann Arbor, MI, May 23–27.

Butler, N., J. Carlisle, and R. Linville. 2012. "Toxicological Summary and Suggested Action Levels to Reduce Potential Adverse Health Effects of Six Cyanotoxins." Sacramento: Office of Environmental Hazard Assessment, California Environmental Protection Agency.

Caldiera, K., and M. E. Wickett. 2003. "Anthropogenic Carbon and Ocean pH." *Nature* 425:365.

Carmichael, W. W. 2001. "Health Effects of Toxin-Producing Cyanobacteria: The CyanoHABs." *Human and Ecological Risk Assessment* 7:1393–1407.

Carmichael, W. W., and I. Falconer. 1993. "Diseases Related to Freshwater Blue-Green Algal Toxins, and Control Measures." In *Algal Toxins in Seafood and Drinking Water*, edited by I. R. Falconer, 187–209. Orlando, FL: Academic Press.

Centers for Disease Control and Prevention. 1996. "Surveillance for Foodborne Disease Outbreaks—United States, 1988–1999." *Morbidity and Mortality Weekly Report* 45 (SS-5):1.

Chorus, I., and J. Bartram. 1999. *Toxic Cyanobacteria in Water: A Guide to Their Public Health Consequences, Monitoring, and Management*. London: E&FN Spon.

Chorus, I., ed. 2012. *Current Approaches to Cyanotoxin Risk Assessment, Risk Management and Regulations in Different Countries*. Dessau Rosslau: Germany Federal Environment Agency.

Clark, R. F., S. R. Williams, S. P. Nordt, and A. S. Manoguerra. 1999. "A Review of Selected Seafood Poisonings." *Journal of the Undersea and Hyperbaric Medicine Society* 26(3):175.

Confalonieri, U., B. Menne, R. Akhtar, K. L. Ebi, M. Hauenque, R. S. Kovats, B. Revich, and A. Woodward. 2007. "Human Health." In *Impacts, Adaptation and Vulnerability Contribution of Working Group II to the Fourth Assessment Report of the Intergovernmental Panel on Climate Change*, edited by M. L. Parry, O. F. Canziani, J. P. Palutikof, P. J. van der Linden, and C. E. Hanson, 391–431. Cambridge: Cambridge University Press.

Darnerud, P. O., G. S. Eriksen, T. Johannesson, P. Larsen, and M. Viluksela. 2001. "Polybrominated Biphenyl Ethers: Occurrence, Dietary Exposure and Toxicity." *Environmental Health Perspectives* 109:49–68.

De Sylva, D. P. 1994. "Distribution and Ecology of Ciguatera Fish Poisoning in Florida, with Emphasis on the Florida Keys." *Bulletin of Marine Science* 54:944–54.

Erdner, D. L., J. Dyble, M. L. Parsons, R. C. Stevens, K. A. Hubbard, M. L. Wrabel, S. K. Moore, et al. 2008. "Centers for Oceans and Human Health: A Unified Approach to the Challenge of Harmful Algal Blooms." *Environmental Health* 7(Suppl. 2):S2.

Epstein, P., T. Ford, and R. Colwell. 1994. "Marine Ecosystems." In *Health and Climate Change*, edited by P. Epstein and D. Sharp, 14–17. London: Lancet.

Falconer, I. 1993. "Measurement of Toxins from Blue-Green Algae in Water and Foodstuffs." In *Algal Toxins in Seafood and Drinking Water*, edited by I. R. Falconer, 165–75. Orlando, FL: Academic Press.

Falconer, I. 1998. "Algal Toxins and Human Health." In *The Handbook of Environmental Chemistry*, vol. 5, edited by J. Hrub, 53–82. Berlin: Springer-Verlag.

Finkel, Z. V., J. Beardall, K. J. Flynn, A. Quigg, T.A.V. Rees, and J. A. Raven. 2010. "Phytoplankton in a Changing World: Cell Size and Elemental Stoichiometry." *Journal of Plankton Research* 32:119–37.

Fleming, L. E., L. Backer, and A. Rowan. 2002. "The Epidemiology of Human Illnesses Associated with Harmful Algal Blooms." In *Neurotoxicology Handbook*, vol. 1: *Natural Toxins of Marine Origin*, edited by D. J. Adams, D. Baden, J. Bloomquist, M. Ehrich, T. Guilarte, and A. Harvey, 363–81. Totowa, NJ: Humana Press.

Fleming, L. E., J. A. Bean, D. Katz, and R. Hammond. 2001. "The Epidemiology of Seafood Poisoning." In *Foodborne Disease Handbook*, volume 4, edited by Y. H. Hui, Do kits, and P. S. Stanfield, 287–310. New York: Marcel Dekker.

Fleming, L. E., D. Kirkpatrick, L. Backer, J. Bean, A. Wanner, D. Dalpra, R. Tamer, et al. 2005. "Initial Evaluation of the Effects of Aerosolized Florida Red Tide Toxins (Brevetoxins) in Persons with Asthma." *Environmental Health Perspectives* 113:650–57.

Florida Department of Health. 2014. "Ciguatera Fish Poisoning." http://www
.floridahealth.gov/diseases-and-conditions/disease-reporting-and-management
/disease-reporting-and-surveillance/_documents/gsi-ciguatera.pdf

Food and Agriculture Organization (FAO). Fisheries and Aquaculture Department.
2010. *The State of World Fisheries and Aquaculture.* Rome: Food and
Agriculture Organization of the United Nations. http://www.fao.org/docrep/013
/i1820e/i1820e00.htm.

Gall, K., and S. Kern. 2012. "Seafood Health Facts." http://seafoodhealthfacts.org
/overview.php#ack

GEOHAB. 2006. *Global Ecology and Oceanography of Harmful Algal Blooms: Harmful Algal Blooms in Eutrophic Systems.* Paris and Baltimore: Intergovernmental
Oceanographic Commission and Scientific Committee on Ocean Research.

Gingold, D. B., M. J. Strickland, and J. J. Hess. 2014. "Ciguatera Fish Poisoning and
Climate Change: Analysis of National Poison Center Data in the United States,
2001–2011." *Environmental Health Perspectives* 122:580–86.

Glibert, P. M., D. M. Anderson, and P. Gentien. 2005 "The Global Complex Phenomena of Harmful Algae." *Oceanography* 18:36–147.

Graham, J. L., K. A. Loftin, and N. Kamman. 2009. "Monitoring Recreational
Freshwaters." *Lakeline* (Summer):18–24.

Hales, S., P. Weinstein, and A. Woodward. 1999. "Ciguatera (Fish Poisoning), El
Niño, and Pacific Sea Surface Temperatures." *Ecosystem Health* 5(1):20–25.

Hallegraeff, G. M., D. M. Anderson, and A. D. Cembella, eds. 1995. *Manual on
Harmful Marine Microalgae.* New York: UNESCO.

Hallegraeff, G. M., M. A. McCausland, and T. K. Brow. 1992. "Early Warning of
Toxic Dinoflagellate Blooms of *Gymnodinium catenatum* in Southern Tasma-
nian Waters." *Journal of Plankton Research* 17:1163–76.

Halstead, B. W., and E. Schantz. 1984. *Paralytic Shellfish Poisoning.* Geneva: World
Health Organization.

Heil, A., and K. A. Steidinger. 2009. "Monitoring, Management and Mitigation of
Kareina Blooms in the Eastern Gulf of Mexico." *Harmful Algae* 8:611–17.

Heymann, D. L., ed. 2004. *Control of Communicable Diseases Manual,* 18th ed.
Washington, DC: American Public Health Association.

Hoagland, P., D. Jin, L. Y. Polansky, B. Kirkpatrick, G. Kirkpatrick, L. E. Fleming,
A. Reich, S. M. Watkins, S. G. Ulmann, and L. C. Backer. 2009. "The Costs of
Respiratory Illnesses Arising from Florida Gulf Coast *Karenia brevis* Blooms."
Environmental Health Perspectives 117:1239–43.

Kirkpatrick, B., L. E. Fleming, L. C. Backer, J. A. Bean, R. Tamer, G. Kirkpatrick,
T. Kane, et al. 2006. "Environmental Exposures to Florida Red Tides: Effects
on Emergency Room Respiratory Diagnoses Admissions." *Harmful Algae*
5:526–33.

Lazensky, B. 2008. "Florida Department of Health, Nassau County Health Department, Investigation of a Cluster of Ciguatera Fish Poisoning Cases (*n* = 13) in
Restaurant Patrons Who Consumed Grouper." Unpublished data.

Lehane, L., and R. J. Lewis 2000. "Ciguatera: Recent Advances But the Risk Remains." *International Journal of Food Microbiology* 61:91–125.

Lewis, N. D. 1986. "Disease and Development: Ciguatera Fish Poisoning." *Social Science and Medicine* 23:983–93.

Lewis, R. J., M. Sellin, M. A. Poli, R. S. Norton, J. K. MacLeod, and M. M. Sheil. 1991. "Purification and Characterization of Ciguatoxins from Moray Eel (*Lycodontis javanicus, Muraenidae*)." *Toxicon* 29:1115–27.

Lipp, E. K., and J. B. Rose. 1997. "The Role of Seafood in Foodborne Disease in the United States of America." *Revue scientifique et technique* 16(2):620.

"Marine Toxins." 2013. Atlanta: National Center of Emerging and Zoonotic Infectious Diseases, Centers for Disease Control. http://www.cdc.gov/nczved /divisions/dfbmd/diseases/marine_toxins/#diseases

MacFadeyn, A., B. M. Hickey, and M.G.G. Foremann. 2005. "Transport of Surface Waters from the Juan de Fuca Eddy Region to the Washington Coast." *Continental Shelf Research* 35:2008–21.

Meironyte, G. D., K. Noren, and A. Bergman. 1999. "Analysis of Polybrominated Diphenyl Ethers in Swedish Human Milk: A Time-Related Trend Study, 1972–1997." *Journal of Toxicology and Environmental Health, Part A* 58:101–13.

Miller, M. A., R. M. Kudela, A. Mekebri, D. Crane, S. C. Oates, M. T. Tinker, M. Staedler, et al. 2010. "Evidence for a Novel Marine Harmful Algal Bloom: Cyanotoxin (Microcystin) Transfer from Land to Sea Otters." *PLoS One* 5(9):e12576. doi:10.1371/journal.pone.0012576

Moore, S. K., N. J. Mantua, B. M. Hickey, and V. L. Trainer. 2009. "Recent Trends in Paralytic Shellfish Toxins in Puget Sound, Relationships to Climate, and Capacity for Prediction of Toxic Events." *Harmful Algae* 8:463–77.

Moore, S. K., V. L. Trainer, N. J. Mantau, M. S. Parker, E. A. Laws, L. C. Backer, and L. E. Fleming. 2008. "Impacts of Climate Variability, Climate Change and Harmful Algal Blooms." *Mini-Monograph: Research in Oceans and Human Health. Environmental Health* 7 (Suppl. 2):S4. PMC 2586717.

Nishitani, T., and K. K. Chew. 1984. "Recent Developments in Paralytic Shellfish Poisoning Research." *Aquaculture* 39:317–29.

Nishiwaki-Matsushima, R., T. Ohta, S. Nishiwaki, M. Suganuma, K. Kohyama, T. Ishikawa, W. W. Carmichael, and H. Fujiki. 1992. "Liver Cancer Promotion by the Cyanobacterial Cyclic Peptide Toxin Microcystin-LR." *Journal of Cancer Research and Clinical Oncology* 118:420–24.

Nylund, K., L. Asplund, B. Jansson, P. O. Jonsson, K. Litzen, and U. Sellstrom. 1998. "Analysis of Some Polyhalogenated Organic Pollutants in Sediment and Sewage Sludge." *Chemosphere* 24:1721–30.

Orr, J. C., V. J. Fabry, O. Aumont, L. Boop, S. C. Doney, R. A. Feely, A. Ganadesikan, N. Gruber, et al. 2005. "Anthropogenic Ocean Acidification over the Twenty-First Century and Its Impact on Calcifying Organisms." *Nature* 437:681–86.

Paerl, H., and J. Huisman. 2009. "Climate Change: A Catalyst for Global Expansion of Harmful Cyanobacterial Blooms." *Environmental Microbiology Reports* 1(1):27–37.

Philipp, R., M. Brown, and F. Francis. 1992. "Health Risks Associated with Recreational Exposure to Blue-Green Algae (Cyanobacteria) When Windsurfing and Fishing." *Health and Hygiene* 13:115–19.

Pilotto, L. C., R. M. Douglas, S. Cameron, M. Beers, G. J. Rouch, P. Robinson, M. Kirk, et al. 1997. "Health Effects of Exposure to Cyanobacteria (Blue-Green Algae) during Recreational Water-Related Activities." *Australian and New Zealand Journal of Public Health* 21:562–66.

Riebesell, U. 2004. "Effects of CO2 Enrichment on Marine Phytoplankton." *Journal of Oceanography* 60:719–29.

Ruff, T. A., and R. J. Lewis. 1994. "Clinical Aspects of Ciguatera: An Overview." *Memoirs of the Queensland Museum* 34(3):609–19.

Schantz, E. 1973. "Seafood Toxicants." In *Toxicants Occurring Naturally in Foods*, edited by Food Protection Committee, 424–47. Washington, DC: National Academy of Sciences.

Sellner, K. G., G. J. Doucette, and G. J. Kirkpatrick. 2003. "Harmful Algal Blooms: Causes, Impacts, and Detection." *Journal of Industrial Microbiology and Biotechnology* 30:383–406.

Senior, V. E. 1960. "Algal Poisoning in Saskatchewan." *Canadian Journal of Comparative Medicine* 24:26–40.

Skulbert, O. M., W. W. Carmichael, G. A. Codd, and R. Skulberg. 1993. "Taxonomy of Toxic Cyanophyceae (Cyanobacteria)." In *Algal Toxins in Seafood and Drinking Water*, edited by I. R. Falconer, 145–64. Orlando, FL: Academic Press.

Spalding, B. 1995. "Better Tests Needed to Meet Goal of Safer Food Supply." *American Society for Microbiology News* 61:639.

Steidinger K. 1993. "Toxic Dinoflagellates." In *Algal Toxins in Seafood and Drinking Water*, edited by I. R. Falconer, 1–28. Orlando, FL: Academic Press.

Stewart, I., A. A. Seawright, and G. T. Shaw. 2008 "Cyanobacterial Poisoning in Livestock, Wild Mammals and Birds—An Overview." *Advances in Experimental Medicine and Biology* 6:613–37.

Stewart, I., P. M. Webb, P. J. Schluter, L. E. Fleming, J. W. Burns Jr., M. Ganta, L. C. Backer, and G. R. Shaw. 2006. "Epidemiology of Recreational Exposure to Freshwater Cyanobacteria: An International Prospective Cohort Study." *BMC Public Health* 6:93.

Tester, P. A. 1994. "Harmful Marine Phytoplankton and Shellfish Toxicity: Potential Consequences of Climate Change." *Annals of the New York Academy of Sciences* 740:69.

Todd, E. 1994. "Emerging Diseases Associated with Seafood Toxins and Other Water-Borne Agents." *Annals of the New York Academy of Sciences* 740:77.

Tozzi, S., O. Schofield, and P. Falkowski. 2004. "Historical Climate Change and Ocean Turbulences as Selective Agents for Two Key Phytoplankton Functional Groups." *Marine Ecology Progress Series* 274:123–32.

Trainer, V. L., and M. Suddleson. 2005. "Monitoring Approaches for Early Warning of Domoic Acid Events in Washington State." *Oceanography* 18:228–37.

Tunik, M. 2011. *Goldfranks's Toxicologic Emergencies*, 9th ed. New York: McGraw-Hill.

University of Georgia. 2012. "Toxic Algae to Blame for Cattle Deaths in Gwinnett County, UGA Determines." http://news.uga.edu/releases/article/toxic-algae-to-blame-for-cattle-deaths-062512/

Van Dolah, F. M. 2000. "Marine Algal Toxins: Origins, Health Effects, and Their Increased Occurrence." *Environmental Health Perspectives* 108(Suppl. 1):133.

Viviani, R. 1992. "Eutrophication, Marine Biotoxins, Human Health." *Science of the Total Environment* (Suppl.):631–62.

World Health Organization. 2003. *Guidelines for safe Recreational Waters, Volume 1—Coastal and Fresh Waters*. Chapter 8. Geneva: World Health Organization.

World Health Organization. 2009. *Protecting Health from Climate Change: Connecting Science, Policy, and People*. Geneva: World Health Organization.

Yu, S.-T. 1995. "Primary Prevention of Hepatocellular Carcinoma." *Journal of Gastroenterology and Hepatology* 10:674–82.

Yu, S.-Z. 1989. "Drinking Water and Primary Liver Cancer." In *Primary Liver Cancer*, edited by Z.-Y. Tang, M.-C. Wu, and S.-S. Xia, 30–37. Berlin: Spring-Verlag.

Yu, S.-Z., Z-Q. Chen, Y-K. Liu, Z-Y. Huang, and Y-F. Zhao. 1989. "The Aflatoxins and Contaminated Water in the Etiological Study of Primary Liver Cancer." In *Mycotoxins and Phycotoxins*, edited by S. Nator, K. Hashimoto, and Y. Ueno, 37–44. Amsterdam: Elsevier.

CHAPTER 7

CLIMATE CHANGE, CARBON DIOXIDE, AND PUBLIC HEALTH

The Plant Biology Perspective

Lewis H. Ziska, Kristie L. Ebi

Because carbon dioxide absorbs and reradiates heat back to the Earth's atmosphere, there is widespread scientific agreement that rising CO_2 level will result in increasing global temperatures (IPCC 2007, 2012). The magnitude and extent of temperature increase and the potential consequences for public health, from undernutrition to the spread of malaria, are the principal theme of this book, as well as the subject of ongoing medical and epidemiological research (Epstein 2005; IPCC 2007).

Some aspects of rising atmospheric CO_2 levels deserve additional scrutiny in the context of public health. Human well-being and even existence are fundamentally dependent on the ability of plants to generate complex carbohydrates and chemical energy from just four basic resources: sunlight, nutrients (e.g., nitrogen, phosphorous), water, and carbon dioxide. At present, approximately 95 percent of all plant species are deficient in the amount of CO_2 needed to operate at maximum efficiency; as a result, the rapid rise in an essential resource (atmospheric CO_2) has increased 23 percent since 1970 and is now at approximately 400 parts per mission by volume (ppmv) is likely to alter many aspects of plant biology—in addition to any concurrent temperature changes resulting from the role of CO_2 as a greenhouse gas (Ziska and Bunce 2006). These global changes in plant biology and physiology can have significant consequences for public health.

Any acknowledgment of these changes should examine their impacts beyond a simple "CO_2 makes plants grow

KEY CONCEPTS

- **Interactions between climate, carbon dioxide (CO_2), and plant biology can directly influence public health (e.g., aerobiology, contact dermatitis).**

- **Similar indirect effects may occur with respect to food security, including nutritional changes and food safety.**

- **Increasing CO_2 may alter plant-based pharmacological and narcotic compounds.**

- **CO_2 and climate can alter food supply and demography of known disease vectors, such as mosquitoes and rodents.**

- **Rising CO_2 and climate may reduce the efficacy of chemical (herbicidal) control, with subsequent environmental and economic harm.**

more" meme. The recognition that CO_2 is a promoter of plant growth has been used by critics of anthropogenic climate change to argue that rising atmospheric CO_2 will lead to an Eden-like plant environment, ignoring, among other likely environmental interactions, that any increase in CO_2 is indiscriminate with respect to which plant species may respond (Idso and Idso 1994; www.co2science.com) and to whether the nutrient content of plants will remain constant (Myers et al. 2014).

In this review, we provide an up-to-date assessment of both CO_2 and temperature as likely drivers of quantitative and qualitative changes in plant function and delineate, wherever possible, the role that such changes are likely to play in the context of public health. We begin with an examination of direct and indirect effects regarding CO_2 and climate, plant biology, and human health. Such effects range in scope from **aerobiology**, to contact dermatitis, to the spread of narcotic plants. Assuming that mitigation efforts in the near term will be limited, we will indicate limitations of current studies and emphasize a number of crucial adaption strategies that will reduce vulnerability to the ongoing challenges associated with climate, plant function, and public health.

Direct Consequences

The role of plant biology in human health may seem somewhat obscure to many public health professionals. Yet there are a number of processes by which plants directly affect human physiology, including aerobiology, contact dermatitis, pharmacology and toxicology, and physical contact (e.g., thorns, spines), among others. All of these are, or will be, affected by the ongoing rise in atmospheric carbon dioxide and subsequent changes in climate.

Aerobiology

One of the most recognized plant-induced health effects is associated with aeroallergens. Contact with plant-based pollen can induce sneezing, inflammation of nose and eye membranes, and wheezing. Complications, from nasal polyps to asthma or permanent bronchial obstructions, can occur in severe cases. Results from a four-year study by Quest Diagnostics (2011) in the United States indicated that sensitivity to ragweed and mold may have increased by 15 and 12 percent, respectively. The same study also indicated that allergies may be affecting 53 percent of children between the ages of two and seventeen. This is consistent with other work by the International Study of Asthma and Allergies in Childhood indicating that the global prevalence of asthma is continuing to increase (Pearce et al. 2007).

The role of rising CO_2 and temperature, or both, in eliciting quantitative or qualitative changes in aeroallergens is still being elucidated. However, sufficient information is now available to recognize that anthropogenic-driven climate change (i.e., CO_2 and temperature) is altering seasonality and beginning to affect the quantitative and qualitative aspects of the three distinct plant-based contributions to allergenic pollen: trees in the spring, grasses and weeds in the summer, and ragweed (*Ambrosia* spp.) in the fall (autumn).

Trees

The number of empirical studies indicate a clear association between anthropogenic climate change and temporal advances in **phenology** as evidenced by early anthesis and pollen shedding in the spring (Fitter and Fitter 2002; Ellwood et al., 2013). For trees, multi-year records have shown earlier floral initiation for oak (*Quercus* species) and birch (*Betula* species) (Emberlin et al., 2002; Garcia-Mozo et al. 2006). Additional studies have projected an advance of pollen initiation of one to three weeks for olive (*Olea europea*) and up to four weeks for Quercus with further warming (Garcia-Mozo et al. 2006).

Research conducted on loblolly pine (*Pinus taeda*) at the Duke University forest using free-air CO_2 enrichment (FACE) demonstrated that elevated CO_2 concentrations (200 ppm above ambient CO_2 levels) resulted in earlier pollen production from younger trees and greater seasonal pollen production (LaDeau and Clark 2006). Consistent with warmer spring temperatures, European pollen data have shown increases in hazel (*Corylus* species) and birch pollen counts in Switzerland and Denmark (Rasmussen 2002; Clot 2003; Frei and Gassner 2008). Currently no data are available regarding warming or CO_2 effects on potential qualitative changes in the allergenicity of tree pollen.

Weeds and Grasses

A number of plant species are recognized as significant sources of allergenic pollen during the summer months. Overall, warmer temperatures and earlier springs are altering pollen production of mugwort (Artemisia species) (Stach et al. 2007), nettle (Frenguelli 2002), and some grasses (Burr 1999; Emberlin et al. 1999). There is an association between pollen production and increasing temperature for other plant species (e.g., *Parietaria*; Ariano, Canonica, and Passalacqua 2010). Recent work

(Albertine et al. 2014) also demonstrates a clear link to rising CO_2 levels and increasing pollen and allergen exposure in timothy grass (*Phleum pratense*).

Ragweed

One of the most studied plant species regarding pollen production is ragweed (*Ambrosia* species). This may in part reflect the large numbers of individuals in the United States and elsewhere who exhibit seasonal ragweed allergies (Burbach et al. 2009; CDC 2011). Indoor studies examining temperature and increased CO_2 as treatment variables indicate consistent stimulation in plant growth and pollen production of common ragweed (*Ambrosia artemisiifolia*) (Ziska and Teasdale 2000; Wan et al. 2002; Wayne et al. 2002) and a potential increase in allergenic content (Singer et al. 2005; El Kelish et al. 2014). Manipulation of both temperature and CO_2 concentration in a glasshouse study to simulate future climate change resulted in earlier flowering, greater floral numbers, and greater pollen production in common ragweed (Rogers et al. 2006).

Because these initial results indicated that common ragweed may respond significantly to anthropogenic climate change and increased CO_2, attempts were made to quantify changes in ragweed biology at greater spatial and temporal scales. To this end, differences in regional microclimate (CO_2/temperature gradient between urban and rural locales) were used as a surrogate of near-term climate change projections to quantify the growth and pollen production of common ragweed for Baltimore, Maryland, and the surrounding environs (Ziska et al. 2003). Data from this study indicated that urban ragweed plants grew faster, flowered earlier, and produced significantly greater above-ground biomass and pollen relative to the same plants growing in a rural location. Similar microclimatic effects of urbanization were linked to longer pollen seasons and earlier floral initiation in European cities (Rodríguez-Rajo et al. 2010). To scale up from regional to continental effects, pollen data collected from the National Allergy Bureau in the United States and the Aerobiology Research Laboratories in Canada were collected to determine whether recent surface warming had resulted in a lengthening of the duration of the ragweed pollen season in North America. An analysis of these data demonstrated that the duration of the season has been increasing since the mid-1990s, but only as a function of increasing latitude, consistent with differential anthropogenic warming as postulated by the IPCC (Ziska et al. 2011) (figure 7.1). While this study did not examine quantitative and qualitative measures, it does suggest that length of exposure is likely to increase with continued anthropogenic warming, particularly in northern latitudes.

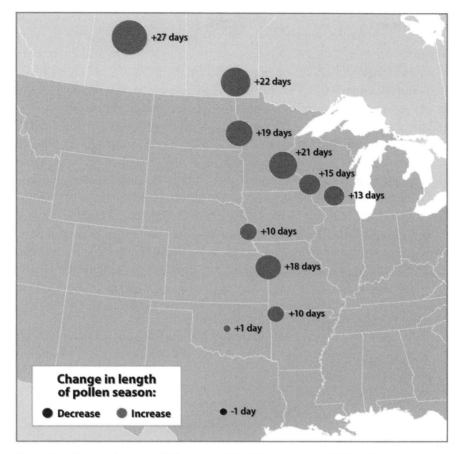

Figure 7.1   Change in the Ragweed Pollen Season, 1995–2011, as a Function of Differential Surface Warming with Latitude

Source: Data are adapted from Ziska et al. (2011) and were updated in 2013. See www.epa.gov/climatechange/science/indicators /society-eco/ragweed.html

Plants and Fungi

It is generally recognized that climate, particularly humidity and precipitation, plays a fundamental role in the induction and spread of allergenic molds (Burch and Levetin 2002). However, it is important to also recognize the role of plants in fungal biology. For example, *Alternaria alternata* is a well-known source of aeroallergens (as spores) with over 350 known plant hosts, including hay. Given that CO_2 and temperature will alter plant (host) biology, a question is how this will alter sporulation of *A. alternate.*

Indirectly, climate change, particularly warming temperatures, could alter the timing of agricultural harvests with subsequent effects on

Alternaria exposure times (Corden and Millington 2001). For example, differences between two UK towns, Derby and Cardiff, in *Alternaria* spore counts were associated with increased cereal production and changes in climate since the 1970s (Corden and Millington, 2001; Corden, Millington, and Mullins 2003). For quaking aspen (*Populus tremuloides*) grown at projected increases of atmospheric CO_2, a significant increase in fungal propagules (including a doubling of *A. alternata*) was observed in the leaf litter (Klironomos et al. 1997). A similar experiment was conducted with timothy grass (*Phleum pratense*) to quantify the effects of recent and projected increases in atmospheric CO_2 (300, 400, 500, and 600 ppm) on the quantity and quality of *Alternaria* spores (Wolf et al. 2010). Results from this study indicated that at 500 and 600 ppm CO_2, *A. alternata* produced nearly three times the number of spores and more than twice the total antigenic protein per plant than at lower CO_2 concentrations. Wolf et al. (2010) suggested that recent and projected increases in CO_2 could increase the carbon to nitrogen ratio in leaves of timothy grass (*Phleum pratense*), with subsequent quantitative and qualitative changes in *A. alternata* sporulation.

Contact Dermatitis

Plants have evolved numerous defensive chemicals, including those associated with contact dermatitis, an immune-mediated (IgE) allergenic response. Plants may also induce **photodermatitis**, a form of allergic contact dermatitis where light is needed to activate the allergen. Contact dermatitis is associated with over one hundred different plant species (e.g., poison ivy, *Toxicodendron radicans*), whereas photodermatitis is associated principally with plant members of the Apiaceal or Umbelliferae family (e.g., giant hogweed, *Heracleum mantegazzianum*). It is estimated that sensitivity to urushiol, the principal allergen in poison ivy, occurs in about two out of every three individuals, and amounts as small as one nanogram (ng) are sufficient to induce a reaction (Tanner 2000). Each year, approximately 300,000 people in the United States suffer from contact with member of the poison ivy family (e.g., poison ivy, oak, and sumac) (Mohan et al. 2006).

How will anthropogenic climate change or rising CO_2 levels, or both, alter the ability of such plants to induce contact dermatitis? Laboratory trials for poison ivy examined the range of growth responses and simulated herbivory (leaf consumption by herbivores) at recent and projected CO_2 changes—300, 400, 500, and 600 parts per million (ppm)—or the approximate CO_2 concentrations that existed during the middle of the twentieth century, the current concentration, and near- and long-term projections for this century, 2050 and 2090, respectively (Ziska et al. 2007). These data indicated that poison ivy can respond to even small (approximately 100 ppm) increases in CO_2 concentration above the mid-twentieth-century carbon dioxide baseline and suggest that its rate of spread, its ability to recover from herbivory, and its production of urushiol may be enhanced in a future, higher CO_2 environment. Outdoor trials of poison ivy using free-air CO_2 enrichment (FACE) technology at Duke University showed that poison ivy responds significantly to projected increases in atmospheric CO_2 (approximately 700 ppm) (Mohan et al. 2006). Interestingly, in addition to growth changes, the ratio of unsaturated to saturated urushiol increased as a function of CO_2 concentration, indicating a more virulent form of urushiol (Mohan et al. 2006). Although information on temperature or temperature-CO_2 interactions is lacking, other known allergenic species such as stinging nettle (*Urtica dioica*) and leafy spurge (*Euphorbia esula*) also showed significant increases in growth in response to recent and projected CO_2 changes (Hunt et al. 1991; Ziska 2003).

Toxicology

In addition to plant-based allergens, plants can produce numerous toxic substances; more than seven hundred plant species are known to be poisonous for human or animal consumption. The amount and location of the poison, as with dermatitis, varies by species; however, some plants, such as poison hemlock (*Conium maculatum*), oleander (*Nerium aleander*), and castor bean (*Ricinus communis*), are sufficiently toxic so that even small quantities can result in death. Accidental ingestion of plant material is recognized as a source of toxic exposure and accounts for nearly 100,000 calls to national poison centers annually (Watson et al. 2004), with approximately 80 percent of plant-related exposures associated with pediatric patients.

At present, little information is available regarding anthropogenic climate-CO_2 impacts on toxicology. One seminal study by Ros Gleadow (Gleadow et al. 2009) indicated that for cassava (*Manihot esculentum*), a primary caloric source for approximately 800 million people globally, rising levels of CO_2 above ambient (550 and 710 ppm CO_2) resulted in nearly doubling the concentration of cyanogenic glycosides in the edible leaves at the highest CO_2 concentration. This suggested that cyanide poisoning could increase as a function of rising atmospheric CO_2 levels. The impact of CO_2 or temperature, or both, on toxicological effects of other plant species has not been examined.

CLINICAL CORRELATES 7.1 GLOBAL FOOD SCARCITY AND THE EFFECTS OF AGROCHEMICALS

Climate change and population growth are increasing demands on the global food supply and increasing reliance on industrialized food production and agricultural chemical use. Research into the long-term health effects of pesticide use lags decades behind widespread use of these compounds. Large studies of the chronic effects of pesticide exposure on children's health have shown links to birth defects, premature birth, intrauterine growth restriction, and several childhood cancers (American Academy of Pediatrics Council on Environmental Health 2012). Many pesticides currently in use are classified as carcinogens by the US Environmental Protection Agency. Expert consensus now holds that there are links between pesticide exposure and neurocognitive development (Kimmel et al. 2005). Prospective studies link early-life exposure to reductions in intelligence quotient and increased rates of attention-deficit hyperactivity disorder and autism (Eckerman et al. 2007; Landrigan et al. 1999).

Unfortunately, there is currently no information on developmental toxicity of over 80 percent of the three thousand chemicals used in US agriculture (Perera 2014). And yet neurodevelopment disorders such as autism, attention deficit disorder, and pervasive development disorder now affect one in six children living in the industrial world (Perera 2014). More research is necessary to untangle the myriad connections between early life exposure and pesticide toxicity, and create regulations that address the severity of the clinical implications of exposure to ensure a safe food supply as we rely more on industrialized food.

Climate change leads to food insecurity, more reliance on industrialized food production, and the use of chemicals with unknown and known detrimental effects on human health.

Physical Contact

Many plants can be associated with physical injury. Spines or other sharp appendages can puncture the skin. Removing or encountering plants such as Canada thistle (*Cirsium arvense*) or puncture vine (*Tribulus terrestris*) can be particularly painful. Physical wounding, however, is usually avoided or minimized by proper protective equipment such as gloves to avoid injury.

As with toxicology, few studies have quantified changes in physical appendages as a function of CO_2 or temperature. One exception is for Canada thistle: data demonstrate that an increase in the number and length of leaf spines as CO_2 increased from preindustrial levels (285 ppm) to projected twenty-first-century levels (721 ppm) (Ziska 2004).

Indirect Consequences

While the direct consequences of CO_2 or in conjunction with rising temperatures are evident with respect to plant biology, additional indirect effects may also be of consequence in any discussion of human health. These effects are not directly induced by plant contact but are associated with secondary consequences and may include such aspects as food security, nutrition, pharmacology, and herbicide use.

Food and Nutrition

Food Security

The interactive role of CO_2 and climatic change on global food security is multifaceted and is likely to include changes in production, distribution, and quality. All three aspects are likely to be affected by CO_2 or climatic changes. (Additional details as to the range and extent of these impacts, as well as potential adaptation measures, can be found in Lobell et al. 2008; Lobell and Burke 2010; and Beddington et al. 2012.)

Although they are complex, water and temperature are among the climatic factors that can significantly affect crop production; both are a concern on the global stage. Water availability, particularly drought, has been a factor in noteworthy reductions in corn, soybean, and wheat production for the United States in 2012 (Gilbert 2012) and Russia in 2010 and 2011 (Wegren 2011). Greater frequency of droughts and extreme precipitation events such as flooding are projected with anthropogenic climate change (IPCC 2012). Irrigation, which is essential to maintaining production of cereal crops with drought, particularly in populous areas (e.g., India, East Asia) may also be at risk as precipitation decreases in many regions and water supply declines as ice and snow reserves diminish in mountainous regions with warming (e.g., Kerr 2007). Record-high spring and summer temperatures observed in the United States during 2012 may also be of concern in agronomic production, as flowering is one of the most thermal-sensitive stages of crop growth (Lobell et al. 2013). Chronic or short-term exposure to higher temperatures during flowering can result in reduced pollen viability, inadequate fertilization, and aborted fruit development (Hatfield et al. 2011). Given the current level of 1 billion individuals who are food insecure and the additional 2 billion who will be added to the global population by 2040, understanding, quantifying, and adapting global agriculture to maintain crop production is a crucial, if underappreciated, aspect of plant biology and public health.

Nutrition

The role of nutrition in all aspects of public health and human wellness is universally acknowledged. As a consequence, it is necessary to also consider the quality, or nutritional aspects, of the food supply in the framework of climate change, CO_2, and plant biology.

As CO_2 increases, photosynthesis requires less nitrogen (i.e., nitrogen use efficiency, the ratio of carbon to nitrogen, or C:N, typically increases). A number of studies have examined the role of rising CO_2 on protein concentration of major crops, including barley, potato, rice, soybean, and wheat (Taub, Miller, and Allen 2008). Overall, among crops examined, a significant decline (about 10 to 15 percent) in protein content was observed if atmospheric CO_2 increases rose to between 540 and 960 ppm (Taub et al. 2008), a range anticipated before the end of this century (IPCC 2007) (figure 7.2). In addition to this dilution of protein levels, rising CO_2 may also reduce water flow through the crop plant due to its physiological effect of closing stomata. As a result, uptake of key micro- and macronutrients from the soil (e.g., iron, zinc, and manganese) may also be negatively affected; micronutrient deficiency is a much larger problem globally than undernutrition (Loladze 2002, 2014; Myers et al. 2014). Conversely, some studies indicate an improvement in some aspects of nutritional quality, such as an increase in antioxidants in strawberries with rising CO_2 (Wang, Bunce, and Maas 2003).

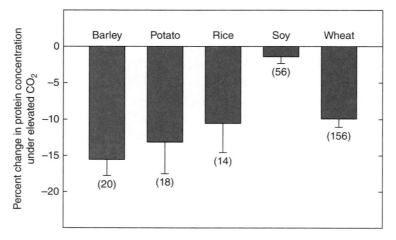

Figure 7.2   Percent Decline in Protein Content of Food Crops at the Elevated CO_2 Concentrations Anticipated by the End of This Century Relative to Ambient CO_2

Source: Adapted from Taub et al. (2008).

Note: Numbers in parentheses represent the number of published studies from which the average and standard error are derived (Taub et al. 2008).

The UN Food and Agriculture Organization estimates that more than 1 billion people worldwide are undernourished (Kennedy, Nantel, and Shetty 2003). Undernutrition generally results from a lack of protein that is needed for muscle development and maintenance, or micronutrients such as iodine, vitamin A, or iron that boost immunity and healthy development. For many populations in the developing world, meat is scarce, and plants provide the primary source of both protein and micronutrients. If, as we expect, rising CO_2 levels decrease the protein concentration or affect the nutritional quality of crops, then it is possible that impoverished areas of the world already threatened by shortages in food supply may face an additional burden of hidden hunger (Lloyd, Kovats, and Chalabi 2011; Myers et al. 2014). Overall, changes in food quality and nutritional value have been well described in the context of CO_2 or climate; however, the focus has been on food production, which, while important, is not always a good indicator of food security.

Pharmacology

Medicine

The use of plants as remedies for human ailments dates to the beginning of civilization (Shultes and Reis 1995). Plants have evolved numerous chemical pathways to protect themselves from viral diseases, fungal pathogens, and herbivores. Diversity in the production of these secondary compounds has been an important pharmacological resource. Although many of these metabolites are now derived synthetically, the World Health Organization (WHO 2002) reported that approximately 3.5 billion people (about half the global population) still relies on plants as a primary source of medicine for health care.

Only a small number of studies have examined how pharmacological compounds could respond to recent or projected increases in atmospheric CO_2 or temperature. Among these, growth of wooly foxglove (*Digitalis lanata*) and production of digoxin were increased at 1,000 ppmv CO_2 relative to ambient conditions (Stuhlfauth and Fock 1990). Production of morphine in wild poppy (*Papaver setigerum*) (Ziska, Panicker, and Wojno 2008) showed significant increases with both recent and projected carbon dioxide concentrations. Growth of St. John's wort (*Hypericum perforatum*) and the concentration of hypericin, a drug used in treatment of depression, were increased when grown at CO_2 concentrations of 1.000 ppm (Zobayed and Saxena 2004). Concurrent rises in temperature or CO_2 increased the production and concentration of atropine and scopolamine in jimson weed (*Datura stromonium*) (Ziska et al. 2005); however, a synergistic effect of CO_2 and temperature on either concentration or production of these compounds was not observed. Overall, such changes in concentration could alter the utility of such substances in regard to their efficacy in human physiology.

Narcotics

Although pharmaceuticals contribute significantly to public health, plants also produce a number of narcotic compounds whose abuse constitutes a significant global health problem including nicotine in tobacco, tetrahydrocannabinol (THC) in *Cannabis* spp., and cocaine chlorohydrate in *Erythoxylum coca*.

Although the growth of narcotic plants can be stimulated by rising CO_2 and temperature (e.g., *Cannabis sativa*; Chandra et al., 2008); few peer-reviewed studies have quantified the impact on the narcotic compound per se. One exception is nicotine in wild tobacco (*Nicotiana* spp.), which was quantified in response to rising CO_2 and temperature (Ziska et al. 2005). In this study increasing CO_2 above the early twentieth-century baseline (approximately 295 ppm) reduced the concentration of nicotine; however, CO_2 stimulated overall plant growth so that while concentration was reduced, production per plant increased (Ziska et al. 2005).

Many of the most used plant compounds are bicyclic alkaloids (e.g., cocaine, nicotine, caffeine, and atropine). It has been suggested (Bryant, Chapin, and Klein 1983) that as CO_2 increases, the resulting increase in the C:N ratio of plant leaves will reduce the concentration of nitrogen-based secondary compounds (e.g., caffeine in coffee) while increasing compounds that have little or no nitrogen (e.g., scopolamine in jimson weed). If true, this implies that concentrations of these compounds could decrease in a warming climate. However, insufficient data exist at present to confirm this hypothesis.

Pesticide Use

Climate-induced changes in pest distribution and populations may exacerbate pest pressures and lead to increases in pesticide use and human exposure to those pesticides. Although the link between pesticide application, exposure, and human health will depend on the chemical used, amount of exposure, genetic predisposition, and other factors, it is reasonable to determine if climate or CO_2 may reduce the efficacy or increase the need for chemical applications.

Temperature and precipitation are known abiotic factors that can affect chemical application rates and overall efficacy (Patterson 1995). There is also increasing evidence that rising CO_2 levels can decrease

Table 7.1   Summary of Changes in Efficacy of Weed Species Response to Herbicide Application at Manufacturers, Recommended Dosage as a Function of CO_2 Concentration

Weed Species	Photosynthetic Pathway	Herbicide (Active Ingredient)	Change in Efficacy?	Reference
Canada thistle (*Cirsium arvense*)	C_3	Glyphosate	Declined	Ziska et al. 2004
Dallisgrass (*Paspalum dilattatum*)	C_4	Glyphosate	Declined	Manea et al. 2011
Lamb's quarters (*Chenopodium album*)	C_3	Glyphosate	Declined	Ziska et al. 1999
Lovegrass (*Eragostis curvula*)	C_4	Glyphosate	Declined	Manea et al. 2011
Quackgrass (*Elytrigia repens*)	C_3	Glyphosate	Declined	Ziska and Teasdale 2000
Red-root pigweed (*Amaranthus retroflexus*)	C_4	Glyphosate	None	Ziska et al. 1999
Rhodes grass (*Chloris gayana*)	C_4	Glyphosate	Declined	Manea et al. 2011
Smut grass (*Sporobolus indicus*)	C_4	Glyphosate	None	Manea et al. 2011

Note: A decline in efficacy indicates that the treated plant survived and continued to grow following herbicide application.

chemical efficacy for the control of annual and perennial weeds (Ziska et al. 1999; Archambault 2007; Manea, Leishman, and Downey 2011) (table 7.1). The basis for a reduction in efficacy with climate is likely related to changes in physical parameters such as increased wind speed and greater frequency of heavy precipitation. A basis for the reduction in efficacy with increasing CO_2 is less clear. At the biological level, increased CO_2 may alter carbon distribution with consequences for translocation (within plant mobility) of the herbicide and potential effects on its chemical efficacy. For example, in Canada thistle, increasing CO_2 resulted in greater carbon allocation to the roots. The increase in the root-to-shoot biomass may have diluted the recommended dosage of glyphosate so that roots were not killed. Because roots of Canada thistle can regenerate the plant asexually, glyphosate efficacy was reduced to zero in an elevated CO_2 environment (Ziska, Faulkner, and Lydon 2004). In addition to the effect of CO_2 on efficacy, there is also evidence that seasonal changes may increase pesticide use. For example, soybeans grown over a north-south transect in the Midwest (Minnesota to Louisiana) showed that pesticide applications increased for soybeans as winters warmed and pest survival over winter increased (Ziska 2014).

Overall, on a global basis, pests, pathogens, and weeds currently consume some 42 percent of growing and stored crops annually (Pimentel 1997), and this figure could escalate as a function of CO_2 or climate disruption. Increased use of petrochemicals for control, combined with reduced efficacy of application, carries additional risks for human and animal health because it could increase the presence of these chemicals in the environment.

CLINICAL CORRELATES 7.2   HEALTH EFFECTS OF FOOD SCARCITY

Global climate change is forecast to intensify global food shortages in vulnerable places. The effects of chronic undernutrition range from physical to cognitive. On a worldwide level, growth stunting, severe wasting, and intrauterine growth retardation together contribute to 2.2 million deaths annually, accounting for 35 percent of mortality of children less than five years of age (Black et al. 2008). Malnutrition has been shown to lead to impaired cognitive development, learning disability, deferment of education, attrition from the workforce, and less decreased lifetime earnings (Hoddinott et al. 2008). Micronutrient deficiencies are pervasive as well and are likely to intensify. Iodine deficiencies result in goiter, hypothyroidism, and developmental disabilities, including severe mental retardation. Insufficient intake of vitamin A is the leading cause of blindness worldwide. Dietary iron deficiency leading to anemia is worsened by chronic parasitic infection and chronic illness that so often accompanies it in resource-poor settings. Folic acid is essential for normal nervous system development, yet is often lacking in diets along with zinc, and both are linked to childhood growth stunting (Alderman and Shekar 2011).

Health effects of chronic undernutrition manifest in myriad ways, ranging from physical to cognitive, and are likely to intensify in the future as a result of climate change.

Uncertainties and Research Priorities

We have thus far reviewed published interactions illustrating the range and scope of plant-based links between anthropogenic perturbations and public health. Further inquiry is warranted because the initial observations are often based on a handful of studies, many of which did not capture the complexity of interactions, address the ambiguity underlying the empirical observation, or explore local interactions that could exacerbate or ameliorate possible negative impacts.

Aerobiology

Studies regarding the role of climate on aeroallergen production, particularly warmer winters and earlier springs, are ongoing. Elucidating the role of warmer winters on **vernalization** and floral production for tree species is critical but often overlooked. In addition, studies on pollen allergen content associated with a changing climate and increased CO_2 levels are needed to help determine changes in the epidemiology of rhinitis and asthma, particularly among children. Integration of these studies with other meteorological factors likely to change, such as ozone, is needed in order to provide regional estimates of the production and dissemination of plant- and fungal-based allergens (Albertine et al. 2014). Such information would also be invaluable in providing clinical and epidemiological knowledge regarding the seasonality and occurrence of allergic disease in the context of climate or CO_2 concentration; as such, this information could facilitate better disease management.

In regard to climate, CO_2, and aeroallergens, research priorities include:

- The development of long-term (multidecadenal) pollen and spore data sets that use consistent methods for quantification, qualification, and monitoring of pollen counts and aeroallergen concentrations at regional and national levels

- Surveillance information from emergency room visits to help clarify the epidemiology of extreme weather events and climate in the context of aeroallergen exposure and asthma

- Increased recognition of the role of plant-based pollen production in international assessments of climate change impacts

- Initiation of urban ecological studies to help identify and manage allergenic plants to minimize aeroallergen exposure

- Additional research to determine potential synergies between aeroallergens and human pollution

- Cooperation and quantitative comparisons between health care professionals and plant biologists to establish a common set of pollen and climate indexes for additional research and modeling efforts

Contact Dermatitis

For plant-based contact dermatitis, additional experimental data on the ubiquity of potential changes in urushiol and similar compounds from other plant species with climate and CO_2 would be crucial in assessing any potential change in contact dermatitis occurrence. Such information should also be collected on plant growth and dissemination under different potential climate- and CO_2-induced scenarios related to the plants' **demography** and range. Warmer temperatures, higher CO_2 concentrations, and longer growing seasons could also facilitate increasing contact with urushiol or similar compounds in urban areas. Such information should also be collected on plant growth and dissemination under different scenarios of potential climate and CO_2 concentrations related to the plants' demography and range.

Secondary Plant Chemistry

From pharmacology to toxicology to nutrition to food allergies (Beggs and Walczyk 2008), it is well established that secondary plant compounds significantly affect human health. It is also clear that rising CO_2 and temperature are, or will, alter the concentration or temporal production of these compounds. However, a number of fundamental research priorities remain to be addressed regarding climate and CO_2. Can we expect toxicological changes in poisonous plants? Will plants that are known sources of either medicine or narcotics change their global distribution in response to climate? Will the concentration or efficacy of the pharmacological compound change? Will allergenic proteins in plants associated with food allergies increase or decrease in response to CO_2?

Food Security

Because of the enormity of and potential vulnerability to food security (access to sufficient, safe, and nutritious food that provides the full range of necessary calories and micronutrients), there are clear and compelling issues related to climate change that have drawn the attention of scientists, the general public, and policymakers. These issues have been extensively examined in a variety of public and academic forums, from the medical community (The Lancet 2009), to the US National Academy of Sciences (Howden et al. 2007), to the international community (IPCC 2007) to business leaders (World Economic Forum, www.weforum.org/issues /agriculture-and-food-security).

Surprisingly however, the role of rising CO_2 in the context of food security is still unclear. Will rising CO_2 alter interactions with drought or flooding? How? Does CO_2 increase vulnerability to rising temperatures by limiting transpirational cooling? Does CO_2 favor weeds over crops, with concomitant reductions in crop yields? Does CO_2 alter susceptibility of crops to pathogens? To insects? Can varieties of wheat or rice be selected that will be able to use additional CO_2 more effectively as a resource to increase seed yields? These are simply a small subset of research priorities that have been recognized but largely, to date, unaddressed at the scientific, modeling, or policy level. A related issue is the fate of cash crops in a changed climate. For subsistence farmers relying on cash crops to purchase agricultural inputs, any change in productivity could affect their ability to continue to feed their families (Ebi et al. 2011)

CLINICAL CORRELATES 7.3   MEDICINES FROM NATURE

Currently more than half of prescribed medications and the majority of medicines approved by the Food and Drug Administration can be traced to natural origins (Grifo 1997). In developing areas of the world, people rely even more directly on natural medicines, in some places deriving as much as 90 percent of their healing substances directly from the local environment (Patwardhan 2005). Habitat destruction and climate change threaten biodiversity and the use of medicines from nature. (See tables 7.2 and 7.3.)

Table 7.2   Examples of Drugs Derived from Natural Sources

Plant	Location	Drug	Use
Willow	Worldwide	Aspirin	Fever and pain
Digitalis purpurea	Eurasia, Africa	Digoxin	Cardiac arrhythmia
Catharanthus roseus	Madagascar	Vinblastine	Hodgkin's lymphoma
Taxus brevifolia	Pacific Northwest	Taxol	Ovarian cancer
Cinchona sp.	Tropical Andes, South America	Quinine	Malaria
Atropa Belladonna	Europe and Asia	Atropine	Cholinergic
Papaver somniferum	Cultivated worldwide	Morphine, codeine	Pain reliever
Curare	Central and South America	Turbocurarine	Nondepolarizing muscle relaxant

Table 7.3   Examples of Noncommercialized, Medically Important Plants

Plant	Location	Uses
Ucaria tormentosa	Tropical forests of South and Central America	Arthritis, rheumatism, gastric ulcers, and wounds
Arnica Montana	North America	Anti-inflammatory
Actaea racemosa	Eastern North America	Premenstrual tension, menopause, anti-inflammatory
Cassia occidentalis	West Africa	Antibacterial/antiparasitic
Pilocarpus	Neotropics of South America	Breast milk inducer, glaucoma, diuretic

Climate change and habitat destruction threaten the availability of natural medicines for local use and for the future development of Western medical cures.

Plant Biology and Disease Vectors

We recognize that plants do not transmit disease. However, it is important to stress that animal reservoirs of disease spread, such as rodents and mosquitoes, rely on plants as a principal food source (although female mosquitoes require blood proteins in order to lay eggs). Given that rising CO_2 can stimulate plant growth, including pollen and seed production, and climate can change plant demography, how will these changes influence disease ecology? For example, a change in climate can influence seed sources for rodents, with consequences for the occurrence and spread of hantavirus (Plowright et al. 2008). Pollen on open ponds can serve as food for mosquito larvae (Ye-Ebiyo, Pollack, and Spielman 2000), but do CO_2-induced increases in pollen production (Ziska and Caulfield 2000) influence mosquito fecundity? Understanding these links, particularly with regard to climate and CO_2 and plant biology and the resulting changes in vector range and disease transmission, remain a little recognized, if highly desirable, research goal.

Conclusion

The potential consequences of a warmer planet in regard to disease outbreaks, air and water quality, food availability, and respiratory illness are well recognized as serious health threats to the global community (IPCC 2007; McMichael and Lindgren 2011; McMichael, Montgomery, and Costello 2012). However, in our estimation, the nexus of climate-CO_2, plant biology, and human health are not well appreciated or evaluated in that context. Yet plant biology affects every aspect of civilization, from air, to water, to clothing, to food, to shelter, to medicine. As this review illustrates, the consequences for public health of climate change and rising CO_2 on plant biology, from aeroallergens to pharmacology to food safety are, and will continue to be, substantial. The hope is that this chapter illustrated the critical nature of these relationships among plants, climate, and health; highlighted critical research areas; and acted as a clear and timely appeal for additional resources to address these challenges.

DISCUSSION QUESTIONS

1. How will CO_2 and temperature alter the US Department of Agriculture's MyPlate?

2. How should CO_2 and temperature changes in plant demographics be considered in the spread of known insect disease vectors (e.g., dengue)?

3. In remote regions that may depend on ethnopharmacological plants for medicine, how will climate change alter public health?

4. How will rising CO_2 and/or air temperature alter the spatial and temporal aspects of plant-based pollen sources? Are there implications for asthma sufferers?

KEY TERMS

Aerobiology: A subset of biology that studies the dynamics of organic particles and small organisms that can be passively transported by air. Aerobiologists are associated with the measuring and reporting of airborne pollen and fungal spores as a public health service.

Demography: The statistical study of living populations in regard to dynamic changes in their size, structure, and distribution in time and space.

Phenology: The study of periodic plant and animal life cycle events and how these are influenced by seasonal and interannual variations in climate.

Photodermatitis: A form of allergic contact dermatitis whereby the allergen is activated by light in order to induce the allergic response.

Vernalization: The biological requirement of cold temperature exposure required by some plants in order to flower in the spring.

References

Albertine, J. M., W. J. Manning, M. DaCosta, K. A. Stinson, M. L. Muilenberg, and C. A. Rogers. 2014. "Projected Carbon Dioxide to Increase Grass Pollen and Allergen Exposure Despite Higher Ozone Levels." *PloS One* 9:e111712.

Alderman, H., and M. Shekar. 2011. "Nutrition, Food Security and Health." In *Nelson Textbook of Pediatrics*, 19th ed., edited by R. M. Kleigman, B. F. Stanton, J. W. St. Geme, N. F. Schor, and R. E. Behrman, 170–78. Philadelphia: Elsevier.

American Academy of Pediatrics Council on Environmental Health. 2012. "Pesticide Exposure in Children." *Pediatrics* 130:2012–57.

Archambault, D. J. 2007. "Efficacy of Herbicides under Elevated Temperature and CO_2." In *Agroecosystems in a Changing Climate*, edited by P.C.D. Newton, R. A. Carran, G. R. Edwards, and P. A. Niklaus, 333–36. Boca Raton, FL: CRC Press.

Ariano, R., G. W. Canonica, and G. Passalacqua. 2010. "Possible Role of Climate Changes in Variations in Pollen Seasons and Allergic Sensitizations during 27 Years." *Annals of Allergy Asthma and Immunology* 104:215–22.

Beddington, J. R., M. Asaduzzaman, M. E. Clark, A. Fernandez Bremauntz, M. D. Guillou, D.J.B. Howlett, et al. 2012. "What Next for Agriculture after Durban?" *Science* 335:289–90.

Beggs, P. J., and N. E. Walczyk. 2008. "Impacts of Climate Change on Plant Food Allergens: A Previously Unrecognized Threat to Human Health." *Air Quality, Atmosphere and Health* 1:119–23.

Black, R. E., L. H. Allen, Z. A. Bhutta, L. E. Caulfield, M. Onis, M. Ezzati, C. Mathers, J. Rivera, and the Maternal and Child Undernutrition Study Group. 2008. "Maternal and Child Undernutrition: Global and Regional Exposures and Health Consequences." *Lancet* 371(9608):234–60.

Bryant, J. P., F. S. Chapin, and D. R. Klein. 1983. "Carbon/Nutrient Balance of Boreal Plants in Relation to Vertebrate Herbivory." *Oikos* 40:357–68.

Burbach, G. J., L. M. Heinzerling, C. Röhnelt, K.-C. Bergmann, H. Behrendt, and T. Zuberbier. 2009. "Ragweed Sensitization in Europe: GALEN Study Suggests Increasing Prevalence." *Allergy* 64:664–65.

Burch, M., and E. Levetin. 2002. "Effects of Meteorological Conditions on Spore Plumes." *International Journal of Biometeorology* 46:107–17.

Burr, M. L. 1999. "Grass Pollen: Trends and Predictions." *Clinical and Experimental Allergy* 29:735–38.

Centers for Disease Control and Prevention (CDC). 2011. "Allergies and Hay Fever." www.cdc.gov/nchs/fastats/allergies.htm

Chandra, S., H. Lata, I. A. Khan, and M. A. Elsohly. 2008. "Photosynthetic Response of *Cannabis sativa l.* to Variations in Photosynthetic Photon Flux Densities, Temperature and CO_2 Conditions." *Physiological and Molecular Biology of Plants* 14:299–306.

Corden, J. M., and W. M. Millington. 2001. "The Long-Term Trends and Seasonal Variation of the Aeroallergen *Alternaria* in Derby, UK." *Aerobiologia* 17:127–36.

Corden, J. M., W. M. Millington, and J. Mullins. 2003. "Long-Term Trends and Regional Variation in the Aeroallergen *Alternaria* in Cardiff and Derby UK: Are Differences in Climate and Cereal Production Having an Effect?" *Aerobiologia* 19:191–99.

Clot, B. 2003. "Trends in Airborne Pollen: An Overview of 21 Years of Data in Neuchâtel (Switzerland)." *Aerobiologia* 19:227–34.

Ebi, K. L., J. Padgham, M. Doumbia, A. Kergna, J. Smith, T. Butt, and B. McCarl. 2011. "Smallholders' Adaptation to Climate Change in Mali." *Climatic Change* 108:423–36.

Eckerman, D. A., L. A. Gimenes, R. C. de Souza, P. R. Lopes Galvão, P. N. Sarcinelli, and J. R. Chrisman. 2007. "Age Related Effects of Pesticide Exposure on Neurobehavioral Performance of Adolescent Farm Workers in Brazil." *Neurotoxicology and Teratology* 29:164–75.

El Kelish, A., F. Zhao, W. Heller, J. Durner, J. B. Winkler, H. Behrendt, C. Traidl-Hoffmann, et al. 2014. "Ragweed (*Ambrosia artemisiifolia*) Pollen Allergenicity: SuperSAGE Transcriptomic Analysis upon Elevated CO_2 and Drought Stress." *BMC Plant Biology* 14:176–90.

Ellwood, E. R., S. A. Temple, R. B. Primack, N. L. Bradley, and C. C. Davis. 2013. "Record-Breaking Early Flowering in the Eastern United States." *PLoS ONE* 8:e53788.

Emberlin, J., M. Detandt, R. Gehrig, S. Jaeger, N. Nolard, and A. Rantio-Lehtimäki. 2002. "Responses in the Start of the Betula (Birch) Pollen Seasons to Recent Changes in Spring Temperatures across Europe." *International Journal of Biometeorology* 46:159–70.

Emberlin, J., J. Mullins, J. Corden, S. Jones, W. Millington, M. Brooke, et al. 1999. "Regional Variations in Grass Pollen Seasons in the UK, Long-Term Trends and Forecast Models." *Clinical and Experimental Allergy* 29:347–56.

Epstein, P. R. 2005. "Climate Change and Human Health." *New England Journal of Medicine* 353:1433–36.

Fitter, A. H., and R.S.R. Fitter. 2002. "Rapid Changes in Flowering Time in British Plants." *Science* 296:1689–91.

Frei, T., and E. Gassner. 2008. "Climate Change and Its Impact on Birch Pollen Quantities and the Start of the Pollen Season: An Example from Switzerland for the Period 1969–2006." *International Journal of Biometeorology* 52:667–74.

Frenguelli, G. 2002. "Interactions between Climatic Changes and Allergenic Plants." *Monaldi Archives for Chest Disease* 57:141–43.

García-Mozo, H., C. Galán, V. Jato, J. Belmonte, C. D. de la Guardia, D. Fernández, M. Gutierrez, et al. 2006. "*Quercus* Pollen Season Dynamics in the Iberian Peninsula: Response to Meteorological Parameters and Possible Consequences of Climate Change." *Annals of Agricultural and Environmental Medicine* 13:209–224.

Gilbert, N. 2012. "Drought Devastates U.S. Maize and Soya Crops." *Nature.* doi:10.1038/nature.2012.11065

Gleadow, R. M., J. R. Evans, S. Mccaffery, and T. R. Cavagnaro. 2009. "Growth and Nutritive Value of Cassava (*Manihot esculenta* Cranz.) Are Reduced When Grown in Elevated CO_2." *Plant Biology* 11:76–82.

Grifo F. 1997. "The Origin of Prescription Drugs." In *Biodiversity and Human Health,* edited by F. Grifo and J Rosenthal, 131–63. Washington, DC: Island Press.

Hatfield, J. L., K. J. Boote, B. A. Kimball, L. H. Ziska, R. C. Izaurralde, D. Ort, A. M. Thomson, and D. Wolfe. 2011. "Climate Impacts on Agriculture: Implications for Crop Production." *Agronomy Journal* 103:351–70.

Hoddinott, J., J. R. Behrman, J. A. Maluccio, J. R. Behrman, R. Flores, and R. Martorell. 2008. "Effect of a Nutrition Intervention during Early Childhood on Economic Productivity in Guatemalan Adults." *Lancet* 371(9610):411–16.

Howden, S. M., J. F. Soussana, F. N. Tubiello, N. Chetri, M. Dunlop, and H. Meinke. 2007. "Adapting Agriculture to Climate Change." *Proceedings of the National Academy of Sciences, USA* 104:9691–96.

Hunt, R., D. W. Hand, M. A. Hannah, and A. M. Neal. 1991. "Response to CO_2 Enrichment in 27 Herbaceous Species." *Functional Ecology* 5:410–21.

Idso, K. E., and S. B. Idso. 1994. "Plant Responses to Atmospheric CO_2 Enrichment in the Face of Environmental Constraints: A Review of the Past 10 Years Research." *Agricultural, Forest Meteorology* 69:153–203.

Intergovernmental Panel on Climate Change (IPCC). 2007. *Climate Change 2007: Impacts, Adaptation and Vulnerability.* Geneva: IPCC Secretariat.

Intergovernmental Panel on Climate Change (IPCC). 2012. *Managing the Risks of Extreme Events and Disasters to Advance Climate Change Adaptation: Special Report of the Intergovernmental Panel on Climate Change.* Cambridge: Cambridge University Press.

Kennedy, G., G. Nantel, and P. Shetty, P. 2003. "The Scourge of 'Hidden Hunger': Global Dimensions of Micronutrient Deficiencies." *Food Nutrition and Agriculture* 32:8–16.

Kerr, R. A. 2007. "Global Warming Coming Home to Roost in the American West." *Science* 318:1859.

Kimmel, C. A., G. W. Collman, N. Fields, and B. Eskenazi. 2005. "Lessons Learned for the National Children's Study from the National Institute of Environmental Health Sciences/US Environmental Protection Agency Centers for Children's Environmental Health and Disease Prevention Research." *Environmental Health Perspectives*, 113:1414–18.

Klironomos, J. N., M. C. Rillig, M. F. Allen, D. R. Zak, K. S. Pregitzer, and M. E. Kubiske. 1997. "Increased Levels of Airborne Fungal Spores in Response to *Populus tremuloides* Grown under Elevated Atmospheric CO_2." *Canadian Journal of Botany* 75:1670–73.

LaDeau, S. L., and J. S. Clark. 2006. "Pollen Production by *Pinus taeda* Growing in Elevated Atmospheric CO_2." *Functional Ecology* 20:541–47.

Lancet Commissions. 2009. "Managing the Health Effects of Climate Change." *Lancet* 373:1693–1733.

Landrigan, P. J., L. Claudio, S. B. Markowitz, G. S. Berkowitz, B. L. Brenner, H. Romero, J. G. Wetmur, et al. 1999. "Pesticides and Inner-City Children: Exposures, Risks, and Prevention." *Environmental Health Perspectives* 107:31–37.

Lloyd, S. J., R. S. Kovats, and Z. Chalabi. 2011. "Climate Change, Crop Yields and Undernutrition: Development of a Model to Quantify the Impact of Climate Scenarios on Child Undernutrition." *Environmental Health Perspectives* 119:1817–23.

Lobell, D. B., and M. B. Burke. 2010. "On the Use of Statistical Models to Predict Crop Yield Responses to Climate Change." *Agricultural and Forest Meteorology* 150:1443–52.

Lobell, D. B., M. B. Burke, C. Rebaldi, M. D. Mastrandrea, W. P. Falcon, and R. L. Naylor. 2008. "Prioritizing Climate Change Adaptation Needs for Food Security in 2030." *Science* 319:607–10.

Lobell, D. B., G. L. Hammer, G. McLean, C. Messina, M. J. Roberts, and W. Schlenker. 2013. "The Critical Role of Extreme Heat for Maize Production in the United States." *Nature Climate Change* 3:497–501.

Loladze, I. 2002. "Rising Atmospheric CO_2 and Human Nutrition: Toward Globally Imbalanced Plant Stoichiometry?" *Trends in Ecology and Evolution* 17:457–61.

Loladze, I. 2014. "Hidden Shift of the Ionome of Plants Exposed to Elevated CO_2 Depletes Minerals at the Base of Human Nutrition." *eLife,* 1–30. doi:10.7554/eLife.02245

Manea, A., M. R. Leishman, and P. O. Downey. 2011. "Exotic C_4 Grasses Have Increased Tolerance to Glyphosate under Elevated Carbon Dioxide." *Weed Science* 59:28–36.

McMichael, A. J., and E. Lindgren. 2011. "Climate Change: Present and Future Risks to Health, and Necessary Responses." *Journal of Internal Medicine* 270:401–13.

McMichael, A. J., H. Montgomery, and A. Costello. 2012. "Health Risks, Present and Future, from Global Climate Change." *British Medical Journal* 344. doi:10.1136/bmj.e1359

Mohan, J. E., L. H. Ziska, W. H. Schlesinger, R. B. Thomas, R. C. Sicher, K. George, and J. S. Clark. 2006. "Biomass and Toxicity Responses of Poison Ivy (*Toxicodendron radicans*) to Elevated Atmospheric CO_2." *Proceedings of the National Academy of Science USA* 103:9086–89.

Myers, S. S., A. Zanobetti, I. Kloog, P. Huybers, A.D.B. Leakey, A. J. Bloom, E. Carlisle, et al. 2014. "Increasing CO_2 Threatens Human Nutrition." *Nature* 510:139–44.

Patterson, D. T. 1995. "Weeds in a Changing Climate." *Weed Science* 43:685–701.

Patwardhan, B. 2005. *Traditional Medicine: Modern Approach for Affordable Global Health.* Geneva: World Health Organization.

Pearce, N., N. Ait-Khaled, R. Besley, J. Malloi, U. Keli, E. Mitchell, and C. Robertson. 2007. "Worldwide Trends in the Prevalence of Asthma Symptoms: Phase III of the International Study of Asthma and Allergies in Childhood (ISAAC)." *Thorax* 62:758–66.

Perera, F. 2014. "Children's Environmental Health: A Critical Challenge of Our Time." *Lancet* 383(9921):943–44.

Pimentel, D. 1997. *Techniques for Reducing Pesticides: Environmental and Economic Benefits.* Chichester, UK: Wiley.

Plowright, R. K., S. H. Sokolow, M. E. Gorman, P. Daszak, and J. E. Foley. 2008. "Causal Inference in Disease Ecology: Investigating Ecological Drivers of Disease Emergence." *Frontiers of Ecology and the Environment* 6:420–49.

Quest Diagnostics Health Trends. *Allergy Report 2011.* Allergies across America. www.questdiagnostics.com/brand/business/healthtrends/allergies/docs/2011_QD_AllergyReport.pdf

Rasmussen, A. 2002. "The Effects of Climate Change on the Birch Pollen Season in Denmark." *Aerobiologia* 18:253–65.

Rodríguez-Rajo, F. J., D. Fdez-Savilla, A. Stach, and V. Jato. 2010. "Assessment between Pollen Seasons in Areas with Different Urbanization Level Related to Local Vegetation Sources and Differences in Allergen Exposure." *Aerobiologia* 26:1–14.

Rogers, C. A., P. M. Wayne, E. A. Macklin, M. L. Mullenberg, C. J. Wagner, P. R. Epstein, and F. A. Bazzaz. 2006. "Interaction of the Onset of Spring and Elevated Atmospheric CO_2 on Ragweed (*Ambrosia artemisiifolia* L.) Pollen Production." *Environmental Health Perspectives* 114:865–69.

Schultes, R. E., and S. V. Reis. 1995. *Ethnobotany: The Evolution of a Discipline.* Portland, OR: Dioscorides Press.

Singer, B. D., L. H. Ziska, D. A. Frenz, D. E. Gebhard, and J. G. Straka. 2005. "Increasing Amb a 1 Content in Common Ragweed (*Ambrosia artemisiifolia*) Pollen as a Function of Rising Atmospheric CO_2 Concentration." *Functional Plant Biology* 32:67–70.

Stach, A., H. García-Mozo, J. C. Prieto-Baena, M. Czarnecka-Operacz, D. Jenerowicz, W. Silny, and C. Galan. 2007. "Prevalence of *Artemisia* Species Pollinosis in Western Poland: Impact of Climate Change on Aerobiological Trends, 1995–2004." *Journal of Allergologia Clinical Immunology* 17:39–45.

Stuhlfauth, T., and H. P. Fock. 1990. "Effect of Whole Season CO_2 Enrichment on the Cultivation of a Medicinal Plant, *Digitalis lanata*." *Journal of Agronomy and Crop Science* 164:168–73.

Tanner, T. 2000. "Rhus (toxicodendron) Dermatitis." *Primary Care* 27:493–501.

Taub, D., B. Miller, and H. Allen. 2008. "Effects of Elevated CO_2 on the Protein Concentration of Food Crops: A Meta-Analysis." *Global Change Biology* 14:565–75.

Wan, S., T. Yuan, S. Bowdish, L. Wallace, S. D. Russell, and Y. Luo. 2002. "Response of an Allergenic Species, *Ambrosia psilostachya* (*Asteraceae*), to Experimental Warming and Clipping: Implications for Public Health." *American Journal of Botany* 89:1843–46.

Wang, S. Y., J. A. Bunce, and J. L. Maas. 2003. "Elevated Carbon Dioxide Increases Contents of Antioxidant Compounds in Field-Grown Strawberries." *Journal of Agriculture and Food Chemistry* 51:4315–20.

Watson, W. A., T. L. Litovitz, W. Klein-Schwartz, G. C. Rodgers, J. Youniss, N. Reid, W. G. Rouse, R. S. Rembert, and D. Borys. 2004. "2003 Annual Report of the American Association of Poison Control Centers Toxic Exposure Surveillance System." *American Journal of Emergency Medicine* 22:335–404.

Wayne, P., S. Foster, J. Connolly, F. A. Bazzaz, and P. R. Epstein, 2002. "Production of Allergenic Pollen by Ragweed (*Ambrosia artemisiifolia* L.) Is Increased in CO_2-Enriched Atmospheres." *Annals of Allergy Asthma and Immunology* 80:669–79.

Wegren, S. K. 2011. "Food Security and Russia's 2010 Drought." *Eurasian Geography and Economics* 52:140–56.

Wolf, J., N. R. O'Neill, C. A. Rogers, M. L. Muilenberg, and L. H. Ziska. 2010. "Elevated Atmospheric Carbon Dioxide Concentrations Amplify *Alternaria alternata* Sporulation and Total Antigen Production." *Environmental Health Perspectives* 118:1223–28.

World Health Organization. 2002. "Traditional Medicine: Growing Needs and Potential." *WHO Policy Perspectives on Medicines* 2:1–6.

Ye-Ebiyo Y., R. J. Pollack, and A. Spielman. 2000. "Enhanced Development in Nature of Larval *Anopheles arabiensis* Mosquitoes Feeding on Maize Pollen." *American Journal of Tropical Medicine and Hygiene* 63:90–93.

Ziska, L. H. 2003. "Evaluation of the Growth Response of Six Invasive Species to Past, Present and Future Atmospheric Carbon Dioxide." *Journal of Experimental Botany* 54:395–404.

Ziska, L. H. 2004. "Influence of Rising Atmospheric CO_2 since 1900 on Early Growth and Photosynthetic Response of a Noxious Invasive Weed, Canada Thistle (*Cirsium arvense*)." *Functional Plant Biology* 29:1387–92.

Ziska, L. H. 2014. "Increasing Minimum Daily Temperatures Are Associated with Enhanced Pesticide Use in Cultivated Soybean along a Latitudinal Gradient in the Mid-Western United States." *PloS One* 9:e98516.

Ziska, L. H., and J. A. Bunce. 2006. "Plant Responses to Rising Carbon Dioxide." In *Plant Growth and Climate Change*, edited by J. Morison Morecroft, 17–47. Oxford: Blackwell.

Ziska, L. H., and F. A. Caulfield. 2000. "Rising CO_2 and Pollen Production of Common Ragweed (*Ambrosia artemisiifolia*), a Known Allergy-Inducing Species: Implications for Public Health." *Australian Journal of Plant Physiology* 27:893–98.

Ziska, L. H., S. D. Emche, E. L. Johnson, K. George, D. R. Reed, and R. C. Sicher. 2005. "Alterations in the Production and Concentration of Selected Alkaloids as a Function of Rising Atmospheric Carbon Dioxide and Air Temperature: Implications for Ethno-Pharmacology." *Global Change Biology* 11:1798–1807.

Ziska, L. H., S. Panicker, and H. L. Wojno. 2008. "Recent and Projected Increases in Atmospheric Carbon Dioxide and the Potential Impacts on Growth and Alkaloid Production in Wild Poppy (*Papaver setigerum* DC.)" *Climatic Change* 91:395–403.

Ziska, L. H., S. S. Faulkner, and J. Lydon. 2004. "Changes in Biomass and Root: Shoot Ratio of Field-Grown Canada Thistle (*Cirsium arvense*), a Noxious, Invasive Weed, with Elevated CO_2: Implications for Control with Glyphosate." *Weed Science* 52:584–88.

Ziska, L. H., D. E. Gebhard, D. A. Frenz, S. Faulkner, and B. D. Singer. 2003. "Cities as Harbingers of Climate Change: Common Ragweed, Urbanization, and Public Health." *Journal of Allergy and Clinical Immunology* 111:290–95.

Ziska, L. H., K. Knowlton, C. Rogers, D. Dalan, N. Tierney, M. A. Elder, W. Filley, et al. 2011. "Recent Warming by Latitude Associated with Increased Length of Ragweed Pollen Season in Central North America." *Proceedings of the National Academy of Sciences USA* 108:4248–51.

Ziska, L. H., R. C. Sicher, K. George, and J. E. Mohan. 2007. "Rising Atmospheric Carbon Dioxide and Potential Impacts on the Growth and Toxicity of Poison Ivy (*Toxidodendron radicans*)." *Weed Science* 55:288–92.

Ziska, L. H., and J. R. Teasdale. 2000. "Sustained Growth and Increased Tolerance to Glyphosate Observed in a C3 Perennial Weed, Quackgrass (*Elytrigia repens* (L.) Nevski), Grown at Elevated Carbon Dioxide." *Australian Journal of Plant Physiology* 27:159–64.

Ziska, L. H., J. R. Teasdale, and J. A. Bunce. 1999. "Future Atmospheric Carbon Dioxide Concentrations May Increase Tolerance to Glyphosate." *Weed Science* 47:608–15.

Zobayed, S., and P. K. Saxena, 2004. "Production of St. John's Wort Plants under Controlled Environment for Maximizing Biomass and Secondary Metabolites." *In Vitro Cell Developmental Biology* 40:108–14.

CHAPTER 8

CLIMATE AND ITS IMPACTS ON VECTOR-BORNE AND ZOONOTIC DISEASES

Charles B. Beard, Jada F. Garofalo, Kenneth L. Gage

Climatologists are in virtual agreement that the climate of our planet is changing as a result of human activities that have rapidly increased levels of greenhouse gases in the atmosphere over the past century. Models developed by the same scientists also predict that the observed climate trends will continue to contribute other unwelcome changes by increasing the frequency of exceptionally severe storms, flooding events, and droughts. Although some disagreement exists about the extent to which these climatic changes have been responsible for recent extreme weather events or how they will manifest, most believe that the changes predicted by current models will continue to pose serious threats to human welfare over the next few decades.

Among the most severe impacts of climate change will be those related to human health. The World Health Organization (WHO) issued a report stating that climate change had led to approximately 150,000 deaths annually by the year 2000 (Institute of Medicine Forum on Microbial Threats 2008). The difficult task of effectively mitigating and adapting to any health-related effects of climate change will be made even more daunting by the fact that the impacts of climate change are likely to have additive, and potentially exacerbating, impacts to human health when combined with other nonclimate impacts, including those associated with ongoing global changes driven by human activities. Unfortunately, the ability to predict how and to what extent climate factors will interact with nonclimate factors to affect human health is made particularly difficult by the lack

KEY CONCEPTS

- **The transmission and distribution of vector-borne and zoonotic diseases (VBZDs) are strongly influenced by environmental conditions, including those affected by climate.**

- **VBZD agents, hosts, and vectors occur in complex ecological communities located within rapidly changing ecosystems.**

- **Climate change acts in conjunction with other drivers of global change to influence human VBZD risks.**

- **Our ability to anticipate and react effectively to the impacts of climate change on VBZDs is greatly hampered by the limited availability of appropriate surveillance, demographic, land use, and environmental data.**

of long-term data sets available on the relationships between human diseases and climate variables. Efforts to predict the effects of climate change on human health are also complicated by the fact that many of the anticipated changes are likely to occur over time scales of thirty or more years. This is especially true for **vector-borne and zoonotic diseases (VBZDs)**, which are expected to increase in incidence and spread to previously disease-free areas in the wake of climate change (Shope 1991; Patz et al. 1996; Gubler and Trent 1993; Epstein 2001; Sutherst 2004; Gage et al. 2008; Mills, Gage, and Khan 2010).

VBZDs are estimated to cause over 300,000 human illnesses every year in the United States. The term *vector borne* means transmitted by mosquitoes, ticks, fleas, and in some cases biting flies, and the term *zoonotic* means harbored by vertebrate animals with potential for spread to humans. Not all vector-borne diseases are zoonotic and not all zoonotic diseases are vector borne. In some cases, vectors transmit pathogens from animal hosts to humans (**Lyme disease**), and in some cases vectors transmit pathogens from human to human (**malaria**). Thousands of zoonotic infections also occur as a result of the nonvector-borne transmission of bacterial, viral, or parasitic pathogens from animals to humans through biting, scratching, inhalation, or ingestion. Some of the latter zoonoses, such as **rabies**, brucellosis, and hantaviral illnesses, are relatively rare in the United States, but others, such as toxoplasmosis, Q fever, and influenza, can account for thousands to many thousands of human infections each year. It is difficult to prevent, control, and predict vector-borne and zoonotic diseases because they involve pathogens, vectors, animal hosts, and humans, each of them affected by climate and nonclimate factors.

In many ways VBZDs are especially susceptible to year-to-year variations in climate and long-term climate change. The fact that arthropod vectors are ectothermic, or cold-blooded, means their body temperature is determined by that of the surrounding environment. This temperature dependency can affect vector behaviors, including host seeking and egg laying, as well as rates of egg development or other aspects of reproduction. The time required for vectors to complete the immature stages of their life cycles is strongly influenced by temperature and can significantly affect vector population dynamics, including the number of vector generations that can be produced in a given transmission season. Temperature also affects the rate at which pathogens reproduce or develop within the vector, an effect that is particularly important because increased temperatures can decrease a pathogen's extrinsic incubation period (EIP), the time required for the pathogen to establish an infection in a blood-feeding vector and then multiply or develop to the point where it can be transmitted during subsequent vector feedings. Temperature often interacts with humidity to determine vector survival. Excessively hot and dry conditions can be particularly deleterious and limit the time that vectors can safely spend questing for hosts. Precipitation can profoundly influence the population dynamics of vectors such as mosquitoes that breed in aquatic habitats and require sufficient standing water for successful egg hatching and development of their larvae and pupae. Because of their influence on the availability of food and suitable habitats, seasonal and long-term changes in precipitation and temperature also can affect the distribution and abundance of the vertebrate hosts of VBZDs, as well as the types and numbers of pathogens they carry.

In this research, however, there is considerable disagreement over the importance of climate change relative to the influence of other nonclimate factors. Some of the other factors include microbial adaptation and change, human susceptibility to infection, socioeconomic factors, human behavior, changing ecosystems, economic development and land use, urbanization, technology and industry, international travel and commerce, vector control measures, war and famine, lack of political will, and intent to harm among others (figure 8.1).

DRIVERS OF DISEASE EMERGENCE

1. Microbial adaptation and change
2. Human susceptibility to infection
3. Climate and weather
4. Changing ecosystems
5. Economic development and land use
6. Human demographics and behavior
7. Technology and industry
8. International travel and commerce
9. Breakdown of public health measures
10. Poverty and social inequality
11. War and famine
12. Lack of political will
13. Intent to harm

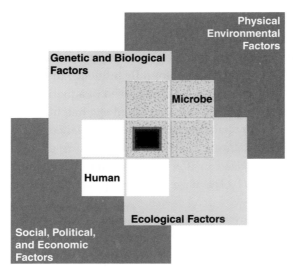

Figure 8.1   Convergence Model for Emerging Diseases
Source: Adapted from Institute of Medicine of the National Academies (2003).

This chapter discusses how climate change might affect the spread and distribution of VBZDs. It also explores how climate change is likely to act in conjunction with other drivers of global change to influence the transmission and complex ecological cycles of the agents responsible for VBZDs. Because of the plethora of VBZDs, we have chosen representative examples to illustrate these topics: malaria, dengue, West Nile virus illness, Lyme disease, and rabies. Finally, we discuss the importance of formulating effective response plans for the recognized effects of climate change on VBZDs. This process necessitates the timely collection of reliable surveillance data on human and animal cases of disease. These data will help identify potential climate-related changes in disease incidence, support the implementation of targeted research to identify areas at greatest risk for VBZD emergence or outbreaks, and create accessible environmental data sets at appropriate spatial and temporal scales for high-risk areas and populations.

CLINICAL CORRELATES 8.1 MALARIA SURVEILLANCE

Strong malaria surveillance systems are fundamental to global eradication efforts. In the setting of climate change, reliable testing is necessary to detect and respond to unusual outbreak trends. The gold standard for malaria testing is microscopy; however, antigen-based rapid diagnostic tests (RTDs) have sensitivities that approach that of the gold standard (95 percent). Barriers to the routine use of RTDs include insufficient numbers of trained health workers, supplying remote locations with testing supplies, and technology that has a limited shelf life. Despite these barriers, there has been a global increase in rate of diagnostic testing from 44 percent in 2010 to 64 percent in 2012 (World Health Organization 2013). Testing is necessary to ensure that medications are used in a manner that prevents drug resistance and ensure that other infections do not go untreated. For example, in a prospective study of nine hundred febrile children presenting to hospitals in northern Tanzania, malaria was the clinical diagnosis in 61 percent, while after testing, the confirmed rate was 1.6 percent. Other acute bacterial zoonotic infections, including brucellosis, leptospirosis, Q fever, and typhus, accounted for 26 percent of infections. The arbovirus chikungunya accounted for 8 percent, while the other causes of fever were unknown (Crump, Morrissey, and Bartlett 2013). As global climate change affects the distribution of zoonotic infections, rapid diagnostic testing and clinical vigilance will be important to detect and mitigate infectious disease outbreaks.

The geographical distributions of malaria and other zoonotic diseases are likely to change as the climate does. Knowledge of these dynamics coupled with clinical vigilance will be necessary to ensure accurate diagnosis and treatment.

Malaria

Etiology

Malaria is a febrile illness caused by protozoan parasites of the genus *Plasmodium* and transmitted by *Anopheles* mosquitoes. After receiving a bite from an infected mosquito, there is an incubation period, typically seven to thirty days, before symptoms appear. Parasites first grow and multiply in liver cells and then move to red blood cells. Symptoms are caused by blood-stage parasites, and at this time the parasite can be transmitted from human to mosquito. The disease is generally categorized as uncomplicated malaria or complicated malaria, a more severe manifestation of the disease; however, the illness is curable if diagnosis and treatment occur promptly. Uncomplicated malaria lasts six to ten hours and consists of a cold stage (chills, shivering), a hot stage (fever, headaches, vomiting, and nausea, and seizures in young children), and a sweating stage (normal temperature with sweats and tiredness). These symptoms may occur every second day (tertian parasites), every third day (quartan parasites), or a patient may have a combination of symptoms, also including body aches. Malaria is categorized as severe when symptoms include serious organ failures and abnormalities in the blood or metabolism (including impaired consciousness, seizure, coma, hemolysis, homoglobinuria, acute respiratory distress syndrome [ARDS], low blood pressure, acute kidney failure, hyperparasitemia, hypoglycemia, and metabolic acidosis).

Of the over one hundred species of the parasite *Plasmodium*, only five can infect humans. The most pathogenic of these is *P. falciparum*, which kills nearly 1 million people per year and is found primarily in Africa (Centers for Disease Control and Prevention 2013d). Malaria is especially dangerous due to high levels of resistance to antimalarial drugs and its ability to cause severe anemia, as well as cerebral malaria, a particularly severe, and often fatal, form of the disease associated with the adherence of *P. falciparum*-infected erythrocytes to the walls of veins in a victim's brain. *P. malariae* is found worldwide and can cause chronic, severe malaria with occasional complications, including nephrotic syndrome. Both *P. vivax*, which is found in parts of Asia, Latin America, and Africa, and *P. ovale*, which is found primarily in Africa and some Pacific islands, have a dormant liver stage, which may lead to relapse several months to years after initial infection. Unlike the above species of *Plasmodium*, which specifically infect humans and are rarely identified in other primates, *P. knowlesi* occurs naturally in Southeast Asia in long-tailed and pig-tailed macaques and represents a zoonotic form of malaria that can be potentially severe in humans, at least in part because of its twenty-four-hour replication cycle, as opposed to the tertian (two-day) replication cycles of *P. falciparum*, *P. vivax*, and *P. ovale*, or the quartan (three-day) cycle of *P. malariae*.

Five species of the Malaria parasite infect humans:

P. falciparum

P. malariae

P. vivax

P. ovale

P. knowlesi

Among the approximately five hundred proposed species of *Anopheles* mosquitoes, about seventy are known to be capable of transmitting human malaria (Garske, Ferguson, and Ghani 2013). While both male and female *Anopheles* feed on sugar, after the mating process, females must seek a blood meal to complete egg development, a process that usually takes two or three days but can be affected by temperature. The progression from egg to larva to pupa to adult is also strongly influenced by temperature, as is the behavior of the blood-seeking female mosquito. Species of *Anopheles* that feed primarily on humans (anthropogenic) and bite indoors (endophagic) tend to have more frequent human contact in an ideal temperature environment and thus have increased vector capacity. The length of time an adult female mosquito survives is particularly important because the longer she lives, the more blood meals she is likely to take. This provides more opportunities for her to become infected and later transmit malaria to susceptible, uninfected hosts.

The relationships among mosquitoes, parasites, and humans are the critical factors in determining malaria transmission. These include mosquito biting frequency, feeding behavior, breeding site availability, and reproduction and survival rates, and the EIP for each species of *Plasmodium*. Each of these relationships is further influenced by climate and nonclimate factors, including temperature, rainfall, humidity, altitude, the ratio of mosquitoes to humans, pathogen resistance to antimalarial drugs, environmental disturbances, and other socioeconomic variables that may limit or enhance human-vector contact (Garske, Ferguson, and Ghani 2013).

For malaria transmission to be successful, a female *Anopheles* must survive long enough after becoming infected (taking initial blood meal) to allow the parasites to complete the extrinsic growth cycle (to mature and become transmittable) and resume the mating and blood seeking cycle.

Linkages to the Climate

On a worldwide basis, malaria is estimated to cause 220 million cases and 660,000 deaths annually, with 80 percent of its burden concentrated in Africa, and these statistics may become even more significant (Garske, Ferguson, and Ghani 2013). The Earth's surface temperature is projected to increase 3.5°C in the next century, which may speed up malaria transmission and mosquito development (Lindsay and Martens 1998). For example, *P. falciparum* cannot complete its growth cycle within an *Anopheles* mosquito at temperatures below 20°C (68°F) and, in general, mosquito survival is negatively associated with exposure to excessively hot or dry conditions (Craig, Snow, and le Sueur 1999; Aboagye-Antwi et al. 2010). A diverse body of evidence describes the known impacts of climate factors on malaria, including numerous studies reporting associations between malaria outbreaks and changing values for various climatic variables, particularly those related to temperature, precipitation, humidity, and fluctuations in climatic cycles or other large-scale global climate phenomena, such as the El Niño Southern Oscillation (ENSO), Indian Ocean Dipole (IOd), and sea surface temperatures (Bouma and Dye 1997; Hashizume, Terao, and Minakawa 2009; Hashizume, Chaves, and Minakawa 2012; Thomson 2010; Mabaso and Ndlovu 2012; Mordecai et al. 2013.

Climate can be used as an indicator of potential outbreaks because climate variability affects the speed of mosquito and parasite proliferation (Lindsay and Martens 1998).

Despite the seemingly large body of evidence indicating that climate change will influence the transmission of the malaria parasite and the incidence of disease, the actual impact of climate change on human cases remains largely controversial (Lafferty 2009; Pascual and Bouma 2009), in part because of differences in interpreting existing data sets and the fact that climate change will not act alone but in conjunction with, and perhaps be of less importance than, other nonclimate factors and regional changes (Reiter 2008; Chaves and Koenraadt 2010).

Malaria in the African Highlands

The introduction of malaria into the Kenyan highlands (Lindsay and Martens 1998) exemplifies how mosquito biology and transmission capabilities can interact with a variety of nonclimate factors to influence malaria transmission and how the quality of data collected may be important to the ability to associate climate change with disease expansion. This case also provides insights into the difficulty in determining the relative importance of climate change compared to other factors affecting the spread of malaria.

In the early twentieth century, malaria was introduced to the Kenyan highlands by soldiers returning from World War I. For centuries, cooler temperatures associated with the higher elevations had provided a defense against malaria by curbing mosquito populations in the highlands; yet at this time, nearly 25 percent of the indigenous population contracted malaria, primarily caused by **Plasmodium falciparum** (Lindsay and Martens 1998). Over the past century, malaria has been rare, but there has been a rise in both epidemic and endemic cases at higher elevations since the 1980s (Lindsay and Martens 1998). For example, in the past thirteen years, western Kenyan epidemics spread from three to fifteen districts and increased from 20 to 60 percent incidence with high morbidity and mortality in all age groups (Githeko and Ndegwa 2001).

Climate change has been a proposed but controversial driver for this malaria resurgence (Thomson 2010). According to some, epidemics in the highlands have worsened due to warming temperatures, which have allowed the mosquitoes to move to higher elevations where, due to lower historical incidence of malaria, human immunity is lower (Lindsay and Martens 1998). However, the putative effects of climate change on malaria resurgence in the highlands are based on analyses of annual epidemic occurrences and their associations with various meteorological factors. Many published models evaluating temperature effects on malaria transmission often ignore diurnal temperature variation and instead use average minimum and maximum temperatures to project the impact of climate change on malaria resurgence (Mabaso and Ndlovu 2012). Models that ignore this diurnal temperature variation may not capture the level of variability in the system and may conceal an observable epidemic-related signal (Reiter 2008; Chaves and Koenraadt 2010; Githeko and Ndegwa 2001). For instance, diurnal temperature fluctuations may influence vector biology and parasite development and propagation, both of which influence transmission of *Plasmodium* to humans (Paaijmans, Read, and Thomas 2009). These models have likely overestimated malaria risk in warmer environments and underestimated risk in cooler environments (Paaijmans, Read, and Thomas 2009). Thus, data must be of the finest resolution possible and collected for all contributing factors when ascertaining the relationship between climate and malaria transmission (Githeko and Ndegwa 2001). Incidentally, in many cases, the projected malaria resurgence may not be precise or in accordance with actual resurgence (Paaijmans, Read, and Thomas 2009; Blanford et al. 2013). Others contend that while climate is an important factor in determining malaria risk, it will likely contribute less to malaria resurgence than other nonclimate factors. For example, in the United States after World War II, malaria was eradicated through the use of intensive DDT applications, effective water management, and measures to minimize human-vector contact (Reiter 2008; Gubler et al. 2001; Levine, Peterson, and Benedict 2004). Effective implementation of these led to eradication of indigenous human malaria transmission in the United States despite the fact that competent *Anopheles* vectors remained pervasive throughout much of the disease's former range, including the southeastern and south-central United States. Because of these past successes, climate change is not projected to result in malaria becoming a major problem in the United States (Reiter 2008; Gubler et al. 2001; Levine, Peterson, and Benedict 2004). Elsewhere, climate-induced migration of

Anopheles will likely contribute only in part to a resurgence of malaria depending on the availability of public health infrastructure that can mitigate human-vector exposure and vector and parasite propagation.

Although the effect of certain climate variables on malaria resurgence in the African Highlands might at first seem straightforward due to the known impacts on mosquito and parasite survival, development, and reproduction, there is uncertainty in attributing the expansion of malaria strictly to climate change (Zhou et al. 2004; Patz et al. 2002, 2005; Hay et al. 2002). This is due to the multitude of nonclimate factors that collectively contribute to the establishment of malaria as an endemic disease in the region, including socioeconomic factors, an increased human population, expanded transportation, types and amount of housing construction, levels of human immunity, inadequate vector control, poor health service infrastructure, increased irrigation and standing water, deforestation, and other changing land use patterns (Lindsay and Martens 1998).

When evaluating the potential impacts of climate change, researchers also should take care to use temperature data appropriate for the given mosquito environment (air, water, inside, outside, hourly, or monthly) and available at the appropriate resolution in order to increase the accuracy of predictions regarding the impacts of all factors on malaria transmission (Garske, Ferguson, and Ghani 2013). Because climate variability affects the speed of mosquito and parasite proliferation and development, it also can be effectively viewed as an indicator of potential outbreaks rather than as an exclusive cause (Lindsay and Martens 1998).

Priorities for mitigating the potential impact of climate change on malaria transmission include initiating activities to prevent the return of *Anopheles*-transmitted malaria in areas where it has been previously eliminated and identifying vulnerable regions at temperate latitudes that have minimal public health infrastructure and are projected to warm disproportionately under future projections of climate change (Patz et al. 2005). More accurate modeling has also been suggested as a means to improve prevention capabilities. This will require the availability of high-quality long-term data sets of both climatological and epidemiological data, which are often not available depending on where and how recently an outbreak has occurred. Inclusion of daily diurnal temperature variation and other high temporal and spatial resolution data in development of these models may also improve understanding of the relationship between vector and parasite and aid in calculating the impacts climate change may have on public health, disease risk, pest populations, and biodiversity loss (Blanford et al. 2013).

CLINICAL CORRELATES 8.2 FOCUSING EFFORTS ON MALARIAL PREVENTION

Malaria has devastating effects on children under the age of five, with an estimated 100,000 deaths per year due to intrauterine growth retardation and over 100,000 deaths in young children arising from primary infection. Morbidity is also high, and chronic infection impairs mental and physical development, ultimately taking a toll on the child's education and subsequent adult productivity (UNICEF 2013). The WHO recommends three prevention strategies to target these high-risk populations in areas with severe malarial burden (van Eijk et al. 2013; Eisele et al. 2012; Cairns et al. 2012):

1. Intermittent preventative treatment in pregnancy

2. Intermittent preventative treatment in infants

3. Seasonal malaria chemoprevention for children aged three to fifty-nine months

These recommendations rely heavily on the medical community to increase the training of skilled health workers and the distribution of medications. At the same time, surveillance is necessary to ensure that labor-intensive efforts are directed where they are needed most.

Malaria is a climate-sensitive disease that continues to cause significant morbidity and mortality in the child population. Global eradication efforts rely on appropriate training of providers and evidence-based use of antimalarial medication.

The Recent Expansion of Dengue

Etiology

Dengue, also known as breakbone fever, is caused by four related viruses (serotypes), referred to as dengue virus (DENV) 1 through 4. The disease is characterized by high fever; severe headache; retro-orbital pain; severe pain in the joints, muscles, and skeleton; mild bleeding; and rash. Symptoms typically appear four to seven days after an infectious mosquito bite and can persist for three to ten days. Disease is usually milder in young persons and those experiencing their first DENV infection. Individuals who recover after infection with one serotype and later are infected with another serotype of DENV are at increased risk of developing the much more serious dengue hemorrhagic fever (DHF) and dengue shock syndrome (DSS). Treatment of dengue patients relies on supportive therapy to ease symptoms and lessen the risk of severe disease. Research is underway to develop a vaccine, but none is currently available for general use. Prevention generally relies on avoiding exposure to the bites of infectious mosquitoes.

Dengue first emerged as a widespread, serious threat to humans in the 1950s (Burek, Gulland, and O'Hara 2008). Currently, at least 125 countries are considered dengue endemic, and estimates of global incidence most often range from 50 to 200 million cases, although recent cartographic approaches suggest about one-third of the world's population is at risk, and the figure could be as high as 400 million (Murray, Quam, and Wilder-Smith 2013). Risks are greatest in tropical areas, especially those experiencing increased urbanization, but temperate regions are also increasingly at risk.

The *Aedes aegypti* mosquito feeds almost exclusively on humans and breeds primarily in cities and villages, where it has benefited greatly from the rapid urbanization now occurring in many developing countries. The mosquito is most active during daylight hours but prefers to feed and rest in sites shaded by trees or in dark areas within buildings.

Linkages to the Climate

The likely impacts of climate change on the spread of mosquito-borne arboviral diseases, including dengue, have been the subject of much recent debate, especially with respect to the relative importance of climate change compared to other drivers of disease spread (Gubler and Trent 1993; Sutherst 2004; Gage et al. 2008; Reiter 2001; Ooi and Gubler 2009; Higa 2011; Thai and Anders 2011). Some have stressed how climate change could affect the distributions of mosquito vectors, development of arboviruses within these vectors, and the onset and duration of transmission seasons (Shope 1991; Epstein 2001; Haines and Patz 2004; Weaver and Reisen 2010). Others have emphasized how nonclimate factors affect the spread of these diseases, including increased urbanization, land and water use changes, shifting agricultural practices, political unrest, demographic shifts, human migration, inefficient public health measures, and other issues. The following discussion examines how these factors could interact with climate change to influence the transmission and geographic spread of DENV.

As was the case for malaria, an understanding of the potential impacts of climate change on the spread of dengue requires knowledge of the biology of the mosquito vectors and its influence on transmission. The primary vector of dengue is the yellow fever mosquito, *Aedes aegypti*, a species that originated in Africa but is now found in the Americas, Asia, Australia, the South Pacific, and Middle East (Higa 2011). This mosquito feeds preferentially on humans and breeds primarily in cities and villages, where it has benefited greatly from the rapid urbanization now occurring in many developing countries. *Ae. aegypti* is most active during daylight hours but prefers to feed and rest in sites shaded by trees or in dark areas within buildings. Those living in natural forest habitats lay their eggs in container tree holes, puddles, or other naturally occurring water-holding structures, while *Ae. aegypti* living in more urbanized areas more often lay their eggs in mud at the edge of puddles or just above the water line in discarded cans, bottles, tires, flower pots, water jugs, or other containers partially filled with water. As water in these sites evaporates, the eggs dry and become resistant to desiccation, often surviving for many weeks to months before rains once again flood the container or puddle where they were laid. Once submerged, the eggs soon hatch, releasing larval mosquitoes that feed on microbes found in the water. Within a few days these larvae grow sufficiently to mature to the pupal stage, from which they will emerge a few days later as adult mosquitoes.

Because *Ae. aegypti* eggs are resistant to desiccation, they can be carried over long distances on various modes of transportation, greatly enhancing the ability of this mosquito to invade new areas. Although this factor, as well as the transportation of larval and pupal stages in water-filled containers, has resulted in the introduction of *Ae. aegypti* into many areas, its permanent distribution has been limited to a zone lying between approximately 40 degrees North and 40 degrees South. This zone includes the southern United States, where *Ae. aegypti* is present year round and maintains permanent breeding populations. Restriction of permanent breeding populations to this particular range of latitudes suggests that climatic factors play a significant role in the distribution of this mosquito, but factors in the human environment also can be important, particularly if human activities provide microhabitats with suitable conditions in an area that is otherwise unfavorable (Jansen and Beebe; Eisen and Moore 2013). *Ae. aegypti* also can temporarily invade higher latitudes, such as those along the mid-Atlantic and New England coasts in the United States but fail to establish permanent populations in these sites because the adult mosquitoes cannot tolerate prolonged exposure to freezing temperatures or overwinter in the egg stage. Nevertheless, these seasonal introductions and temporary breeding during the warmer months of the year can threaten human health, as demonstrated by the occurrence of multiple summer outbreaks of dengue and yellow fever (another arboviral illness transmitted by *Ae. aegypti*) in eighteenth-century Philadelphia, a city that experiences below-freezing temperatures in winter months and is unsuitable for the long-term persistence of this mosquito or the diseases it transmits (Shope 1991; Gubler et al. 2001; Ooi and Gubler 2009).

Another mosquito, *Ae. albopictus* (Asian tiger mosquito), is less efficient at transmitting DENV and usually serves as a secondary vector in areas where its distribution coincides with that of *Ae. aegypti* (Higa 2011). However, in sites where *Ae. aegypti* are absent, *Ae. albopictus* can act as a primary vector of dengue. The significance of *Ae. albopictus* as a dengue vector is likely to increase as its geographic range continues to expand far beyond its original Asian homeland into parts of North and South America, Europe, and Africa (Higa 2011; Rezza 2012). Frequently these range expansions have occurred as the result of viable eggs being transported in used tires or other container habitats. In addition to used tires, eggs also are laid in bamboo stumps, tree holes, flower vases, and other natural or man-made container habitats. Once laid, the eggs of certain strains of *Ae. albopictus* can undergo a winter diapause, allowing this mosquito to overwinter and become established in temperate regions with winters too cold for the survival of *Ae. aegypti*. The increased temperatures brought on by climate change are likely to increase the range of suitable habitat available to this mosquito. *Ae. albopictus* are also much less host specific than *Ae. aegypti*, feeding not only on humans but also on a wide variety of amphibians, reptiles, birds, and mammals found in domestic and forested environments, a factor that might reduce its role in dengue transmission but poses a threat for the transmission of other arboviruses of zoonotic origin. Unlike the yellow fever mosquito, Asian tiger mosquitoes prefer to seek blood meals outdoors, usually at dawn and dusk. They also tend to rest in vegetation rather than buildings, which explains their relative abundance in suburban and rural areas compared to the more urban dwelling *Ae. aegypti*.

The *Ae. albopictus* (Asian tiger mosquito) usually serves only as a secondary vector of dengue in areas where its distribution coincides with that of *Ae. aegypti*. However, where the latter species is absent, such as in certain areas of Japan, *Ae. albopictus* acts as the primary vector of dengue despite the fact that it is less efficient at transmitting DENV than *Ae. aegypti*.

Climatic variability, including periods of increased rainfall, unusual temperatures, elevated relative humidity, vapor pressure, and oscillations in climatic cycles, such as the ENSO, are known to affect dengue transmission, as well as the survival, development, host seeking, and reproduction of the mosquito vectors (Gubler et al. 2001; Reiter 2001; Thai and Anders 2011; Jansen and Beebe 2010). For example, in New Caledonia, the likelihood of dengue outbreaks over a four-decade period was found to depend on maximal temperature and relative humidity thresholds (Descloux et al. 2012). In Singapore, time-lagged values for mean weekly temperature and mean relative humidity were correlated with reports of dengue cases (Earnest, Tan, and Wilder-Smith 2012). Dengue transmission in the South Pacific was associated not only with rainfall and temperature but also with the values for ENSO and the Southern Oscillation Index (SOI) (Hales et al. 1999). ENSO, as well as rainfall, temperature, and humidity, also was linked to dengue in Vietnam (Thai et al. 2010), although a study in Puerto Rico found only weak relationships of ENSO, climate, and dengue incidence (Johansson, Cummings, and Glass 2009).

Although increased rainfall and elevated temperatures are often cited as factors promoting the spread of mosquito-borne diseases, not all studies have shown this to be the case or that climate factors contribute significantly only in some situations (Hay et al. 2000; Cazelles et al. 2005). Increased temperatures also can lead to decreased adult mosquito survival when low humidity conditions prevail, a circumstance likely to be encountered in arid tropical and temperate areas at least on a seasonal basis. *Ae. aegypti* abundance in Bangkok, Thailand, was found to depend not on rainfall amounts but rather on the refilling of container habitats in domestic environments by the city's human residents (Ooi and Gubler 2009). Others have stressed the difficulties encountered in determining the contributions of potential causal mechanisms (Cazelles et al. 2005). By using wavelet analysis to investigate the occurrence of dengue cases in Thailand from 1983 to 1997, these authors found that some specific dengue outbreaks reported between 1986 and 1992 were indeed associated with El Niño events, but other outbreaks occurring through the entire period of the study did not exhibit this relationship and were thought to be due to the influence of local factors.

Sustained climate change, as opposed to year-to-year climatic variability, will result in long-term changes in rainfall, temperature and humidity, or vapor pressure values that could influence dengue transmission and the geographic range of the mosquito vectors of DENV. Obviously this could occur as a result of climate change affecting the development of DENV within *Ae. aegypti* and *Ae. albopictus* or by altering environments in such a way that poor habitats become suitable for supporting populations of these vectors. For example, an increase in average winter temperatures could allow *Ae. aegypti* to persist in areas where it has been introduced in the past but failed to become established because of its inability to survive freezing temperatures (Shope 1991). Research in Japan suggests that rising temperatures also will result in poleward expansions of the range of the more cold-tolerant *Ae. albopictus* (Higa 2011). Rising temperatures also can be expected to decrease mosquito generation times by accelerating larval growth rates, an effect that could increase the number of potential vectors available to acquire and transmit DENV in a given area. A third effect of increasing temperatures will be a decrease in the EIP. Typically the EIP in dengue-endemic areas would be about eight to twelve days (Centers for Disease Control and Prevention 2013b). In one study the EIP for infected mosquitoes was twelve days at 30°C but only seven days when these insects were held at 32°C to 35°C (Watts et al. 1987).

Although a difference of a few days in the EIP for DENV-infected mosquitoes might seem trivial, it can significantly affect the rate at which infectious mosquitoes appear in local vector populations, a factor that can significantly influence the rate at which dengue spreads among humans. This seemingly simple relationship between temperature, decreased EIPs, and the spread of dengue is likely to be more complex than it first appears, however, because the expected positive correlation between the effects of increased temperatures on EIPs and levels of transmission is likely to be offset to at least some extent by the negative impacts of increased temperatures on daily survivorship of the mosquito vectors. In another study, the recent global distribution of dengue was shown by logistic regression modeling to depend strongly on climate, and the climatic variable that contributed most significantly to the fit of the final model, which exhibited 89 percent accuracy, was long-term vapor pressure, a variable that is likely to affect the survival and activity of *Ae. aegypti* and *Ae. albopictus* mosquitoes (Hales et al. 2002). As its authors noted, this study provides good evidence that climatic factors influence the global distribution of dengue, but did not attempt to examine the many human factors that might influence dengue transmission and distribution.

Despite abundant evidence that climate can influence mosquito biology and dengue transmission, a general consensus seems to exist that climate change is likely to be of secondary importance in many instances to other anthropogenic-driven environmental changes, especially when those changes act in combination with other global changes and inefficient public health measures (Reiter 2001; Ooi and Gubler 2009). Among the most influential of these factors are the increasing trend of urbanization in the tropics, the migration of susceptible persons from rural areas to those becoming more urbanized, and the transport of infected persons and mosquitoes carrying one or more of the four strains of dengue virus from one region to another. Also important is the number of persons in a population who have acquired immunity following exposure to one or more strains of DENV, a factor that can reduce the number of hosts who are susceptible to dengue and therefore capable of developing the high-level viremias required to infect feeding mosquitoes and sustain local transmission of the disease.

Human behaviors, styles of home and building construction, and the use of air-conditioning are also significant because they can act to reduce contact between infectious mosquitoes and susceptible humans.

During recent dengue outbreaks along the US-Mexico border, infection with DENV was more prevalent on the Mexican side of the border. This is presumably because of the greater use of air-conditioning on the US side of the border, which resulted in more persons remaining indoors where they were far less likely to be bitten by infectious mosquitoes than those living in nearby Mexican communities that had fewer air-conditioned homes (Reiter et al. 2003). Also contributing to the reduced risk on the US side of the border was the presence of effective sanitary sewers and piped household water supplies that acted to lower mosquito numbers and the likelihood of humans being bitten by infected mosquitoes. Availability of air-conditioning in homes is clearly related to the economic well-being of individuals, and the economic status of different regions and countries is often mentioned as a factor influencing the incidence of mosquito-borne diseases. One suggested that although climate change was likely to increase dengue risk worldwide, its impact will depend significantly on the economic conditions of at-risk countries. Specifically these authors found that rising gross domestic product per capita is likely to result in decreased dengue risks by 2050 even in the face of projected climate changes (Astrom et al. 2012).

Because the maintenance and expansion of *Ae. agypti* populations depends on the presence of sufficient numbers of container habitats, the storage of water in domestic environments by persons living in relatively arid or drought-stricken areas also can significantly increase risk by providing container breeding habitats for vector mosquitoes. In one study in Australia, where the disease is endemic in Queensland but not in the more temperate state of New South Wales, it was determined that climatic variables were likely to affect dengue risk in the latter state only indirectly as a result of the use of water storage containers to augment the limited water supplies available to homes and businesses during droughts or in anticipation of projected periods of water shortage (Beebe et al. 2009). Those who recommend caution when predicting the effects climate change will have on the spread of dengue to new areas also point to the fact that dengue repeatedly has caused outbreaks in temperate zone cities only to disappear soon after its introduction. The spread of dengue to these cities occurred not as a result of climate change but rather through the transport of infectious mosquitoes or people into cities with large numbers of susceptible persons and seasonally abundant *Ae. aegypti* populations.

CLINICAL CORRELATES 8.3 CLINICAL IMPLICATIONS OF HUMAN MOVEMENTS AND VECTOR-BORNE ILLNESS

Climate change is likely to cause mass movements of people—from rural areas into urban zones, as well as migrations across country lines. Therefore, clinicians worldwide must have a high index of suspicion for the appearance of nonendemic diseases. For example, the West Nile virus first made its appearance in Uganda in 1937 and then spread to Tunisia and Israel before appearing in New York City. The spread of this virus, as well as others such as Ebola and avian influenza A (H5N1) exemplify the interconnectedness of our environment and highlight the need for international communication about the appearance of infectious vector-borne diseases.

Climate change and resulting mass human movement mean that clinicians must be alert to the possibility of infectious diseases appearing in unexpected places.

The Sudden Emergence of West Nile Virus–Associated Illnesses

Etiology

Unlike DENV, **West Nile virus (WNV)** is a viral vector-borne zoonotic agent associated primarily with birds and transmitted by certain species of *Culex* mosquitoes that feed on these vertebrates. It was first isolated in the West Nile region of Uganda in 1937, and in the decades following, its identification appeared to cause only a mild febrile disease in humans. In the 1990s, however, outbreaks of WNV disease occurred in many Mediterranean countries and Russia, causing hundreds of cases and the deaths of perhaps 4 or 5 percent of those infected (Tsai et al. 1998). This outbreak was followed in 1999 by the first report of WNV disease in the Western Hemisphere when WNV appeared unexpectedly in New York City. The virus was probably spread by infected birds or mosquitoes (Petersen and Hayes 2008), although some have speculated it could have been carried by an infected person who traveled to New York City from Tel Aviv, Israel, where WNV cases had recently occurred. While it must be admitted that virus isolates from infected persons in the Israeli outbreak appeared highly similar, if not identical, to those first identified in US patients, humans are not considered a likely source of the New York outbreak because they fail to develop the high viremias required to efficiently infect mosquitoes with WNV. Regardless of how it first arrived in the United States, WNV took less than five years to spread from the Atlantic to Pacific states and parts of southern Canada, presumably as a result of local or migratory movements of infected birds (Petersen and Hayes 2008). During the decade following its introduction, WNV and seropositive hosts also were identified in the Caribbean and Central and South America.

To date, evidence of WNV infection has been identified in roughly 65 species of mosquitoes and 320 bird species in the United States, and many more species of mosquitoes and birds elsewhere around the world, although only a few of these are significant vectors or amplifying or reservoir hosts, respectively. The rapid dispersion of WNV across southeastern Europe, the eastern Mediterranean, and the Americas provides a classic example of the ability of an emerging vector-borne disease to spread explosively in the presence of susceptible host populations, efficient vectors, and favorable environmental conditions.

Serological surveys from recent outbreaks suggest about 80 percent of WNV infections are asymptomatic. Among persons experiencing illness, symptoms typically include high fever, chills, headache, rash, myalgia, and nausea that last for three to five days (Petersen and Hayes 2008; Petersen, Brault, and Nasci 2013; Centers for Disease Control and Prevention 2013a; Nasci et al. 2001). In less than 1 percent of cases, more severe neuroinvasive illness develops with one or more of the following symptoms: neck stiffness, stupor, disorientation, coma, tremors, convulsions, muscle weakness, vision loss, numbness, and paralysis. Neuroinvasive disease also can occur with differing combinations of encephalitis, meningitis, or myelitis, as well as flaccid paralysis of respiratory muscles and limbs. These severe symptoms can last for several weeks, or the neurological effects can be permanent. Risk of severe illness is greatest in those over fifty years of age and the elderly are particularly at risk for severe neurological disease. Humans and other vertebrates that survive infection have lifelong immunity, and it is believed that high levels of herd immunity can decrease epidemic spread of the disease even when environmental and epidemiological conditions are otherwise favorable.

Since its introduction in 1999, WNV infections have caused more than thirty thousand cases of illness in the United States, ranking second only to Lyme disease in incidence among vector-borne diseases reported in this country. Human infections are usually acquired in the late summer and early fall following a spring-to-summer buildup of infection among competent mosquito vectors that acquire their infections primarily from certain species of birds that act as amplifying hosts. The primary vectors of WNV in the United States are species of the genus *Culex* that feed preferentially on birds but bite mammals when avian hosts are absent or few in numbers (Petersen and Hayes 2008; Andreadis 2012). These mosquitoes include *Culex pipiens pipiens* in the North, *Cx. pipiens quinquefasciatus* in southern states, *Cx. nigripalpus* in the Southeast, and *Cx. tarsalis* in the western states. The primary vector in eastern Canada is *Cx. pipiens pipiens*, whereas *Cx. tarsalis* plays this role in the western part of that country. Important amplifying hosts include members of the crow family, house sparrows, American robins, and other birds (Komar 2003; Reisen and Brault 2007).

The seasonal cycle of WNV transmission in temperate North America begins in the spring when birds are nesting, thus providing a large number of susceptible avian hosts on which infectious *Culex* mosquitoes can feed. Birds that develop high-level viremias following infection can act as amplifying hosts for infecting female mosquitoes (Petersen, Brault, and Nasci 2013). If these feeding mosquitoes are competent vectors, they will support development of the virus and can eventually become infective and feed on multiple birds before dying, thus furthering the spread of WNV. When this amplification cycle involves certain highly susceptible species of birds such as crows, mortality among those birds can be quite high, as was frequently noted following the invasion of WNV into the New York City area and other localities in the United States (Komar 2003).

As the transmission season progresses, the bird breeding season comes to an end, and young birds fledge, often leaving the area to start their seasonal migrations to the tropics. Some believe a proportion of these migrating birds remain infected with WNV and therefore act as potential reservoirs of infection. As the year progresses and the number of available bird hosts begins to decline due to seasonal migration, it also has been reported that *Cx. tarsalis* can shift its feeding activities to mammals in mid- to late summer (Kent et al. 2009), a fact that increases risk of WNV infection for the humans and other mammals on which these mosquitoes feed.

The seasonal cycle of WNV in temperate North America begins in the spring when birds are nesting, thus providing a large number of susceptible avian hosts on which infectious *Culex* mosquitoes can feed. Important amplifying hosts include members of the crow family, house sparrows, robins, and certain wading birds. Individuals of bird species that develop a high level of the virus in their blood following infection can act as amplifying hosts for infecting other mosquitoes. As the number of bird hosts begin to decline, the *Culex* vectors start to shift their feeding activities to mammals in late summer and early fall, a fact that increases risk of WNV infection for humans and other mammalian mosquito hosts fed on by these mosquitoes.

Linkages to the Climate

The effects of climatic variability on the transmission cycle of the WNV and the occurrence of WNV-related illnesses have been the subject of much discussion. In general, temperature and precipitation are reported to be the strongest predictors of regional WNV activity and human risk (Johnson and Sukhdeo 2013; Landesman et al. 2007; Pecoraro et al. 2007; Ruiz et al. 2010; Soverow et al. 2009; Chen et al. 2012). In the northern United States and southern Canada, WNV successfully invaded and spread quickly among bird hosts when summer temperatures were above normal (Reisen and Brault 2007; Ruiz et al. 2010). Increased temperatures during the spring and summer months when mosquitoes are actively reproducing will increase the growth rates of the immature stages and decrease the time required for egg development, thereby increasing mosquito populations. In addition, higher-than-normal temperatures could increase viral replication rates and therefore increase the opportunities that regionally adaptive mutations will appear among WNV strains. All else being equal, viral loads in mosquitoes also can be expected to increase as the rate of viral replication increases, a result that should enhance dissemination of WNV through host populations (Johnson and Sukhdeo 2013; Soverow et al. 2009; Dohm, O'Guinn, and Turell 2002; Reisen, Fang, and Martinez 2006; Kilpatrick et al. 2008; Paz and Albersheim 2008).

Vector abundance is thought to be a critical factor for supporting high rates of mosquito infection and increased levels of WNV transmission among amplification hosts and to humans or other dead-end hosts likely to suffer illness following infection. Optimal conditions for the reproduction of *Cx. pipiens* mosquitoes appear to occur when periods of heavy spring rainfall are followed by warm, dry summer temperatures (Brault 2009). The growth of *C. pipiens* and *C. restuans* populations in Ontario, Canada, could be predicted by time-lagged temperature and precipitation data (Wang, Ogden, and Zhu 2011). Specifically, mosquito abundance depended on the occurrence of temperatures in excess of 9°C (the threshold temperature for mosquito activity), and precipitation levels measured thirty-five days previously. In one Illinois study, increased temperature, as measured by cumulative high temperature differences, was the primary factor distinguishing years with higher rates of WNV infection in mosquitoes and WNV-caused illness in humans from those years that experienced lower rates for these variables (Ruiz et al. 2010).

The impacts of warmer-than-normal summer temperatures on WNV transmission are not limited to North America, as Platonov et al. (2008) noted a similar situation for WNV outbreaks in Russia. Similarly, although disease occurrence coincided closely with population distribution in Israel,

risk tended to escalate around a metropolitan heat island. Positive temperature anomalies reportedly increased the abundance of mosquitoes and led
to greater disease spread among humans in these areas, suggesting that
extreme heat in early spring promoted increases in vector populations that
resulted a few weeks later in WNV infections in humans (Paz 2006; Paz and
Albersheim 2008). In New York's Suffolk County, increased WNV infection rates in mosquitoes were associated with wetter-than-normal winters,
warmer-and-wetter-than-normal springs, and drier-than-average summers (Shaman, Harding, and Campbell 2011). During 2007, an outbreak of
WNV illness occurred on the Great Plains of the northern United States
and southern Canada when unusually heavy spring and summer (May-July)
rains and very hot summer temperatures were followed by warmer-than-
normal fall temperatures, a sequence of events that reportedly resulted in
increased availability of breeding habitats and prolonged seasonal activity
for *Cx. Tarsalis* mosquitoes (Artsob et al. 2009).

Temperature and precipitation are reported to be the strongest climatic predictors of regional
transmission and human risk of WNV.

Studies of the interannual variability of WNV infection rates in mosquitoes and illness in humans or other animals suggest that climatic
variables are important but rarely exert their effects on transmission in a
simple linear fashion. Instead, climate is most likely to act in concert with
other environmental or human-related variables. For example, although
increased spring rainfall might favor the eventual buildup of *Cx. pipiens
populations* to levels that later in the year will result in higher-than-normal
rates of WNV transmission, exceptionally heavy rains can cause flushing of
mosquito eggs from larval habitats, a process that will decrease mosquito
numbers (Ruiz et al. 2010). In Italy the time-lagged abundance of *C. pipiens*
mosquitoes in an area that had experienced previous WNV outbreaks was
positively correlated with temperature and negatively correlated with rainfall; the negative correlation with rainfall was presumed to be due to a flushing effect or perhaps that sites filled by excessive rainfall were unattractive
to female mosquitoes as sites for laying their eggs (Ruiz et al. 2010). Others
have suggested that periods of reduced precipitation and actual drought
can increase risks of WNV outbreaks, as observed in the United States,
southeastern Europe, Russia, and Israel (Johnson and Sukhdeo 2013; Ruiz
et al. 2010). Presumably this occurs because drought conditions can result
in the concentration of water into sites such as storm drains that become

increasingly eutrophic and stagnate, creating conditions that are highly attractive to egg-laying female *Cx. Pipiens* mosquitoes and favorable for the rapid growth of mosquito larvae.

Drought also could increase local rates of WNV transmission by causing birds to concentrate near remaining water sources, thereby increasing the likelihood susceptible birds will come into contact with infected mosquitoes using these sites for breeding or other purposes. In one New Jersey study, county-level drought conditions were associated with an increase in the numbers of blood-fed *Culex* mosquitoes and greater "vector community competence" compared to the following year, which was milder and wetter (Johnson and Sukhdeo 2013). At the state level, drought also was reported to exert a positive influence on the amplification of WNV, with increased temperatures in June and July, and accompanying summer decreases in precipitation, being strongly correlated with increases in yearly WNV infection rates in mosquitoes over the nine-year period from 2003 to 2011. This observation led these authors to conclude that below-average precipitation is a better predictor of WNV activity than above-average precipitation.

In contrast to these studies, Soverow et al. (2009) used surveillance data reported to the Centers for Disease Control and Prevention from 2001 to 2005 and a case-crossover study design to investigate how certain temperature, precipitation, and humidity variables were associated with WNV disease in humans in the United States. The authors concluded that heavy precipitation, warmer temperatures, and elevated humidity were associated with increased rates of human WNV infection. Among their findings, it was found that a 29 to 66 percent increase in WNV infections occurred among humans within one week of a heavy rainfall, an effect that lasted for an additional two weeks. A twenty-millimeter increase in cumulative weekly precipitation was associated with a less dramatic 4 to 8 percent increase in WNV infection rates over the subsequent two weeks.

Sustained climate change will also affect the distribution and transmission of WNV and the illnesses it causes. Although temperatures in the southern United States are always sufficiently warm during the summer months to sustain viral amplification for long periods, this is not always the case in the northern United States and southern Canada, suggesting temperature could be a limiting factor for further WNV spread in these northern regions, and sustained increases in average summer temperatures could favor the spread and long-term establishment of WNV in these more northerly regions. The minimum temperature at which a WNV strain will develop in mosquitoes is reportedly 14.7°C. Above this temperature and within the range of temperatures allowing mosquito survival, viral reproduction increases in a linear fashion. A northward displacement of the isotherm matching this threshold temperature for viral development in mosquitoes might allow WNV to exist at increasingly higher latitudes, although other climate-independent factors, such as the decreasing day lengths that signal the approach of autumn and induce winter diapause in *Culex* mosquitoes, will present a temperature-independent limit to the northward expansion of the vector and therefore the virus. Nevertheless, numerous studies have suggested that greater-than-normal temperatures favored the northward expansion of the range of WNV, presumably because such warmer-than-normal summers resulted in an extended transmission season with greater viral amplification in local bird populations and the consequent infection of large numbers of mosquito vectors (Reisen and Brault 2007).

In addition to the presence of a naive and highly susceptible community of birds, highly competent *Culex* vectors and perhaps warmer-than-normal temperatures following the introduction of WNV, the rapid spread of this virus also was enhanced by its ability to overwinter in infected mosquitoes (Nasci et al. 2001). Prior to the appearance of WNV in North America, another WNV strain was identified in eastern Europe and the Mediterranean region that had increased virulence for birds, enabling this or similar strains to replicate to high densities in avian hosts, a factor that increases the likelihood that mosquitoes feeding on these birds will become infected with WNV. The appearance of new WNV phenotypes can be expected to occur fairly frequently because of the rapid rates at which RNA viruses characteristically evolve (Reisen and Brault 2007). The appearance of another WNV strain that could disseminate more rapidly and with greater efficiency at elevated temperatures than the strain first identified in New York City also suggests that incubation temperatures for the virus in its mosquito vectors is an important selective factor (Brault 2009). Another variant, first recognized in Texas only two years after the initial appearance of WNV in the United States in 1999, exhibited a shorter EIP in *C. pipiens* than was observed in the same mosquitoes infected with a strain typical of those first isolated in this country (Artsob et al. 2009; Moudy et al. 2007). Because of its reduced EIP, this variant can be expected to have more opportunities to be transmitted over a given period of time, a selective advantage that apparently enabled it to become the dominant North American genotype by 2003 (Pesko and Ebel 2012). The impact of a reduced EIP is likely to be even more significant when warmer-than-normal summers prolong the WNV transmission season, a circumstance that will occur more frequently in the event of global warming.

Clearly WNV transmission and the associated risks of human illnesses resulting from infection with this virus are influenced strongly by climatic variability. Actual climate change is expected to result in some expansion of WNV to higher latitudes, where the virus is likely to encounter highly susceptible host populations and competent mosquito vectors, perhaps setting the stage for serious outbreaks among humans and other hosts. It should be remembered, however, that temperature is only one factor affecting the distribution of WNV and its ability to cause outbreaks. In some instances, such as in the tropics, temperatures remain high, but WNV outbreaks are limited by other factors. Clearly much remains to be learned about the relative importance of and interactions between climatic variables, such as increased temperatures, and other factors that could influence human WNV risk, including those related to land and water use, agricultural practices, human behaviors, home construction, the use of air-conditioning, or other socioeconomic and environmental variables.

Lyme Disease in the United States

Etiology

Lyme disease is a tick-borne spirochetal infection caused by *Borrelia burgdorferi* sensu stricto in the United States and Europe, along with the related spirochetes, *B. afzelii* and *B. garinii*, in Europe and Asia. Other closely related tick-borne spirochetes have been described, but their significance as human pathogens remains uncertain. *B. burgorferi* is maintained in nature in a zoonotic cycle that involves small rodents and birds as reservoirs for the spirochete, ticks in the genus *Ixodes* (*I. scapularis* and *pacificus* in the United States and *I. ricinus* and *I. persulcatus* in Europe and Asia, respectively) as vectors, and a variety of large and small mammals and birds, which serve as host for the tick vectors. Humans are infected when bitten by infected *Ixodes* ticks. Symptoms typically include fever, headache, fatigue, and erythema migrans, a characteristic skin rash that appears at the site of the initial tick bite and often resembles a target bull's eye. If treated promptly with appropriate antibiotics, patients usually recover quickly and without complications. If unrecognized or treated improperly, however, the spirochetes can spread to the joints, where they can cause arthritis, and to the heart and nervous system, which can result in more serious complications.

In 2012, Lyme disease was the seventh most commonly reported infectious disease and the most frequently reported vector-borne disease in the United States.

Lyme disease, also referred to as Lyme borreliosis, was first recognized as a clinical entity in the late 1970s in coastal Connecticut, appearing in a cluster of juvenile rheumatoid arthritis cases (Steere et al. 1977). Tick-bite-associated rash illness cases were also reported from Wisconsin during the same period (Scrimenti 1970). It was not until the early 1980s, however, that the etiological agent *B. burgdorferi* was discovered in ticks from Shelter Island, New York (Burgdorfer et al. 1982). Since that time, Lyme disease cases have been increasing steadily in the United States, in number and geographic distribution.

Currently, over thirty thousand cases of Lyme disease are reported each year in the United States, making it the nation's seventh most commonly reported infectious disease in 2012 and the most frequently reported vector-borne disease. Over 95 percent of these cases occur in fifteen states located primarily in the northeastern and upper midwestern regions of the United States, where *I. scapularis* ticks are common and bite humans. Fewer (about 100 to 150 cases per year) cases occur annually in the Pacific coast region, where the tick vector is *I. pacificus.* Lyme disease is relatively uncommon in the southern United States despite the presence of *I. scapularis* in many areas of the southeast and south-central states. This is primarily due to two factors associated with host preferences of southern *I. scapularis* populations: that larval ticks often feed on lizards, which are incompetent hosts for *Borrelia,* and that nymphal ticks, which are small and difficult to detect, rarely bite humans in this region of the country.

Larval ticks feed on lizards in some parts of the country, but lizards are incompetent hosts for *Borrelia.*

This increase in Lyme disease cases, a trend also seen for the other major nationally notifiable tick-borne diseases, has resulted in efforts over the last few decades aimed at determining the drivers of tick-borne disease emergence in the United States (Hoen et al. 2009). Clearly these drivers are multifactorial, involving changes in land use patterns, demographics, and human behavior. It is likely that Lyme disease was broadly enzootic throughout portions of the northern United States during pre-colonial days, but with widespread clearing of land for agricultural purposes, the causative agent of the disease apparently was pushed back into local pockets or refuges, where sufficient populations of deer or other large mammals remained to support survival of tick vector (*I. scapularis*) populations (Margos et al. 2012). Continuation of the Industrial

Revolution in the United States during the 1900s resulted in the movement of rural populations to more urbanized areas and increased reforestation of previously cultivated regions of the northern United States, a trend that was followed in the second half of the century by the suburbanization of much of the secondary growth forest found on lands that previously were farmed.

Linkages to the Climate

Reforestation, overabundant deer, increased tick populations, and suburban encroachment on wooded areas in the northeastern and Upper Midwest states have led collectively to increased tick exposures and a subsequent increase in Lyme disease in residents of these regions. Although this series of events provides a plausible explanation for the emergence of this disease in the northeastern United States, some concern has been raised about how its rate of spread and geographic range will be influenced by climate change. It is not unreasonable to suspect that climate change could affect both the distribution of *B. burgdorferi* and the human risk of acquiring this disease. Clearly the survival, reproduction, and behavior of the *Ixodes* ticks that transmit *B. burgorferi* are strongly influenced by the abiotic environment, with water stress and temperature significantly influencing mortality in off-host tick populations (Needham and Teel 1991; Brownstein, Holford, and Fish 2005; Bertrand and Wilson 1996).

The image most people bring to mind when asked about ticks is one where the ectoparasites are attached to and sucking blood from a host, such as a human or dog. Only a small portion of a typical tick's life cycle (about 2 percent) is actually spent on the host, however (Brownstein, Holford, and Fish 2003). Because ticks spend only limited time on hosts, they are likely to be exposed as eggs, larvae, nymphs, and adults to varying and potentially harmful environmental conditions (Bertrand and Wilson 1996). For example, hot, dry conditions can increase mortality, especially among larvae, nymphs, or adults as they leave the more stable and high-humidity microclimates found in leaf litter or moist soil in order to quest for hosts. *Ixodes* ticks responsible for transmitting *B. burgdoreri* and other closely related spirochetes are especially vulnerable, requiring at least 80 percent relative humidity to prevent death by desiccation (Gray et al. 2009). Egg hatching success for ticks also decreases markedly at low temperatures (10°C or lower) (Dorr and Gothe 2001). Because ticks are poikilothermic (cold-blooded), their metabolic activity, development, hatching success, and oviposition behavior are influenced by changes in ambient temperatures (Bertrand and Wilson 1996; Dorr and Gothe 2001).

Drivers of Lyme borreliosis are multifactorial. They include climate and nonclimate factors: reforestation, overabundant deer, increased tick populations, suburban encroachment on wooded areas, and increased human exposure to ticks, as well as temperature and precipitation.

Models of future climate change and environmental factors affecting tick distributions have been used to predict the impact of a changing climate on the distribution of Lyme borreliosis in the United States (Brownstein, Holford, and Fish 2005) and in southern Canada (Ogden et al. 2008). Outputs of these models show the geographical range of the tick vectors and subsequent areas at risk for Lyme disease significantly expanding, primarily as a result of a northward expansion into areas such as southern Canada, which were previously too cold for maintenance of *I. scapularis* populations. These models also have suggested that the southern limit of this tick's geographical range will retract, resulting in its disappearance of *I. scapularis* from some areas within the southeastern and south-central states of the United States. Although this prediction could eventually prove true, it should be noted that the distribution and frequency of Lyme disease have increased recently not only northward into Canada but also southward along the mid-Atlantic coast (Diuk-Wasser et al. 2012; Centers for Disease Control and Prevention 2013c), driven presumably by factors other than climate change.

Lyme disease is maintained in a complex cycle involving ticks, multiple mammal and bird species, and humans. While reforestation, increasing biodiversity, and expanding deer populations have been proposed as significant drivers in the emergence of Lyme and other tick-borne diseases over the last fifty years at larger spatial scales, it is likely that at local scales, habitat fragmentation and reduced biodiversity have contributed to increased disease risk (Margos et al. 2012; Allan, Keesing, and Ostfeld 2003; Wood and Lafferty 2013). The challenge that must be addressed is in determining how climate variability and disruption interact with the numerous and diverse factors, both ecological and epidemiologic and at local and regional scales, that contribute to Lyme disease transmission and subsequent disease emergence.

Strategies for mitigating the potential impact of climate change on Lyme disease emergence in the United States and Canada should include the development of high-resolution models that can be used for projecting changes in spatial and temporal risk that will occur as a result of climate change. Both field and laboratory research should be conducted to determine how various environmental factors influence vector-pathogen-host interaction and subsequent pathogen transmission. Long-term vector and reservoir surveillance programs should be established to detect zoonotic activity prior to the occurrence of human illness. Education of both the general public and health care providers in areas of anticipated disease expansion will help raise the awareness of risk. Finally, there should also be greater investment in routine disease reporting and surveillance activities and the capacity for local vector control response measures so that when diseases occur in areas where they had not been previously known to exist, cases will be detected quickly and responded to appropriately.

Rabies in Wild Carnivores and Bats

Etiology

Rabies, a disease that is virtually always fatal in humans without prompt postexposure prophylaxis, is caused by infection with the rabies virus (RABV) and a few related viruses within the genus *Lyssavirus* of the family Rhabdoviridae (Warrell and Warrell 2004). Transmission of rabies virus depends on exposure to infectious nervous system tissue or saliva, an event that typically occurs when victims are bitten by a rabid animal. Once the rabies virus enters a susceptible mammalian host through a bite wound, it multiplies and spreads along peripheral nerves until it reaches the central nervous system, including the brain. From the brain, it can spread elsewhere in the body along other peripheral nerve pathways, eventually causing the distinctive symptoms of the disease (Beran 1994).

Acute, early symptoms of rabies virus infection in humans typically last two to ten days and include weakness, discomfort, fever, or headache. Later clinical symptoms include prickling or itching sensation at the site of bite, cerebral dysfunction, anxiety, confusion, agitation, delirium, abnormal behavior, hallucinations, and insomnia. Eventually the rabies virus appears in the infected host's saliva, rendering its bite infectious for other susceptible animals.

Rabies infection is particularly dangerous because of the virtually symptom-free incubation period (weeks to months), which can allow highly mobile hosts to carry the virus over long distances, and the low chance for survival once symptoms do become apparent. Luckily, vaccines and postexposure prophylaxis to prevent human rabies have been available for over one hundred years. Fatalities continue to occur, however, because people fail to seek postexposure prophylaxis or sometimes because available rabies vaccines fail to protect against certain regional strains of RABV or related *Lyssaviruses*, including those that are present in some developing countries (Warrell and Warrell 2004). Worldwide, rabies occurs in more than 150 countries and causes an estimated fifty-five thousand to seventy thousand deaths annually (Hatz, Kuenzli, and Funk 2012).

Rabies prevention can be highly effective by promoting the removal of stray dogs, providing vaccinations to domestic dogs, and avoiding contact with animals that may be dangerous.

CLINICAL CORRELATES 8.4 COMPLEXITY OF ZOONOTIC DISEASE TRANSMISSION

Zoonotic pathogens account for 61 percent of all infectious pathogens and 60 percent of emerging infectious diseases (Utzinger and Keiser 2006). Anthropogenic land use patterns, climate change, hydrological cycle changes, and urbanization influence transmission of these pathogens by altering the ecologic niches of the vector and host, changing community structure, and altering behavior of vectors, hosts and humans (Gottdenker et al. 2014). Such complexity makes it difficult to predict whether changing climates will lead to increased or decreased disease incidence (Mutero et al. 2004). What we do know is that immunology and physiology play a large role in determining the severity of infection as well as its further transmission. Poor nutrition, environmental stress, and prior immunological exposure all contribute to the robustness of the human host's defense and determine parasitic, bacterial, and viremic loads and thus how contagious a patient will become (Beldomenico and Begon 2010). Malnutrition and chronic diseases are widespread in both the industrialized and developing world and thus play an integral part in the spread of zoonotic pathogens.

The manifestation of disease from climate-sensitive zoonotic pathogens is influenced by the baseline health of communities and individuals.

Linkages to the Climate

According to the Fourth Assessment report of the Intergovernmental Panel on Climate Change (IPCC), warmer temperatures, increased rainfall, summer droughts, and an increased frequency of extreme weather events will be seen throughout much of North America as a result of climate change (Greer, Ng, and Fisman 2008). These conditions are forecast to be most severe in extreme (Arctic) latitudes and are anticipated to directly influence the distribution and incidence of infectious diseases, including rabies (Greer, Ng, and Fisman 2008; Parkinson and Butler 2005; Kim et al. 2014). In midlatitude regions, climate-driven increases in temperature will lengthen summer seasons and are expected to increase populations of certain mammalian hosts that carry rabies (Greer, Ng, and Fisman 2008). As the frequency and density of infected and susceptible rabies hosts increase, the duration of the transmission season will lengthen, and more frequent outbreaks can be expected (Greer, Ng, and Fisman 2008). The geographical range covered by rabies hosts normally found only in tropical or subtropical areas may also see a poleward expansion encouraged by increasing average temperatures. The following paragraphs discuss how the spread of rabies might be affected by climate change in the Arctic and red foxes in Alaska, raccoon dogs and red foxes in northeastern Europe, and vampire bats (*Desmodus rotundus*) in Latin America.

Rabies transmission in Alaska follows a strong seasonal trend that peaks in winter and spring among both arctic foxes (*Vulpes lagopus*) and red foxes (*Vulpes vulpes*), the two main reservoirs of the disease in the state (Greer et al. 2008; Kim et al. 2014; see figure 8.2). The effects of climatic and seasonal factors on rabies transmission are more severe at higher latitudes and have been shown to disproportionately affect arctic foxes (Kim et al. 2014). More specifically, as average maximum and minimum temperatures increase, the number of rabid arctic foxes is likely to decrease, while viral transmission among red foxes is likely to increase, a conclusion supported by probabilistic modeling (Kim et al. 2014). If predicted warming trends continue, the primary reservoir of rabies is likely to switch from arctic foxes

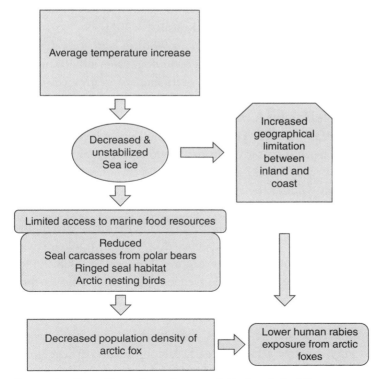

Figure 8.2 Climate Effect on Human Exposure to Rabies from the Arctic Fox
Source: Blanford et al. (2013).

to red foxes (Kim et al. 2014). This will likely alter the geographical range of rabies in Alaska, an outcome with potentially significant implications for human health and the potential spillover of the disease into domestic dogs.

A better understanding of the dynamics of lemming populations is still needed (Kim et al. 2014) because these rodents are a major food source for foxes living at high latitudes. Their annual population fluctuations exert considerable influence on fox population dynamics and are likely to affect the transmission of rabies among arctic and red foxes and therefore may have an impact on human rabies risk (Kim et al. 2014). Arctic foxes and red foxes also serve as rabies hosts in the Russian Arctic, and climate change is expected to increase the spread of rabies in this region as well (Revich, Tokarevich, and Parkinson 2012).

Cases of rabies in red foxes and raccoon dogs (*Nyctereutes procyonoides*) in northeastern Europe provide other interesting examples of how the spread of rabies could be influenced by climate change. The red fox is native to Eurasia and North America, where it has proven quite adaptable and remains widespread in many areas, including those considered semirural or urbanized. In contrast, the raccoon dog, although also quite adaptable, is an invasive species that has spread throughout much of northeastern Europe following its introduction from eastern Asia into western Russia in the first half of the twentieth century (Kauhala and Kowalczyk 2011).

At present, the red fox remains the main wildlife host for rabies in Europe, but the expanding range of the raccoon dog, especially in northeastern Europe, is raising concern because of its increasing importance as a rabies host in the region. These concerns are amplified by predictions that global warming will lead to the further spread of raccoon dogs in northern Europe. One of the areas of greatest concern is Finland, which has been rabies free in part because the country's fox densities are too low to maintain a fox-to-fox transmission cycle. Modeling studies indicate that the introduction of another competent wildlife rabies host, such as the raccoon dog, could dramatically change this situation by raising the density of rabies hosts and creating a two-host reservoir system. This would permit the virus to be maintained indefinitely in Finland, a result that appeared extremely unlikely when the virus circulated among only one reservoir host (Singer et al. 2008, 2009). Although foxes remain active all year, as do raccoon dogs living in the warmer portions of Europe, populations of the raccoon dogs will undergo hibernation in the colder, subarctic latitudes of northeastern Europe, perhaps affecting their ability to spread and maintain rabies. Laboratory studies demonstrate that the incubation period for rabies is greatly prolonged and pathogenicity is reduced in hibernating rodents, thus delaying the onset of illness in these animals until they awaken from hibernation (Botvinkin, Gribanova, and

Nikifirova 1983). Presumably the rabies virus will behave similarly in hibernating raccoon dogs (Cerkasskij 1980; Holmala and Kauhala 2006).

Modeling results indicate that when rabies incubation periods are lengthened during hibernation, the likelihood of the virus persisting is greatly strengthened because it allows raccoon dogs to survive through the winter before becoming symptomatic. Under this scenario, infected raccoon dogs could wake from hibernation in the spring and live for a sufficient length of time to transmit rabies to other susceptible hosts before dying of the disease (Singer et al. 2009). However, increased temperatures caused by global warming could deter raccoon dogs from entering hibernation. At present, the effect that such a change in hibernation behavior is likely to have on rabies virus transmission remains uncertain, but it could be significant. If a population of rabies-infected raccoon dogs did not enter hibernation, they would likely have less time to transmit the virus before they died of the disease, but other factors could also be important. Lack of hibernation also could significantly affect the population dynamics of raccoon dogs because starvation during hibernation is a major source of mortality among raccoon dog juveniles (Singer et al. 2009).

Clearly, terrestrial carnivores such as dogs, foxes, raccoons, and skunks are critical hosts for maintaining certain strains of rabies viruses in nature. Although dogs remain the most significant source of exposure for human rabies, the ability of these animals to spread the rabies virus over long distances can be limited by the presence of geographical barriers, such as large rivers, oceans, mountain ranges, deserts, or other landscape features that are too rugged or extensive to simply cross by walking or swimming. Dispersal also can be impeded by the presence of large swaths of land that contain insufficient food, water, or shelter to sustain these animals during their attempts to reach more suitable habitats. Bats, another important group of rabies hosts, are unique among mammals because of their ability to fly, a trait that enables them to cross quickly over many of the geographical barriers or areas of unsuitable habitat that frequently prove impassable to their terrestrial relatives. Indeed, many bat species travel over long distances during seasonal migrations or in attempts to find suitable roosts or foraging sites. Such dispersal flights might become more common as climate change forces various bat species to leave areas that were previously suitable but no longer meet their environmental requirements. Unfortunately, as climate change forces bats to search for new habitats, they are likely to spread the rabies virus to areas that previously had little or no rabies risk.

The potential impacts of climate change on the dispersal and distribution of bats is worth noting because of the emerging role these animals are likely to play in spreading not only strains of the actual rabies virus, but also other recently identified viruses that belong to the same genus (*Lyssavirus*) and reportedly are capable of causing illnesses indistinguishable from rabies (Warrell and Warrell 2004). Bats also have been identified recently as hosts for other dangerous viral pathogens, including Marburg, Ebola, SARS-coronavirus, Hendra, and Nipah viruses (Hayman et al. 2012; Wood et al. 2012), and it is likely that climate change will affect the spread of these viruses in ways that are similar to its impact on rabies transmission. Many bats living in temperate regions also undergo hibernation, the duration and timing of which can be affected by climate change. Hibernation can, as noted for raccoon dogs, result in prolonged incubation periods for rabies viruses in infected bats, thus providing a mechanism for overwintering of the virus in these hosts (George et al. 2011).

Most of the world's bats, including nearly all of those considered important hosts of rabies and related viruses, are either insectivorous or frugivorous. Vampire bats represent an interesting exception to this statement, using their exceptionally large and sharp incisors to slice skin and blood vessels so they can feed on the blood of other mammalian species, including cattle, horses, other ungulates, and occasionally, humans. This blood feeding habit provides vampire bats not only with a source of nutrition but also excellent opportunities to acquire and transmit rabies viruses. Among the three known species of vampire bats (*Desmodus rotundus, Diaemus youngi,* and *Diphylla ecaudata*), the most widespread and significant as a rabies host is the common vampire bat (*D. rotundus*), which is found from northern Mexico to Uruguay and the northern regions of Chile and Argentina.

Rabies transmission by *D. rotundus* represents a significant threat not only to humans but also to the cattle industry in Latin America (Lee, Papes, and Van den Bussche 2012). Due to rabies, many places in Latin America face substantial decreases in milk production, increased risk of secondary infection, and difficulties in predicting future risk of infection (Lee et al. 2012). In order to investigate this last issue, investigators used ecological niche modeling, current cattle density estimates, and data from the A2, A1B, and the B1 climate scenarios from the IPCC for the years 2030, 2050, and 2080 to forecast the future distribution of *D. rotundus* throughout the Americas, a finding that should be highly correlated with the areas likely to be at risk for vampire bat–related rabies exposures (Intergovernmental Panel on Climate Change Data Distribution Centre n.d.). The IPCC has constructed four narrative storylines for world regions and the Earth during the twenty-first century. Each storyline is unique, based on the relationships between, and the evolution of, the forces that drive greenhouse gas and aerosol emissions, as well as various levels of demographic, social, economic, technological, and environmental developments. From these four storylines, forty scenarios were developed, all equally plausible. The five climate variables that contributed most significantly to the development of the model investigating risk for infection were precipitation seasonality, temperature seasonality, precipitation of the wettest month, precipitation of the driest month, and mean temperature of the coldest month.

At present, suitable habitat for the common vampire bat exists in most of Mexico and Central America, as well as certain areas in Venezuela, Guyana, the Brazilian highlands, western Ecuador, northern Argentina, and east of the Andes in Peru, Bolivia, and Paraguay. Based on the results of their model, additional habitat, and presumably increased rabies risk, is expected to appear in these same areas as well as parts of French Guyana, Suriname, Venezuela, and Colombia (Lee et al. 2012). Despite the range of expansions predicted above, it is interesting to note that these bats are not expected to expand their range into the United States or the southern reaches of South America, presumably because of their inability to tolerate temperatures below 15°C or sustained humidity values greater than 45 percent (Lee et al. 2012). It is hoped that predictions such as these can aid in focusing prevention activities and decreasing the risk of human infection.

Undoubtedly the changing epidemiology of rabies will present other as yet unrecognized challenges to understanding how climate change and other global changes will affect the spread of this virus. The lack of integrated long-term data on this disease, as well as detailed predictions about the geographically variable changes in climate that will occur at smaller spatial scales than those currently available in global climate change models, also make it difficult to model and predict the regional effects that climate change will have on rabies transmission. It appears clear, however, that changes in temperature and seasonality are already affecting the geographical distribution of rabies as well as the potential reservoirs of the viruses causing this disease (Burek et al. 2008; Greer et al. 2008; Kim et al. 2014; Lee et al. 2012). Obviously rabies-endemic countries will need to maintain comprehensive surveillance for this disease and compare these data to those on climate change and other associated environmental or human-driven changes now occurring in many parts of the world in order to provide acceptable estimations of rabies risk in these nations.

Conclusion

Climate change is likely to act in concert with other environmental and anthropogenic factors to increase the transmission and risk of infectious disease. These interactions are best understood within the context of the Institute of Medicine's (IOM) (2008) convergence model for disease emergence. According to the model, disease emergence is driven by a number of overlapping factors or determinants that collectively influence the interaction between humans and pathogens. Climate and weather are listed as one of the thirteen specific drivers that the IOM report lists (figure 8.1): physical environmental factors; social, political, and economic factors; genetic and biological factors; and ecological factors. It is noteworthy that climate variability has an impact on many of these. Due to the interactive nature of the determinants of disease, without years of longitudinally collected data, it is much more difficult to link annual disease trends to climate change than it is to link individual outbreak events to weather patterns, such as mild winters, early springs and warm summers, or an ENSO event.

It is still uncertain how much climate variability contributes to human-pathogen exposure; however, certain trends have become apparent. Sustained increases in average temperatures due to climate change are likely to cause infectious disease transmission to spread to higher elevations and latitudes and may support long-term establishment and spread of VBZD. This is because increased temperatures speed the rate that vectors and pathogens mature and replicate. It is essential to understand the interactions of the climate (ENSO, relative humidity, temperature, and rainfall) with other nonclimate factors and across different geographical locations in order to prepare effectively for the effects on infectious disease occurrence.

The trends mentioned in this chapter have helped to clarify the limitations in data and identify what is needed to assist infectious disease mitigation moving forward. Undeniably, prevention efforts need to be strengthened. First, an anticipatory framework that uses predictive disease models to show temporal associations between weather and disease trends needs to be developed. Such models can help shape public health investments for the future and can also be used to identify areas of habitat likely to harbor disease or reservoir hosts. Prevention measures, such as local vector control, ought to be implemented from within localities. In conjunction, large-scale public health infrastructure needs to support these local efforts by establishing state control measures for their establishment or funding mechanisms for their maintenance (e.g., requiring canine vaccinations for rabies and decreasing the number of stray dogs in an area). Refining routine disease surveillance will ensure that there are high-quality and long-term data sets available for use in predictive disease models. Surveillance is needed for disease cases, vectors, reservoir hosts, and the determinants of disease. Reporting systems also require further development to promote a more streamlined and consistent approach to quantifying disease risk and disseminating warning messages. In addition, scientists should strive for consensus regarding their methodology of data collection and its application to research; this will encourage consistency and progress. Ultimately, using high-resolution models to project spatial and temporal disease risk based on specific weather indexes and environmental drivers will help to anticipate the effects that climate variability may have on the spread of infectious diseases. Once disease risk has been estimated, the next generation of vector-borne and zoonotic disease specialists can be trained more accurately for what is expected to come.

DISCUSSION QUESTIONS

1. Describe EIP and why it is temperature dependent.
2. What is the general consensus among scientists as to the role of climate change in dengue expansion?
3. What climactic factors contribute to a heightened incidence of West Nile fever?
4. List one of the factors that contributed to the emergence of tick-borne disease in the United States in the past few decades.
5. How is climate change projected to affect rabies?

KEY TERMS

Dengue: A mosquito-borne disease, also known as breakbone fever, of many tropical and sub-tropical regions caused by four related dengue viruses.

Lyme disease: A tick-borne spirochetal infection caused by the bacteria *Borrelia burgdorferi* in the United States and Europe and by *Borrelia afzelii* and *Borrelia garinii* in Europe and Asia.

Malaria: A febrile illness caused by protozoan parasites of the genus *Plasmodium* and transmitted by *Anopheles* mosquitoes.

Plasmodium falciparum: The most pathogenic of the five *Plasmodium* species that can infect humans, estimated to kill nearly 1 million people per year and found primarily in Africa.

Rabies: The disease caused by infection with the rabies virus and a few related viruses within the genus *Lyssavirus* of the family Rhabdoviridae. Transmission depends on exposure to infectious nervous system tissue or saliva, an event that typically occurs when victims are bitten by a rabid animal.

Vector-borne and zoonotic diseases (VBZD): Vector-borne diseases are carried and transmitted by vectors, organisms (usually a mosquito, tick, or flea) that carry and transmits an infectious pathogen into another living organism. A zoonotic disease is an animal disease that can be transmitted to human beings. VBZD is used in this chapter to refer to diseases that are both vector borne and zoonotic. It should not be inferred that all diseases that are either vector borne or zoonotic are necessarily both.

West Nile virus (WNV): A zoonotic agent that belongs to the genus *Flavivirus*. It is associated primarily with birds and is transmitted by certain species of mosquitoes of the genus *Culex* that feed on these vertebrates.

References

Aboagye-Antwi, F., A. Guindo, A. S. Traoré, H. Hurd, M. Coulibaly, S. Traoré, and F. Tripet. 2010. "Hydric Stress-Dependent Effects of *Plasmodium falciparum* Infection on the Survival of Wild-Caught *Anopheles gambiae* Female Mosquitoes." *Malaria Journal* 9:243. http://www.malariajournal.com/content/9/1/243

Allan, B. F., F. Keesing, and R. S. Ostfeld. 2003. "Effect of Forest Fragmentation on Lyme Disease Risk." *Conservation Biology* 17:267–72.

Andreadis, T. G. 2012. "The Contribution of *Culex pipiens* Complex Mosquitoes to Transmission and Persistence of West Nile Virus in North America." *Journal of the American Mosquito Control Association* 28(4 Suppl.):137–51.

Artsob, H., D. J. Gubler, D. A. Enria, M. A. Morales, M. Pupo, M. L. Bunning, and J. P. Dudley. 2009. "West Nile Virus in the New World: Trends in the Spread and Proliferation of West Nile Virus in the Western Hemisphere." *Zoonoses and Public Health* 56:357–69.

Astrom, C., J. Rocklöv, S. Hales, A. Beguin, V. Louis, and R. Sauerborn. 2012. "Potential Distribution of Dengue Fever under Scenarios of Climate Change and Economic Development." *Ecohealth* 9:448–54.

Beebe, N. W., R. D. Cooper, P. Mottram, and A. W. Sweeney. 2009. "Australia's Dengue Risk Driven by Human Adaptation to Climate Change." *PLoS Neglected Tropical Diseases* 3(5):e429.

Beldomenico, P., and M. Begon. 2010. "Disease Spread, Susceptibility and Infection Intensity: Vicious Circles?" *Trends in Ecology and Evolution* 25(1):21–27.

Beran, G. W. 1994. "Rabies and Infections by Rabies-Related Viruses." In *Handbook of Zoonoses*, 2nd ed., edited by G. Beran, 307–57. Boca Raton, FL: CRC Press.

Bertrand, M. R., and M. L. Wilson. 1996. "Microclimate-Dependent Survival of Unfed Adult *Ixodes scapularis* (Acari: Ixodidae) in Nature: Life Cycle and Study Design Implications." *Journal of Medical Entomology* 33(4):619–27.

Blanford, J. I., S. Blanford, R. G. Crane, M. E. Mann, K. P. Paaijmans, K. V. Schreiber, and M. B. Thomas. 2013. "Implications of Temperature Variation for Malaria Parasite Development across Africa." *Scientific Reports* 3:1300.

Botvinkin, A. D., L. Gribanova, and T. A. Nikifirova. 1983. [Experimental rabies in the raccoon dog]. *Zh Zhurnal mikrobiologii, epidemiologii, i immunobiologii* 12:37–40.

Bouma, M. J., and C. Dye. 1997. "Cycles of Malaria Associated with El Niño in Venezuela." *Journal of the American Medical Association* 278:1772–74.

Brault, A. C. 2009. "Changing Patterns of West Nile Virus Transmission: Altered Vector Competence and Host Susceptibility." *Veterinary Research* 40(2):43.

Brownstein, J. S., T. R. Holford, and D. Fish. 2003. "A Climate-Based Model Predicts the Spatial Distribution of the Lyme Disease Vector *Ixodes scapularis* in the United States." *Environmental Health Perspective* 111:1152–57.

Brownstein, J. S., T. R. Holford, and D. Fish. 2005. "Effect of Climate Change on Lyme Disease Risk in North America." *Ecohealth* 2(1):38–46.

Burek, K. A., F. M. Gulland, and T. M. O'Hara. 2008. "Effects of Climate Change on Arctic Marine Mammal Health." *Ecological Applications* 18(2 Suppl.):S126–34.

Burgdorfer, W., A. G. Barbour, S. F. Hayes, J. L. Benach, E. Grunwaldt, and J. P. Davis. 1982. "Lyme Disease: A Tick-Borne Spirochetosis?" *Science* 216:1317–19.

Cairns, M., A. Roca-Feltrer, T. Garske, A. L. Wilson, D. Diallo, P. J. Milligan, et al. 2012. "Estimating the Potential Public Health Impact of Seasonal Malaria Chemoprevention in African Children." *Nature Communications* 6:881.

Cazelles, B., M. Chavez, A. J. McMichael, and S. Hales. 2005. "Nonstationary Influence of El Niño on the Synchronous Dengue Epidemics in Thailand." *PLoS Medicine* 2(4):e106.

Centers for Disease Control and Prevention. 2013a. *West Nile.* Atlanta, GA: CDC.

Centers for Disease Control and Prevention. 2013b. *Dengue.* Atlanta, GA: CDC.

Centers for Disease Control and Prevention. 2013c. *Lyme Disease.* Atlanta, GA: CDC.

Centers for Disease Control and Prevention. 2013d. *Malaria.* Atlanta, GA: CDC.

Cerkasskij, V. L. 1980. "The Role of the Raccoon Dog in the Epizootiology of Rabies." *Rabies Bulletin Europe* 3:11–14.

Chaves, L. F., and C. J. Koenraadt. 2010. "Climate Change and Highland Malaria: Fresh Air for a Hot Debate." *Quarterly Review of Biology* 85(1):27–55.

Chen, C-C., T. Epp, E. Jenkins, C. Waldner, P. S. Curry, and C. Soos. 2012. "Predicting Weekly Variation of *Culex tarsalis* (Diptera: Culicidae) West Nile Virus Infection in a Newly Endemic Region, the Canadian Prairies." *Journal of Medical Entomology* 49(5):1144–53.

Craig, M. H., R. W. Snow, and D. le Sueur. 1999. "A Climate-Based Distribution Model of Malaria Transmission in Sub-Saharan Africa." *Parasitology Today* 15:105–11.

Crump, J., A. Morrissey, et al. 2013. "Etiology of Severe Non-Malaria Febrile Illness in Northern Tanzania: A Prospective Cohort Study." *PLoS Neglected Tropical Disease* 7(7):e2324. doi: 10.1371/journal.pntd.0002324

Descloux, E., M. Mangeas, C. E. Menkes, M. Lengaigne, A. Leroy, T. Tehei, L. Guillaumot, et al. 2012. "Climate-Based Models for Understanding and Forecasting Dengue Epidemics." *PLoS Neglected Tropical Diseases* 6(2):e1470.

Diuk-Wasser, M. A., A. G. Hoen, P. Cislo, R. Brinkerhoff, S. A. Hamer, M. Rowland, R. Cortinas, et al. 2012. "Human Risk of Infection with *Borrelia burgdorferi*, the

Lyme Disease Agent, in Eastern United States." *American Journal of Tropical Medicine and Hygiene* 86:320–37.

Dohm, D. J., M. L. O'Guinn, and M. J. Turell. 2002. "Effect of Environmental Temperature on the Ability of *Culex pipiens* (Diptera: Culicidae) to Transmit West Nile Virus." *Journal of Medical Entomology* 39(1):221–25.

Dorr, B., and R. Gothe. 2001. "Cold-Hardiness of *Dermacentor marginatus* (Acari: Ixodidae)." *Experimental and Applied Acarology* 25:151–69.

Earnest, A., S. B. Tan, and A. Wilder-Smith. 2012. "Meteorological Factors and El Niño Southern Oscillation Are Independently Associated with Dengue Infections." *Epidemiology and Infection* 140:1244–51.

Eisele, T. P., D. A. Larsen, P. A. Angleqicz, J. Keating, J. Yukich, A. Bennett, P. Hutchinson, and R. W. Steketee. 2012. "Malaria Prevention in Pregnancy, Birth Weight, and Neonatal Mortality: A Meta-Analysis of 32 National Cross-Sectional Datasets in Africa." *Lancet Infectious Diseases* 12:942–49.

Eisen, L., and C. G. Moore. 2013. "*Aedes* (Stegomyia) *aegypti* in the Continental United States: A Vector at the Cool Margin of Its Geographical Range." *Journal of Medical Entomology* 50:467–78.

Epstein, P. R. 2001. "Climate Change and Emerging Infectious Diseases." *Microbes and Infection* 3:747–54.

Gage, K. L., T. R. Burkot, R. J. Eisen, and E. B. Hayes. 2008. "Climate and Vector-Borne Diseases." *American Journal of Preventative Medicine* 35:436–50.

Garske, T., N. M. Ferguson, and A. C. Ghani. 2013. "Estimating Air Temperature and Its Influence on Malaria Transmission across Africa." *PLoS One* 8(2):e56487.

George, D. B., C. T. Webb, M. L. Farnsworth, T. J. O'Shea, R. A. Bowen, D. L. Smith, T. R. Stanley, L. E. Ellison, and C. E. Rupprecht. 2011. "Host and Viral Ecology Determine Bat Rabies Seasonality and Maintenance." *Proceedings of the National Academy of Sciences of the United States of America* 108:10208–13.

Githeko, A. K., and W. Ndegwa. 2001. "Predicting Malaria Epidemics in the Kenyan Highlands Using Climate Data: A Tool for Decision Makers." *Global Change and Human Health* 2(1):54–63.

Gottdenker, N., D. Streicker, C. Faust, and C. R. Carroll. 2014. "Anthropogenic Land Use Change and Infectious Diseases: A Review of the Evidence." *Ecohealth* 11:619–32.

Gray, J. S., H. Dautel, A. Estrada-Pena, O. Kahl, and E. Lindgren. 2009. "Effects of Climate Change on Ticks and Tick-Borne Diseases in Europe." *Interdisciplinary Perspectives on Infectious Diseases* 2009:1–12. doi:10.1155/2009/593232

Greer, A., V. Ng, and D. Fisman. 2008. "Climate Change and Infectious Diseases in North America: The Road Ahead." *Canadian Medical Association Journal* 178:715–22.

Gubler, D. J., P. Reiter, K. L. Ebi, W. Yap, R. Nasci, and J. A. Patz. 2001. "Climate Variability and Change in the United States: Potential Impacts on Vector- and Rodent-Borne Diseases." *Environmental Health Perspectives* 109(Suppl. 2): 223–33.

Gubler, D. J., and D. W. Trent. 1993. "Emergence of Epidemic Dengue/Dengue Hemorrhagic Fever as a Public Health Problem in the Americas." *Infectious Agents and Disease* 2:383–93.

Haines, A., and J. A. Patz. 2004. "Health Effects of Climate Change." *Journal of the American Medical Association* 291(1):99–103.

Hales, S., P. Weinstein, Y. Souares, and A. Woodward. 1999. "El Niño and the Dynamics of Vectorborne Disease Transmission." *Environmental Health Perspectives* 107:99–102.

Hales, S., N. de Wet, J. Maindonald, and A. Woodward. 2002. "Potential Effect of Population and Climate Changes on Global Distribution of Dengue Fever: An Empirical Model." *Lancet* 360:830–34

Hashizume, M., L. F. Chaves, and N. Minakawa. 2012. "Indian Ocean Dipole Drives Malaria Resurgence in East African Highlands." *Scientific Reports* 2:269.

Hashizume, M., T. Terao, and N. Minakawa. 2009. "The Indian Ocean Dipole and Malaria Risk in the Highlands of Western Kenya." *Proceedings of the National Academy of Sciences of the United States of America* 106:1857–62.

Hatz, C. F., E. Kuenzli, and M. Funk. 2012. "Rabies: Relevance, Prevention, and Management in Travel Medicine." *Infectious Disease Clinics of North America* 26:739–53.

Hay, S. I., J. Cox, D. J. Rogers, S. E. Randolph, D. I. Stern, G. D. Shanks, M. F. Myers, and R. W. Snow. 2002. "Climate Change: Regional Warming and Malaria Resurgence—Reply." *Nature* 420:628–28.

Hay, S. I., M. F. Myers, D. S. Burke, D. W. Vaughn, T. Endy, N. Ananda, G. D. Shanks, et al. 2000. "Etiology of Interepidemic Periods of Mosquito-Borne Disease." *Proceedings of the National Academy of Sciences of the United States of America* 97:9335–39.

Hayes, E. B., N. Komar, R. S. Nasci, S. Montgomery, D. R. O'Leary, and G. L. Campbell. 2005. "Epidemiology and Transmission Dynamics of West Nile Virus Disease." *Emerging Infectious Diseases* 11:1167–73.

Hayman, D. T., A. R. Fooks, J. M. Rowcliffe, R. McCrae, O. Restif, K. S. Baker, D. L. Horton, et al. 2012. "Endemic Lagos Bat Virus Infection in *Eidolon helvum*." *Epidemiology and Infection* 140:2163–71.

Higa, Y. 2011. "Dengue Vectors and Their Spatial Distribution." *Tropical Medicine and Health* 39(4 Suppl.):17–27.

Hoen, A. G., G. Margos, S. J. Bent, M. Duik-Wasser, A. Barbour, K. Kurtenbach, and D. Fish. 2009. "Phylogeography of *Borrelia burgdorferi* in the Eastern United States Reflects Multiple Independent Lyme Disease Emergence Events." *Proceedings of the National Academy of Sciences of the United States of America* 106:15013–18.

Holmala, K., and K. Kauhala. 2006. "Ecology of Wildlife Rabies in Europe." *Mammal Review* 36(1):17–36.

Institute of Medicine of the National Academies. 2003. *Microbial Threats to Health Emergence, Detection, and Response*. Washington, DC: National Academies Press.

Institute of Medicine Forum on Microbial Threats. 2008. *Global Climate Change and Extreme Weather Events: Understanding the Contributions to Infectious Disease Emergence: Workshop Summary.* Washington, DC: National Academies Press.

Intergovernmental Panel on Climate Change Data Distribution Centre. n.d. "SRE Emission Scenarios." Accessed June 4, 2015, at http://sedac.ipcc-data.org/ddc /sres/.

Jansen, C. C., and N. W. Beebe. 2010. "The Dengue Vector *Aedes aegypti*: What Comes Next." *Microbes and Infection* 12:272–79.

Johansson, M. A., D.A.T. Cummings, and G. E. Glass. 2009. "Multiyear Climate Variability and Dengue-El Niño Southern Oscillation, Weather, and Dengue Incidence in Puerto Rico, Mexico, and Thailand: A Longitudinal Data Analysis." *PloS Medicine* 6(11).

Johnson, B. J., and M. V. Sukhdeo. 2013. "Drought-Induced Amplification of Local and Regional West Nile Virus Infection Rates in New Jersey." *Journal of Medical Entomology* 50:195–204.

Kauhala, K., and R. Kowalczyk. 2011. "Invasion of the Raccoon Dog *Nyctereutes procyonoides* in Europe: History of Colonization, Features behind Its Success, and Threats to Native Fauna." *Current Zoology* 5:584–98.

Kent, R., L. Juliusson, M. Weissmann, S. Evans, and N. Komar. 2009. "Seasonal Blood-Feeding Behavior of *Culex tarsalis* (Diptera: Culicidae) in Weld County, Colorado, 2007." *Journal of Medical Entomology* 46:380–90.

Kilpatrick, A. M., M. A. Meola, R. M. Moudy, and L. D. Kramer. 2008. "Temperature, Viral Genetics, and the Transmission of West Nile Virus by *Culex pipiens* Mosquitoes." *PLoS Pathogens* 4(6):e1000092.

Kim, B. I., J. D. Blanton, A. Gilbert, L. Castrodale, K. Hueffer, D. Slate, and C. E. Rupprecht. 2014. "A Conceptual Model for the Impact of Climate Change on Fox Rabies in Alaska, 1980–2010." *Zoonoses Public Health* 61(1):72–80.

Komar, N. 2003. "West Nile Virus: Epidemiology and Ecology in North America." *Advances in Virus Research* 61:185–234.

Lafferty, K. D. 2009. "The Ecology of Climate Change and Infectious Diseases." *Ecology* 90:888–900.

Landesman, W. J., B. F. Allan, B. Langerhans, T. M. Knight, and J. M. Chase. 2007. "Inter-Annual Associations between Precipitation and Human Incidence of West Nile Virus in the United States." *Vector Borne and Zoonotic Diseases* 7:337–43.

Lee, D. N., M. Papes, and R. A. Van den Bussche. 2012. "Present and Potential Future Distribution of Common Vampire Bats in the Americas and the Associated Risk to Cattle." *PLoS One* 7(8):e42466.

Levine, R. S., A. T. Peterson, and M. Q. Benedict. 2004. "Distribution of Members of *Anopheles quadrimaculatus* say s.l. (Diptera: Culicidae) and Implications for Their Roles in Malaria Transmission in the United States." *Journal of Medical Entomology* 41:607–13.

Lindsay, S. W., and W. J. Martens. 1998. "Malaria in the African Highlands: Past, Present and Future." *Bulletin of the World Health Organization* 76(1):33–45.

Mabaso, M. L., and N. C. Ndlovu. 2012. "Critical Review of Research Literature on Climate-Driven Malaria Epidemics in Sub-Saharan Africa." *Public Health* 126:909–19.

Margos, G., J. I. Tsao, S. Castillo-Ramirez, Y. A. Girard, S. A. Hamer, A. G. Hoen, R. S. Lane, S. L. Raper, and N. H. Ogden. 2012. "Two Boundaries Separate *Borrelia burgdorferi* populations in North America." *Applied Environmental Microbiology* 78:6059–67.

Mills, J. N., K. L. Gage, and A. S. Khan. 2010. "Potential Influence of Climate Change on Vector-Borne and Zoonotic Diseases: A Review and Proposed Research Plan." *Environmental Health Perspectives* 118:1507–14.

Mordecai, E. A., K. P. Paaijmans, L. R. Johnson, C. Balzer, T. Ben-Horin, E. deMoor, A. McNally, et al. 2013. "Optimal Temperature for Malaria Transmission Is Dramatically Lower Than Previously Predicted." *Ecology Letters* 16(1):22–30.

Moudy, R. M., M. A. Meola, L-L. Morin, G. D. Ebel, and L. D. Kramer. 2007. "A Newly Emergent Genotype of West Nile Virus Is Transmitted Earlier and More Efficiently by Culex Mosquitoes." *American Journal of Tropical Medicine and Hygiene* 77:365–70.

Murray, N.E.A., M. B. Quam, and A. Wilder-Smith. 2013. "Epidemiology of Dengue: Past, Present, and Future Prospects." *Clinical Epidemiology* 5:299–309.

Mutero, C. M., C. Kabutha, V. Kimani, L. Kabuage, G. Gitau, J. Ssennyonga, J. Githure, et al. 2004. "A Transdisciplinary Perspective on the Links between Malaria and Agroecosystems in Kenya." *Acta Tropica* 89:171–86.

Nasci, R. S., H. M. Savage, D. J. White, J. R. Miller, B. C. Cropp, M. S. Godsey, A. J. Kerst, P. Bennet, K. Gottfried, and R. S. Lanciotti. 2001. "West Nile Virus in Overwintering Culex Mosquitoes, New York City." *Emerging Infectious Diseases* 7:742–44.

Needham, G. R., and P. D. Teel. 1991. "Off-Host Physiological Ecology of Ixodid Ticks." *Annual Review of Entomology* 36:659–81.

Ogden, N. H., M. Bigras-Poulin, C. J. O'Callaghan, I. K. Barker, L. R. Lindsay, A. Maarouf, et al. 2005. "A Dynamic Population Model to Investigate Effects of Climate on Geographic Range and Seasonality of the Tick *Ixodes scapularis*." *International Journal for Parasitology* 3:375–89.

Ogden N. H., S. O. Laurie, and I. K. Barker. 2008. "Risk Maps for Range Expansion of the Lyme Disease Vector, *Ixodes scapularis*, in Canada Now and with Climate Change." *International Journal of Health Geographics* 7:24. doi:10.1186/1476–072X-7-24

Ogden, N. H., L. R Lindsay, K. Hanincova, I. K. Barker, M. Bigras-Poulin, D. F. Charron, A. Heagy, et al. 2008. "Role of Migratory Birds in Introduction and Range Expansion of *Ixodes scapularis* Ticks and of *Borrelia burgdorferi* and *Anaplasma phagocytophilum* in Canada." *Applied and Environmental Microbiology* 74:1780–90.

Ooi, E. E., and D. J. Gubler. 2009. "Global Spread of Epidemic Dengue: The Influence of Environmental Change." *Future Virology* 4:571–80.

Paaijmans, K. P., A. F. Read, and M. B. Thomas. 2009. "Understanding the Link between Malaria Risk and Climate." *Proceedings of the National Academy of Sciences of the United States of America* 106:13844–49.

Parkinson, A. J., and J. C. Butler. 2005. "Potential Impacts of Climate Change on Infectious Diseases in the Arctic." *International Journal of Circumpolar Health* 64:478–86.

Pascual, M., and M. J. Bouma. 2009. "Do Rising Temperatures Matter?" *Ecology* 90:906–12.

Patz, J., D. Campbell-Lendrum, T. Holloway, and J. A. Foley. 2005. "Impact of Regional Climate Change on Human Health." *Nature* 438:310–17.

Patz, J., P. R. Epstein, T. A. Burke, and J. M. Balbus. 1996. "Global Climate Change and Emerging Infectious Diseases." *Journal of the American Medical Association* 275:217–23.

Patz, J., M. Hulme, C. Rosenzweig, T. D. Mitchell, R. A. Goldberg, A. K. Githeko, S. Lele, et al. 2002. "Climate Change: Regional Warming and Malaria Resurgence." *Nature* 420(6916):627–28.

Paz, S. 2006. "The West Nile Virus Outbreak in Israel (2000) from a New Perspective: The Regional Impact of Climate Change." *International Journal of Environmental Health Research* 16:1–13.

Paz, S., and I. Albersheim. 2008. "Influence of Warming Tendency on *Culex pipiens* Population Abundance and on the Probability of West Nile Fever Outbreaks (Israeli Case Study: 2001–2005)." *Ecohealth* 5(1):40–48.

Pecoraro, H. L., H. L. Day, R. Reineke, N. Stevens, J. C. Withey, J. M. Marzluff, and J. S. Meschke. 2007. "Climatic and Landscape Correlates for Potential West Nile Virus Mosquito Vectors in the Seattle Region." *Journal of Vector Ecology* 32(1):22–28.

Pesko, K. N., and G. D. Ebel. 2012. "West Nile Virus Population Genetics and Evolution." *Infection, Genetics and Evolution* 12:181–90.

Petersen, L. R., A. C. Brault, and R. S. Nasci. 2013. "West Nile Virus: Review of the Literature." *Journal of the American Medical Association* 310:308–15.

Petersen, L. R., and E. B. Hayes. 2008. "West Nile Virus in the Americas." *Medical Clinics of North America* 92:1307–22.

Platonov, A. E., M. V. Fedorova, L. S. Karan, T. A. Shopenskaya, O. V. Platonova, and V. I. Zhuravlev. 2008. "Epidemiology of West Nile Infection in Volgograd, Russia, in Relation to Climate Change and Mosquito (Diptera: Culicidae) Bionomics." *Parasitology Research* 103 (Suppl. 1):S45–53.

Reisen, W., and A. C. Brault. 2007. "West Nile Virus in North America: Perspectives on Epidemiology and Intervention." *Pest Management Science*, 63:641–46.

Reisen, W. K., Y. Fang, and V. M. Martinez. 2006. "Effects of Temperature on the Transmission of West Nile Virus by *Culex tarsalis* (Diptera: Culicidae)." *Journal of Medical Entomology* 43:309–17.

Reiter, P. 2001. "Climate Change and Mosquito-Borne Disease." *Environmental Health Perspectives* 109(Suppl. 1):141–61.

Reiter, P. 2008. "Global Warming and Malaria: Knowing the Horse before Hitching the Cart." *Malaria Journal* 7(Suppl. 1):S3. doi:10.1186/1475–2875–7-S1-S3

Reiter, P., S. Lathrop, M. Bunning, B. Biggerstaff, D. Singer, T. Tiwari, L. Baber, et al. 2003. "Texas Lifestyle Limits Transmission of Dengue Virus." *Emerging Infectious Diseases* 9(1):86–89.

Revich, B., N. Tokarevich, and A. J. Parkinson. 2012. "Climate Change and Zoonotic Infections in the Russian Arctic." *International Journal of Circumpolar Health* 71:18792. http://dx.doi.org/10.3402/ijch.v71i0.18792

Rezza, G. 2012. "*Aedes albopictus* and the Reemergence of Dengue." *BMC Public Health* 12:72.

Ruiz, M. O., L. F. Chaves, G. L. Hamer, T. Sun, W. M. Brown, E. D. Walker, L. Haramis, T. L. Goldberg, and U. D. Kitron. 2010. "Local Impact of Temperature and Precipitation on West Nile Virus Infection in *Culex* Species Mosquitoes in Northeast Illinois, USA." *Parasites and Vectors* 3:19.

Scrimenti, R. J. 1970. "*Erythema chronicum migrans*." *Archives of Dermatology* 102(1):104–105.

Shaman, J., K. Harding, and S. R. Campbell. 2011. "Meteorological and Hydrological Influences on the Spatial and Temporal Prevalence of West Nile Virus in Culex Mosquitoes, Suffolk County, New York." *Journal of Medical Entomology* 48:867–75.

Shope, R. 1991. "Global Climate Change and Infectious Diseases." *Environmental Health Perspectives* 96:171–44.

Singer, A., K. Kauhala, K. Holmala, and G. C. Smith, 2008. "Rabies Risk in Raccoon Dogs and Foxes." *Developments in Biologicals* 131:213–22.

Singer, A., K. Kauhala, K. Holmala, and G. C. Smith. 2009. "Rabies in Northeastern Europe: The Threat from Invasive Raccoon Dogs." *Journal of Wildlife Diseases* 45:1121–37.

Soverow, J. E., G. A. Wellenius, D. N. Fisman, and M. A. Mittleman. 2009. "Infectious Disease in a Warming World: How Weather Influenced West Nile Virus in the United States (2001–2005)." *Environmental Health Perspectives* 117:1049–52.

Steere, A. C., S. E. Malawista, J. A. Hardin, S. Ruddy, P. W. Askenase, and W. A. Andiman. 1977. "*Erythema chronicum migrans* and Lyme Arthritis: The Enlarging Clinical Spectrum." *Annals of Internal Medicine* 86:685–98.

Sutherst, R. W. 2004. "Global Change and Human Vulnerability to Vector-Borne Diseases." *Clinical Microbiology Reviews* 17:136–73.

Thai, K.T.D., and K. L. Anders. 2011. "The Role of Climate Variability and Change in the Transmission Dynamics and Geographic Distribution of Dengue." *Experimental Biology and Medicine* 236:944–54.

Thai, K.T.D., B. Cazelles, N. V. Nruyen, L. T. Vo, M. F. Boni, J. Farrar, C. P. Simmons, H. R. van Doorn, and P. J. de Vries. 2010. "Dengue Dynamics in Binh Thuan Province, Southern Vietnam: Periodicity, Synchronicity and Climate Variability." *PLoS Neglected Tropical Diseases* 4(7):e747.

Thomson, A. J. 2010. "Climate Indices, Rainfall Onset and Retreat, and Malaria in Nigeria." *Journal of Vector Borne Diseases* 47:193–203.

Tsai, T. F., F. Popovici, C. Cernescu, G. L. Campbell, and N. I. Nedelcu, for the Investigative Team. 1998. "West Nile Encephalitis Epidemic in Southeastern Romania." *Lancet* 352:767–71.

UNICEF Division of Policy and Strategy. 2013. "World Malaria Day: Invest in the Future, Defeat Malaria." New York: United Nations.

Utzinger, J., and J. Keiser. 2006. "Urbanization and Tropical Health—Then and Now." *Annals of Tropical Medicine and Parasitology* 100:517–33.

van Eijk, A. M., J. Hill, D. A. Larsen, J. Webster, R. W. Steketee, T. P. Eisele, et al. 2013. "Coverage of Intermittent Preventive Treatment and Insecticide-Treated Nets for the Control of Malaria during Pregnancy in Sub-Saharan Africa: A Synthesis and Meta-Analysis of National Survey Data, 2009–11." *Lancet Infectious Diseases* 12:1029–42.

Wang, J., N. H. Ogden, and H. Zhu. 2011. "The Impact of Weather Conditions on *Culex pipiens* and *Culex restuans* (Diptera: Culicidae) Abundance: A Case Study in Peel Region." *Journal of Medical Entomology* 48:468–75.

Warrell, M. J., and D. A. Warrell. 2004. "Rabies and Other Lyssavirus Diseases." *Lancet* 363:959–69.

Watts, D. M., D. S. Burke, B. A. Harrison, R. E. Whitmire, and A. Nisalak. 1987. "Effect of Temperature on the Vector Efficiency of *Aedes aegypti* for Dengue 2 Virus." *American Journal of Tropical Medicine and Hygiene* 36(1):143–52.

Weaver, S. C., and W. K. Reisen. 2010. "Present and Future Arboviral Threats." *Antiviral Research* 85:328–45.

Wood, C. L., and K. D. Lafferty. 2013. "Biodiversity and Disease: A Synthesis of Ecological Perspectives on Lyme Disease Transmission." *Trends in Ecology and Evolution* 28:239–47.

Wood, J. L., M. Leach, L. Waldman, H. MacGregor, A. R. Fooks, K. E. Jones, O. Restif, et al. 2012. "A Framework for the Study of Zoonotic Disease Emergence and Its Drivers: Spillover of Bat Pathogens as a Case Study." *Philosophical Transactions of the Royal Society B* 367:2881–92.

World Health Organization. 2013. *World Malaria Report 2013.* Geneva: WHO.

Zhou, G. F., N. Minakawa, A. K. Githeko, and G. Yan. 2004. "Association between Climate Variability and Malaria Epidemics in the East African Highlands." *Proceedings of the National Academy of Sciences of the United States of America* 101:2375–80.

CHAPTER 9

ADDRESSING THE CHALLENGES OF CLIMATE CHANGE TO FOOD SECURITY, SAFETY, AND NUTRITION

Cristina Tirado

Climate change, and the consequent global environmental change, can have significant impacts on food and water security and eventually on **undernutrition**, particularly in developing countries in the sub-Sahara and in Southeast Asia. Climate change and variability affect all four dimensions of food security: food availability, stability of food supplies, access to food, and food utilization.

Climate change and variability affect the key underlying causes of undernutrition: household food access, access to maternal and child care and feeding practices, and environmental health and health access. Undernutrition in turn undermines resilience to shocks and the coping mechanisms of vulnerable populations, lessening their capacities to resist and adapt to the consequences of climate change.

Climate change may have direct and indirect impacts on their occurrence of food safety hazards at various stages of the food chain, from primary production to consumption. It may affect underlying drivers of food safety such as agriculture, crop production and plant health, animal production and animal health, fisheries and aquaculture, food trade, distribution, and consumer behavior. These impacts in turn have substantial public health, economic, and social consequences.

KEY CONCEPTS

- **Climate change and variability can affect all the dimensions of food security, food availability, nutrient content, stability of food supplies, access to food, and food utilization.**

- **Climate change has an impact on the key underlying causes of undernutrition: household food access, access to maternal and child care and feeding practices, health access, and environmental health.**

- **Impacts on the occurrence of food safety hazards can be affected at various stages of the food chain from production to consumption.**

- **Food and agriculture systems and dietary preferences influence greenhouse gas emissions.**

KEY CONCEPTS (*CONTINUED*)

• A combination of nutrition-sensitive adaptation and mitigation measures, supported by research and technological development, increased policy coherence, and institutional and cross-sectoral collaboration, can contribute to address the threats to food security, safety, and nutrition from climate change.

• Sustainable food production, sustainable food consumption, and food waste reduction have benefits to nutrition, health, and the environment.

Climate Change and Food Security: Impacts on Availability, Stability, Access, and Food Utilization

Climate change and variability affect all four dimensions of food security: food availability (production and trade), stability of food supplies, access to food, and food utilization (Schmidhuber and Tubiello 2007; Food and Agriculture Organization 2008a; Tirado, Cohen et al. 2010a). In addition food security depends not only on climate, environmental, and socioeconomic impacts but also on changes to trade flows, stocks, and food aid policy.

Climate Change Impacts on Food Availability: Food Production and Trade

Food Crops Production

Agricultural output in developing countries is expected to decline by 10 to 20 percent by 2080, depending on whether there are beneficial effects from carbon dioxide fertilization (Easterling et al. 2007; Vermeulen et al. 2012; Porter et al. 2014). Climate change and variability impacts on food production will be mixed and vary regionally. Globally, the potential for food production is projected to increase, with increases in local average temperature over a range of 1°C to 3°C, but above this, it is projected to decrease. Evidence from models from the Fourth IPCC Assessment suggests that moderate local increases in temperature (1°C to 3°C), along with associated carbon dioxide increase and rainfall changes, can have small beneficial impacts on the production of major rain-fed crops (maize, wheat, rice) and pastures in mid- to high-latitude regions. However, in seasonally dry and tropical regions, even slight warming (1°C to 2°C) reduces yield. Further warming (above a range of 1°C to 3°C) has increasingly negative impacts on global food production in all regions (Easterling et al. 2007; Porter et al. 2014). (See figure 9.1.)

While the United States will be less affected than some other countries (Gregory, Ingram, and Brklacich 2005; Lloyd, Kovats, and Chalabi 2011), the nation will not be immune. For example, Alaskan natives have unique dietary patterns and will confront shortages of key foods (Brubaker et al. 2011).

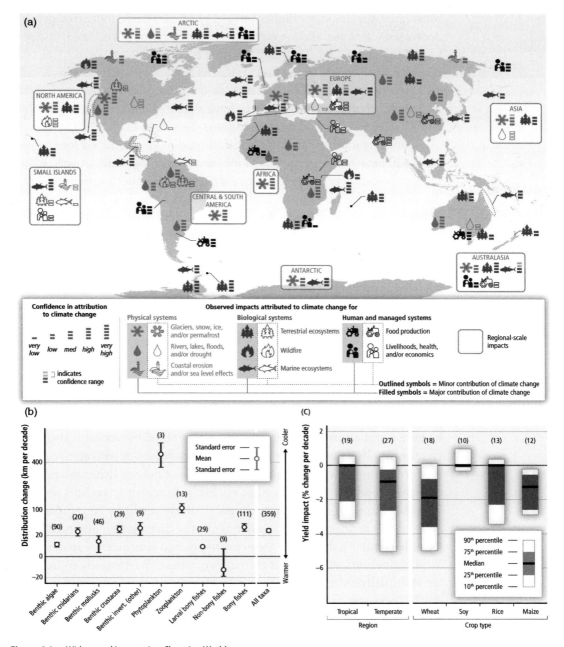

Figure 9.1   Widespread Impacts in a Changing World

Source: IPCC

Impacts on Nutrients' Content of Food Crops

Elevated atmospheric carbon dioxide is associated with decreased nitrogen concentration and results in a reduction in protein concentration for most crops (Taub, Miller, and Allen 2008). Under elevated carbon dioxide, most plant species show higher rates of photosynthesis, increased growth, decreased water use, and lowered tissue concentrations of nitrogen and protein (Taub et al. 2008; Taub 2010). Rising atmospheric carbon dioxide concentration affects protein concentration of wheat grain, which decreases by 12.7 percent at elevated carbon dioxide conditions (Fernando et al. 2012). Elevated carbon dioxide is likely to have a greater impact on grain protein levels under warmer and drier conditions (Fernando et al. 2012).

Concentrations of atmospheric carbon dioxide predicted for the year 2100 will have major implications for plant physiology and growth. Rising carbon dioxide over the next century is likely to affect both agricultural production and food quality and is likely to decrease the protein concentration of many human plant foods. The nutrient content of crops is also projected to decline, with reduced levels of nutrients such as calcium, iron, zinc, vitamins, and sugars (Idso and Idso 2001). For example, grains that use the C3 pathway of photosynthesis (such as wheat and rice) and legumes (such as soybeans and field peas) have lower concentrations of zinc and iron when grown under field conditions at the elevated atmospheric carbon dioxide concentration predicted for the middle of this century (Myers et al. 2014). C3 crops other than legumes also have lower concentrations of protein, whereas crops that use the C4 pathway of photosynthesis, such as maize, sugar cane, millet, and sorghum, seem to be less affected (Myers et al. 2014).

Fisheries and Aquaculture Production

Fisheries and aquaculture production are affected by seawater warming, change of salinity, and water acidification. Increases in seawater temperature are leading to changes in the distribution of marine fisheries and community interactions (Hollowed et al. 2013). Brackish water species from delicate estuarine ecosystems are particularly sensitive to temperature and salinity changes. Regional changes in the distribution and productivity of particular fish species are expected due to continued warming, and local extinctions will occur at the edges of ranges, particularly in freshwater and diadromous species such as salmon or sturgeon (Easterling et al. 2007). Increases in atmospheric carbon dioxide are raising ocean acidity, which affects calcification processes, coral reef bleaching, and the balance of the food web (UK Royal Society 2005). Global warming will confound the impact of natural variation on fishing activity and complicate management. The sustainability of the fishing industries of many countries will depend on increasing flexibility in bilateral and multilateral fishing agreements, coupled with international stock assessments and management plans (Easterling et al. 2007; Food and Agriculture Organization 2008a; Tirado et al. 2010a).

Food Trade

Trade in cereal crops, livestock, and forestry products is projected to increase in response to climate change, with increased dependence on food imports for most developing countries. Exports of temperate zone food products to tropical countries will rise, while the reverse may take place in forestry in the short term (Easterling et al. 2007; Porter et al. 2014). Climate change has impacts on the stability of primary production, food manufacturing, and trade (Food and Agriculture Organization [FAO] 2008a).

Climate Change Impacts on Food Stability and Access

Changes in the patterns of extreme weather events such as floods, cyclones, and hurricanes will affect the stability of, as well as access to, food supplies. Modeling studies suggest that the increasing frequency of crop loss due to these extreme events may overcome positive effects of moderate temperature increases (Easterling et al. 2007; Porter et al. 2014). For forests, elevated risks of fires, insect outbreaks, wind damage, and other forest-disturbance events are projected. This change in frequency of extreme events such as floods is likely to have a disproportionate impact on food stability and access, particularly for smallholder farmers and artisanal fishers (Easterling et al. 2007). Food insecurity and loss of livelihood may be exacerbated by the loss of cultivated land and nursery areas for fisheries through inundation and coastal erosion in low-lying areas affecting food stability and access (Hollowed et al. 2013).

Climate-related animal and plant pests and diseases and alien invasive aquatic species will reduce the stability of the production system and the stability of food stocks. Food access will be affected through reduction of income from animal production, reduction of yields of food and cash crops, lowered forest productivity, and changes in aquatic populations, as well as increased costs of control (FAO 2008b). Climate change and variability influence the contamination of food with noninfectious hazards such as biotoxins (e.g., mycotoxins or marine toxins) and chemicals and environmental contaminants such as dioxins or heavy metals, which may have an impact on food and animal feed stability and access. For example, droughts, floods, and higher temperatures heighten crop susceptibility to fungal attack, which facilitates mycotoxin contamination of animal and human food crops and reduces the stability of food and animal feed stocks.

Climate change impacts on the stability of primary production affect food safety. Emerging hazards in primary production could influence the design of the safety management systems required to control those hazards and ensure the safety of the final product. In addition, rising average temperatures could increase hygiene risks associated with storage and distribution of food commodities, affecting food stability and access (Tirado et al. 2010b).

Food Prices

Food prices have an impact on food access of households by limiting the acquisition of appropriate foods for a nutritious diet and the purchasing power of food aid programs. Climate variability and change will likely contribute substantially to rising food prices (Cline 2007). Temperature increases of more than 3°C may cause prices to increase by up to 40 percent (Easterling et al. 2007). Food insecurity increases with rising food prices (Brown et al. 2007; Hertel and Rosch 2010); in such situations, people cope by turning to nutrient-poor but calorie-rich foods or they endure hunger, with consequences ranging from micronutrient **malnutrition** to obesity (Bloem, Semba, and Kraemer 2010).

Climate Change and Food Utilization

Food utilization refers to the ability to absorb and use food nutrients and is related to individual health status, water and food sanitation, and food and water safety, among other factors. Climate change may affect health outcomes and food utilization with additional malnutrition consequences. Populations in water-scarce regions are likely to face decreased water availability, particularly in the subtropics, with implications for the consumption of safe food and drinking water. Flooding and increased precipitation are likely to contribute to increased incidence of infectious and diarrheal diseases. The risk of emerging zoonosis may increase due to changes in the survival of pathogens in the environment; changes in migration pathways, carriers, and vectors; and changes in the natural ecosystems.

Climate change plays an important role in the spatial and temporal distribution of vector-borne diseases such as malaria. Malaria affects food availability, access, and utilization of humans as well as of livestock. Climate change will have mixed effects on malaria distribution. In the long term, the geographical range in some areas will contract due to the lack of the necessary humidity and water for mosquito breeding. Elsewhere, the geographical range of malaria will expand and the transmission season may change. It is estimated that in Africa, climate change will increase the number of person-months of exposure to malaria by 16 to 28 percent by 2100 (McMichael 2004).

Most of the projected climate-related disease burden will result from increases in diarrheal diseases and malnutrition. Diarrheal diseases particularly affect nutrient absorption and food utilization. Associations between monthly temperature and diarrheal episodes and between extreme rainfall events and monthly reports of outbreaks of waterborne disease have been reported worldwide. Higher temperatures have been associated with increased episodes of diarrheal disease in adults and children in Peru, where diarrheal reports increased 8 percent for each degree of temperature increase (Checkley et al. 2000). Climate change is projected to increase the burden of diarrheal diseases in low-income regions by approximately 2 to 5 percent in 2020 and will affect low-income populations already experiencing a large burden of disease (Campbell-Lendrum, Prüss-Üstün, and Corvalan 2003).

Climate Change and Food Safety

Climate change may have direct and indirect impacts on their occurrence of food safety hazards at various stages of the food chain, from primary production to consumption. It may affect underlying drivers of food safety such as agriculture, crop production and plant health, animal production and animal health, fisheries and aquaculture, food trade, food distribution, consumer behavior, and so on. All food-borne pathogens and their associated diseases can be potentially affected by climate change (European Centre for Disease Prevention and Control 2007).

Microbiological Food Contamination and Associated Food-Borne Diseases

Climate-related factors such as temperature and precipitation changes have an impact on microbial population; the environment; the emergence, persistence, and patterns of occurrence of bacteria, viruses, and parasites in animals and foods; and the corresponding patterns of food-borne and waterborne disease (e.g., viral and bacterial diarrheal episodes, salmonellosis, vibriosis, shigellosis, cryptosporidiosis) (Food and Agriculture Organization 2008b; Tirado et al. 2010b). (See table 9.1 on page 276.) These climate factors have an impact on the emergence, redistribution, and changes in the incidence and intensity of plant and animal diseases and pest infestations, all of which could affect food-borne diseases and zoonoses (Food and Agriculture Organization 2008b; Tirado et al. 2010b). The interactions between climate and microbiological food-borne disease are complex since climatic factors can affect the sources and modes of transmission, the growth and survival of pathogens in the environment, and the food matrix, among others. (These complex interactions have been reviewed in detail by Food and Agriculture Organization 2008b).

Bacterial Food Contaminants and Foodborne Diseases

Time series analysis studies on the impacts of climate change on food-borne diseases have focused mostly on salmonellosis and campylobacteriosis in Europe, Canada, and Australia. Food-borne diseases such as salmonellosis have been found to increase by 12 percent for each degree increase in weekly or monthly temperature above 6°C ambient temperature (Kovats et al. 2004).

Increased ocean temperatures are leading to increased densities of *Vibrio* spp. in shellfish and have been linked with large diarrheal outbreaks (Zimmerman et al. 2007; Paz et al. 2007). Risk of infection is influenced by temperature, precipitation, and accompanying changes in salinity with freshwater runoff, addition of organic carbon or other nutrients or changes in pH, and sea-level rise (Food and Agriculture Organization 2008b; Tirado, et al. 2010b; Martinez-Urtaza et al. 2010). These factors affect the geographic and temporal range of *Vibrio* spp. In countries with endemic cholera, temperature-based models suggest a relationship between the disease and temperature (Reyburn et al. 2011).

Parasitical Agents and Food-Borne Diseases

There is a causal relationship between climate change and emerging parasitic diseases (Poulin and Mouritsen 2006). Temperature and other climatic variables have direct and indirect effects on parasite transmission, and this makes it difficult to predict how climate change may affect any given parasites or their hosts. Several studies in different geographical regions in the United States and Europe show that climate-related variability, such as intense rainfall and changes in precipitation, affect the incidence of parasitical food-borne and waterborne diseases transmitted by protozoan parasites such as cryptosporidiosis and giardiasis (Curriero et al. 2001; European Centre for Disease Prevention and Control 2007, 2012). While these diseases are generally waterborne, they can be also transmitted by contaminated foods such as raw vegetables. Increased temperature may affect the transmission cycle of trematodes (Poulin and Mouritsen 2006). Important zoonotic food-borne trematode infections affect more than 40 million people per year worldwide, and more than 50 percent of the global burden of food-borne trematodes is in Southeast Asia and West Pacific (World Health Organization/Food and Agriculture Organization 2002). Food-borne trematodes are transmitted by the consumption of raw or undercooked freshwater fish, crabs, crayfish, and plants and may affect aquaculture products. Food-borne trematodes of public health significance in Asia-include trematodes from Fasciola, Fasciolopsis, Clonorchis, Opisthorchis, Paragonimus,

Haplorchis, and Metagonimus. Small increases in air and water temperature forecast by many climate models will not only influence the geographical distribution of trematodes but may also promote the proliferation of their infective stages in many ecosystems (Poulin and Mouritsen 2006).

Food Contamination with Biotoxins

Climate change and variability influence food contamination with biotoxins such as marine toxins and mycotoxins that affect human health and food and animal feed safety and utilization.

Harmful Algal Blooms and Safety of Fishery Products

Increased seawater temperature and other climate-related changes exacerbate eutrophication, causing phytoplankton growth and increased frequencies of harmful algal blooms (HABs) (Edwards et al. 2006; Food and Agriculture Organization 2008b). Accumulation of marine toxins by filter feeders and the subsequent consumption of these products by humans have serious health implications.

A number of human illnesses are caused by ingesting seafood (primarily shellfish) contaminated with natural toxins produced by HAB organisms; these include amnesic shellfish poisoning (ASP), diarrhetic shellfish poisoning (DSP), neurotoxic shellfish poisoning (NSP), azaspiracid shellfish poisoning (AZP), paralytic shellfish poisoning (PSP), and ciguatera fish poisoning and cyanobacteria poisoning. These toxins may cause respiratory and digestive problems, memory loss, seizures, lesions and skin irritation, or even fatalities in fish, birds, and mammals (including humans) (Anderson, Glibert, and Burkholder 2002; Sellner, Doucette, and Kirkpatrick 2003). Some of these toxins can be acutely lethal, and are some of the most powerful natural substances known; in addition, no antidote exists to any HAB toxin (Glibert et al. 2005).

Because these toxins are tasteless, odorless, and heat and acid stable, normal screening and food preparation procedures will not prevent intoxication if the fish or shellfish is contaminated (Baden, Fleming, and Bean 1995; Fleming et al. 2006).

In addition to human health effects, HABs also have detrimental economic impacts due to closure of commercial fisheries, public health costs, and other related environmental and sociocultural impacts (Hallegraeff 2010; NOAA–CSCOR 2008; Trainer and Suddleson 2005).

Climate change impacts on harmful algal blooms and marine toxins and health impacts have been covered in chapter 6.

Table 9.1 Examples of Microbiological Agents That Could Be Affected by Climate Change and Variability and Mode of Transmission to Humans

Bacteria	Host	Mode of Transmission to humans
Salmonella	Poultry and pigs	Fecal/oral
Campylobacter	Poultry	Fecal/oral
Vibrio Spp.	Shellfish, fish	Fecal/oral
E. coli O157	Cattle and other ruminants	Fecal/oral
Anthrax Clostridium	Livestock and wild birds	Ingestion of spores through environmental routes, water, soil and feeds
		Associated with outbreaks after droughts
Yersinia	Birds and rodents with regional differences in the species of animal infected; pigs are a major reservoir	Handling pigs at slaughter is a risk to humans
Listeria monocytogenes	Livestock	In the Northern Hemisphere, listeriosis has a distinct seasonal occurrence in livestock, probably associated with feeding of silage
Leptospira	All farm animal species	Leptospirae shed in urine to contaminate pasture, drinking water, and feed

Virus	Host	Mode of transmission to humans
Rift Valley fever virus	Multiple species of livestock and wildlife	Blood or organs of infected animals (handling of animal tissue), unpasteurized or uncooked milk of infected animals, mosquito, hematophagous flies
Nipah virus	Bats and pigs	Directly from bats to humans through food in the consumption of date palm sap; Infected pigs present a serious risk to farmers and abattoir workers
Hendra virus	Bats and horse	Secretions from infected horses
Hantavirus	Rodents	Aerosol route from rodents; Outbreaks from activities such as clearing rodent-infested areas and hunting
Hepatitis E virus	Wild and domestic animals	Fecal/oral, pig manure is a possible source through contamination of irrigation water and shellfish
Encephalitis tick-borne virus	Sheep, goats	Unpasteurized milk

Parasite	Host	Mode of transmission to humans
Tapeworm *Cysticercus bovis*	Cattle	Fecal/oral
Liver fluke	Sheep, cattle	Eggs are excreted in feces
Protozoan parasites		
Toxoplasma Gondii	Cats, pigs, sheep	Cat feces are a major source of infection; handling and consuming raw meat from infected sheep and pigs
Cryptosporidium	Cattle, sheep	Fecal/oral transmission; waterborne; (00) cysts are highly infectious and with high loadings, livestock feces pose a risk to animal handlers
Giardia	Cattle, cats, dogs	Fecal/oral transmission; waterborne

Sources: Food and Agriculture Organization (2008b); Tirado, Clarke et al. (2010b).

Toxigenic Fungi and Mycotoxin Contamination

Climate change and variability can affect infection of crops by toxigenic fungi, the growth of these fungi, and the production of mycotoxins. This may have consequences for food and feed safety. Droughts, floods, and higher temperatures affect crop susceptibility to fungal attack, which facilitates mycotoxin contamination of animal and human food crops (Food and Agriculture Organization 2008b).

Mycotoxins are naturally occurring substances produced by toxigenic fungi that commonly grow on a number of crops (e.g., corn, nuts) and cause adverse health outcomes such as cancer, immunosuppression, or acute toxicity when humans and animals consume them. Some mycotoxins such as aflatoxins are carcinogenic and are a public health concern. Human dietary exposure to mycotoxins can be directly through consumption of contaminated crops and through livestock that have consumed contaminated feed. Evidence suggests that aflatoxins are a likely cause of linear growth retardation in children (Khlangwiset, Shephard, and Wu 2011; Smith, Stoltzfus, and Prendergast 2012).

The Emerging Risks Unit of the European Food Safety Authority (2012) has identified changing patterns in mycotoxin contamination in cereals such as wheat, maize, and rice due to climate change as a potential emerging hazard. In particular, aflatoxins, which are frequent in tropical and subtropical areas, may become a concern in Europe. *Aspergillus flavus* and *A. parasiticus,* the main aflatoxin producers, are xerophilic fungi. With climate change and expected increasing temperature and decreasing rain, these fungi may find conditions that are more suitable for their development. Predictions showed a reduction in season length and an advance in flowering and harvest dates leading to an enlargement of the crop growing areas toward northern Europe, mainly for maize and rice, because earlier ripening could occur in these areas. The risk of *A. flavus* contamination was expected to increase in maize, in both the 2°C and 5°C scenarios, to be very low in wheat, and to be absent in rice (European Food Safety Authority 2012).

Environmental Contaminants and Chemical Residues in the Food Chain

Climate-related extreme weather events and environmental changes may lead to chemical contamination of food with environmental pollutants and chemical residues. Climate change may challenge animal and plant health management practices, and this may have consequences on the presence of chemical pesticides and drug residues in foods (Tirado, Clarke et al. 2008b).

Environmental Contaminants

Floods, droughts, and other climate-related transport mechanisms for chemical contaminants such as persistent organic pollutants (POPs) and dioxins contribute to the dispersion or accumulation of chemical contaminants on soils, crops, animal feeds, and foods.

Changes in Complex Transport Pathways of Contaminants in the Arctic   Delicate and important ecosystems such as the Arctic have complex contaminant pathways that are affected by climate change (Arctic Climate Impact Assessment 2004)—for example, the northern freshwater ecosystems in which persistent organic pollutants (POPs), metals, and radionuclides have been widely distributed by long-range atmospheric transport from other regions during the past fifty years (ACIA 2004). Transports and transfers are altered by climate change and are very likely to result in enhanced bioaccumulation of contaminants in fish and other aquatic animals, particularly POPs and mercury (ACIA 2004) leading to increased risk of high dietary exposure to POPs in particular to local and indigenous populations (Kuhnlein 2003).

Increasing ocean temperatures may influence human exposure to environmental contaminants through fishery products. Temperature increases in the North Atlantic are projected to increase rates of mercury methylation in fish and marine mammals, thus increasing human dietary exposure to methyl mercury (Booth and Zeller 2005). Ocean warming increases methylation of mercury by 3 to 5 percent for each 1°C rise in water temperature and subsequent uptake of methyl mercury in fish and mammals (Booth and Zeller 2005). Chemical food contamination may lead to recommendations to limit consumption of locally produced food in order to protect human health, thus reducing the dietary options of rural communities and indigenous peoples and compromising their traditional diets.

Pesticides and Other Chemical Residues

Climate change may affect pest developmental rates and numbers of pest generations per year, pest mortality due during winter months, or host plant susceptibility to pests (Food and Agriculture Organization 2005). It has been suggested that a general warming trend will increase both insect pest numbers and their range in the United States (US Department of Agriculture, 2008). Pesticides that are commonly used now could in fact be no longer appropriate to the new agricultural scenario of climate-plant-environment, compromising the application of good agriculture practices (Tirado, Clarke et al. 2010b). Climate-related changes on practices of crop production could lead to new or increased use of agrochemicals, presenting new challenges for risk assessment and risk management. Many pesticides have limited activity in dry conditions (Muriel et al. 2001), probably requiring higher dose levels or more frequent applications to protect crops. In addition, there is some evidence of faster degradation of pesticides due to higher temperatures (Bailey 2004). This may have implications for the implementation of good agriculture practices and integrated pest management programs to respond to problems associated with established pests (Tirado et al. 2010b). Climate-related changes in ecological conditions, increased crop pests, and suitability of new areas to potential pests may lead to the misuse or abuse of pesticide use, contribute to environmental contamination with pesticide residues, and lead to increased residues in crops (Food and Agriculture Organization 2008b).

Veterinary Drug Residues

Climate change may result in changes in the incidence of food-borne zoonoses and animal pests and possibly increased use of veterinary drugs (Food and Agriculture Organization 2008b). New diseases in aquaculture could also result in increased chemical use. Consequently there may be higher and even unacceptable levels of pesticide and veterinary drugs in foods (Food and Agriculture Organization 2008b).

Bluetongue and Rift Valley fever, as well as tick-borne livestock diseases, will be strongly influenced by climate change (Easterling et al. 2007; Porter et al. 2014). Climate may also have a direct or indirect influence on the onset of complex bacterial syndromes, such as bovine mastitis, that usually require antibiotic treatment and may lead to an increase in residues in foods. Concerns associated with aquaculture in a warming environment include a greater susceptibility to disease, introduction of pathogens and antibiotic-resistant pathogens, heavy use of antibiotics, and environmental contamination with chemicals.

Climate change and variability therefore pose a challenge to pest and disease control measures based on established good agriculture practices and good veterinary practices and good aquaculture practices with potential implications for the presence of chemical residues (pesticides or antibiotics) in the food chain and thus requiring strengthened controls for veterinary residues in foods (Food and Agriculture Organization 2008b; Tirado et al. 2010b.

Agriculture Impacts on Climate Change

The agriculture sector is a major source of greenhouse gas (GHG) emissions. Agriculture, land use, and waste account for some 35 percent of the GHG emissions that contribute to climate change (Stern 2006). The expansion of livestock and biofuel sectors plays a major role in deforestation and land degradation and thereby contributes to climate change. The agriculture and livestock sectors contribute from 7 to 18 percent of total global anthropogenic emissions of GHG (Steinfeld et al. 2006; Hristov, Johnson, and Kebreab 2014). This is attributable to carbon dioxide emissions resulting from agriculturally induced deforestation, emissions of nitrous oxide (N_2O) from livestock manure and urine, and application of nitrogen-containing fertilizers to soils and emissions of methane (CH_4) from ruminant digestion, anaerobic soil, and rice cultivation, for example.

Systemic reforms in rice production, through adoption of methods such as systems of rice intensification, can generate tremendous gains in sustainability by transforming a process that feeds nearly half the world's population into one with significant reductions in water demand, methane gas emissions, and nitrogen fertilizer inputs (Africare 2010). Additional emissions of carbon dioxide from fossil fuel results from the whole food continuum, such as food transport, storage, cold chain (including the use of refrigerant gases) processing, and food waste. Food waste is roughly one-third of food produced for human consumption; about 1.3 billion tonnes per year gets lost or wasted globally, the equivalent of 6 to 10 percent of human-generated GHG emissions (Gustavsson et al. 2011; Vermeulen et al. 2012).

Biofuel Production Challenges for Food Security and Nutrition

Climate change mitigation is critical to limit the impact of climate change on food and nutrition security. However, there are mitigation strategies that could also increase food and nutrition insecurity. In particular, the production of certain biofuels can have a negative impact on food production and nutrition of vulnerable groups (Food and Agriculture Organization 2008a; Tirado, Cohen et al. 2010a). Biofuel production requires large amounts of natural resources (arable land, water, labor) that often are diverted from the cultivation of food crops, or if not, increase pressures on deforestation (Food and Agriculture Organization 2008a; Tirado et al. 2010b). Local and global food availability may subsequently be reduced, leading to shortages in markets and associated food price increases (Food and Agriculture Organization 2008a). The production of biofuels made from food crops (e.g., maize, sugarcane) can have an impact on food security in a number of ways (Rosegrant 2008; Food and Agriculture Organization 2008a). Research is underway to develop cellulosic biofuels from low-value nonfood crops such as grasses or wood, but these substances are more difficult to process than starch or sugar crops and it is not clear that their production will expand significantly in the near future (Food and Agriculture Organization 2008c).

Biofuel production can have negative impacts on food security and nutrition through increased GHG emissions that may result from burning forests to clear land for crop cultivation, as well as through direct effects on health and sanitation and reduced food availability and associated price effects. One major problem is diversion of food and feed crops to biofuel production, as returns to biofuel production are often greater than the returns a farmer might get were the same crops sold for food or nonbiofuel crops (Trostle 2008). Such practices can reduce food availability and may consign food and feed production to less productive land, thus reducing yields and food security and raising food prices. In relation to such effects, the International Food Policy Research Institute (IFPRI) estimates that rising bioenergy demand accounted for 30 percent of the increase in weighted average grain prices between 2000 and 2007. The impact was 39 percent of the real increase in maize prices (Rosegrant 2008). Furthermore, Food and Agriculture Organization (2008d) analysis found global expenditures on imported foodstuffs in 2007 rose by about 29 percent above the record of the previous year. The bulk of the increase was accounted for by rising prices of imported cereals and vegetable oils—commodity groups that feature heavily in biofuel production.

A rise in the food bill for households that are net buyers of food may lead to the substitution of starchy staples for micronutrient-rich animal source foods, legumes, processed foods, fruits, and vegetables. Extremely poor people will experience decreased calorie consumption (Food and Agriculture Organization 2008e). Decreased overall food consumption in terms of calories, as well as of other essential nutrients including protein, fat, and micronutrients, can lead to weight loss; impaired developmental, mental and physical growth in children; and either subclinical or clinical micronutrient deficiency in all age groups (Food and Agriculture Organization 2008e). IFPRI projects that in 2020, if biofuel production proceeds at or exceeds its current pace, calorie availability will decline and child malnutrition will increase substantially, particularly in sub-Saharan Africa (Rosegrant et al. 2008).

Climate Change and Undernutrition

Climate change affects all the key drivers of undernutrition, including food security and household food access, access to proper maternal and child care and feeding practices, and environmental health and health access (Easterling et al. 2007; Costello et al. 2009; Nelson 2009; Food and Agriculture Organization 2008a; UNICEF 2007; Parry et al. 2009; Tirado et al. 2010a; Lloyd et al. 2011; Tirado et al. 2013). At the same time undernutrition undermines climate resilience and the climate adaptation capacity of vulnerable populations.

Pathways through Which Climate Change Affects Nutrition

Climate extremes, variability, and change influence maternal and child undernutrition and its three key determinants: household food access, maternal and child care and feeding practices, and access to health services and environmental health (Tirado et al. 2013; see figure 9.2). These three key determinants are shaped in turn by other factors, such as livelihoods; formal and informal institutions; economic and political structures; and resources and structural transformations.

In addition to its impact on agriculture, food systems, and food security, climate change has negative effects on the nutritional value of plant foods. Elevated carbon dioxide results in a reduction in protein concentration and other nutrients in many human plant crops (Taub et al. 2008; Taub 2010; Fernando et al. 2012; Myers et al. 2014). The distinction between food security and nutrition security is emphasized in the framework outlined in figure 9.2

According to the IPCC Assessment Reports 4th and 5th, if current trends continue, it is estimated that 200 million to 600 million more people will suffer from hunger by 2080 (Yohe et al. 2007). Calorie availability in 2050 is likely to decline throughout the developing world, resulting in an additional 24 million undernourished children, 21 percent more than in a world with no climate change, almost half of whom would be living in sub-Saharan Africa (Nelson et al. 2009; Parry et al. 2009).

Furthermore, it has been projected that climate change will lead to a relative increase in moderate stunting of 1 percent to 29 percent in 2050 compared with a future without climate change (Lloyd et al. 2011). Climate change will have a greater impact on rates of severe stunting, which are estimated to increase by 23 percent (in central sub-Saharan Africa) to 62 percent (in South Asia) (Lloyd et al. 2011). There is also growing appreciation of the social upheaval and damage to population health that may arise from the interaction of large-scale food insecurity, population dislocation, and conflict.

Nutrition-Sensitive Climate Change Adaptation

Direct Nutrition Interventions to Build Resilience to Climate Change Impacts

Direct nutrition interventions can contribute to reducing vulnerability and building resilience to climate change consequences. The 2008 and 2013 *Lancet* series on efficacious nutrition interventions and a World Bank study

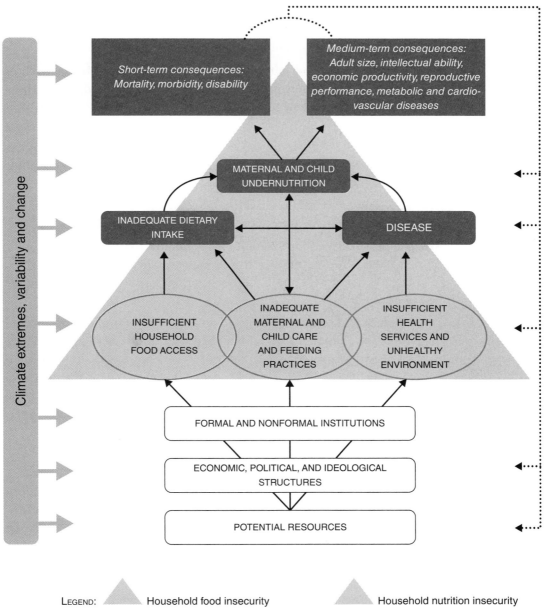

Figure 9.2   Framework Illustrating the Pathways through Which Climate Change Affects Nutrition
Source: Tirado et al. (2013).

on the programmatic feasibility and cost-effectiveness of these interventions led to the identification of a package of highly cost-effective interventions, concentrating on the window of opportunity for children under two years of age but including some components with broader benefits, including for maternal undernutrition (Horton and Shekar 2010; Bhutta et al. 2008).

These evidence-based high-return nutrition investments include:

- Promotion of good nutrition, care, and hygiene practices, such as breastfeeding, complementary feeding for infants beyond six months of age, improved hygiene practices including handwashing, and deworming programs

- Micronutrient supplementation for young children and their mothers (e.g., periodic vitamin A supplements and therapeutic zinc supplements for diarrhea management)

- Provision of micronutrients through food fortification for all (e.g., salt iodization, iron fortification)

- Therapeutic feeding for malnourished children with special foods, including the prevention or treatment for moderate undernutrition and the treatment of severe undernutrition with ready-to-use therapeutic foods

Food assistance must be targeted directly to meet immediate food and nutritional requirements of vulnerable people, increase their productive potential and adaptive capacity, and protect them from climate-related disasters. Food assistance can be delivered, for instance, by the provision of school meals (school feeding), labor-based safety nets, or cash-based intervention such as vouchers.

Sustainable, Climate-Resilient, and Nutrition-Sensitive Agricultural Development

Sustainable climate-resilient and nutrition-sensitive agricultural development is fundamental to reducing undernutrition and, along with the health- and care-based approaches, to improving nutrition security in a changing climate (Parry et al. 2009; Tirado et al. 2013). In order to be sustainable, nutrition-sensitive climate change adaptation strategies must be suitable for the local needs, microclimate, and sociocultural context. Appropriate crops, seeds, and agricultural techniques differ by region, making low-cost, socially feasible interventions at the local level heavily context dependent.

Climate change instills greater urgency to find more sustainable, resilient, and efficient ways of producing, trading, distributing, and consuming diversified agricultural food products. Producing more food does not necessarily lead to better access to a healthy and balanced diet or to an improved nutritional status of those who need it most (Sheeran 2010). In Kenya and in the Philippines, for example, the adoption of cash crops expanded food supply and doubled the household incomes of small farmers, but studies showed that children's energy intake increased only from 4 to 7 percent and that child undernutrition was little changed because households tended to spend extra income on less but more expensive higher-quality foods and other basic needs (Hawkes and Ruel 2006).

As part of the climate adaptation process, developing countries need to enhance the quantity and nutritional quality and dietary diversity of agricultural food production for local consumption. Sustainable climate-resilient and nutrition-sensitive agricultural development is fundamental to reducing undernutrition and, with the health- and care-based approaches, improving nutrition security in a changing climate (Parry et al. 2009; Tirado et al. 2013). In this context, agricultural policies must go beyond staples and increase the availability and affordability of a diverse range of nutritious food (e.g., vegetables, fruits, legumes, animal and dairy products, small fish, underutilized nutrient-rich indigenous foods).

There is a need for a greater emphasis on the nutritional quality and dietary diversity of agricultural food production for local consumption in the developing country context. Climate-resilient agriculture should be nutrition sensitive and health promoting (see table 9.2) and contribute to improving dietary diversity and nutrition by supporting, among others (Parry et al. 2009):

- Agriculture and family farming extension services promoting better crop and food production diversity (including aquaculture) and biodiversity for improved nutrition
- Integrated agroforestry systems, in particular in areas with traditional agroforestry knowledge, that reduce deforestation and promote the sustainable exploitation of nutrient-rich nonwood forest products (which are also available to buffer in times of staple dietary shortages and failed harvests)
- Integrated farming systems exploiting the synergies of horticulture, aquaculture, and small livestock rearing to reduce waste and expenses on agricultural inputs and increase food production diversity
- Good agriculture and good veterinary practices to prevent food safety problems that affect health, nutrition security, and growth such as diarrheal and zoonotic diseases and contamination with aflatoxins, pesticides, and other chemicals
- Better use of weather and climate variability information to manage climate-related risks for agriculture, forestry, and fishery and enhancing the effectiveness of food and nutrition insecurity surveillance and early warning systems and their linkages to early response mechanisms

In addition, education, communication for development, and social marketing strategies that strengthen local food systems and promote cultivation and consumption of local micronutrient-rich foods, research and development programs for the breeding of selected crops and livestock with enhanced nutritional quality, and improved postharvest management (food storage, transformation, handling and processing) to reduce losses in terms of quantity and nutrients content also contribute to nutrition security (Parry et al. 2009).

Agricultural policies must go beyond staples and increase the availability and affordability of a diverse range of nutritious food (vegetables, fruits, legumes, animal and dairy products, small fish, underused nutrient-rich indigenous foods). Agricultural policies should help the poor by enhancing and sustaining people's ability to procure and use the amount and variety of food required to be active and healthy. Policies must also be gender sensitive: the majority of small-scale farmers are women who are balancing their childcare responsibilities and farming every day. Particular attention should be given to strategies to reduce the workload of women, taking into account the repercussions on the nutrition and care of children (Save the Children UK 2009). Agricultural investment in sustainable, climate-resilient, gender-sensitive, and nutrition-sensitive development can contribute to reducing undernutrition among children under five years of age. The International Assessment of Agricultural Knowledge, Science and Technology for Development report (IAASTD) recommended reversing top-down transfers of technology and replacing them with bottom-up, participatory, farmer-oriented innovations (McIntyre 2009).

Access to Maternal and Child Care, Reproductive Health Services, Safe Water and Sanitation Systems, and Adequate, Safe Food

There is a need for additional investment and planning to address the new challenges posed by climate change to health and nutrition related issues (WHO 2008). Maternal and child health care need to be implemented successfully and provide universal health coverage and access, including access to reproductive health services and family planning. Important actions for minimizing maternal and child health and nutrition impacts from climate change include (WHO 2008; Food and Agriculture Organization 2008b; Inter-Agency Standing Committee 2009):

- Strengthening public health systems and basic clinical care systems, including the availability of essential drugs

- Enhancing local capacities to address public health emergencies

- Strengthening surveillance systems of infectious disease

- Improving the use of early warning systems by the health sector

♦   Addressing known environmental risk factors and water-related diseases

♦   Integrating nutrition and hygiene education in interventions for the treatment of severe malnutrition, diarrheal illness, and other common childhood illnesses

♦   Strengthening surveillance and control of food hazards and food-borne disease by food control and health authorities

There are benefits of providing access to reproductive health services, including modern family planning, to improve child and maternal health, and therefore nutrition security, through birth spacing while reducing population growth, energy use, and consequent climate-altering pollutant emissions over time (Smith et al. 2014). Greater emphasis needs to be placed on protecting the health of vulnerable groups, more particularly young children and pregnant and lactating women. The critical role of the nutritional status of adolescent girls and women prior to conception and interpregnancy intervals needs to be specifically addressed. Rural communities and urban areas with high levels of maternal and child undernutrition, as well as communities with high infectious disease burdens from malaria, tuberculosis, and HIV, deserve specific attention.

Social Protection Schemes That Have Proven Effective in Addressing Undernutrition and Building Resilience

Droughts or other climate-related shocks frequently force poor families to resort to negative coping strategies (e.g., reduction of the quality, safety, and quantity of their meals; reduction of the expenditures on health and education; sale of productive asset). These coping strategies generally increase the risk of undernutrition (World Food Programme et al. 2009) in the short or medium-term, and women and children are the first to be affected. Food security and nutrition-related social protection mechanisms, including safety nets, can help vulnerable households become less exposed, less sensitive, and more adaptive to a range of shocks (Beddington 2011). They can be powerful instruments to link risk reduction and immediate protection measures with efforts to build long-term resilience among the most vulnerable groups (Davies et al. 2009), more specifically young children and their mothers. Given the critical role that women play in the nutrition of children, transfers should be delivered through gender-sensitive mechanisms.

Short-term emergency or seasonal safety nets can avoid irreversible losses in human capital, reduce the incidence of negative coping mechanisms, and protect the family's access to sufficient, nutritious, and safe food. Food and cash-for-work programs prevent poor farmers from selling off their few productive assets during crises, thereby protecting development gains. Social cash transfers, generally delivered by governments on a permanent basis, can help poor families reduce their vulnerability and may also directly influence nutritional status. Conditional cash transfer programs in Colombia, Mexico, and Nicaragua decreased stunting rates by 7, 10, and 5.5 percentage points, respectively (Adato and Hoddinott 2007). Labor-based productive safety nets and pro-poor insurance schemes can allow poor farmers to protect their productive assets and gain access to investment opportunities that they would otherwise miss.

School-based approaches (e.g., school feeding programs, school gardens, nutrition education) can support child nutrition through improved diets and food and nutrition education and provide a platform for addressing child health. When children are reached during the critical period between conception and two years of age, the irreversible and intergenerational effects of undernutrition can be hindered. Later in life, school-based approaches may support child nutrition through improved diets and food and nutrition education and provide a platform for addressing child health.

In view of recurrent disasters, there is also growing demand for more predictable, flexible, and long-term safety nets that take into account climate risks (Davies et al. 2009). Innovative examples of climate risk management have already been developed and could be scaled up and replicated. One example is the Livelihoods, Early Assessment and Protection (LEAP) project in which the World Food Programme, supported by the World Bank, has assisted the government of Ethiopia in the development of a comprehensive national weather risk management framework. LEAP links Ethiopia's Productive Safety Net Program to a contingency fund. Based on the weather index, tailored LEAP software estimates the costs of scaling up the program, allowing for a timely response in case of droughts or floods (Hazell et al. 2010).

Empowerment and Social Participation within Climate-Resilient and Nutrition-Sensitive Community-Based Development

Empowerment and social participation of women and other vulnerable groups is necessary throughout the decision-making, planning, and implementing processes. Investments for community food and nutrition security should (World Food Programme et al. 2009):

* Target strengthened legal rights and equal access to resources, including land, for both women and men

* Support responsive institutions grounded in the local context

* Expand and improve education and livelihood options

- Support gender dynamics, gender equality, and girls' education

- Enhance local capacities by building on local, indigenous, and traditional knowledge with institutions at all levels

- Create a restored, diversified natural resource base and ensure that populations have the capacities and means for a sustainable management of their natural resources

In addition to a rural focus, attention has to be given to urban and periurban areas. The food supply in these areas can be put at risk by climate change hazards (e.g., as a result of the interruptions of supply channels). These perturbations can have an important impact on the growing urban and periurban populations, in particular the poorest and most vulnerable living in precarious conditions in slums, with no access to social protection or safety nets. Young children, adolescent girls, and pregnant and nursing women in rural, urban, and periurban areas should receive specific attention.

Nutrition-Sensitive Community-Based Disaster Risk Reduction and Management

With increasing risks of climate-related disasters, there is a need to better protect those who are already food and nutrition insecure by developing nutrition-sensitive disaster risk-reduction strategies and risk management practices. There is a reservoir of important indigenous and traditional knowledge in hazard-prone communities. Policymakers and practitioners should capitalize on this existing knowledge and promote the positive local risk management and coping strategies. In line with the Hyogo Framework of Action (UN International Strategy for Disaster Reduction 2005) key areas would be participatory, nutrition-focused risk assessments and risk-reduction plans; effective nutrition surveillance and early warning systems, coupled with early response mechanisms; disaster preparedness for effective response to adverse hazard events and capacity to address nutrition emergencies; contingency planning and stockpiling emergency nutrition supplies; and building resilience of food- and nutrition-insecure communities to disasters (table 9.2; UN International Strategy for Disaster Reduction 2005). The potential of innovative microinsurance schemes targeting food- and nutrition-insecure households should be explored. Quality climate risk and early warning information should be accessible to communities, with a special focus on women, to decision makers and humanitarian stakeholders at all levels. These stakeholders should improve their ability to prepare for and provide early responses to disasters, food, and nutrition crises. They should also be ready to cope with increased demand for support in light of the increasing frequency and severity of climate-related hazards.

Table 9.2 Nutrition–Sensitive Adaptation and Mitigation Strategies in the Agricultural Sector

Adaptation Strategies	Initiatives	Cobenefit: Nutrition and Health	Cobenefit: Environment
Sustainable agricultural development	Family farming and homesteads	Provides vegetables throughout the year Increases production for self-consumption Improves soil fertility and crop yield Creates employment opportunities Builds household sufficiency and increased dietary intake	Enhances soil fertility Improves moisture retention Reduces runoff Prevents soil erosion Climate-resistant crops can mitigate climate effects
	Integrated farming systems	Increases climate resilience Increases dietary diversity and micronutrient intake Increases livelihood diversification	Enhances soil fertility Prevents soil erosion Increases biodiversity
	Integrated agroforestry systems	Increases biodiversity and micronutrient intake Enhances soil fertility and decreases soil erosion	Reduces deforestation Increases biodiversity Serves as protective barriers Reduces runoff Enhances local temperature regulation
	Promotion of crop and food production diversity	Increases biodiversity and micronutrient intake	Increases biodiversity and enhances soil fertility
Food safety	Adoption of good practices within food safety, agriculture, livestock, and aquaculture production sectors: Good Agriculture/Veterinary Practices, Good Husbandry/Aquaculture Practices, Good Hygiene Practices	Promotes safe storage and good hygiene	Decreases food waste
Disaster-risk reduction and risk management	Mangrove repopulation and risk management	Mangroves are sources of diverse food, fuel, medicinal plants, and so on	Protect against sea surges and coastal erosion Protect fisheries Increase biodiversity
	Aqui-silviculture systems		
	Tapping into indigenous knowledge		Promotes climate resilience

Agroforestry	Improved crop and grazing land management to increase soil carbon sequestration; costs may be offset by public or private sponsorships	Increased soil carbon sinks Improved supply of fodder for fish and livestock Increased supply of fuel wood Improved soil fertility and water supply Increased diversity in diets Multiple harvests at different times of the year	Increased soil carbon sequestration
Systems of Rice Intensification	Efficient rice cultivation methodology that yields greater rice output with lower labor, chemical, and water inputs	Higher crop yields improve food security and household nutrition	Lower labor inputs reduce related emissions Improved nitrogen fertilizer management reduce nitrous oxide emissions
Sustainable livestock production	Integrated approaches to farming and livestock rearing	High biological value protein improves children's nutrition and development	Sustainable intensification reduces effects on deforestation, pasture degradation, and resource use Improved diets reduce fermentation in ruminants' digestive systems and improve manure and biogas management
	Anaerobic digestion of livestock waste to produce biogas		Small-scale anaerobic digesters used as a source of cooking gas in place of other higher emissions

Source: Tirado et al. (2015).

Nutrition-Sensitive Climate Change Mitigation

Climate change mitigation measures need to be put in place urgently in all the sectors in order to reduce the diverse impacts of climate change, including on food and nutrition security. The agriculture sector substantially contributes to GHG emissions worldwide and therefore offers a significant potential for mitigation (Steinfeld et al. 2006; Smith et al. 2007). One of the most potent GHGs is methane, emitted in the digestive processes and manure of ruminant livestock. The mitigation potential of reduced methane emissions from the agricultural sector is estimated at 17 to 40 percent (UN Framework Convention on Climate Change 2011). Agriculture, in particular livestock production, is also a driver in deforestation, whose climate impacts are thus often considered in the agricultural context (Friel et al. 2009).

Climate change mitigation in the agriculture sector calls for pro-poor and sustainable strategies that avoid compromising food and nutrition security (Food and Agriculture Organization et al. 2008a; Tirado, Cohen et al. 2010a; Consultative Group on International Agricultural Research 2009). The lower-middle-income countries (LMIC) face the challenge of investing more in agriculture and ensuring food and nutrition security for their populations and strengthening the resilience of their food production systems to climate change, while also reducing emissions from agriculture. Specific low net greenhouse emissions agricultural development pathways can help achieve this triple objective in LMICs, in particular agroecological food production systems, low external input agricultural systems, and integrated agroforestry and silvo-pastoral systems (Food and Agriculture Organization 2008a; Steinfeld et al. 2006). The Climate Change, Agriculture and Food Security research program (CCAFS) of the Consultative Group for International Agricultural Research (CGIAR) and the Climate Smart Agriculture initiative proposed by the Food and Agriculture Organization and the World Bank promote these triple-win development pathways (Consultative Group on International Agricultural Research 2009; Liniger et al. 2011; Food and Agriculture Organization 2010; World Bank 2010). The CCAFS also promotes the development of pro-poor climate change mitigation measures by enhancing the capacity of the effective capacity of poor to benefit from carbon financing (UN Framework Convention on Climate Change 2011).

Agriculture-related strategies and nonagricultural mitigation measures that bring benefits in terms of sustainable food production, enhanced food production per unit of energy, land, and water resources consumed, as well as enhanced access to nutritional foods and to health in LMIC, should be encouraged, tested, and scaled up. Nonagricultural mitigation measures include the diffusion of the low-emission stove technology for burning local biomass fuels, which can reduce the risk of respiratory conditions in young children. Strategies to reduce the production and consumption of foods from animal origin would help to prevent GHG emissions while benefiting the health of adults in countries consuming high amounts of products from animal origin (Friel et al. 2009). Mitigation strategies that aim to reduce the carbon footprint from the whole food sector through sustainable food production, sustainable food consumption, and food waste reduction should be explored and encouraged. Recognition that climate change mitigation strategies, nutrition, and health are intertwined should lead to a more systematic assessment of the health and nutrition impacts of mitigation strategies and more integrated solutions and policies. Such approaches can be more cost-effective, more equitable, and socially attractive. They can generate greater overall benefits for food and nutrition security, health, and climate protection.

Implications of Dietary Patterns to Climate and Nutrition

In very low-income settings, better access to animal products may be essential to improving nutrition among groups lacking access to diverse food sources. Livestock production is also a critical component of income and food security among many rural populations, including the rural poor. But at the same time, many high- and middle-income countries are facing an epidemic of obesity that is also fueled in part by increased consumption of animal products (Friel et al. 2009). Global trends in meat consumption and livestock production have an impact on the environment and climate change but can also have profound long-term impacts on production, availability, and pricing of certain basic food commodities. Some one-third of agricultural cropland is devoted to the production of feed for livestock (Food and Agriculture Organization 2009; Steinfeld et al. 2006). As a result of this and other factors, production of certain kinds of animal protein, particularly beef, are more greenhouse gas-intensive per unit than cultivation of alternative plant-based protein sources (Carlsson-Kanyama and Gonzalez 2009) and thus contribute comparatively more to climate change. In a world of finite land, water, and energy resources, the expected trends of continued rapid growth in global livestock production may constrain investments of land, water, and resources into alternative sources of nutritionally rich and diverse food crops. Imbalances in agricultural production patterns are inevitably going to be reflected in an imbalance on the dinner plate. These in turn may perpetuate trends of obesity in middle- and high-income countries but also constrain the ability of nutritionally vulnerable groups to both cultivate and purchase nutritionally rich, diverse diets more affordably (UN Environment Programme 2009; McMichael et al. 2007).

Patterns of human consumption over time have shown a steady shift in diet preferences as incomes increase and socioeconomic shifts, such as urbanization, occur. In general, the per capita levels of cereals consumption decline with increasing income, whereas that of meat increases (Msangi and Rosegrant 2012). Consumption of high-income countries is growing far beyond the world average, while the growth in dynamic economies such as China and Brazil account for much of what is observed in East Asia and the Latin America region.

The options for mitigation are not as straightforward, however, when it comes to changing human consumption patterns as for technological efficiency in conversion or energy generation. The instruments that policymakers have to influence household-level consumption choices are not nearly as direct as those that might influence industries or the decisions of political entities that control their regulation. The decrease in feed grain consumption that would result from a shift in preferences that lowered growth in per capita meat consumption in high-income countries could be as large as 5 percent, when compared to the baseline case, and could be as high as a 14 percent decrease in feed grain consumption if the fast-growing economies (and consumer cultures) of China and Brazil were also to exhibit a shift from the expected growth in meat consumption (Msangi et al. 2011). This would have implications for food market prices, price-driven nutrition outcomes, and even land use changes, which have direct impacts on GHG emissions from agriculture, as reflected in a comprehensive study for the EU region (Westhoek et al. 2011).

Sustainable diets have been recommended to address malnutrition, ecosystems degradation, and biodiversity loss caused at least in part by changes in dietary patterns (Food and Agriculture Organization 2010). Sustainable diets contribute to the promotion of food biodiversity, including traditional foods of indigenous peoples.

Cobenefits of Sustainable Food Production, Sustainable Food Consumption, and Food Waste Reduction

Sustainable food production, sustainable food consumption, and food waste reduction have been proposed as strategies to direct consumers' choices toward healthier and more sustainable food patterns while reducing emissions in the agriculture and food sectors (Tirado el al. 2013).

The steadily increasing global demand for meat and animal products, particularly in developed countries and in the urban developing world, presents a set of different but equally complex challenges for climate change mitigation, agriculture, and nutrition (Food and Agriculture Organization 2013). Global trends in meat consumption and livestock production have an impact on the environment and climate change but can also have profound long-term impacts on the production, availability, and pricing of certain basic food commodities. In 2005 roughly one-third of the world's cereal harvest was fed to livestock (Food and Agriculture Organization 2013). This in turn has certain long-term impacts on the availability and price of basic commodities and access to nutritionally diverse food sources (Friel et al. 2009).

There are many cobenefits of mitigating against climate change and improving health, particularly noncommunicable diseases, at the same time. These cobenefits include shifting diets in rich countries to less red meat and dairy products and redesigning communities to promote active transport and therefore physical activity (Smith et al. 2014). Strategies to reduce the production and consumption of fats from animal origin could help to prevent GHG emissions while benefiting the health of adults in countries consuming high amounts of products from animal origin (Friel et al. 2009). Countries such as Sweden have included sustainability criteria in the revision of their national dietary guidelines. Further research is necessary to measure the health, environmental, and financial cobenefits of sustainable diets and sustainable food consumption.

Food waste is a huge problem globally, but the underlying reasons differ by region. While food waste in high-income countries is dominated by consumer waste, developing countries have high losses at the postharvest and processing stages due to spoilage. Factors leading to food spoilage include lack of modern transport and storage infrastructure, as well as financial, managerial, and technical limitations in difficult climatic conditions (Venkat 2011; Gustavsson et al. 2011). These issues should be addressed by the agriculture, food, and environmental health sectors within a climate adaptation and mitigation frameworks and supported by agriculture extension programs.

Policy Coherence and Good Governance for Climate Change and Nutrition

A number of policy, institutional, and governance issues have considerable influence on food and nutrition security. Reaching and sustaining food and nutrition security in a changing climate requires a multisectoral approach involving nutrition, agriculture, health, and social protection. There are also important links to education, water supply, and sanitation, as well as to cross-cutting issues like gender equality, governance, and state fragility.

The cross-sectoral nature of nutrition, the impacts and threats of climate change, and the potential negative implications of climate change mitigation actions on nutrition call for increased policy coherence and institutional and cross-sectoral collaboration at local, national, and international levels. Mechanisms that ensure this policy coherence between food and nutrition security, development, adaptation, and mitigation objectives should be explored and implemented at all levels. Effective cross-sectoral planning and solutions should be facilitated by joint efforts and partnerships among communities and local stakeholders, governmental and public agencies, the UN agencies, civil society, the private sector, and academia. It is necessary to strengthen the capacities of the various stakeholders involved in direct nutrition interventions, food production and access, and social protection systems and also improve their ability to prepare for and respond to disasters.

Many low- and medium-income countries lack the adequate institutional framework and human resources to implement nutrition-based agendas (Benson 2008). Special efforts are needed to raise awareness on nutrition and climate change among decision makers and policymakers, strengthen national capacities, and bridge the gaps among sectoral institutions. At the international level, there is a need for policy coherence and cooperation to eradicate undernutrition in all its forms (Food and Agriculture Organization 2008a; Tirado et al. 2010a), including both undernutrition and overnutrition.

Stakeholders involved in climate change discussions should draw on support from the UN Standing Committee on Nutrition and other related international institutions and initiatives, such as the Committee on World Food Security (CFS). There is a gap between affected communities and the national and multilateral debates, and it is necessary to better link the local-level experience to the national and international climate change agendas for adaptation and mitigation to succeed.

Mechanisms that ensure policy coherence between food and nutrition security, development, adaptation, and mitigation objectives should be explored and implemented at all levels. It is necessary to improve collaboration and communication among stakeholder to develop coherent and coordinated nutrition-aware institutional and policy frameworks at local, national, and international levels to address the impacts of climate change on nutrition.

The current climate change negotiation process at the UN Framework Convention on Climate Change, the adaptation efforts and the work toward the sustainable development goals, and the post-2015 development agenda offer a unique opportunity to take key actions needed to protect nutrition in a comprehensive way. Further multisectoral efforts, leadership, and political will are required to integrate nutrition sensitive actions into sustainable development efforts in view of the post-2015 development agenda. Applying a human rights approach to adapt to and mitigate the impacts of climate change on health food security and nutrition is essential to advance the agenda toward climate-resilient sustainable development.

Conclusion

Climate change and the consequent global environmental change can have significant impacts on food and water security and eventually on undernutrition, particularly in developing countries in the sub-Sahara and in Southeast Asia. Climate change and variability affect all four dimensions of food security: food availability, stability of food supplies, access to food, and food utilization.

Climate change and variability have an impact on the key underlying causes of undernutrition: household food access, access to maternal and child care and feeding practices, and environmental health and health access. Undernutrition in turn undermines resilience to shocks and the coping mechanisms of vulnerable populations, lessening their capacities to resist and adapt to the consequences of climate change.

Climate change may have direct and indirect impacts on their occurrence of food safety hazards at various stages of the food chain from primary production to consumption. It may affect underlying drivers of food safety such as agriculture, crop production and plant health, animal production and animal health, fisheries and aquaculture, food trade, distribution, and consume behavior. These impacts in turn have substantial public health, economic, and social consequences.

Climate change mitigation is critical to limit the impact of climate change on food security and nutrition. However, mitigation strategies could also increase food and nutrition insecurity. In particular, the production of certain biofuels from food crops can have a negative impact on food production and nutrition of vulnerable groups. Similarly, the steadily increasing global demand for meat and animal products, particularly in developed countries and the urban developing world, presents a set of different but equally complex challenges for mitigation, agriculture, and nutrition.

A combination of nutrition-sensitive adaptation and mitigation measures, supported by research and technological development, nutrition-smart investments, increased policy coherence, and institutional and cross-sectoral collaboration, can contribute to address the threats to food and nutrition security and safety from climate change. Sustainable food production, sustainable food consumption, and food waste reduction have cobenefits to nutrition, health, and the environment. These measures should be further analyzed and integrated within development strategies and programs.

CLINICAL CORRELATES 9.1 THE GLOBAL NUTRITION TRANSITION, DUAL-BURDEN DISEASE HOUSEHOLDS, AND CLIMATE CHANGE

Global climate change has a direct impact on agriculture and the cost and availability of food. Stark differences exist between rich and poor nations in terms of the prevalence of various diseases; communicable diseases and malnutrition predominate in developing countries, whereas noncommunicable diseases such as diabetes, cancer, and cardiovascular disease are more common in developed countries (Doak et al. 2005). However, this phenomenon is rapidly changing in low- to middle-income countries, where there is now a trend toward the existence of both types of disease within the same household (Popkin et al. 2012). Malnourished children live alongside mothers who suffer from obesity, diabetes, and cardiovascular disease, causing a dual burden.

The current nutrition transition is a shift from a diet rich in legumes, vegetables, and coarse grains, which have a low carbon footprint, to a diet high in refined carbohydrates, sugars, fats, and animal source foods. The forces shaping this transition are thought to be food prices, demographic shifts from rural to urban lifestyles, the commercialization and packaging of food, and lifestyle changes in developing regions (Popkin 1999). Researchers forecast that the impact of this transition will be epidemic levels of obesity throughout the world. From 1988 to 1998 alone, the prevalence of obesity increased from 2.3 percent to 19.6 percent (Popkin and Doak 1998). Estimates predict that by 2030, there will be approximately 2.16 billion overweight and 1.12 billion obese adults (Kelly et al. 2008). The obesity epidemic will take a tremendous toll on health care systems in transitioning countries. Providers will have to shift their expertise and resources toward caring for the comorbidities associated with obesity, such as diabetes and cardiovascular disease, while at the same time addressing the needs of those suffering from diseases related to communicable diseases and malnutrition.

Global climate change is affecting food availability and lifestyle choices, thus shifting the prevalence of diseases worldwide.

CLINICAL CORRELATES 9.2 NUTRITION AND INFECTION

Experts estimate that one-third of the world population is infected with some form of intestinal helminth parasite at all times (Warren et al. 1993). Helminth infections have been correlated with impaired physical and cognitive growth and development in children (Fernando et al. 1983).

Ascuris lumbricoides, Trichuris trichiuru, Schistosoma species, and other hookworms colonize the intestinal lining. Colonization prevents the absorption of nutrients and causes a chronic inflammatory state, diarrhea, and blood-loss anemia (Stephenson 1987). Helminth life cycles involve periods of dormancy in the environment and are likely to be affected by changing global climates. Researchers propose that either the infection itself or the secondary manifestations of malnutrition, stunting, and anemia have effects on cognition and learning among infected children. These findings bring urgency to the need to develop proper treatment and surveillance of infections among communities living in poverty.

Most public health programs have targeted infection through improved hygiene and handling of food and human waste or through chemotherapeutic drugs. Recently studies looking at the effects of improved nutrition suggest that dietary intake of micronutrients such as vitamin A, vitamin B12, vitamin C, riboflavin, zinc, selenium, and iron all have immunomodulating functions (Cunningham-Rundles et al. 2005) and may affect the course of parasitic disease (Papier et al. 2014). Thus, a positive feedback situation emerges whereby dietary malnutrition increases risk for parasitic infection, which itself furthers the extent of the malnutrition through malabsorption. A new clinical approach to eradication of infection could focus on intervening in micronutrient deficiencies while at the same time employing the use of chemotherapeutic agents and public health measures.

Helminth infections are a prevalent climate-sensitive illness that has wide-reaching implications for human health. Clinicians must be aware of the complicated ways that these infections take root and affect the lives of communities in poverty and be well versed in treatment options.

CLINICAL CORRELATES 9.3 NUTRITION, MICROFINANCE, AND WOMEN'S EMPOWERMENT IN THE ERA OF CLIMATE CHANGE

Climate change is likely to alter the price and availability of food in the future and thus is important to household nutrition. When resources are finite within a household or community, the decision of how and when to allocate finances to food and health is crucial. Resource-poor communities are most susceptible to scarcity and should be a focus of programs to build resilience.

Empowering women and addressing gender inequalities is part of the UN Millennium Development Plan and may be directly linked to health and nutrition. Gender inequalities exist in many contexts. They range from impaired access to education and ability to exhibit self-determination to household decision-making power. To quantify household power, Mizan (1995) provides an index that qualifies the amount of influence a woman has on decisions of food purchase, education and marriage of children, expenses on medication for self and husband, purchase and sale of land, and more (Pitt et al. 2003). Prior studies have shown that when women have higher levels of household power, the overall health of children improves, likely because of changes in allocation of resources toward purchasing food and health care. The effects of microloans made directly to women in Bangladesh through Grameen Bank have shown that the length of participation in this loan program is directly correlated to increases in women's household power. Microfinance directed to women may have a positive effect on resource allocation, thereby building resilience in communities most vulnerable to the food and resource spikes.

Empowering women is an evidence-based method to build resilience in communities at risk of resource and nutrition scarcity.

CLINICAL CORRELATES 9.4 INFECTIOUS GASTROINTESTINAL PATHOGENS IN FOOD SUPPLIES

All infectious foodborne diseases are potentially affected by climate change (European Centre for Disease Prevention and Control 2007). Pathogens that have been identified as a priority for routine monitoring include salmonellosis, campylobacteriosis, vibriosis, listeriosis, and other parasitic infections and viral diarrheal syndromes. Observational studies suggest increasing rates of infection are possible with climate change. For example, recent analysis of human salmonellosis showed that cases increased by 5 to 10 percent for each 1 degree Celsius increase in average weekly temperature (Kovats et al. 2004). Higher temperatures, sea level elevation, and precipitation may all have an impact on water microflora such as *Vibrio* spp. (Tirado et al. 2010b). In addition, studies suggest that climate-related variability in rainfall and temperature may affect the transmission of cryptosporidiosis and giardiasis, both of which can be transmitted by contaminated foods such as raw vegetables (Tirado et al. 2010b). Infections with these and other gastrointestinal pathogens are a leading cause of morbidity and mortality worldwide, and thus clinicians must be aware of these changing disease dynamics.

Pathogens that cause infectious gastrointestinal disease are likely to be affected by climate change.

CLINICAL CORRELATES 9.5 FLOODING AND ENVIRONMENTAL CONTAMINATION

Severe weather events are associated with flooding and release of toxins from contained sources that have the potential to enter the human food chain and affect food safety. For example, following the 2002 floods in central Europe, monitoring programs traced the toxic compounds polychlorinated dibenzo-p-dioxins and dibenzifluranes from breached containers into soils and into the food chain via cow milk (Umlauf et al. 2005). Floodwaters from Hurricane Katrina caused oil spillage from storage tanks as well as spillage of pesticides, metals, and stored hazardous waste that were untraced, and thus their impact unknown (Manuel 2006). The significance these toxins have to human health is unclear; however, it is a field that deserves monitoring and intervention in order to ensure a safe food supply, especially during disasters.

Extreme weather and flooding may cause release of toxins from storage containers that have **the potential to enter the food chain and adversely affect human health.**

DISCUSSION QUESTIONS

1. What are the implications of rising carbon dioxide on plant physiology and growth, fisheries, and food trade?

2. Explain the correlation between pesticide use and climate change.

3. Explain how social protection schemes are effective in addressing undernutrition and building community resilience. List some of the community-based development steps that the author recommends.

4. List and discuss some of the direct nutrition interventions that the author recommends.

KEY TERMS

Malnutrition: As used by UNICEF, refers to both undernutrition and overnutrition.

Undernutrition: UNICEF defines undernutrition as "the outcome of insufficient food intake (hunger) and repeated infectious diseases. Undernutrition includes being underweight for one's age, too short for one's age (stunted), dangerously thin (wasted), and deficient in vitamins and minerals (micronutrient malnutrition.)"

References

Adato, M., and J. Hoddinott. 2007. *Conditional Cash Transfer Programs: A "Magic Bullet" for Reducing Poverty?* Washington, DC: International Food Policy Research Institute.

Africare, Oxfam America, WWF-ICRISAT Project. 2010. *More Rice for People, More Water for the Planet.* Hyderabad, India: WWF-ICRISAT Project.

Anderson, D. M., P. M. Glibert, and J. M. Burkholder. 2002. "Harmful Algal Blooms and Eutrophication: Nutrient Sources, Composition, and Consequences." *Estuaries* 25:704–26.

Arctic Climate Impact Assessment. (ACIA). 2004. "Impacts of a Warning Arctic: Arctic Climate Impact Assessment. ACIA Overview Report". Cambridge: Cambridge University Press.

Baden, D., L. E. Fleming, and J. A. Bean. 1995. "Marine Toxins." In *Handbook of Clinical Neurology: Intoxications of the Nervous System Part II: Natural Toxins and Drugs,* edited by F. A. deWolff, 141–75. Amsterdam: Elsevier Press.

Bailey, S. W. 2004. "Climate Change and Decreasing Herbicide Persistence." *Pest Management Science* 60:158–62.

Beddington, J. 2011. "The Future of Food and Farming: Challenges and Choices for Global Sustainability." www.bis.gov.uk/assets/bispartners/foresight/docs/food-and-farming/11–546-future-of-food-andfarming-report.pdf

Benson, T. D. 2008. *Improving Nutrition as a Development Priority: Addressing Undernutrition within National Policy Processes in Sub-Saharan Africa.* Washington, DC: International Food Policy Research Institute.

Bhutta, Z. A., T. Ahmed, R. E. Black, S. Cousens, K. Dewey, E. Giugliani, B. A. Haider, et al. 2008. "What Works? Interventions for Maternal and Child Undernutrition and Survival." *Lancet* 371:417–40.

Bloem, M. W., R. D. Semba, and K. Kraemer. 2010. "Castel Gandolfo Workshop: An Introduction to the Impact of Climate Change, the Economic Crisis, and the Increase in the Food Prices on Malnutrition." *Journal of Nutrition* 140:132S-35S. doi:10.3945/jn.109.112094

Booth, S., and D. Zeller. 2005. "Mercury, Food Webs, and Marine Mammals: Implications of Diet and Climate Change for Human Health." *Environmental Health Perspectives* 113:521–26.

Brown, M. E., C. C. Funk, G. Galu, and R. Choularton. 2007. "Earlier Famine Warning Possible Using Remote Sensing and Models." *Transactions of the American Geophyscal Union* 88:381–82.

Brubaker, M., J. Berner, R. Chavan, and J. Warren. 2011. "Climate Change and Health Effects in Northwest Alaska." *Global Health Action,* 4:1–5.

Campbell-Lendrum, D., A. Prüss-Üstün, and C. Corvalan 20030. *Climate Change and Human Health: Risks and Responses*, edited by A. McMichael, D. Campbell-Lendrum, C. Corvalan, K. Ebi, A. Githeko, J. Scheraga, and A. Woodward, 133–59. Geneva: WHO/WMO/UNEP.

Carlsson-Kanyama, A., and A. D. Gonzalez. 2009. "Potential Contributions of Food Consumption Patterns to Climate Change." *American Journal of Clinical Nutrition* 89(5):1704S.

Checkley, W., L. D. Epstein, R. H. Gilman, D. Figueroa, R. I. Cama, J. A. Patz, and R. E. Black. 2000. "Effects of El Niño and Ambient Temperature on Hospital Admissions for Diarrhoeal Diseases in Peruvian Children." *Lancet* 355:442-50.

Cline, W. R. 2007. *Global Warming and Agriculture: Impact Estimates by Country.* Washington, DC: Center for Global Development and Peterson Institute for international Economics.

Consultative Group on International Agricultural Research. 2009. *Climate, Agriculture and Food Security: A Strategy for Change.* Washington, DC: Consultative Group on International Agricultural Research.

Costello, A., M. Abbas, A. Allen, S. Ball, S. Bell, R. Bellamy, S. Friel, et al. 2009. "Managing the Health Effects of Climate Change." *Lancet* 373:1693–1733.

Cunningham-Rundles, S., D. F. McNeeley, and A. Moon. 2005. "Mechanisms of Nutrient Modulation of the Immune Response." *Journal of Allergy and Clinical Immunology* 115:119–28.

Curriero, F., J. A. Patz, J. B. Rose, and S. Lele. 2001. "The Association between Extreme Precipitation and Waterborne Disease Outbreaks in the United States, 1948–1994." *American Journal of Public Health* 91:1194–99.

Davies, M., B. Guenther, J. Leavy, T. Mitchell, and T. Tanner. 2009. "Climate Change Adaptation, Disaster Risk Reduction and Social Protection: Complementary Roles in Agriculture and Rural Growth?" IDS Working Paper 320:01–37. Brighton, UK: Communication Unit, Institute of Development Studies.

Doak, C. M., L. S. Adair, M. Bentley, C. Monteiro, and B. M. Popkin. 2005. "The Dual Burden Household and the Nutrition Transition Paradox." *International Journal of Obesity* 29:129–36.

Easterling, W. E., P. Aggarwal, P. Batima, K. Brander, L. Erda, S. Howden, A. Kirilenko, et al. 2007. *Food, Fibre and Forest Products. Climate Change 2007: Impacts, Adaptation and Vulnerability. Contribution of Working Group II to the Fourth Assessment Report of the Intergovernmental Panel on Climate Change*, edited by M. L. Parry, 273–313. Cambridge: Cambridge University Press.

Edwards, M., D. G. Johns, S. C. Leterme, E. Svendsen, and A. J. Richardson. 2006. "Regional Climate Change and Harmful Algal Blooms in the Northeast Atlantic." *Limnology and Oceanography* 51:820–29.

European Centre for Disease Prevention and Control. 2007. *Meeting Report.* Environmental Change and Infectious Disease Workshop. Stockholm, March 29–30.

European Centre for Disease Prevention and Control. 2012. *Assessing the Potential Impacts of Climate Change on Food and Waterborne Diseases in Europe.* Stockholm: ECDPC.

European Food Safety Authority 2012. "Modelling, Predicting and Mapping the Emergence of Aflatoxins in Cereals in the EU due to Climate Change." EFSA-Q-2009–00812, Parma, Italy.

Fernando M. A., and S. Balasuriya. 1983. "Effect of *Ascaris lumbricoides* Infestation on Growth of Children." *Indian Pediatrics* 20:721–31.

Fernando, N., J. Panozzo, M. Tausz, R. Norton, G. Fitzgerald, and S. Seneweer. 2012. "Rising Atmospheric Carbon Dioxide Concentration Affects Mineral Nutrient and Protein Concentration of Wheat Grain." *Food Chemistry* 133:1307–11.

Fleming, L. E., K. Broad, A. Clement, E. Dewailly, S. Elmir, A. Knap, S. A. Pomponi, et al. 2006. "Oceans and Human Health: Emerging Public Health Risks in the Marine Environment." *Marine Pollution Bulletin* 53:545–60.

Food and Agriculture Organization. 2005. "Special Event on Impact of Climate Change, Pests and Diseases on Food Security and Poverty Reduction."

Background document to the 31st Session of the Committee on World Food Security. ftp://ftp.fao.org/docrep/fao/meeting/009/j5411e.pdf

Food and Agriculture Organization. 2008a. *Impact of Climate Change and Bioenergy on Nutrition,* by M. J. Cohen, C. Tirado, N. L. Aberman, and B. Thompson. Rome: Food and Agricultural Organisation of the United Nations and International Food Policy Research Institute, Rome.

Food and Agriculture Organization. 2008b. "Food Safety and Climate Change." FAO Conference on Food Security and the Challenges of Climate Change and Bioenergy. Rome: FAO.

Food and Agriculture Organization. 2008c. "Expert Meeting on Bioenergy Policy, Markets and Trade and Food Security and Global Perspectives on Fuel and Food Security Options for Decision Makers." Rome: FAO February. http://www.fao.org/fileadminuser_upload/foodclimate/presentations/EM56/OptionsEM56.pdf

Food and Agriculture Organization. 2008d. *The State of Food and Agriculture 2008.* Rome: FAO.

Food and Agriculture Organization. 2008e. *The State of Food Insecurity in the World, 2008.* Rome: FAO. ftp://ftp.fao.org/docrep/fao/011/i0291e/i0291e00.pdf

Food and Agriculture Organization. 2009. *The State of Food Insecurity in the World 2009.* Rome: Electronic Publishing Policy and Support Branch Communication Division, FAO.

Food and Agriculture Organization. 2010. *"Climate Smart" Agriculture: Policies, Practices and Financing for Food Security, Adaptation and Mitigation.* Rome: FAO.

Food and Agriculture Organization. 2013. *The State of Food and Agriculture: Food Systems for Better Nutrition.* Rome: FAO.

Friel, S., A. D. Dangour, T. Garnett, K. Lock, Z. Chalabi, I. Roberts, A. Butler, et al. 2009. "Public Health Benefits of Strategies to Reduce Greenhouse-Gas Emissions: Food and Agriculture." *Lancet* 374:2016–25.

Glibert, P. M., D. M. Anderson, P. Gentien, E. Granéli, and K. G. Sellner. 2005. "The Global, Complex Phenomena of Harmful Algal Blooms." *Oceanography* 18:136–47.

Gregory, P. J., J.S.I. Ingram, and M. Brklacich. 2005. "Climate Change and Food Security." *Philosophical Transactions of the Royal Society B: Biological Sciences* 360:2139–48.

Gustavsson, J., C. Cederberg, U. Sonesson, R. Van Otterdijk, and A. Meybeck. 2011. *Global Food Losses and Food Waste.* Rome: Food and Agriculture Organization.

Hallegraeff, G. M. 2010. "Ocean Climate Change, Phytoplankton Community Responses and Harmful Algal Blooms: A Formidable Predictive Challenge." *Journal of Phycology* 46:220–35.

Hawkes, C., and M. T. Ruel. 2006. "Agriculture and Nutrition Linkages—old lessons and new Paradigms." "In *Understanding the links Between Agriculture and Health. 2020 Vision Focus 13*, edited by C. Hawkes and M. T. Ruel Washington, DC: International Food Policy Research Institute.

Hazell, P., J. Anderson, N. Balzer, A. H. Clemmensen, U. Hess, and F. Rispoli. 2010. *Potential for Scale and Sustainability in Weather Index Insurance for Agriculture and Rural Climate Change and Nutrition Livelihoods*. Rome: International Fund for Agricultural Development and World Food Programme.

Hertel, T. W., and S. D. Rosch. 2010. "Climate Change, Agriculture, and Poverty." *Applied Economic Perspectives and Policy* 32:355–85.

Hristov, A. N., K. A. Johnson, and E. Kebreab. 2014. "Livestock Methane Emissions in the United States." *PNAS* 111:E1320.

Hollowed, A. B., M. Barange, R. Beamish, K. Brander, K. Cochrane, K. Drinkwater, M. Foreman, et al. 2013. "Projected Impacts of Climate Change on Marine Fish and Fisheries." *ICES Journal of Marine Science* 70:1023–37. doi:10.1093/icesjms/fst081

Horton, S., and M. Shekar. 2010. *Scaling Up Nutrition: What Will It Cost?* Washington, DC: World Bank.

Idso, S. B., and K. E. Idso. 2001. "Effects of Atmospheric Carbon Dioxide Enrichment on Plant Constituents Related to Animal and Human Health." *Environmental and Experimental Botany* 45:179–99.

Inter-Agency Standing Committee. 2009. *Protecting the Health of Vulnerable People from the Humanitarian Consequences of Climate Change and Climate Related Disasters*. Bonn, Germany: UN Framework Convention on Climate Change.

Kelly, T., W. Yang, C. S. Chen, K. Reynolds, and J. He. 2008. "Global Burden of Obesity in 2005 and Projections to 2030." *International Journal of Obesity* 32:1431–37.

Khlangwiset, P., G. S. Shephard, and F. Wu. 2011. "Aflatoxins and Growth Impairment: A Review." *Critical Reviews in Toxicology* 41:740–55.

Kovats, S., S. Edwards, S. Hajat, B. Armstrong, K. Ebi, and B. Menne. 2004. "The Effect of Temperature on Food Poisoning: Time Series Analysis in 10 European Countries." *Epidemiology Infection* 132:443.

Kuhnlein, H. V. 2003. "Micronutrient Nutrition and Traditional Food Systems of Indigenous Peoples." *Food, Nutrition and Agriculture* 32:33–39.

Liniger, H. P., R. M. Studer, C. Hauert, and M. Gurtner. 2011. *Sustainable Land Management in Practice: Guidelines and Best Practices for Sub-Saharan Africa*. Rome: Food and Agriculture Organization.

Lloyd, S. J., R. S. Kovats, and Z. Chalabi. 2011. "Climate Change, Crop Yields, and Undernutrition: Development of a Model to Quantify the Impact of Climate Scenarios on Child Undernutrition." *Environmental Health Perspectives* 119:1817.

Manuel, J. 2006. "In Katrina's Wake." *Environmental Health Perspectives* 114(1):32–39.

Martinez-Urtaza, J., J. C. Bowers, J. Trinanes, and A. DePaola. 2010. "Climate Anomalies and the Increasing Risk of *Vibrio Parahaemolyticus* and *Vibrio Vulnificus* Illnesses." *Food Research International* 43:1780–90.

McIntyre, B. D. 2009. *International Assessment of Agricultural Knowledge, Science and Technology for Development, IAASTD*. Washington, DC: Island Press.

McMichael, A. 2004. "Climate Change." In *Comparative Quantification of Health Risks: Global and Regional Burden of Disease due to Selected Major Risk Factors*, vol. 2, edited by M. Ezzati, A. Lopez, A. Rodgers, and C. Murray, 1543–1649. Geneva: World Health Organization.

McMichael, A. J., J. W. Powles, C. D. Butler, and R. Uauy. 2007. "Food, Livestock Production, Energy, Climate Change, and Health." *Lancet* 370:253–63.

Mizan, A. N. 1995. *In Quest of Empowerment: The Grameen Bank Impact on Women's Power and Status*. London: University Press.

Msangi, S., and M. W. Rosegrant. 2011. "Feeding the Future's Changing Diets: Implications for Agricultural Markets, Nutrition and Policy." IFPRI 2020 Conference Paper 3. New Delhi: International Food Policy Research Institute.

Msangi, S., and M. W. Rosegrant. 2012. "Feeding the Future's Changing Diets: Implications for Agricultural Markets, Nutrition and Policy." In *Reshaping Agriculture for Nutrition and Health*, edited by S. Fan and R. Pandya-Lorch, 65–71. Washington, DC: International Food Policy Research Institute.

Muriel, P., T. Downing, M. Hulme, R. Harrington, D. Lawlor, D. Wurr, C. J. Atkinson, et al. 2001. *Climate Change and Agriculture in the United Kingdom*. London: Ministry of Agriculture, Fisheries and Forestry.

Myers, S. S., A. Zanobetti, I. Kloog, P. Huybers, A. Leakey, A. J. Bloom, E. Carlisle, et al. 2014. "Increasing Carbon Dioxide Threatens Human Nutrition." *Nature* 510:139–42.

Nelson, G. C. 2009. *Climate Change: Impact on Agriculture and Costs of Adaptation*. Washington, DC: International Food Policy Research Institute.

National Oceanic and Atmospheric Administration, Center for Sponsored Coastal Ocean Research. 2008. "Economic Impacts of Harmful Algal Blooms (HABs)." Fact sheet. http://www.cop.noaa.gov/stressors/extremeevents/hab/current/HAB_Econ.html

Papier, K., G. M. Williams, R. Luceres-Catubig, F. Ahmed, R. M. Olveda, D. P. McManus, D. Chy, et al. 2014. "Childhood Malnutrition and Parasitic Helminth Interactions." *Clinical Infectious Disease* 59:234–43.

Parry, M., A. Evans, M. W. Rosegrant, and T. Wheeler. 2009. *Climate Change and Hunger: Responding to the Challenge*. Washington, DC: International Food Policy Research Institute.

Paz, S., N. Bisharat, E. Paz, O. Kidar, and D. Cohen. 2007. "Climate Change and the Emergence of *Vibrio vulnificus* Disease in Israel." *Environmental Research* 103:390-96.

Pitt, M., S. R. Khandker, O. H. Chowdhury, and S. Millimet. 2003. "Credit Programs for the Poor and the Health Status of Children in Rural Bangladesh." *International Economic Review* 44(1):87–118.

Popkin, B. M. 1999. "Urbanization, Lifestyle Changes and the Nutrition Transition." *World Development* 27:1905–16.

Popkin, B. M., L. Adair, and S. W. Ng. 2012. "Now and Then: The Global Nutrition Transition: The Pandemic Obesity in Developing Countries." *Nutrition Review* 70(1):3–21.

Popkin, B. M., and C. M. Doak. 1998. "The Obesity Epidemic Is a Worldwide Phenomenon." *Nutrition Reviews* 56:106–14.

Porter, J. R., L. Xie, A. J. Challinor, K. Cochrane, S. M. Howden, M. M. Iqbal, D. B. Lobell. et al. 2014. "Food Security and Food Production Systems." In *Climate Change 2014: Impacts, Adaptation, and Vulnerability. Contribution of Working Group II to the Fifth Assessment Report of the Intergovernmental Panel on Climate Change,* edited by C. B. Field, V. R. Barros, D. Dokken, K. J. Mach, M. D. Mastrandrea, T. E. Bilir, M. Chatterjee, et al., 485–533. Cambridge: Cambridge University Press.

Poulin, R., and Mouritsen, K. N. 2006. "Climate Change, Parasitism and the Structure of Intertidal Ecosystems." *Journal of Helminthology* 80:183–91.

Reyburn, R., D. R. Kim, M. Emch, A. Khatib, L. von Seidlein, and M. Ali. 2011. "Climate Variability and the Outbreaks of Cholera in Zanzibar, East Africa: A Time Series Analysis." *American Journal of Tropical Medicine and Hygiene* 84:862–69. doi:10.4269/ajtmh.2011.10–0277

Rosegrant, M. W. 2008. "Biofuels and Grain Prices: Impacts and Policy Responses." Statement prepared for presentation to the Committee on Homeland Security and Governmental Affairs, US Senate.

Rosegrant, M. W., T. Zhu, S. Msangi, and T. Sulser. 2008. *Global Scenarios for Biofuels: Impacts and Implications.* Washington, DC: International Food Policy Research Institute.

Save the Children UK. 2009. "Hungry for Change: An Eight-Step, Costed Plan of Action to Tackle Global Child Hunger." London: Save the Children Fund.

Schmidhuber, J., and F. N. Tubiello. 2007. "Global Food Security under Climate Change." *Proceedings of the National Academy of Sciences* 104(50):19703–708.

Sellner, K. G., G. J. Doucette, and G. J. Kirkpatrick. 2003. "Harmful Algal Blooms: Causes, Impacts and Detection." *Journal of Industrial Microbiology and Biotechnology* 30:383–406.

Sheeran, J. 2010. "How to End Hunger." *Washington Quarterly* 33(2):3–16.

Smith, K. R., A. Woodward, D. Campbell-Lendrum, D. D. Chadee, Y. Honda, Q. Liu, J. Olwoch, et al. 2014. "Human Health: Impacts, Adaptation, and Co-Benefits." In *Climate Change 2014: Impacts, Adaptation, and Vulnerability. Part A: Global and Sectoral Aspects. Contribution of Working Group II to the Fifth Assessment Report of the Intergovernmental Panel on Climate Change,* edited by C. B. Field, V. R. Barros, D. Dokken, K. J. Mach, M. D. Mastrandrea, T. E. Bilir, M. Chatterjee et al., 709–54. Cambridge: Cambridge University Press.

Smith, L. E., R. J. Stoltzfus, and A. Prendergast. 2012. "Food Chain Mycotoxin Exposure, Gut Health, and Impaired Growth: A Conceptual Framework." *Advances in Nutrition* 3:526–31.

Smith, P., D. Martino, Z. Cai, D. Gwary, H. Janzen, P. Kumar, B. McCarl, et al. 2007. "Agriculture, Climate Change 2007: Mitigation." In *Contribution of Working Group III to the Fourth Assessment Report of the Intergovernmental Panel on Climate Change,* edited by M. L. Parry, O. F. Canziani, J. P. Palutikof, P. J. van der Linden, and C. E. Hanson, 498–540. Cambridge: Cambridge University Press.

Steinfeld, H., P. Gerber, T. Wassenaar, V. Castel, and C. de Haan. 2006. *Livestock's Long Shadow: Environmental Issues and Options: The Livestock, Environment and Development (LEAD) Initiative.* Rome: FAO.

Stephenson, L. 1987. *The Impact of Helminth Infections on Human Nutrition.* London: Taylor and Francis.

Stern, N. 2006. *Stern Review on the Economics of Climate Change.* Cambridge: Cambridge University Press.

Taub, D. 2010. "Effects of Rising Atmospheric Concentrations of Carbon Dioxide on Plants." *Nature Education Knowledge* 3(10):21.

Taub, D. R., B. Miller, and H. Allen. 2008. "Effects of Elevated Carbon Dioxide on the Protein Concentration of Food Crops: A Meta-Analysis." *Global Change Biology* 14:565–75.

Tirado, M. C., M. Cohen, N. Aberman, J. Meerman, and B. Thompson. 2010a. "Addressing the Challenges of Climate Change and Biofuel Production for Food and Nutrition Security." *Food Research International* 43:1729–44.

Tirado, M. C., A. Amadeo, K. Chen, and A. Mascareñas. 2015. Climate Smart Nutrition. Rome: FAO. [in press].

Tirado, M. C., R. Clarke, L. A. Jaykus, A. McQuatters-Gollop, and J. M. Frank. 2010b. "Climate Change and Food Safety: A Review." *Food Research International* 43:1745–65.

Tirado, M. C., P. Crahay, L. Mahy, C. Zanev, M. Neira, S. Msangi, D. Costa Cohitinio, and A. Mueller. 2013. "Climate Change and Nutrition: Creating a Climate for Nutrition Security." *Food and Nutrition Bulletin* 34:4.

Trainer, V. L., and M. Suddleson. 2005. "Monitoring Approaches for Early Warning of Domoic Acid Events in Washington State." *Oceanography* 18:228–37.

Trostle, R. 2008. *Global Agricultural Supply and Demand: Factors Contributing to the Recent Increase in Food Commodity Prices.* Washington, DC: US Department of Agriculture, Economic Research Service.

Umlauf, G., G. Bidoglio, E. Christoph, J. Kampheus, F. Krüger, D. Landmann, A. J. Schultz, et al. 2005. "The Situation of PCDD/Fs and Dioxin-Like PCBs after the Flooding of River Elbe and Mulde in 2002." *Acta Hydrochimica et Hydrobiologica* 33:543–54.

UK Royal Society. 2005. *Ocean Acidification due to Increasing Atmospheric Carbon Dioxide.* Cardiff: Clyvedon Press.

UN Environment Programme. 2009. *The Environmental Food Crisis: The Environment's Role in Averting Future Food Crises.* Nairobi, Kenya.

UN Framework Convention on Climate Change. 2011. "Fact Sheet: Reducing Emissions from Deforestationin Developing Countries." Bonn, Germany.

UN International Strategy for Disaster Reduction (UNISDR). 2005. *Hyogo Framework for Action, 2005–2015: Building the Resilience of Nations and Communities to Disasters (HFA).* Geneva: UNISDR.

UNICEF. 2007. *Climate Change and Children.* www.unicef.org/publications/files /Climate_Change_and_Children.pdf

US Department of Agriculture. 2008. *Synthesis and Assessment Product 4.3, USDA. The Effects of Climate Change on Agriculture, Land Resources, Water Resources and Biodiversity in the United States.* Washington, DC: US Department of Agriculture.

Venkat, K. 2011. "The Climate Change and Economic Impacts of Food Waste in the United States." *International Journal of Food System Dynamics* 2:431–46.

Vermeulen, S. J., P. K. Aggarwal, A. Ainslie, C. Angelone, B. M. Campbell, A. J. Challinor, J. W. Hansen, et al. 2012. "Options for Support to Agriculture and Food Security under Climate Change." *Environmental Science and Policy* 15:136–44.

Warren, K., D.A.P. Bundy, R. Anderson, A. R. Davis, D. A. Henderson, D. T. Jamison, N. Prescott, and A. Senft. 1993. "Helminth Infection." In *Disease Control Priorities in Developing Countries*, edited by D. T. Jamison, W. Mosley, A. Measham, and J. Bobadilla, 131–60. Oxford: Oxford Medical Publications.

Westhoek, H., T. Rood, M. van den Berg, J. Janse, D. Nijdam, M. Reudink, and E. Stehfest. 2011. "The Protein Puzzle: The Consumption and Production of Meat, Dairy and Fish in the European Union." *European Journal of Food Research and Review* 1:124–44.

World Bank. 2010. *The Hague Conference on Agriculture, Food Security and Climate Change Opportunities and Challenges for a Converging Agenda: Country Examples.* Hague, Netherlands: World Bank.

World Food Programme, Caritas, CARE, Food and Agriculture Organization, IFRC, Oxfam, Save the Children, World Health Organization, and World Vision. 2009. *Climate Change, Food Insecurity and Hunger: Key Messages for UNFCCC Negotiators.* Rome: World Food Program.

World Health Organization and Food and Agriculture Organization. 2002. "Report of the Joint WHO/FAO Workshop on Food-Borne Trematode Infections in Asia." Regional office for the Western Pacific Ha Noi, Vietnam, November 26–28.

Yohe, G. W., R. D. Lasco, Q. K. Ahmad, N. W. Arnell, S. J. Cohen, C. Hope, et al. 2007. "Perspectives on Climate Change and Sustainability." In *Climate Change 2007: Impacts, Adaptation and Vulnerability, Contribution of Working Group II to the Fourth Assessment Report of the Intergovernmental Panel on Climate Change*, edited by M. L. Parry, O. F. Canziani, J. P. Palutikof, P. J. van der Linden, and C. E. Hanson, 811–41. Cambridge: Cambridge University Press.

Zimmerman, M., A. DePaola, J. C. Bowers, J. A. Krantz, J. L. Nordstrom, C. N. Johnson, and D. J. Grimes. 2007. "Variability of Total and Pathogenic *Vibrio parahaemolyticus* Densities in Northern Gulf of Mexico Water and Oysters." *Applied and Environmental Microbiology* 73:7589–96.

CHAPTER 10

CLIMATE CHANGE AND POPULATION MENTAL HEALTH

Abdulrahman M. El-Sayed, Sandro Galea

Since the late nineteenth century, global surface temperatures have increased by about 0.74°C, and the rate of global warming per decade over the past fifty years is nearly twice as high as that for the past one hundred years combined (Field et al. 2014). These increases have demonstrably changed the Earth's climate, with serious implications for human well-being. For example, over the past two decades, the number of natural disasters on record has doubled from nearly two hundred to greater than four hundred annually (Guterres 2008).

Climate change is therefore among the most important issues facing the global community today. As what were once thought to be long-term effects of climate change begin to demonstrate themselves in the short term, understanding the causes and consequences of this challenge takes on particular urgency. Among the most serious and direct consequences of climate change will be its toll on human health. From the latent increase in ambient temperature to the increasing severity and frequency of natural disasters, the changing environment will have clear implications for the potentially harmful conditions to which humans are exposed and to our capacity to cope with these exposures.

Among the most important health sequelae of climate change will be the rising burden of mental disorders. Already, mental disorder results in substantial morbidity and financial cost worldwide. The World Health Organization's (WHO) latest Global Burden of Disease report, for example, ranked depression among the top three most prevalent causes of disability in the world, accounting for the highest single proportion of life

KEY CONCEPTS

- **There are several mechanisms by which climate change affects population mental health, including natural disasters, forced migration, conflict over scarce resources, and physical comorbidity.**

- **The burden of psychopathology resulting from climate change is borne disproportionately by the poor and marginalized who lack the resources to protect themselves.**

- **Climate change and population psychopathology have shared causes and consequences that should be considered in policy conversations about either individually.**

years lived with disability worldwide (Hyman et al. 2006; Mathers, Fat, and Boerma 2008). Panic disorder and self-inflicted injury, often occurring secondary to depression, also ranked high on the WHO list (Mathers et al. 2008). In the United States alone, nearly 50 percent of adults have experienced a mood or anxiety disorder at some point in their lives. Mental disorders are also profoundly expensive, imposing substantial costs, direct and indirect, on individuals, families, industries, and health systems, alike (Luppa et al. 2007).

In this chapter, we explore the mechanisms by which climate change may influence global mental health. We then discuss how climate change can contribute to deepening inequalities in global mental health. We conclude with a discussion regarding the reciprocal mechanisms by which mental disorder may potentiate climate change.

CLINICAL CORRELATES 10.1 TRAUMA AND THE FABRIC OF SOCIETY

When major disasters create psychosocial trauma, individuals and relational structures among communities and families have the potential to become strained. Research has examined the prevalence of stress disorders following disasters and found that not all individuals are affected equally. While many experience acute stress immediately following events, only some go on to develop long-term and debilitating conditions (Litz 2004). Furthermore, despite the negative connotations of stress, some investigations have found that when individuals are able to adapt after trauma, new opportunities, deeper compassion for others, and strengthened spirituality can be the rewards (Tedeschi and Calhoun 1996). What factors contribute to an individual's ability to adapt and evolve? Researchers have found that communication and trusting relationships may counter feelings of helplessness and meaninglessness in the setting of trauma (Walsh 2007). Therefore, perhaps disaster management must encompass mechanisms to nurture stronger community ties as a way to instill resilience.

Landau and Saul (2004) outline the following helpful themes for building community in the wake of a disaster: (1) enhance social connectedness and information and resource sharing, (2) encourage involvement in collective storytelling and validation of the trauma and response with the goal of shared meaning, (3) reestablish the rhythms and routines of life and engage in collective healing rituals, and (4) arrive at a positive vision of the future with renewed hope. Healers and leaders can work within their communities to foster these processes at many levels by raising awareness, arranging community meetings, and nurturing an open and compassionate attitude towards distress in others.

Mitigation of climate-related disasters must consider the psychological effects that trauma has on communities. Clinicians and other community leaders can serve as leaders in rehabilitation efforts.

Mechanisms

There are several mechanisms, both direct and indirect, by which climate change may influence global mental health, as indicated in figure 10.1. First, climate change will increase the frequency and severity of natural disasters: wind storms, flooding, and drought (Aumann, Ruzmaikin, and Teixeira 2008; Murray and Ebi 2012). More frequent disasters will increase exposure to trauma that may threaten mental health, as well as harm the material well-being of victims of natural disasters. Second, climate change will destroy landscapes, ecosystems, and habitats, thereby destroying dependent ways of life, affecting a wide variety of agricultural pursuits and ethnic, cultural, and religious traditions. Third, climate change will intensify global competition for resources, which could increase the rate and consequences of global conflict. Fourth, climate change will have important influences on physical health, which will in turn increase the burden of mental comorbidity. We discuss each of these mechanisms in turn.

Natural Disasters

One of the most important implications of climate change for human health is the increase in the frequency and severity of natural disasters. Over the past two decades alone, the number of natural disasters on record has doubled (Guterres 2008). A recent study by researchers at the National Aeronautics and Space Agency (NASA) demonstrated that at the present rate of global climate change, the frequency of severe storms can be

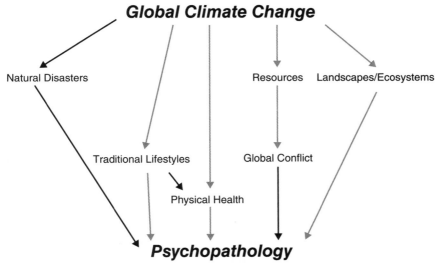

*Black arrows indicate increases while blue arrows indicate decreases in variables to which arrows point.

Figure 10.1   A Mechanistic Map Relating Global Climate Change and Psychopathology

expected to increase at 6 percent per decade (Aumann et al. 2008; Murray and Ebi 2012). The severity of these storms is also increasing. For example, one study tracked the volume of the heaviest rainfall over a twenty-four-hour period each year over half a century in the Northern Hemisphere and showed that that volume was increasing with time, suggesting that climate change is increasing the severity of climate events (Min et al. 2011). Moreover, a substantial proportion of climate-related natural disasters will occur at the coasts, where hurricanes, tropical storms, and tsunamis wreak their greatest havoc.

Compounding the increasing frequency and severity of natural disasters are demographic changes in the global population. First, the population continues to grow exponentially. In this regard, the human cost of natural disasters will increase simply because there will be more people to suffer them. Second, migratory patterns over the past several decades, both within and between countries, have been toward coastal regions. In 2010, over half of the US population lived in counties below the coastal watershed. And the National Oceanic and Atmospheric Administration (NOAA) estimates that the US coastal population will reach 133 million by 2020—nearly four times larger than it was in 1980 (33 million) (Culliton 1998). Globally, 44 percent of the world's population lives within 150 kilometers of a coast, and net coastal migration totals approximately 50 million annually (Culliton 1998). This trend increases the human burden of climate change by placing both larger absolute and relative components of the population in zones particularly vulnerable to natural disasters.

As the frequency and severity of natural disasters increase, their mental health sequelae will as well. Victims of natural disasters are at high risk for several mental health problems. A large literature documents the high burden of **posttraumatic stress disorder (PTSD)** after disasters (Galea, Nandi, and Vlahov 2005; Neria, Nandi, and Galea 2008). For example, the prevalence of PTSD following the 2010 Haiti earthquake was 25 percent (Cerdá et al. 2013). Similarly, following Hurricane Katrina, the prevalence of PTSD among residents of the twenty-three southernmost counties in Mississippi was 23 percent (Galea et al. 2008). Beyond PTSD, exposure to natural disasters can carry other deleterious mental health risks as well. For example, along with the substantial burden of PTSD, the burden of **major depressive disorder (MDD)** in Haiti was nearly 30 percent (Cerdá et al. 2013).

Natural disasters take the lives of loved ones, destroy homes and workplaces, and obliterate livelihoods. While the bulk of psychopathologic sequelae of disasters may occur in their immediate to short-term aftermath, their long-term implications are not to be overlooked. In the aftermath of Hurricane Katrina, for example, one study demonstrated that the prevalence of both suicidal ideation and severe mental illness among survivors nearly tripled among respondents between five months and one year following the disaster (Kessler et al. 2008). The investigators found that unresolved hurricane-related stresses accounted for over 60 percent of the increase in suicidality and nearly 90 percent of the increase in severe mental illness. In this regard, chronic stressors, or life circumstances that are difficult to cope with, the residual of natural disasters, may have important long-term implications for the burden of psychopathology as survivors struggle to cope with difficult new realities. As the frequency and severity of disasters increase and greater relative and absolute numbers of people are exposed to them, it is clear that the mental health sequelae of natural disasters caused by climate change will be an important mechanism through which the changing environment will influence mental health.

CLINICAL CORRELATES 10.2 PHYSICAL PAIN AND PSYCHOLOGICAL TRAUMA

Natural disasters can result in significant physical and emotional trauma. The symptoms of trauma can be expressed in many forms, which may complicate accurate clinical diagnosis and compound existing medical comorbidities, especially chronic pain. Some experts in the field of trauma have begun to unravel the ways in which culture informs the expression of psychological distress. The Harvard Program for Refugee Trauma has employed behavioral health specialists to design unique screening tools for six countries in order to detect PTSD in various cultures. They have found in many cases that neurological, somatic, and visceral pains become physical manifestations of psychological trauma. The severe pain that patients report is a real experience for them, regardless of any organic cause recognized by biomedicine.

Experts point out that a large barrier to patient treatment is the fact that health care professionals often shy away from asking patients about their history of trauma because they "believe they won't have the tools or the time to help survivors once they've elicited their history" (Mollica 2004). However, this history is imperative and will possibly become more so in the future. Recent studies through the Veterans Administration have shown the value of proper identification and treatment of PTSD. It is estimated that up to 70 percent of veterans who live with chronic pain have PTSD, and up to 80 percent of those with PTSD suffer from refractory chronic pain (Kip et al. 2013). Research has shown that treatment of PTSD statistically lowers a patient's perception of pain (Plagge et al. 2013), improving quality of life and decreasing dependence on narcotic pain medications. To prepare for the future and better address the already heavy burden of trauma in society, medical schools and professional organizations can design curricula to incorporate practical education on detecting, discussing, and managing trauma.

Climate change has the potential to result in widespread physical and psychological trauma. Thus, clinicians must be well versed in properly diagnosing and treating stress syndromes.

Forced Migration

Climate change will cause substantial changes in the ways in which populations interact with their surroundings as those surroundings change as a result of iterative disasters as well as slow, creeping alterations to microenvironments the world over. These changes will include the loss of coastal environments as the polar ice caps continue to melt and the sea level continues to rise, and changes in the crop potential of agricultural lands important to human survival. In this regard, a substantial proportion of the mental health consequences of climate change will result from the forced migration of communities to new contexts as their habitats and livelihoods degrade and the resulting vulnerabilities to which these communities will be exposed.

Glaciers and the polar ice caps are melting (Paul, Frey, and Le Bris 2011). It is clear that this will have serious implications for coastal communities as the ocean literally engulfs coastal human habitats (Solomon et al. 2009). The vulnerability of inhabitants of particular environmental regions to climate change is already well established. For example, Briguglio (1995) demonstrated that small island states were particularly vulnerable to natural disasters. Moreover, coastal residents, particularly in low-income countries, are disproportionately poor, suggesting they will already lack access to viable alternatives (McGranahan, Balk, and Anderson 2007). Mountain communities may also be vulnerable given that glaciers provide freshwater resources to such communities. Social scientists have warned of the potential for forced migration and deep exploitation of poor coastal communities in highly vulnerable countries such as Bangladesh (Poncelet et al. 2010). While the displacement of coastal communities is likely to occur over the course of several decades, climate change in this regard is a serious potential cause of forced migration in the future.

The loss of the habitat is not the only migratory force that climate change will create. Irreversible desertification in areas that had been arable and supported generations of agricultural families is also occurring (Lobell et al. 2008; Williams, Jackson, and Kutzbach 2007) as dry-season rainfall continues to drop (Solomon et al. 2009). This will force communities away from their ancestral homelands in an effort to find new means of self-support. This type of forced migration has already begun to occur in several countries in sub-Saharan Africa, where it is estimated that nearly 65 percent of arable land has degraded (Grote and Warner 2010).

Moreover, there is clear evidence that climate variability over the past several decades has had tangible effects on crop yields in various contexts. For example, one study showed that decreases in total precipitation during the warm half of the year were associated with decreases in the yield of winter wheat and maize production in a heavily agricultural context in Bulgaria (Alexandrov and Hoogenboom 2000). The influences of these climate-change-related outcomes on the communities that rely on these contexts is clear. One case study follows the migration of nomadic peoples in remote drylands of Ethiopia resulting from climate-related droughts (Meze-Hausken 2004). Similarly, in the last half of the twentieth century, social scientists tracked the movement of heads of household in southern Sudan in relation to climatic events, suggesting that poor agricultural yields have forced male heads of household to leave the countryside for the city in search of wage labor opportunities (Afolayan and Adelekan 1999; McLeman and Smit 2006). Similar findings were noted among communities in Burkina Faso (Henry, Schoumaker, and Beauchemin 2004).

These findings do not uniquely affect low-income settings. For example, one study suggests that crop yields in Mexico may be an important contributor to cross-border emigration to the United States (Feng, Krueger, and Oppenheimer 2010). Moreover, studies have suggested that US crop yields stand to suffer substantial losses with climate change as well (Schlenker and Roberts 2009), potentiating the trend toward coastal migration within the United States as agricultural life becomes even less tenable.

Forced migration has several important consequences for mental health. First, migration itself—and the implicit requirement to adapt socially, financially, and structurally to a new context—is a powerful stressor. Second, the vast majority of those forced to migrate have few social or economic resources to leverage in their new contexts, and therefore they are vulnerable to deep exploitation, which itself carries tremendous mental health consequences. Compounding this potential is that much of the forced migration resulting from climate change will move agricultural communities whose skills will be ill matched for the employment opportunities available in the contexts to which they are migrating.

Several studies have considered the mental health consequences of migration. One study, for example, found the rate of PTSD among Somali and Rwandan refugees in African refugee settlements to be nearly 50 percent (Onyut et al. 2009). A systematic review of the literature measuring the prevalence of depression and anxiety among labor migrants and refugees found that 20 percent of labor migrants around the world were depressed and 21 percent suffered anxiety disorders (Lindert et al. 2009). Rates of depression and anxiety among refugees were nearly twice as high (Lindert et al. 2009).

The same study found that the income of the country in which migrant laborers migrated was an important modifier of the risk for depression and anxiety—the higher income the country, the lower the likelihood of adverse outcomes (Lindert et al. 2009). In this regard, the literature is also clear that resources available for coping are an important predictor of the mental health risks of forced migration. One systematic review of the literature concluded that although migration is associated with a substantial amount of stress, the translation of this stress to adverse mental health was a consequence of the coping resources available (Bhugra 2004). Coping is highly influenced by the structural and legal obstacles in contexts into which communities migrate (Lindert et al. 2008). Unfortunately, it is clear that in many circumstances, forced migrants very quickly exhaust available resources and are "otherized" by the communities into which they migrate (Grove and Zwi 2006).

For those reasons, forced migrants are often victims of exploitation, including economic and sexual exploitation and human trafficking (Andrees and Belser 2009; Belser 2005; Decker et al. 2009). This exploitation can have important mental health consequences. For example, one study showed that exploitation-related trauma was associated with higher risk for adverse mental health outcomes among trafficked women (Hossain et al. 2010). Similarly, the prevalence of depression, anxiety, and suicidality among Mexican migrant workers is high (Hiott et al. 2008; Hovey 2000; Hovey and Magaña 2003; Sullivan and Rehm 2005).

Among the most important mental health consequences of climate change, therefore, will be the community migration it forces. In uprooting coastal communities that lose their homes and agricultural communities whose lands erode, climate change will expose large communities to migration-associated stressors, such as acculturation and exploitation, which will have deleterious consequences for population mental health.

Economics, Geopolitics, and Violent Conflict

As climate change progresses, the relative availability of commodities will shift, heightening competition for natural resources that are already scarce. This competition is likely to be a geopolitically destabilizing force, increasing the chances of violent conflict as geopolitical actors vie for access to increasingly important commodities (Barnett and Adger 2007; Homer-Dixon 1994; Klare 2002).

Changing demand for freshwater is among the most important potential climate-related causes of conflict. As the rate of drought increases, access to freshwater for drinking and irrigation will be at a premium. At the same time, however, climate change is likely to alter the courses of rivers and the accessibility of other freshwater sources (Klare 2002; Mearns and Norton 2010; Tir and Stinnett 2012). Social scientists have demonstrated that water scarcity increases the likelihood of armed conflict (Tir and Stinnett

2012). One study, for example, demonstrated that deviations in rainfall in either direction—expected to increase as climate change follows its current course—were associated with increasing incidence of violent events on the African continent (Hendrix and Salehyan 2012). Other important commodities over which conflict is likely to occur include oil, food, arable land, and fisheries (Klare 2002; Mearns and Norton 2010; Adano et al. 2012; Allison et al. 2009).

Armed conflict is among the most important causes of severe mental trauma and resulting psychopathology among both combatants and civilians. For example, in a longitudinal study of active and reserve soldiers returning from the Iraq war, 20 percent of active-duty soldiers and 40 percent of reservists met screening requirements for care from a mental health professional (Milliken, Auchterlonie, and Hoge 2007). A similar study among over 100,000 veterans of the US wars in Iraq and Afghanistan found that nearly one in four was diagnosed with a mental disorder (Seal et al. 2007).

More problematic are the mental health consequences among civilian victims of conflict. For example, one study among Kosovar Albanians following the 1998–1999 war in Kosovo showed that over 17 percent reported symptoms that met criteria for PTSD. Particularly affected were those who had firsthand exposure to traumatic events and those who had been internally displaced during the war (Cardozo et al. 2000). Another study assessed the prevalence of PTSD among over thirteen hundred adult survivors of the civil war in Liberia nearly two decades following the end of the conflict and found that 50 percent of the study sample was affected (Galea et al. 2010).

The mental health consequences of war are particularly pronounced in children. For example, one study among children in Gaza who had experienced siege by Israeli forces found the prevalence of PTSD to be 73 percent (Thabet and Vostanis 1999). Alarmingly high prevalence of psychopathology also has been documented among children in other war-torn contexts (Dyregrov et al. 2000). The consequences last into adulthood. Several studies have demonstrated that exposure to childhood trauma increases the risk for adulthood psychopathology (Widom 1999; Widom, DuMont, and Czaja 2007). For example, one study found that separation from parents during wartime increased risk of depressive symptoms in adulthood (Pesonen et al. 2007).

Conflict is, in this way, an important mechanism by which climate change will increase the burden of mental disorders. Climate change then stands to increase the scarcity of important natural resources, such as food, freshwater, and oil, and, as a consequence, increase violent conflict and subject millions to the horrors of war, as well as its mental health sequelae.

Physical Health

Among the most important determinants of psychopathology is poor physical health. Those with chronic physical maladies have substantially higher risk for mood and anxiety disorders and, in some circumstances, suicidality. For example, one study of a nationally representative US sample showed that the risk of psychopathology was up to four times higher in those with chronic pain than those without (McWilliams, Cox, and Enns 2003). In another study, 35 percent of those with chronic back or neck pain had comorbid psychopathology (Von Korff et al. 2005). One study assessed the relation between chronic disease diagnoses and suicidality in the elderly and found that several diseases, including chronic obstructive lung disorder, congestive heart failure, seizure disorder, moderate pain, and severe pain, were predictive of suicide risk (Juurlink et al. 2004).

Each of the mechanisms by which climate change may directly contribute to population psychopathology that we have previously discussed—natural disasters, forced migration, and violent conflict—will also increase physical morbidity. The physical morbidity associated with these mechanisms will act as a multiplier of the mental health burden of climate change. Not only will these mechanisms provide acute and chronic stressors that directly lead to mental disorder, but their physical sequelae will act as chronic stressors that indirectly contribute to mental disorder as well.

We illustrate this point through one specific example. One condition that may be particularly important for the transmission of mental health is obesity. First, it is clear that obesity and mental disorder are syndemic, meaning that they potentiate one another and disproportionately among certain vulnerable populations. The literature about the directionality of the relationship suggests that obesity is more likely to cause depression than depression is to cause obesity (although many studies have demonstrated that depression may also increase subsequent risk for obesity as well) (Faith et al. 2011). Climate change could increase the population burden of obesity through several mechanisms (Blaine 2008). First, climate change has the potential to reduce physical activity (Townsend et al. 2003). As ambient temperatures increase, the viability of outdoor recreational activity will diminish. Moreover, concomitant with the trend toward urbanization, access to and availability of green space is likely to decrease with climate change as well. Climate change may also influence population dietary patterns (Parry, Rosenzweig, and Livermore 2005). As larger swathes of arable land deteriorate, the price of food is likely to increase. This may drive the consumption of high-caloric-density foods, particularly among the poor. In this regard, the consumption of refined carbohydrates and fats, important drivers of obesity, is likely to increase. With obesity comes a host of other high-burden diseases, including hypertension, diabetes, cardiovascular disease, chronic pain conditions, and several types of cancers (Must et al. 1999). Therefore, climate change may contribute to increased population mental disorder through an increase obesity and its chronic disease sequelae.

CLINICAL CORRELATES 10.3 STRESS AND PHYSICAL HEALTH: IMPLICATIONS FOR CURRENT AND FUTURE GENERATIONS

Stress is a common complaint in our society. It may be conceived of as the passing of a mental, emotional, or physiological threshold after which a person can no longer cope and adapt (Haushofer and Fehr 2014). On a physiological level, stress is mediated through the production of the hormone cortisol in the adrenal glands. Higher levels of cortisol have been correlated with poor physical health, manifested through decreased immune function, high blood pressure, reproductive disturbances (Damti et al. 2008), and more. In an era of global climate change, stress levels are expected to be rising due to the real and perceived threats of drought, famine, severe weather, overpopulation, and forced migration, for example. In a study of Kenyan farmers subject to drought conditions, cortisol levels were found to be significantly elevated (Chemin, De Laat, and Haushofer 2013). In another study, unemployment and job insecurity were found to have an impact on the neuroendocrine and immune systems (Arnetz et al. 1991).

Even perceived stress may have negative health implications. In one study, participants who reported that stress was affecting their health were found to be twice as likely to suffer a heart attack as those who believed that stress had no effect on their physical well-being (Nabi et al. 2013).

Higher stress levels have implications for current as well as future generations. For example, women living in war-torn regions of the Democratic Republic of the Congo experience high levels of stress during pregnancy that may directly influence birth weight and lead to epigenetic modification of the glucocorticoid receptor NR3C1 of the infant (Rodney and Mulligan 2014). These epigenetic changes could affect how the child responds to stress and thus his or her long-term health profile. Clinicians will be faced with these health implications of stress at all levels of care and must learn how to advise patients.

Climate change causes real and perceived threats of food scarcity, job insecurity, natural disasters, and more. Stress has wide-reaching effects on health that clinicians must be able to promptly and accurately diagnose and treat.

A Disproportionate Burden

Climate change will have broad influences on population mental health through several important mechanisms, including the anticipated increase in natural disasters, forced migration, violent conflict, and assaults on physical health. These mechanisms have in common the limitations they impose on the availability of important resources—limitations that create emotional and psychological stressors in the population as communities attempt to cope with their scarcity. In that respect, lack of resources is a unifying theme in the translation of climate change to mental disorder. It should be no surprise, then, that the mental health influence of climate change will disproportionately affect the poor and marginalized.

This follows decades of social epidemiological theory explaining disproportionalities in the burden of public health exposures (Link and Phelan 1996; Phelan and Link 2005). The health consequences of such exposures, like climate change, are never borne equally because higher socioeconomic status affords people the means to insulate themselves from these exposures through access to knowledge, money, capital, power, social connectedness, and prestige (Link and Phelan 1996; Phelan and Link 2005). It follows that these resources can be used to insulate against potentially harmful exposures, regardless of what they are. An understanding of the mechanisms through which climate change may affect population mental health makes it clear that in each circumstance, socioeconomic resources could mitigate potentially harmful effects.

For example, the population health effects of natural disasters are not borne equally. In most coastal cities and towns, for instance, the rich occupy the high ground, while the poor and minorities generally live in low-lying areas more vulnerable to storm damage (Cutter and Emrich 2006; Kusenbach, Simms, and Tobin 2010). To illustrate, the devastation of Hurricane Katrina is known to have disproportionately affected low-income blacks in New Orleans because they were most likely to live in the low-lying center of the city, while higher-income whites generally occupied suburbs on higher ground (Snyder 2005). Following the storm, 53 percent of black residents reporting "losing everything," compared to just 19 percent of white residents (Gallup 2006). Moreover, because government officials provided no means of public transportation out of New Orleans prior to Katrina's landfall, evacuation was dependent on car ownership: 33 percent of blacks (and 52 percent of poor blacks) in the city had no car, as compared to 10 percent of whites (Berube and Raphael 2005). It follows that on exposure to Katrina's ravages, black race and lower income predicted higher risk for PTSD (Galea et al. 2007).

Similarly, forced migration is one means by which climate change may influence population mental health. However, climate change is likely to force migration because it may degrade the agricultural viability of lands and associated livelihoods for communities that rely on these for sustenance.

Forced migration is, in this way, a function of the lack of wealth, influence, or transferrable skill sets that enable self-support—a function of poverty and marginalization. What is more, the potentially negative consequences of forced migration, such as exploitation and abuse, are tied implicitly to the absence of resources that force individuals into potentially exploitative situations to begin with. The costs of war are also disproportionately borne on the poor. Conflict is more common in lower-income contexts because of poverty and direct dependence on natural resources for survival (Elbadawi and Sambanis 2000). Moreover the consequences of war are more devastating among the poor, who often lack the ability to escape conflict and for whom relative losses are more pronounced. There is also clear evidence that physical health is a function of socioeconomic position (Dalstra et al. 2005; Winkleby et al. 1992), suggesting that the influence of climate change on physical health, as well as the mental health burden it mediates, is likely to bear more strongly on the poor as well.

Given that low socioeconomic position is itself a stressor that promotes mental disorder (Zimmerman and Katon 2005), the disproportionate influence of climate change on the mental health of the poor is concerning. As much of the mental health consequence of climate change will be borne by the poor and marginalized, a particular focus on the mental health of this population is warranted as the consequences of climate change ensue.

Conclusion

Throughout this chapter, we have discussed several mechanisms by which climate change may influence mental health and how the consequences of these mechanisms would fall inequitably across the socioeconomic continuum. We discuss how natural disasters resulting from climate change will create traumatic stressors that will harm population mental health. Similarly climate change will degrade arable lands and swallow coastal regions, challenging communities that have occupied those contexts and forcing them to migrate in search of new livelihoods, in the process exposing them to stressors that will have negative consequences for their mental well-being. Global competition over resources depleted by climate change, such as arable land and foodstuffs, oil, and freshwater, will inspire violent conflict with hazardous consequences for mental health. And finally, climate change will increase physical morbidity and the subsequent mental disorder that accompanies it as more people struggle with the realities of chronic disease. Importantly, the consequences of climate change will not be equitable. Because each of these mechanisms functions through the changing availability of resources, those who have the least will suffer most.

While we have focused here on the unidirectional influence of climate change on mental health, it is important to recognize that the relationship between climate change and mental health may also share common causes. Consumerism is a determinant of adverse mental health, as higher consumerism in highly inequitable societies is thought to mediate the relation between income inequality and mental disorder (Pickett, James, and Wilkinson 2006; Pickett and Wilkinson 2010). The overconsumption associated with consumerism is also a clear driver of climate change as the excess combustion of fossil fuels and the overconsumption of greenhouse-gas emitting foods (estimated to be responsible for up to 30 percent of emissions; Garnett 2009) fuels consumerist lifestyles. In that respect, materialism and overconsumption may concomitantly drive both climate change and population psychopathology.

Solutions must take into account all of the mechanisms by which the two pathologies are related. In that respect, understanding the reciprocal mechanisms by which mental pathology may drive climate change, as well as the common causes of both, may yield insight into avenues to mitigate the concomitant pathologies. In the end, the question of human well-being is intimately tied to the Earth that we share, and its well-being is a consequence of our own. Without a full appreciation of that reciprocity, attempts to intervene on either are likely to be ineffectual.

DISCUSSION QUESTIONS

1. What can be done, if anything, to mitigate the population mental health consequences of climate change?

2. Are some of the mechanisms relating climate change to mental health more amenable to intervention than others? If so, which? And why?

3. Why will the burden of population mental health resulting from climate change be unequal, and what can be done to address this?

KEY TERMS

Major depressive disorder (MDD): A mood disorder characterized by a pervasive and persistent sense of hopelessness and despair.

Posttraumatic stress disorder (PTSD): A mental health condition triggered by a terrifying event—war, disaster, or physical or emotional trauma.

References

Adano, W. R., T. Dietz, K. Witsenburg, and F. Zaa. 2012. "Climate Change, Violent Conflict and Local Institutions in Kenya's Drylands." *Journal of Peace Research* 49(1):65–80.

Afolayan, A., and I. Adelekan. 1999. "The Role of Climatic Variations on Migration and Human Health in Africa." *Environmentalist* 18:213–18.

Alexandrov, V., and G. Hoogenboom. 2000. "The Impact of Climate Variability and Change on Crop Yield in Bulgaria." *Agricultural and Forest Meteorology* 104:315–27.

Allison, E. H., A. L. Perry, M. C. Badjeck, W. N. Adjer, K, Brown, D. Conway, A. S. Halls, G. M. Pilling, J. D. Reynolds, N. L. Andrew, and N. K. Dulvy. 2009. "Vulnerability of National Economies to the Impacts of Climate Change on Fisheries." *Fish and Fisheries* 10:173–96.

Andrees, B., and P. Belser. 2009. *Forced Labor: Coercion and Exploitation in the Private Economy.* Boulder, CO: Lynne Rienner.

Arnetz, B. B., S. O. Brenner, L. Levi, R. Hjelm, I. L. Petterson, J. Wasserman, B. Petrini, et al. 1991. "Neuroendocrine and Immunologic Effects of Unemployment and Job Insecurity." *Psychotherapy and Psychosomatics* 55(2–4):76–80.

Aumann, H. H., A. Ruzmaikin, and J. Teixeira. 2008. "Frequency of Severe Storms and Global Warming." *Geophysical Research Letters* 35(19):L19805.

Barnett, J., and M. N. Adger. 2007. "Climate Change, Human Security and Violent Conflict." *Political Geography* 26:639–55.

Belser, P. 2005. "Forced Labour and Human Trafficking: Estimating the Profits." (Working paper 42). Social Science Research Networks, International Labour Office, Geneva, Switzerland.

Berube, A., and S. Raphael. 2005. *Access to Cars in New Orleans.* Washington, DC: Brookings Institution.

Bhugra, D. 2004. "Migration and Mental Health." *Acta Psychiatrica Scandinavica* 109:243–58.

Blaine, B. 2008. "Does Depression Cause Obesity? A Meta-Analysis of Longitudinal Studies of Depression and Weight Control." *Journal of Health Psychology* 13:1190–97.

Briguglio, L. 1995. "Small Island Developing States and Their Economic Vulnerabilities." *World Development* 23:1615–32.

Cardozo, B. L., A. Vergara, F. Agani, and C. A. Gotway. 2000. "Mental Health, Social Functioning, and Attitudes of Kosovar Albanians following the War in Kosovo." *JAMA* 284:569–77.

Cerdá, M., M. Paczkowski, S. Galea, K. Nemethy, C. Péan, and M. Desvarieux. 2013. "Psychopathology in the Aftermath of the Haiti Earthquake: A Population-Based Study of Posttraumatic Stress Disorder and Major Depression." *Depression and Anxiety* 30:413–24.

Chemin, M., J. De Laat, and J. Haushofer. 2013. "Negative Rainfall Shocks Increase Levels of the Stress Hormone Cortisol among Poor Farmers in Kenya." http://ssrn.com/abstract=2294171 or http://dx.doi.org/10.2139/ssrn.2294171

Culliton, T. J. 1998. "Population: Distribution, Density, and Growth." In *State of the Coast Report*. Silver Spring, MD: NOAA. http://state-of-coast.noaa.gov/bulletins/html/pop_01/pop.html

Cutter, S. L., and C. T. Emrich. 2006. "Moral Hazard, Social Catastrophe: The Changing Face of Vulnerability along the Hurricane Coasts." *Annals of the American Academy of Political and Social Science* 604(1):102–12.

Dalstra, J. A., A. E. Kunst, C. Borrell, E. Breeze, E. Cambois, G. Costa, J. J. Geurts, et al. 2005. "Socioeconomic Differences in the Prevalence of Common Chronic Diseases: An Overview of Eight European Countries." *International Journal of Epidemiology* 34:316–26.

Damti, O. B., O. Sarid, E. Sheiner, T. Zilberstein, and J. Cwikel. 2008. [Stress and distress in infertility among women]. *Harefuah* 147(3):256–60.

Decker, M. R., S. Oram, J. Gupta, and J. G. Silverman. 2009. "Forced Prostitution and Trafficking for Sexual Exploitation among Women and Girls in Situations of Migration and Conflict: Review and Recommendations for Reproductive Health Care Personnel." In *Women, Migration, and Conflict*, edited by S. F. Martin and J. Torman, 63–86. New York: Springer.

Dyregrov, A., L. Gupta, R. Gjestad, and E. Mukanoheli. 2000. "Trauma Exposure and Psychological Reactions to Genocide among Rwandan Children." *Journal of Traumatic Stress* 13(1):3–21.

Elbadawi, E., and N. Sambanis. 2000. "Why Are There So Many Civil Wars in Africa? Understanding and Preventing Violent Conflict." *Journal of African Economies* 9:244–69.

Faith, M., M. Butryn, T. Wadden, A. Fabricatore, A. Nguyen, and S. Heymsfield. 2011. "Evidence for Prospective Associations among Depression and Obesity in Population-Based Studies." *Obesity Reviews* 12(5):e438–53.

Feng, S., A. B. Krueger, and M. Oppenheimer. 2010. "Linkages among Climate Change, Crop Yields and Mexico–US Cross-Border Migration." *Proceedings of the National Academy of Sciences* 107:14257–62.

Field, C. B., V. R. Barros, K. Mach, and M. Mastrandrea. 2014. *Climate Change 2014: Impacts, Adaptation, and Vulnerability.* Working Group II to the Fifth Assessment Report of the Intergovernmental Panel on Climate Change

Galea, S., C. R. Brewin, M. Gruber, R. T. Jones, D. W. King, L. A. King, R. J. McNally, et al. 2007. "Exposure to Hurricane-Related Stressors and Mental Illness after Hurricane Katrina." *Archives of General Psychiatry* 64:1427–34.

Galea, S., A. Nandi, and D. Vlahov. 2005. "The Epidemiology of Post-Traumatic Stress Disorder after Disasters." *Epidemiologic Reviews* 27(1):78–91.

Galea, S., P. C. Rockers, G. Saydee, R. Macauley, S. T. Varpilah, and M. E. Kruk. 2010. "Persistent Psychopathology in the Wake of Civil War: Long-Term Post-traumatic Stress Disorder in Nimba County, Liberia." *American Journal of Public Health* 100:1745.

Galea, S., M. Tracy, F. Norris, and S. F. Coffey. 2008. "Financial and Social Circumstances and the Incidence and Course of PTSD in Mississippi during the First Two Years after Hurricane Katrina." *Journal of Traumatic Stress* 21:357–68.

Gallup. 2006. "One in Three New Orleans Residents Lost Everything Following Hurricane." Washington, DC: Gallup.

Garnett, T. 2009. "Livestock-Related Greenhouse Gas Emissions: Impacts and Options for Policy Makers." *Environmental Science and Policy* 12(4):491–503.

Grote, U., and K. Warner. 2010. "Environmental Change and Migration in Sub-Saharan Africa." *International Journal of Global Warming* 2(1):17–47.

Grove, N. J., and A. B. Zwi. 2006. "Our Health and Theirs: Forced Migration, Othering, and Public Health." *Social Science and Medicine* 62:1931–42.

Guterres, A. 2008. "Climate Change, Natural Disasters and Human Displacement: A UNHCR Perspective." Geneva: UN High Commissioner for Refugees. http://www.unhcr.org/4901e81a4html

Haushofer, J., and E. Fehr. 2014. "On the Psychology of Poverty." *Science* 344(6186):862–67.

Hendrix, C. S., and I. Salehyan. 2012. "Climate Change, Rainfall, and Social Conflict in Africa." *Journal of Peace Research* 49(1):35–50.

Henry, S., B. Schoumaker, and C. Beauchemin 2004. "The Impact of Rainfall on the First Out-Migration: A Multi-Level Event-History Analysis in Burkina Faso." *Population and Environment* 25:423–60.

Hiott, A. E., J. G. Grzywacz, S. W. Davis, S. A. Quandt, and A. Arcury. 2008. "Migrant Farmworker Stress: Mental Health Implications." *Journal of Rural Health* 24(1):32–39.

Homer-Dixon, T. F. 1994. "Environmental Scarcities and Violent Conflict: Evidence from Cases." *International Security* 1994:5–40.

Hossain M., C. Zimmerman, M. Abas, M. Light, and C. Watts. 2010. "The Relationship of Trauma to Mental Disorders among Trafficked and Sexually Exploited Girls and Women." *American Journal of Public Health* 100:2442–49.

Hovey, J. D. 2000. "Acculturative Stress, Depression, and Suicidal Ideation in Mexican." *Cultural Diversity and Ethnic Minority Psychology* 6(2):134.

Hovey, J. D., and C. G. Magaña. 2003. "Suicide Risk Factors among Mexican Migrant Farmworker Women in the Midwest United States." *Archives of Suicide Research* 7:107–21.

Hyman, S., D. Chisholm, R. Kessler, V. Patel, and H. Whiteford. 2006. "Mental Disorders." In *Disease Control Priorities Related to Mental, Neurological, Developmental and Substance Abuse Disorder,* 1–20. http://whqlibdoc.who.int/publications/2006/924156332x_eng.pdf.

Juurlink, D. N., N. Herrmann, J. P. Szalai, A. Kopp, and D. A. Redelmeier. 2004. "Medical Illness and the Risk of Suicide in the Elderly." *Archives of Internal Medicine* 164:1179–84.

Kessler, R. C., S. Galea, M. J. Gruber, N. A. Sampson, R. J. Ursano, and S. Wessely. 2008. "Trends in Mental Illness and Suicidality after Hurricane Katrina." *Molecular Psychiatry* 13:374–84.

Kip, K., L. Rosenzweig, D. Hernandez, A. Shuman, D. M. Diamond, S. A. Girling, K. L. Sullivan, et al. 2013. "Accelerated Resolution Therapy for Treatment of Pain Secondary to Symptoms of Combat-Related Posttraumatic Stress Disorder." *European Journal of Psychotraumatology* 5:240–66.

Klare, M. T. 2002. "The Deadly Nexus: Oil, Terrorism, and America's National Security." *Current History—New York Then Philadelphia* 101:414–20.

Kusenbach, M., J. L. Simms, and G. A. Tobin. 2010. "Disaster Vulnerability and Evacuation Readiness: Coastal Mobile Home Residents in Florida." *Natural Hazards* 52(1):79–95.

Landau, J., and J. Saul. 2004. "Family and Community Resilience in Response to Major Disaster." In *Living beyond Loss: Death in the Family,* 2nd ed., edited by F. Walsh and M. McGoldrick, 285–309. New York: Norton.

Lindert, J., O. S. Ehrenstein, S. Priebe, A. Mielck, and E. Brähler. 2009. "Depression and Anxiety in Labor Migrants and Refugees: A Systematic Review and Meta-Analysis." *Social Science and Medicine* 69:246–57.

Lindert, J., M. Schouler-Ocak, A. Heinz, and S. Priebe. 2008. "Mental Health, Health Care Utilisation of Migrants in Europe." *European Psychiatry* 23:14–20.

Link, B. G., and J. C. Phelan. 1996. "Understanding Sociodemographic Differences in Health: The Role of Fundamental Social Causes." *American Journal of Public Health* 86:471–73.

Litz, B. 2004. *Early Intervention for Trauma and Traumatic Loss.* New York: Guilford Press.

Lobell, D. B., M. B. Burke, C. Tebaldi, M. D. Mastrandrea, W. P. Falcon, and R. L. Naylor. 2008. "Prioritizing Climate Change Adaptation Needs for Food Security in 2030." *Science* 319:607–10.

Luppa, M., S. Heinrich, M. C. Angermeyer, H.-H. König, and S. G. Riedel-Heller. 2007. "Cost-of-Illness Studies of Depression: A Systematic Review." *Journal of Affective Disorders* 98(1):29–43.

Mathers, C., D. M. Fat, and J. Boerma. 2008. *The Global Burden of Disease: 2004 Update.* Geneva: World Health Organization.

McGranahan G., D. Balk, and B. Anderson. 2007. "The Rising Tide: Assessing the Risks of Climate Change and Human Settlements in Low Elevation Coastal Zones." *Environment and Urbanization* 19(1):17–37.

McLeman, R., and B. Smit. 2006. "Migration as an Adaptation to Climate Change." *Climatic Change* 76(1–2):31–53.

McWilliams, L. A., B. J. Cox, and M. W. Enns. 2003. "Mood and Anxiety Disorders Associated with Chronic Pain: An Examination in a Nationally Representative Sample." *Pain* 106:127–33.

Mearns, R., and A. Norton. 2010. *Social Dimensions of Climate Change: Equity and Vulnerability in a Warming World.* Washington, DC: World Bank.

Meze-Hausken, E. 2004. "Contrasting Climate Variability and Meteorological Drought with Perceived Drought and Climate Change in Northern Ethiopia." *Climate Research* 27:19–31.

Milliken, C. S., J. L. Auchterlonie, and C. W. Hoge. 2007. "Longitudinal Assessment of Mental Health Problems among Active and Reserve Component Soldiers Returning from the Iraq War." *JAMA* 298:2141–48.

Min, S.-K., X. Zhang, F. W. Zwiers, and G. C. Hegerl. 2011. "Human Contribution to More-Intense Precipitation Extremes." *Nature* 470:378–81.

Mollica, R. 2004. "Surviving Torture." *New England Journal of Medicine* 351:5–7.

Murray, V., and E. L. Ebi. 2012. "IPCC Special Report on Managing the Risks of Extreme Events and Disasters to Advance Climate Change Adaptation (SREX)." *Journal of Epidemiology and Community Health* 66:759–60.

Must, A., J. Spadano, E. H. Coakley, A. E. Field, G. Colditz, and W. H. Dietz. 1999. "The Disease Burden Associated with Overweight and Obesity." *JAMA* 282:1523–29.

Nabi, H., M. Kivimäki, G. D. Batty, M. J. Shipley, A. Britton, E. J. Brunner, J. Vahtera, C. Lemogne, A. Elbaz, and A. Singh-Manoux. 2013. "Increased Risk of Coronary Heart Disease among Individuals Reporting Adverse Impact of Stress on Their Health: The Whitehall II Prospective Cohort Study." *European Heart Journal* 34:2967–705.

Neria, Y., A. Nandi, and S. Galea. 2008. "Post-Traumatic Stress Disorder following Disasters: A Systematic Review." *Psychological Medicine* 38:467–80.

Onyut, L. P., F. Neuner, V. Ertl, E. Schauer, M. Odenwald, and T. Elbert. 2009. "Trauma, Poverty and Mental Health among Somali and Rwandese Refugees Living in an African Refugee Settlement: An Epidemiological Study." *Conflict and Health* 3(6):90–107.

Parry, M., C. Rosenzweig, and M. Livermore. 2005. "Climate Change, Global Food Supply and Risk of Hunger." *Philosophical Transactions of the Royal Society B: Biological Sciences* 360:2125–38.

Paul, F., H. Frey, and R. Le Bris. 2011. "A New Glacier Inventory for the European Alps from Landsat TM Scenes of 2003: Challenges and Results." *Annals of Glaciology* 52:144–52.

Pesonen, A-K., K. Räikkönen, K. Heinonen, E. Kajantie, T. Forsén, and J. G. Eriksson. 2007. "Depressive Symptoms in Adults Separated from Their Parents as Children: A Natural Experiment during World War II." *American Journal of Epidemiology* 166:1126–33.

Phelan, J. C., and B. G. Link. 2005. "Controlling Disease and Creating Disparities: A Fundamental Cause Perspective." *Journals of Gerontology Series B: Psychological Sciences and Social Sciences* 60(Special Issue 2):S27-S33.

Pickett, K. E., O. W. James, and R. G. Wilkinson. 2006. "Income Inequality and the Prevalence of Mental Illness: A Preliminary International Analysis." *Journal of Epidemiology and Community Health* 60:646–47.

Pickett, K. E., and R. G. Wilkinson. 2010. "Inequality: An Underacknowledged Source of Mental Illness and Distress." *British Journal of Psychiatry* 197:426–28.

Plagge, J., M. W. Lu, T. I. Lovejoy, A. I. Karl, and S. Dobscha. 2013. "Treatment of Comorbid Pain and PTSD in Returning Veterans: A Collaborative Approach Utilizing Behavioral Activation." *Pain Medicine* 14:1164–72.

Poncelet, A., F. Gemenne, M. Martiniello, and H. S. Bousett. 2010. "A Country Made for Disasters: Environmental Vulnerability and Forced Migration in Bangladesh." In *Environment, Forced Migration and Social Vulnerability*, edited by T. Afifi and J. Jäger, 211–22. New York: Springer.

Rodney, N. C., and C. J. Mulligan. 2014. "A Biocultural Study of the Effects of Maternal Stress on Mother and Newborn Health in the Democratic Republic of Congo." *American Journal of Physical Anthropology* 155:200–209.

Schlenker, W., and M. J. Roberts. 2009. "Nonlinear Temperature Effects Indicate Severe Damages to US Crop Yields under Climate Change." *Proceedings of the National Academy of Sciences* 106:15594–98.

Seal, K. H., D. Bertenthal, C. R. Miner, S. Sen, and C. Marmar. 2007. "Bringing the War Back Home: Mental Health Disorders among 103,788 US Veterans Returning from Iraq and Afghanistan Seen at Department of Veterans Affairs Facilities." *Archives of Internal Medicine* 167:476–82.

Snyder, M. G. 2005. "It Didn't Begin with Katrina." *Shelterforce Online*, 143. http://www.nhi.org/online/issues/143/beforekatrina.html

Solomon, S., G. K. Plattner, R. Knutti, and P. Friedlingstein. 2009. "Irreversible Climate Change due to Carbon Dioxide Emissions." *Proceedings of the National Academy of Sciences* 106:1704–1709.

Sullivan, M. M., and R. Rehm. 2005. "Mental Health of Undocumented Mexican Immigrants: A Review of the Literature." *Advances in Nursing Science* 28:240–51.

Tedeschi, R. G., and L. G. Calhoun. 1996. "The Posttraumatic Growth Inventory: Measuring the Positive Legacy of Trauma." *Journal of Traumatic Stress* 9:455–71.

Thabet, A.A.M., and P. Vostanis. 1999. "Post-Traumatic Stress Reactions in Children of War." *Journal of Child Psychology and Psychiatry* 40:385–91.

Tir, J., and D. M. Stinnett. 2012. "Weathering Climate Change: Can Institutions Mitigate International Water Conflict?" *Journal of Peace Research* 49:211–25.

Townsend, M., M. Mahoney, J. Jones, K. Ball, J. Salmon, and C. Finch. 2003. "Too Hot to Trot? Exploring Potential Links between Climate Change, Physical Activity and Health." *Journal of Science and Medicine in Sport* 6(3):260–65.

Von Korff, M., P. Crane, M. Lane, D. L. Miglioretti, G. Simon, K. Saunders, P. Stang, N. Brandenburg, and R. Kessler. 2005. "Chronic Spinal Pain and Physical–Mental Comorbidity in the United States: Results from the National Comorbidity Survey Replication." *Pain* 113:331–39.

Walsh, F. 2007. "Traumatic Loss and Major Disasters: Strengthening Family and Community Resilience." *Family Process* 46(2):207–27.

Widom, C. S. 1999. "Posttraumatic Stress Disorder in Abused and Neglected Children Grown Up." *American Journal of Psychiatry* 156(8):1223–29.

Widom, C. S., K. DuMont, and S. J. Czaja. 2007. "A Prospective Investigation of Major Depressive Disorder and Comorbidity in Abused and Neglected Children Grown Up." *Archives of General Psychiatry* 64:49–56.

Williams, J. W., S. T. Jackson, and J. E. Kutzbach. 2007. "Projected Distributions of Novel and Disappearing Climates by 2100 AD." *Proceedings of the National Academy of Sciences* 104:5738–42.

Winkleby, M. A., D. E. Jatulis, E. Frank, and S. P. Fortmann. 1992. "Socioeconomic Status and Health: How Education, Income, and Occupation Contribute to Risk Factors for Cardiovascular Disease." *American Journal of Public Health* 82:816–20.

Zimmerman, F. J., and W. Katon. 2005. "Socioeconomic Status, Depression Disparities, and Financial Strain: What Lies behind the Income-Depression Relationship?" *Health Economics* 14:1197–15.

PART 3

THE PUBLIC HEALTH APPROACH
TO CLIMATE CHANGE

CHAPTER 11

IMPROVING THE SURVEILLANCE OF CLIMATE-SENSITIVE DISEASES

Pierre Gosselin, Diane Bélanger, Mathilde Pascal, Philippe Pirard, Christovam Barcellos

Health surveillance is a key step for the management of any health issue, as it provides data and knowledge useful for short- and long-term prevention. Historically health surveillance systems have been developed for specific diseases. In the case of climate-sensitive diseases, the design of a surveillance system must take into account the variety of possible health end points, the spatiotemporal dynamics, and the interactions of environmental and social risk factors (World Health Organization 2013a; Public Health Agency of Canada 2011). Yet the development of new technologies offers new perspectives for integrated, dynamic surveillance systems.

Rapid technological developments over the past twenty years, mainly in geomatics and the Internet, have led to the development of high-performing large- and small-scale surveillance systems (e.g., at the city level). Some countries have elaborate systems, but this is still the exception. This chapter draws from the available gray and scientific literature on the topic and presents examples best known to us from their own countries' experiences (Canada, France, Brazil) and through sharing of information with other national and international institutes (United States, Europe, Africa, Asia). We examine the topic of surveillance under four topics: **environmental monitoring, health surveillance** for climate risks, decision making from surveillance information, and future improvements to be promoted.

Our thanks to Ray Bustinza (INSPQ), Olivier Gagnon and Philippe Gachon (Environment Canada), and Marie-France Sottile (Ouranos) for providing useful sources and references and for their review of some parts of the chapter. We gratefully acknowledge partial funding from Fonds vert of the Quebec government and IRIACC-FACE program of the IDRC.

KEY CONCEPTS

- Some diseases can be directly attributed to climate change such as vector-borne disease, heat illness, and extreme weather traumatic injury. Others are indirectly related, such as mental illness, malnutrition, and exacerbations of cardiopulmonary disease.

- The health sector uses the word *surveillance* for diseases and their determinants, while the environmental sector prefers the word *monitoring* when measuring pollutants or environmental conditions of interest. The concept is the same—to measure indicators linked to health risk in order to make informed decisions for intervention and influencing public policy.

- The World Health Organization (2013a) defines a risk factor as "any attribute, characteristic or exposure of an individual that increases the likelihood of developing a disease or injury" and "social determinants of health are the conditions in which people are born, grow, live, work and age, including the health system." In the case of climate change, risk

Scientific knowledge about the links among meteorology, climate, and health problems has also increased rapidly in the past ten to fifteen years, as has our knowledge about the links among environmental risks, social inequalities, and diseases (or health). This knowledge is still rather incomplete, particularly for anything related to weather extremes, and some complete components of human activity are measured only poorly or not at all, as is the case with the implementation of emergency measures in the field or even the impact of behavior awareness campaigns. Much still remains to be done.

One of the specific characteristics of climate change is its occurrence over long periods of time, which necessitates the use of time series over several decades. While such series are relatively available in the field of natural sciences, it is completely different for deaths, health problems, individual or institutional behaviors, or exposure measurement. Several influences are in fact at work with humans, from genetics to neighborhoods. A number of jurisdictions in developed countries use a conceptual model for surveillance based on the one proposed in 2002 by several American health organizations (figure 11.1),

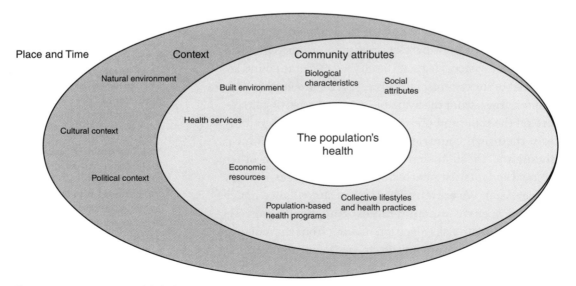

Figure 11.1   A Conceptual Model of Influences on the Population's Health

Source: Department of Health and Human Services Data Council, Centers for Disease Control and Prevention, National Center for Health Statistics, National Committee on Vital and Health Statistics (2002).

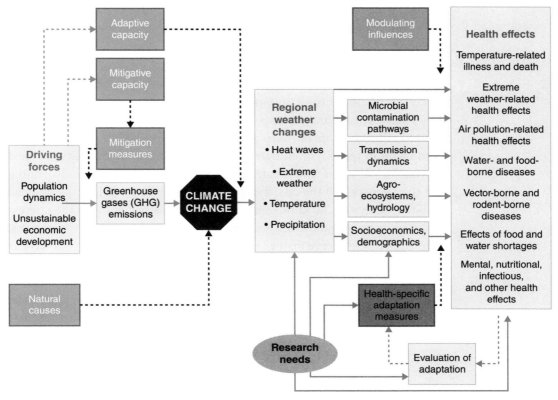

Figure 11.2   WHO's Conceptual Model for Climate Change and Health
Source: Confalonieri et al. (2007).

which clearly illustrates the complexity of the task. It plainly shows that climate is only one of the operative factors, among dozens of others. The possible impacts of climate change on health and the factors that modulate them are summarized in figure 11.2. These logical models well illustrate the need for nesting any climate-change surveillance system within a national or regional surveillance system, considering the many interactions among the variables of interest.

Environmental Monitoring

In surveillance applied to environmental health, exposure measurement is often neglected or imprecise. The same is true for everything related to climate or weather, our concern here. For example, during a heat wave, the objective is to measure heat exposure and correlate it with the deaths that occurred in a city. Many studies use one or two stations available in a city and average the temperatures during the few days of the heat wave. However, temperatures vary with the type of residence and the floor on which a person lives, the availability and use of air-conditioning, and the presence of parks or other cooler locations nearby, and these differences can be as much as 10°C to 15°C within a city or a building. This therefore involves a differential classification bias, as epidemiologists call it, because the risk of exposure to excessive heat is far from uniformly distributed in a city.

Interest therefore focuses on the climate, generally defined over a period of thirty years or more, and on the weather, which covers the short and medium terms. For climate, two sources of data are mainly used: past chronological series from weather stations, of variable duration depending on the country and the city, as well as future or historical modeling (also called reanalysis). The same tools are used for weather, but with the interest focused on the few days or weeks preceding the actual day for the stations, while the models serve instead to prepare forecasts for the next few days or the next season.

The weather series to be used over long periods should be previously homogenized. This process consists of examining all the changes that the measuring stations have undergone during past decades, estimating their impacts, and correcting the series to take them into account. For example, if a weather station is moved or if the measurement technology is modified, part of the series often has to be adjusted by a few degrees following this change. The station density will also be crucial in determining the reliability of exposure measurement. Generally stations measuring only temperature and precipitation are the most common, while those that include measurement of wind, humidity, snow cover, or solar radiation are usually less common. Many studies thus choose to use only temperature as the variable (average, maximum, minimum, with calculated variables such as degree days); the precipitation variable varies much more in space than the temperature, and its use will have to take this into account.

One of the most important adaptations for reducing the health impacts of weather extremes continues to be a good warning system based on weather forecasts. It then becomes important to know well the reliability of the forecasts and the scientific basis of a warning threshold. Public health workers and other users of weather data should consult World Meteorological Organization guides on this subject (2000, 2013).

Other analyses of weather data may be necessary for surveillance. Thus, the danger linked to urban heat islands will vary with the precipitation received (or not) in the days preceding a heat wave. But certain hazards appear slowly, such as droughts. These situations require meteorological expertise to be interpreted and determine whether to initiate specific health surveillance. Interinstitutional collaboration becomes vital in these situations at the local and regional levels or the continental level. Interesting examples of such collaboration should be mentioned, such as the North American Drought Monitor system encompassing Canada, the United States, and Mexico (National Oceanic and Atmospheric Administration 2013b) and the American National Hurricane Center, which covers the Americas from Peru in the south to Newfoundland in the north, passing through the Caribbean on its way (National Oceanic and Atmospheric Administration 2013a).

Anticipating the future main health determinants that will be driven by climate change is crucial to reinforce societal resilience to climate change and orient future surveillance programs that are relevant for public health. Modeling allows future climates to be simulated, based on greenhouse gas evolution scenarios, which are themselves based on socioeconomic scenarios. These scenarios have been established by the Intergovernmental Panel on Climate Change (IPCC; 2000) in the past few years and are periodically updated. There are now many global circulation models (GCM) (approximately sixty currently; PCMDI 2013), and their spatial resolution varies from very gross tiles of 400 kilometers by 400 kilometers up to the so-called regional models of 5 kilometers by 5 kilometers or smaller. Depending on their initial base of development, these models may have biases (e.g., hot or cold) and perform better for certain variables than others; regional climate models (RCM) have more limitations due to their huge calculation requirements, which reduces their uses (Christensen et al. 2007). Improvements are therefore still desirable for precipitation and extratropical hurricanes (Randall et al. 2007), and certain variables, such as hydrometeorological extremes, remain difficult to simulate (IPCC 2012).

Good practice recommendations now exist for validating and using these GCM (IPCC 2010). These models are impressive in their sophistication and their capacity to simulate long-term trends and averages. They now include complex atmospheric chemistry, the carbon cycle, dynamic vegetation, and oceanic biochemistry. For this reason, GCM are now often called earth system models. In a practical way for surveillance, however, no single simulation of GCM should be used to simulate future health impacts. Current recommendations in this regard are to average several simulations of models well mastered by researchers in order to simulate more realistic future health impacts; this approach is, however, still rather unusable with RCM. Historical reanalysis also allows certain biases to be corrected as needed by comparing backward simulations to historical weather data.

In general, future climate simulations, and therefore dealing with the 2050 or 2080 horizons, are mainly useful in research for establishing base levels and the recent evolution in diseases. Otherwise they are not greatly used in surveillance, which is focused instead on the short or medium term. These simulations nevertheless will be useful for deciding on the relative importance of various diseases in the future, their likely economic consequences, and, consequently, the need to implement enhanced surveillance programs now—for example, for some mosquitoes, algae, or animals with infectious potential that can migrate into new zones.

Another characteristic of environmental monitoring applicable to this field is the more frequent use than elsewhere of satellite and geospatial data. Satellite images can be useful for identifying urban heat islands or characterizing ecological niches suitable for outbreaks of vectors such as insects or animals. Levels of atmospheric pollution can also be estimated from these images for cities lacking a monitoring system or during large brush fires, or even for following major floods in quasi-real time. Together with the appropriate geospatial data, these data often prove vital in establishing certain **vulnerabilities**. This field requires high-level skills that are mainly found in central research organizations and universities, but unfortunately infrequently in health networks, which limits their use.

CLINICAL CORRELATES 11.1   MALARIA EARLY WARNING SYSTEMS

The transmission of malaria through *Anopheles* mosquitoes is strongly linked to climate conditions. Predicting epidemic outbreaks of malaria in relation to environmental conditions has therefore become an area of intense research. Malaria early warning systems combine elements of early detection of epidemics (case surveillance), early warning (based on monitoring meteorological data), and long-range climate modeling (Cox and Abeku 2007). As opposed to endemic malaria, which occurs in populations that have some immune resistance to the parasite, epidemics occurring in immune-naive communities have more disastrous health consequences with higher rates of morbidity and mortality. The health impacts of accurate prediction of epidemics appear promising. A recent model developed by Thomson and colleagues (2006) is able to predict epidemic occurrence with reasonable certainty and lead times greater than one month and at times five months (Thomson et al. 2006). Advocates for early warning systems urge that precise prediction models give policymakers and health officials the time necessary to protect vulnerable populations in a proactive versus a reactive way. The question now is whether the models are sound enough to put into practice as they remain quite variable in precision for various countries (Zinszer et al. 2012) and if policymakers are willing to respond.

Malaria early warning systems combine case surveillance with long-range climate modeling to allow clinicians and policymakers to proactively prepare for outbreaks.

Health Surveillance for Climate Risks

There is no international or global surveillance system for risks related to climate change. Some essential elements have already been compiled or estimated, such as deaths related to natural catastrophes (World Health Organization and World Meteorological Organization 2012), and several warning systems for these same catastrophes have been created or enhanced in the past fifteen years worldwide. Zoonotic or vector-borne infectious diseases are monitored as well, including those that are climate sensitive (Gubler 2008; Jones et al. 2008). Other regions, such as numerous countries in Africa, must still link weather warning systems and health warning systems, mainly for some serious diseases such as malaria (Cox and Abeku 2007). The remainder are initiatives of a few countries or some states and provinces within countries, and these initiatives are often limited to problems related to heat waves.

At the American federal level, the Environmental Health Tracking Program of the Centers for Disease Control and Prevention (2013) is probably one of the most developed systems in the environmental health world. For climate-related risks, it allows the online consultation of interactive maps of four vulnerability indicators available in each state and county; however, human vulnerabilities are limited in it. The other existing systems for infectious diseases (including those related to climate, such as dengue and West Nile virus, for example) or for other relevant diseases complete the heat component. A recent addition from the US Global Change Research Program is MATCH (Metadata Access Tool for Climate and Health). This clearinghouse of publicly available metadata and sources of monitoring and surveillance data sets is an online tool for researchers and public health specialists. More integrated systems for all the climatic hazards exist at finer scales, such as the one implemented by the Institut national de santé publique du Québec. This system provides data from several sources in real or quasi-real time (Toutant et al. 2011), and currently serves end users of the regional and central health agencies in the province. The indicators used in this system, presented in table 11.1, were established through the literature review process, consultations with users, and in relation to the availability of data.

The SUPREME System in Québec, Canada

After conducting a detailed needs analysis, the Quebec National Institute for Public Health developed and implemented in 2010 the SUPREME system, an integrated web application leveraging open source software for the real-time surveillance and prevention of the impacts of extreme meteorological events on public health. Its first field use involved heat waves. This decision-support system is based on open source software and is composed of four modules through its climate change and health portal: data acquisition and integration, risk analysis and alerts, mapping application, and information dissemination. The system is available to health specialists (and others) through a secure web information portal and provides access to automated real-time weather warnings, health data (admissions to emergency rooms and hospitals, deaths, ambulance calls, info-health calls on specific topics), and various mapping data used for conducting prevention activities and launching emergency measures. The system does not hold all these data; it simply connects frequently to existing databases through web services, thus providing the most recent available information.

Its health indicators vary depending on the climatic hazard of interest and include both **risk factors** and **health determinants** (table 11.1). These indicators are available at the dissemination area level, which is the smallest stable census area in Canada (average of seven hundred people). Using the portal's functions, any user can parameterize each of the indicators, for example, by selecting only a subset of age groups (say, seventy-five years and up), or a category of housing conditions, and launch a query that will return the list of all the dissemination areas that correspond to the selected multicriteria analysis (e.g., areas with a proportion of deprived households of 20 percent or more, located within an urban heat island, with a proportion of immigrants above 50 percent), thus allowing better targeting for emergency preparedness and the use of appropriate languages for further communication. The query result can be visualized using the mapping application.

The system was included in the 2012 Medical Devices and eHealth Solutions Compendium of innovative health technologies for low-resource settings of the World Health Organization. It is also being adapted in Morocco and Niger within the IRIACC-FACE research program funded by the International Development Research Centre (Canada).

Systems such as these present several benefits besides the alert function, including that of data availability to prioritize the risks and document the impacts within a region or a country; multicriteria analysis tools can be useful for this. Another approach is to use indexes to follow some groups of behaviors, as proposed in a recent adaptation index to heat (Bélanger et al. 2015). Several systems also allow the rapid evaluation of the health impact of an extreme, such as the number of deaths and emergency room visits after a heat wave or a flood (Medeiros et al. 2010). An original approach is also used in some countries where the information can be more complex to obtain, such as in Amazonia. In this way, various groups of the population that possess an often intimate knowledge about the territory and

Table 11.1   Examples of Indicators Used in the SUPREME System (Québec, Canada) for Heat, Cold, and Flooding

Health Indicators	Hazard Indicators	Context Indicators	Warnings
Heat			
A dynamic and parameterizable graph presents, by health region, the temperatures, the number of events per day and the average for the displayed period, of the following indicators: • Daily deaths, all causes (and specific causes) • Daily hospitalizations, all causes (and specific causes) • Daily admissions to emergency rooms, all causes (and specific causes) • Daily ambulance transports, all causes • Info-Health calls "'oppressive heat"[a] • Info-Health calls "heat-related illness" (cardiovascular problems; respiratory problems; thermoregulation) The period of interest can be parameterized within the limits of data availability. A map displays in real time the: • Steps in the intervention plan implemented by the health regions during a heat episode	The following indicators are presented by weather region (WR): • Maximum (minimum) temperature observed in the last three days • Maximum (minimum) temperature forecast for the next three days • Weighted average of the forecast maximum (minimum) temperatures • Extreme heat thresholds of the maximum and minimum temperatures • Maximum humidex index observed in the last three days • Maximum humidex index forecast for the next three days • Number of days per year by health region and WR where the daily maximum and minimum temperatures simultaneously reached the extreme heat thresholds	Parameterizable spatial data presented by dissemination area (mapping): • Spatial density of population suffering from chronic diseases (index) • Distribution of the population by age (classes of five years) • Distribution of people sixty-five years of age and older living alone • Spatial population density • Social and material deprivation index • Air-conditioning level estimated by electrical consumption • Location of swimming pools • Location of cooling centers • Location of green spaces • Heat islands (20 meter resolution) • Cool areas (20 meter resolution)	• Extreme heat wave with risk of excess mortality (when the weighted forecast values for the next three days for maximum and minimum temperatures for a WR reach the extreme heat thresholds specific to a given health region) • Day of oppressive heat (when for a WR, the forecast values for the next 24 hours for the maximum temperature reach 30°C and the humidex index reaches 40°) • Summer smog (when the air quality, based on the concentrations of tropospheric ozone and fine particulates is forecast as poor for WR)
Cold			
A dynamic and parameterizable graph presents, by health region, the temperatures, the number of events per day and the average for the displayed period, of the following indicators: • Daily deaths, all causes (and specific causes)	The following indicators are presented by WR: • Maximum (minimum) temperature observed in the last three days • Maximum (minimum) temperature forecast for the next three days	Parameterizable spatial data presented by dissemination area (mapping): • Spatial density of people suffering from chronic diseases (index)	• Wind chill (when the combined effect of air temperature and wind velocity could produce frostbite on exposed skin)

(*continued*)

Table 11.1 (*Continued*)

Health Indicators	Hazard Indicators	Context Indicators	Warnings
• Daily hospitalizations, all causes (and specific causes) • Daily admissions to emergency, all causes (and specific causes) • Daily ambulance transports, all causes • Info-Health calls "'cardiovascular problems" • Info-Health calls "'respiratory problems" • The period of interest can be parameterized within the limits of data availability	• Number of days per year by health region and by WR where the minimum temperature was below 20°C • Number of days per year by health region and by WR where the minimum temperature was below 30°C	• Distribution of the population by age (classes of five years) • Distribution of people sixty-five years of age and older living alone • Social and material deprivation index • Distribution of residences according to need for major repairs • Location of temporary lodging in the event of disaster • Location of educational institutions • Location of day cares • Location of health services institutions • Location of public low-cost housing	• Winter smog (when the air quality, based on the concentrations of tropospheric ozone and fine particulates, is forecast as poor for WR)

Flood

A dynamic and parameterizable graph presents, by health region, the temperatures, the number of events per day and the average for the displayed period, of the following indicators: • Daily deaths, all causes (and specific causes) • Daily hospitalizations, all causes (and specific causes) • Daily admissions to emergency, all causes (and specific causes) • Daily ambulance transports, all causes • Info-Health calls "Injury" • Info- Health calls "Gastrointestinal problems'" • Info-Health calls "respiratory problems"	The following indicator is presented by WR: • Rainfall forecasts for the next 24 hours • Torrential rain thresholds (50 mm or more in less than 24 hours in summer and 25 mm or more in winter) Map presenting, in relation to the values of the levels or flows of stations for several streams, the different flood thresholds by administrative region, as established by the appropriate authorities: • Normal • Surveillance threshold • Minor flood • Average flood • Major flood	Parameterizable spatial data presented by dissemination area (mapping): • Spatial density of people suffering from chronic diseases • Distribution of the population by age (classes of five years) • Distribution of people sixty-five years of age and older living alone • Spatial population density • Social and material deprivation index • Distribution of landed immigrants • Distribution of people speaking neither English nor French	• Major flood

Table 11.1   *(Continued)*

Health Indicators	Hazard Indicators	Context Indicators	Warnings
• The period of interest can be parameterized within the limits of data availability	• Flood-prone area (2, 20, 100 years) • Floodway zones	• Location of temporary lodging in the event of disaster • Location of educational institutions • Location of day care centers • Location of health services institutions • Location of public low-cost housing	

ªDissemination area: smallest area in the Canadian census (average of 700 people) with stable boundaries.

risks of weather-related diseases can be used for collecting surveillance information.

The Experience of the Brazilian Climate and Health Observatory

The Brazilian Climate and Health Observatory project is making information on climate and health available online (www.climasaude.icict.fiocruz.br) where data originating from different sources can be accessed on a common platform. This technology is innovative in that it allows users to make consultations that simultaneously use distributed data, that is, data generated and maintained by different institutions (Vera et al. 2010). The information technology (IT) and the information content were agreed on by the participating institutions, researchers, and representatives of government and civil society in workshops during which a consensual platform was approved by data producers and data users.

The possible impacts of climate changes on health were initially assessed by a group of public health researchers, resulting in a list of **climate-sensitive diseases**. Vector-borne diseases (Lowe et al. 2012), respiratory and cardiovascular diseases, waterborne diseases, and a variety of health problems resulting from prolonged drought (Carmo et al. 2010) or floods, such as hunger and infant mortality, were selected for monitoring by the observatory (Barcellos et al. 2009).

The debate on climate change drivers, impacts on public health, and adaptation actions need to be a democratic process that allows participation by different social actors with guidance toward motivating changes with short-, medium- and long-term effects. In the observatory project, participation is proposed as a path leading to integration between citizens, researchers, and public health administrators so as to enable interactions with other individuals within the community to develop reflective discussions and propose new ways of understanding the process of climate change. Participation is a skill that should be learned and perfected, and this requires a process of knowledge construction among the people involved so that reliable and easy-to-understand information channels can be opened.

In seeking interaction among administrators, researchers, citizens, and health care professionals and managers, their different academic training, languages and interests need to be taken into consideration. Citizens, even without links to any institution, can supply the observatory with information on extreme meteorological events and with new data giving warnings about the population's health conditions by means of the "live database." The intention with this database is to allow insertion and publication of georeferenced information in the format of text, images, or external links. In addition, comments on news items or research conducted under the coordination of the observatory are encouraged. The observatory's various workshops held in different regions of the country have included participation from organizations within local and national civil society.

Furthermore, the project has acted as a means of assembling researchers interested in the debate on the effects of climate change on health. The workshops held within the project have made it possible to identify and mobilize researchers who could contribute to understanding the relationships between climate and health. Recent occurrences of extreme events, such as the torrential rainfall on the coastal mountain range of the state of Rio de Janeiro, the fluctuations in river levels in the Amazon region, and the intensification of vegetation burning in the arc of deforestation have raised awareness among researchers and citizens regarding the need for preventive action to reduce the impact of climate-related natural disasters.

Nevertheless, the long-term and indirect effects of climate change on health, such as expansion of the incidence of vector-borne diseases, remain rather unexplored by researchers and rarely publicized by the media. This makes it difficult to bring citizens into the debate on the long-term effects of climate change and the possible measures for adapting to these changes.

The results from studies under development at the sentinel sites have shown how climatic factors influence the transmission of waterborne diseases in Manaus; how atmospheric pollution associated with vegetation burning influences respiratory diseases in the states of Rondônia and Mato

Grosso; and how rainfall and temperatures affect vector-borne diseases like dengue. These studies may promote a greater depth of debate on the effects of climate change on health, and on the role of health care services, primarily within the Brazilian National Health System (SUS), in reducing these impacts.

Risk Mapping Approaches

Some risk mapping approaches carried out by WHO (2013a) in several regions of the world (Europe, eastern Mediterranean, Africa) are interesting and useful for monitoring natural disasters. Online interactive maps are available for several climate-related risks, and these maps can be integrated into national systems. The methodologies used are documented as well. The European Centre for Disease Prevention and Control (2013a, 2013b) has produced various distribution maps for vectors (ticks, mosquitoes, sandflies) for Europe and coordinates a well-organized network on emerging and vector-borne diseases, which encourages countries in human surveillance, of course, but also entomological surveillance. Similar work is being discussed or implemented in Asia and in the Americas (Beatty et al. 2010), mainly about encephalitides (such as West Nile virus) or dengue. Other countries are focusing more on food safety and are establishing or improving forecasting systems for food crops, mainly in Central America and the Andean countries (El Consejo andino de ministros de relaciones exteriores 2010).

Several European countries, including France and the United Kingdom, operate highly developed surveillance systems for following the impacts in real or quasi-real time. The Institut de veille sanitaire français, in partnership with Météo-France, publishes heat and cold watch maps using meteorological forecasts to anticipate extreme events and initiate preventative actions (surveillance, care, social support, and communications). The warning levels were defined in partnership by the Institut de veille sanitaire français (2013) and the Ministry of Health. During the episodes, syndromic surveillance is used to check the real-time evolution of the situation, and if needed to reorient the preventative measures. Public Health England presents a similar approach, focused mainly on heat and cold, while preparing for other short-term risks. We should mention the existence, as in other European countries, of syndromic surveillance systems developed in emergency rooms (daily data for serious cases, on a sentinel basis; Public Health England 2013) and in family medical clinics (weekly data that can be mobilized on a daily basis in an emergency) which can support decision making (see Clinical Correlations 11.3).

Syndromic Surveillance for the Analysis of Extreme Weather Events in France

Every day, as of July 1, 2012, the French syndromic surveillance system SurSaUD (Surveillance sanitaire des urgences et des décès, health surveillance of emergencies and deaths) centralizes the data from 394 emergency services (visits by cause and age) of 59 associations of emergency doctors (medical data from city emergency rooms) and from 3,000 communes collecting mortality data. This represents close to 50 percent of the activity of emergency services in France, 90 percent of the activity of SOS Médecins, and 80 percent of daily deaths (Josseran et al. 2008).

When the expected health effects are well documented, the indicators to be followed can be defined a priori as, for example, in the case of heat waves. From the impacts documented in the literature, and mainly from a significant increase in mortality that can be associated with a slight or moderate increase in the care-use indicator, the indicators retained for surveillance during heat waves in France are mortality, emergency room visits (all causes, and for heat stroke and dehydration), and the use of emergency doctors (management of emergencies outside an institution). Experience with these data since 2004 has shown that trips to emergency rooms for heat stroke have been extremely sensitive to temperature but have represented a modest number of cases. The other care-use indicators varied little during heat waves, but this could mask a greater impact on mortality, which would be visible later, due to the time lag in obtaining mortality data (Pascal et al. 2012). This is why heat wave alerts are based on temperature forecasts (which make it possible to anticipate preventive actions), not on health data.

It might also be interesting to implement a rather lax or nonrigorous health surveillance when there is no prior assumption about the expected health effects. For example, analysis of the motives for emergency room use, as consulted in a doctor's notes at the Mont-de-Marsan hospital, revealed a high number of visits linked to the use of a chainsaw in the month after Tropical Storm Klaus, which hit the Landes forest department in 2009: twenty-nine episodes compared to six during the same month in the previous year (Verrier, Motreff, and Pirard 2011). In all cases, when interest focuses on fine geographical scales, analysis of the indicators chosen a priori or not is limited to a description, because the low number of cases would result in the statistical identification of only very large peaks.

Pollens and Allergies

Other interesting and recently implemented realizations address allergenic pollens and their spatial monitoring. In 2011, France created the

Observatoire de l'ambroisie, an observatory for ragweed, whose invasion, promoted by several factors, including the changing climate, particularly affects this country and others in Europe (Hungary, Croatia). Plans to control this plant and monitor its pollen have been in place for some time (Ministère des affaires sociales et de la santé 2013). Generalizing this approach to the European territory is proposed, given the increase in related allergies (Oswalt and Marshall 2008). The situation is similar in North America with respect to the increase in the plant's territory and allergies (Ziska et al. 2011).

We are therefore, practically worldwide, busy developing the aspects that will be included in more integrated systems for the final user, who is often responsible for all types of emergencies and must therefore look almost everywhere for the information that he or she needs. With a scientific watch, new aspects established by scientific research can be included as our knowledge improves.

CLINICAL CORRELATES 11.2   BARRIERS AND ADVANCES IN WEST NILE VIRUS SURVEILLANCE: LESSONS FROM THE 2012 EPIDEMIC IN DALLAS, TEXAS

West Nile is a mosquito-transmitted, climate-sensitive disease that causes a spectrum of illness from a viral syndrome to severe neuro-invasive disease (Centers for Disease Control and Prevention n.d.). After a period of relative dormancy in the continental United States, it made an epidemic comeback in Dallas County in 2012. In the months prior to the epidemic, researchers in Dallas County regularly checked dispersed mosquito traps, monitoring the local "vector index," an estimate of the prevalence of West Nile virus–infected mosquitoes (Chung et al. 2013). Historical reference informed a threshold index after which clinical cases of infection would likely appear. This threshold was crossed in May 2012, and warnings were issued to area physicians to be on high alert for viral syndromes associated with neurological complaints. Increased testing resulted, and the first cases were detected in early June. Although systems accurately predicted the epidemic, areal spraying did not begin until August 2012, when the bulk of infections had already occurred and death rates began to escalate. What caused this delay was likely prolonged laboratory testing times to confirm diagnosis and delays in action on behalf of public health officials, perhaps secondary to unfamiliarity with the validity of early detection systems. Physicians and health officials must work more closely in the future to make better use of surveillance systems to orchestrate timely responses and avoid unnecessary morbidity and mortality.

Early surveillance programs for West Nile virus are sensitive enough to predict outbreaks of disease. Clinicians and public health officials must increase their cooperation and communication to bring this knowledge to meaningful place in clinical practice.

Decision Making from Surveillance Information

Epidemiological surveillance has the ultimate goal of supporting the implementation of effective public health policies by providing useful information for decision making. The type of surveillance implemented for a given subject will therefore depend on the nature of the information considered useful for answering the decision makers' questions. In the case of climatic hazards, surveillance can contribute to decision making by helping in the management of health emergencies, evaluating the effectiveness of the prevention and adaptation measures, identifying and ranking the hazardous situations and the needs for adaptation, and communicating the health effects of climate change. We review those categories in detail.

Help in Health Emergency Management

Surveillance has a major role to play in anticipation, follow-up, and rapid evaluation during unusual episodes presenting risks to the population's health (Pirard, Pascal, and Motreff 2012). For example, these could be extreme weather events such as heat waves and storms and their consequences, such as floods. Different surveillance tools can be used during the event and its aftermath to help organize immediate relief, longer-term management, and prevention.

During the Warning

During the event, the priority is to identify the affected populations and provide warnings about potential health effects. This involves a rapid synthesis of the available information through simple surveillance systems, if possible preexisting and not requiring the involvement of the clinicians in the health system (or other organizations such as civil protection authorities) who must instead focus on taking charge of the victims. Syndromic health surveillance systems, based on the collection of nonspecific care-use data, can be particularly useful. Follow-up on care-use data, such as emergency room visits, allows unusual variations to be detected and early warnings to be provided, since these data can be descriptively analyzed rapidly during the event. Statistical methods can also be used to initiate a warning when an abnormal increase is observed in the number of cases in relation to a reference value. Several methods exist for choosing the reference value, but in all cases, the statistical warning must be confirmed by an analysis of the situation by an epidemiologist, directly linked to the source of the data (e.g., emergency physicians). In fact, these systems provide access to a large number of data that can be erroneous and are difficult to interpret. One can easily be drowned in a flood of syndromic information, ineffective for rapid decision making.

Information can also be collected directly from the victims, notably by means of simple questionnaires, on the condition that this does not interfere with the care work. This can be useful for identifying the people using the implemented support mechanisms (e.g., psychological management units) and for helping in the evolution of these support tools. Some specific preexisting surveillance systems can also be mobilized, in particular, surveillance systems for poisoning or infection.

With the development of new computer tools, the issue in surveillance will be to successfully integrate data originating from sources as varied as those described above, together with other sources of mainly environmental information, and to develop techniques allowing rapid translation of the mass of data thus collected into useful decision-making information.

After the Warning

In the aftermath of the event, surveillance must help to identify the possible long-term effects, as well as the risk factors or social determinants (World Health Organization 2013b), in order to orient prevention for future events. The implemented methods are then very different from syndromic surveillance and correspond to more classic epidemiological studies. Thus, the impact of extreme events on mental health over the short and long terms has been identified on several occasions by surveys using health information systems (Six et al. 2002; Motreff et al. 2013) or cross-sectional surveys (Verger et al. 2003). As well, time-series analyses of heat waves allow quantification of the impacts after an event and help define warning thresholds for the construction of warning systems (Fouillet et al. 2006). Case control studies provide more detailed information about the risk factors, and their results can be translated into concrete action in heat wave prevention plans or similar plans for other hazards. The development of long-range epidemiological studies after these events is therefore an important issue for managing populations and improving prevention; other studies pertaining to management, behavioral aspects, or health economics often show a high relevance for prevention too.

Effectiveness of Prevention and Adaptation Measures

Evaluation of the effectiveness of the prevention measures used to deal with climatic hazards, and in particular extreme meteorological events, is still a rather unexplored field. Existing initiatives mainly focus on heat waves and comparisons of the impacts of different events. When a reduction in mortality is observed, as, for, example, in France in 2006 compared to 2003 (Fouillet et al. 2006), a possible explanation might be the effectiveness of prevention. However, statistical analysis of extreme events is made difficult by their scarcity, and the comparison of the impacts of two equally extreme and equally different heat waves as those in 2003 and 2006 must be interpreted with caution. Also, this type of approach gives rather global information for the general population and focuses on the most serious health events. It does not provide information on the causes of the observed differences. If mortality is higher after a plan is implemented, does this mean that the plan was not well implemented, that the measures were not followed by the population, that they were followed but were ineffective, or even that they were followed and were effective but that an additional unexpected risk occurred besides the original risk covered by the measures? Only studies closest to the affected sites and questioning the population and the professionals in the field can answer these questions. These studies could mobilize more disciplines than just epidemiology, and health surveillance alone cannot provide the answer.

In the case of climate change where environmental hazards will evolve over time and the sociodemographic characteristics of the populations will change at the same time, reflection about the concept of vulnerability is particularly interesting. Among the many definitions proposed in the scientific literature, *vulnerability* seen as "a function of individual sensitivity, exposure, and the capacity to adapt" (Hinkel 2011) offers perspectives in terms of surveillance. Could the evolution of the populations at risk, their exposure, their adaptive behavior, undergo surveillance, and the evolution of the health effects that one is trying to avoid be compared?

Identification and Ranking of Hazardous Situations

Decision makers are often disadvantaged in dealing with the complexity of the impacts of climate change and by the dozens of health risks that can be identified by the reports (e.g., some twenty risks and several dozen associated effects identified in Canada; Health Canada 2008). Surveillance has a role to play in helping to identify and rank these risks by providing information mainly on the current incidence. Information on the real exposures of the population and the meteorological impacts on these exposures would also be valuable but is rarely produced. For this, for example, large repeated cross-sectional surveys interested in lifestyles, dietary behaviors, or other aspects could be used as a basis.

CLINICAL CORRELATES 11.3   FAMINE EARLY WARNING SYSTEMS AND CLIMATE CHANGE

According to the National Climate Assessment in 2013, "Climate change is expected to threaten both food production and certain aspects of food quality... Food insecurity increases with rising food prices. In such situations, people cope by turning to nutrient-poor but calorie-rich foods, and/or they endure hunger, with consequences ranging from micronutrient malnutrition to obesity."

This statement implies far-reaching consequences for domestic and global health and nutrition security. How can we prepare for such impacts? Famine early warning systems are a proactive way to address threats to food insecurity. Remote sensing systems, numerical modeling of geographical information systems as well as satellite vegetation index imagery, can be used to forecast crop yields (Verdin et al. 2005) and thus predict where food shortage may appear. However, shortage of food does not necessarily imply a food crisis. Livelihood analysis scrutinizes the link between shortage and crisis by examining the relative importance of certain food crops, as well as sources of income of an area's inhabitants, and uses modeling to predict how a food shortage will affect an area (Grillo 2009). (For more information see FEWS NET for live monitoring of famine crisis worldwide: http://www.fews.net.)

Policy planners, clinicians, and public health officials can prepare for and intervene in current and future humanitarian crises using this real-time system.

Famine early warning systems predict where famine may occur using climate and anthropologic models. Information from these models may be used to target resources to food-vulnerable areas.

Communication

Communication about the health effects of climate change could prompt politicians and the population to take this theme into account better (Maibach, Roser-Renouf, and Leiserowitz 2008; Maibach et al. 2010) and to become even more involved in greenhouse gas emission control. Health impact assessment is one of the most promising tools for helping in this communication, because it allows the results from scientific studies to be transcribed into local data from health and environmental surveillance and different intervention scenarios to be compared (Medina et al. 2013).

Future Improvements to Be Promoted

As often happens in surveillance, the technology is available and rapidly evolving, and its costs constantly dropping, particularly if open source software is used and a distributed data architecture is established that allows each institution to retain ownership of its data, while sharing the components that can be useful to others, according to established modalities. Each institution therefore remains responsible for controlling the quality of the data made available and respecting confidentiality, if relevant. Vulnerability to a given risk, after all, can be defined at a much lower cost on a spatial basis (such as a census area or a postal code) compared to the use of individual data, and allows effective action by the authorities. With this approach, many conflicts can be resolved and risks reduced while ensuring that updated data are always used and consulted by easy-to-establish automated web services at the desired frequency. Provision must also be made for the possibility of parameterizing the data according to the users' preferences (often changing) to take into account the evolution in knowledge and future regulatory requirements. Generalization of these technological approaches will therefore be a desirable improvement over the short term.

Surveillance tools such as these have important organizational consequences that must not be ignored. In fact, intervention thresholds based on risk levels must be established (and rigorously justified), periodic analyses and postevent reports planned, and continuing education sessions organized. However, the benefits dominate in such a process: good surveillance tools allow discussion on common bases, and a fruitful harmonization of approaches and practices generally ensues. Surveillance reports are facilitated by this and allow a better justification and promotion of the adaption to climate change. While the initial implementation can prove demanding for the first or second hazard of interest, what follows is much easier. One must therefore start modestly and build gradually.

Several practitioners in surveillance believe that there is no need to create a specific system for climate change, and they are probably correct. In view of the numerous indicators needed in this subject, priority should be given to supplementary analyses specific to climate-related variables, the improved surveillance of known climate-sensitive diseases and their determinants, and nesting formally those surveillance systems within larger national systems. In the case of climate-sensitive diseases, risk factors of interest for public health will be mostly social and environmental factors linked to exposure to extreme meteorological events and their consequences.

Connectivity with nonhealth institutions remains particularly vital for effective action. This approach also allows a sharing of all types of data rather than duplication. Several tasks await us, however, to complete the list of health problems requiring surveillance and to develop proven methodologies. We should mention that very little research exists on the health of workers exposed to high levels of heat outside plants (e.g., cooks, forestry workers) and at higher risk during heat waves. Mental health problems increase the risk of mortality and morbidity in some contexts, but there is still little solid scientific knowledge about this. Still relating to the psychological component, major disasters (where people lose loved ones, their work or their homes) are a surveillance challenge that some researchers are beginning to tackle, mainly to better recognize posttraumatic stress disorder when it occurs and to offer the appropriate clinical and preventative services. Finally, there is as yet little interest in the various individual and organizational behaviors that are prescribed on all websites: Who puts them into everyday practice? Are they effective? What are the determinants facilitating their adoption? The barriers? Are the emergency plans appropriate and updated? These few unanswered questions illustrate the need for a research effort that can support surveillance as another important direction to be taken.

Finally, surveillance must normally support the activities of public and private organizations that can take action in hazard prevention and emergency preparedness. The next priority will therefore be one of knowledge transfer between field practitioners who can have an impact on health, and the realm of clinician and public health. While physicians, nurses, psychologists, and pharmacists treat disease most of the time, those who can keep us healthy are instead engineers, land use planners, environmentalists or politicians, as well as environmental, civil protection, and public health authorities. The ultimate purpose of surveillance systems is to properly inform all these people and to orient them towards useful solutions.

Conclusion

Health surveillance in relation to climate change presents several challenges worldwide. A number of countries have already implemented systems mainly relating to heat and cold waves, and are preparing their approach for other hazards. Systems relating to infectious diseases must also integrate climatic considerations. However, much remains to be done.

DISCUSSION QUESTIONS

1. How can surveillance contribute to the promotion of greater environmental justice for the hazards related to climate change?

2. Is the spatial scale used for surveillance important? What are its actual impacts on the observed phenomena?

3. The new technologies can improve the public's participation in data collection for surveillance. Do you believe that this aspect is important to develop in the future?

4. Population displacement following extreme weather events becomes often permanent for a good proportion. Hurricane Katrina hit New Orleans in 2005 and was identified as the first climate change–related ecological migration in a developed country. Would you support such a statement?

KEY TERMS

Climate-sensitive diseases: Diseases that can be directly related to the climate and sensitive to it, with others only indirectly.

Health determinants: According to WHO, "the conditions in which people are born, grow, live, work and age, including the health system."

Health surveillance; environmental monitoring: Different terms but the same concept of measuring over time certain indicators. The health sector uses *surveillance* and the environment sector *monitoring*. The indicators relate to the hazards, exposure to these hazards, known health problems, and the related determinants or risk factors, in order to identify the problems, follow their evolution, support interventions, and influence public policies.

Risk factor: According to WHO, "any attribute, characteristic or exposure of an individual that increases the likelihood of developing a disease or injury."

Vulnerabilities: A function of individual sensitivity, exposure, and the capacity to adapt. Vulnerabilities can be established for geographical areas (e.g., flood-prone areas) or for groups of people based on their characteristics (risk factors and/or determinants).

References

Barcellos, C., A.M.V. Monteiro, C. Corvalan, H. C. Gurgel, M. S. Carvalho, P. Artaxo, S. Hacon, and V. Ragoni. 2009. "Mudanças climáticas e ambientais e as doenças infecciosas: cenários e incertezas para o Brasil." [Climate and Environment change and Infections Diseases: Scenarios and Uncertainties for Brazil]. *Epidemiologia e Serviços de Saúd* 18:285–304.

Beatty, M. E., A. Stone, D. W. Fitzsimons, J. N. Hanna, S. K. Lam, S. Vong, M. G. Guzman, et al. 2010. "Best Practices in Dengue Surveillance: A Report from the Asia-Pacific and Americas Dengue Prevention Boards." *PLoS Neglected Tropical Diseases* 4(11):e890. PM:21103381.

Bélanger, D., B. Abdous, P. Gosselin, and P. Valois. 2015. "An Adaptation Index to High Summer Heat Associated with Adverse Health Impacts in Deprived Neighborhoods." *Climatic Change* (May 25). http://link.springer.com/article/10.1007/s10584–015–1420–4

Carmo, C. N., S. Hacon, K. M. Longo, S. Freitas, E. Ignotti, A. Ponce de Leon, and P. Artaxo. 2010. "Association between Particulate Matter from Biomass Burning and Respiratory Diseases in the Southern Region of the Brazilian Amazon." *Revista Panamerica de Salud Publica* 27(1):10–66.

Centers for Disease Control and Prevention. 2013. "Environmental Health Tracking Program." http://ephtracking.cdc.gov/showAbout.action

Centers for Disease Control and Prevention. n.d. "West Nile Virus: Symptoms and Treatment." http://www.cdc.gov/westnile/symptoms/index.html

Christensen, J., B. Hewitson, A. Busuioc, A. Chen, X. Gao, I. Held, R. Jones, et al. 2007. "Regional Climate Projections." In *Climate Change 2007: The Physical Science Basis,* edited by S. Solomon, D. Qin, M. Manning, Z. Chen, M. Marquis, K. B. Avert, M. Tignor, and H. L. Miller, 847–940. Cambridge: Cambridge University Press.

Confalonieri, U., B. Menne, R. Akhtar, K. L. Ebi, M. Hauengue, R. S. Kovats, B. Revich, and A. Woodward. 2007. "Human Health." In *Climate Change 2007: Impacts, Adaptation and Vulnerability. Contribution of Working Group II to the Fourth Assessment Report of the Intergovernmental Panel on Climate Change,* edited by M. L. Parry, O. F. Canziani, J. P. Palutikof, P. J. van der Linden and C. E. Hanson, 391–431. Cambridge: Cambridge University Press.

Chung, W. M., C.M.S.N. Buseman, S. Joyner, S. M. Hughes, T. B. Fomby, J. P. Luby, and R. W. Haley. 2013. "The 2012 West Nile Encephalitis Epidemic in Dallas, Texas." *JAMA* 310:297–307.

Cox, J., and T. A. Abeku. 2007. "Early Warning Systems for Malaria in Africa: From Blueprint to Practice." *Trends in Parasitology.* 23:243–46. PM:17412641.

Department of Health and Human Services Data Council, Centers for Disease Control and Prevention, National Center for Health Statistics, and National Committee on Vital and Health Statistics. 2002. *Shaping a Health Statistics Vision for the 21st Century,* 9. Hyattsville, MD: National Center for Health Statistics.

El Consejo andino de ministros de relaciones exteriors. 2010. "DECISION 742. Programa Andino para Garantizar la Seguridad y Soberanía Alimentaria y Nutricional—SSAN." [Andino Program to Ensure Security and Food Sovereignty and Nutrition]. http://andina.vlex.com/vid/decision-742–214155739

European Centre for Disease Prevention and Control 2013a. "Emerging and Vector-borne Diseases Programme." http://www.ecdc.europa.eu/en/activities/diseaseprogrammes/emerging_and_vector_borne_diseases/Pages/index.aspx

European Centre for Disease Prevention and Control 2013b. "Guidelines for the Surveillance of Invasive Mosquitoes in Europe." http://ecdc.europa.eu/en/publications/Publications/TER-Mosquito-surveillance-guidelines.pdf

Fouillet, A., G. Rey, F. Laurent, G. Pavillon, S. Bellec, C. Guihenneuc-Jouyaux, J. Clavel, E. Jougla, and D. Hemon. 2006. "Excess Mortality Related to the August 2003 Heat Wave in France." *International Archives of Occupational and Environmental Health* 80(1):16–24. PM:16523319.

Grillo, J. 2009. "Application of the Livelihood Zone Maps and Profiles for food Security Analysis and Early Warning." USAID. http://www.fews.net/sites/default/files/uploads/Guidance_Application%20of%20Livelihood%20Zone%20Maps%20and%20Profiles_final_en.pdf

Gubler, D. J. 2008. "The Global Threat of Emergent/Reemergent Vector-Borne Diseases." In *Vector-Borne Diseases: Understanding the Environmental, Human Health, and Ecological Connection*, edited by P. W. Atkinson, 3–46. Washington, DC: Institute of Medicine, National Academies Press.

Health Canada 2008. *Human Health in a Changing Climate: A Canadian Assessment of Vulnerabilities and Adaptive Capacity.* Ottawa: Government of Canada. http://www.2degreesc.com/Files/CCandHealth.pdf

Hinkel, J. 2011. "Indicators of Vulnerability and Adaptive Capacity: Towards a Clarification of the Science-Policy Interface." *Global Environmental Change* 21:198–208.

Institut de Veille Sanitaire. 2013. "Climat et santé." http://www.invs.sante.fr/Dossiers-thematiques/Environnement-et-sante/Climat-et-sante

Intergovernmental Panel on Climate Change. 2000. "IPCC Special Report: Summary for Policymakers." http://www.ipcc.ch/pdf/special-reports/spm/sres-en.pdf

Intergovernmental Panel on Climate Change. 2010. *Meeting Report of the Intergovernmental Panel on Climate Change Expert Meeting on Assessing and Combining Multi Model Climate Projections.* https://www.ipcc-wg1.unibe.ch/publications/supportingmaterial/IPCC_EM_MultiModelEvaluation_MeetingReport.pdf

Intergovernmental Panel on Climate Change. 2012. *Managing the Risks of Extreme Events and Disasters to Advance Climate Change Adaptation: A Special Report of Working Groups I and II of the Intergovernmental Panel on Climate Change.* Cambridge: Cambridge University Press.

Jones, K. E., N. G. Patel, M. A. Levy, A. Storeygard, D. Balk, J. L. Gittleman, and P. Daszak. 2008. "Global Trends in Emerging Infectious Diseases." *Nature* 451:990–93. 18288193.

Josseran, L., A. Fouillet, N. Caillere, M. Pascal, D. Ilef, and P. Astagneau. 2008. "Syndromic Surveillance and Climate Change, a Possible Use?" *Advances in Disease Surveillance* 5:106.

Lowe, R., T. C. Bailey, D. B. Stephenson, T. E. Jupp, R. J. Graham, C. Barcellos, and M. S. Carvalho. 2012 . "The Development of an Early Warning System for Climate-Sensitive Disease Risk with a Focus on Dengue Epidemics in Southeast Brazil." *Statistics in Medicine* 32:864–83. doi:10.1002/sim.5549

Maibach, E. W., M. Nisbet, P. Baldwin, K. Akerlof, and G. Diao. 2010. "Reframing Climate Change as a Public Health Issue: An Exploratory Study of Public Reactions." *BMC Public Health* 10:299. PM:20515503.

Maibach, E. W., C. Roser-Renouf, and A. Leiserowitz. 2008. "Communication and Marketing as Climate Change-Intervention Assets a Public Health Perspective." *American Journal of Preventative Medicine* 35:488–500. 18929975.

Medeiros, H., M. Pascal, A.-C. Viso, and S. Medina, 2010. *Conference Proceedings of the Workshop on Public Health Surveillance and Climate Change.* http://opac .invs.sante.fr/doc_num.php?explnum_id=109

Medina, S., F. Ballester, O. Chanel, C. Declercq, and M. Pascal. 2013. "Quantifying the Health Impacts of Outdoor Air Pollution: Useful Estimations for Public Health Action." *Journal of Epidemiology and Community Health* 67(6):480–83. doi:10.1136/jech-2011–200908

Ministère des Affaires sociales et de la santé, République française. 2013. "Ambroisie à feuille d'armoise: Coordonnons la lutte contre cette plante allergisante et envahissante." [Ambrosia artemisiifolia: Coordinating the Fight Against Plant Invasion and Allergenicity]. http://www.sante.gouv.fr/ambroisie-a-feuille-d-armoise-coordonnons-la-lutte-contre-cette-plante-allergisante-et-envahissante.html

Motreff, Y., P. Pirard, S. Goria, B. Labrador, C. Gourier-Fréry, J. Nicolau, A. Le Tertre, and C. Chan-Chee. 2013. "Increase in Psychotropic Drug Deliveries after the Xynthia Storm, France, 2010." *Prehospital and Disaster Medicine* 28(5):428–33.

National Oceanic and Atmospheric Administration. 2013a. "National Hurricane Center." http://www.nhc.noaa.gov/?atlc

National Oceanic and Atmospheric Administration. 2013b. "North American Drought Monitor." http://www.ncdc.noaa.gov/temp-and-precip/drought /nadm/

Oswalt, M. L., and G. D. Marshall. 2008. "Ragweed as an Example of Worldwide Allergen Expansion." *Allergy Asthma and Clinical Immunology* 4:130135. PM:20525135.

Pascal, M., K. Laaidi, V. Wagner, A. B. Ung, S. Smaili, A. Fouillet, C. Caserio-Schonemann, and P. Beaudeau. 2012. "How to Use Near Real-Time Health Indicators to Support Decision-Making during a Heat Wave: The Example of the French Heat Wave Warning System." *PLoS Currents* 4:e4f83ebf72317d.

PCMDI (Program for Climate Model Diagnosis and Intercomparison). 2013. "Earth System Grid Federation." http://pcmdi9.llnl.gov/esgf-web-fe/live

Pirard, P., M. Pascal, and Y. Motreff. 2012. "Gestion des événements climatologiques extrêmes: nécessité d'une réponse épidémiologique intégrée et planifiée dans l'organisation de la réponse sanitaire et sociale." [Management of Extreme Weather Events: The Need for Integrated Epidemiological and Planned Response in the Organization of Health and Social Response]. *Bulletin Epidemiologique Hebdomadaire* 12–13:151–55.

Public Health Agency of Canada. 2011. "What Determines Health?" http://origin .phac-aspc.gc.ca/ph-sp/determinants/#key_determinants

Public Health England. 2013. "Emergency Department Syndromic Surveillance System (EDSSS)." http://www.hpa.org.uk/Topics/InfectiousDiseases/InfectionsAZ /RealtimeSyndromicSurveillance/SyndromicSystemsAndBulletinArchive/EDSSS/

Randall, D., R. Wood, S. Bony, R. Colman, T. Fichefet, J. Fyfe, V. Kattsov, A. Pitman, et al. 2007. "Climate Models and Their Evaluation." In *Climate Change 2007: The Physical Science Basis*, edited by S. Solomon, D. Qin, M. Manning, Z. Chen, M. Marquis, K. B. Avery, M. Tignor, and H. L. Miller, 589–662. Cambridge: Cambridge University Press.

Six, C., K. Mantey, F. Franke, L. Pascal, and P. Malfait. 2002. *Étude des conséquences psychologiques des inondations à partir des bases de données de l'Assurance maladie.* [*Study of the Psychological Consequences of Flooding from the Health Insurance Database*]. Paris: Institut national de veille sanitaire.

Thomson, M. C., F. J. Doblas-Reyes, S. J. Mason, R. Hagedorn, S. J. Connor, T. Phindela, A. P. Morse, and T. N. Palmer. 2006. "Malaria Early Warnings Based on Seasonal Climate Forecasts from Multi-Model Ensembles." *Nature* 439:576–79.

Toutant, S., P. Gosselin, D. Belanger, R. Bustinza, and S. Rivest. 2011. "An Open Source Web Application for the Surveillance and Prevention of the Impacts on Public Health of Extreme Meteorological Events: The SUPREME System." *International Journal of Health Geographics* 10:39. doi:10.1186/1476–072X-10–39

Vera, C., M. Barange, O. P. Dube, L. Goddard, D. Grigg, N. Kobysheva, E. Odada, et al. 2010. "Needs Assessment for Climate Information on Decadal Timescales and Longer." In *Procedia Environmental Sciences*, vol. 1, edited by M.V.K. Sivakumar, B. S. Nyenzi, and A. Tyagi, 275–86. Geneva: Elsevier.

Verdin, J., C. Funk, G. Senay, and R. Choularton. 2005. "Climate Science and Famine Early Warning." *Philosophical Transactions of the Royal Society B* 360:2155–68.

Verger, P., M. Rotily, C. Hunault, J. Brenot, E. Baruffol, and D. Bard. 2003. "Assessment of Exposure to a Flood Disaster in a Mental-Health Study." *Journal of Exposure Analysis and Environmental Epidemiology* 13:436–42. PM:14603344.

Verrier, A., Y. Motreff, and P. Pirard. 2011. "Encadré 1—Surveillance épidémiologique activée lors de la tempête Klaus." [Box 1—Epidemiological Monitoring of Storm Klaus]. In *Surveillance épidémiologique* [Epidemiological Monitoring], edited by P. Astagneau and T. Ancelle. Paris: Lavoisier.

World Health Organization. 2013a. "Risk Factors." http://www.who.int/topics /risk_factors/en/index.html

World Health Organization. 2013b. "Social Determinants of Health." http://www .who.int/social_determinants/en/index.html

World Health Organization and World Meteorological Organization. 2012. "Atlas of Health and Climate." http://www.who.int/globalchange/publications/atlas /report/en/index.html.

World Meteorological Organization. 2000. "Guidelines on Performance Assessment of Public Weather Services." http://www.wmo.int/pages/prog/amp/pwsp /pdf/TD-1023.pdf.

World Meteorological Organization. 2013. "Survey of Common Verification Methods in Meteorology." http://www.cawcr.gov.au/projects/verification /Stanski_et_al/Stanski_et_al.html.

Zinszer, K., A. D. Verma, K. Charland, T. F. Brewer, J. S. Brownstein, Z. Sun, and D. L. Buckeridge. 2012. "A Scoping Review of Malaria Forecasting: Past Work and Future Directions." *BMJ Open* 2(6):e001992. doi:10.1136 /bmjopen-2012–001992

Ziska, L., K. Knowlton, C. Rogers, D. Dalan, N. Tierney, M. A. Elder, W. Filley, J. Shropshire, et al. 2011. "Recent Warming by Latitude Associated with Increased Length of Ragweed Pollen Season in Central North America." *Proceedings of the National Academy of Sciences (USA)* 108:4248–51. PM:21368130.

CHAPTER 12

CLIMATE AND HEALTH VULNERABILITY ASSESSMENTS

A Practical Approach

Diarmid Campbell-Lendrum, Joy Guillemot, Kristie L. Ebi

Human-induced climate change poses a fundamental risk to human health and well-being. In the short to medium term, however, much of the potential health impact of climate change can be avoided through a combination of strengthening key health system functions and targeted improvements in management of specific risks presented by a changing climate. Policymakers from around the world have recognized this challenge. At levels of health policymaking, from the World Health Assembly, through regional groupings, to the national and community levels, the health community has begun to organize its response by assessing and addressing the health risks of climate change.

The critical first step in this process is to carry out a **health vulnerability and adaptation assessment**. This allows countries to assess which populations are most vulnerable to different kinds of health effects, identify weaknesses in the systems that should protect them, and specify interventions to respond. Assessments can also improve evidence and understanding of the linkages between climate and health within the assessment area, serve as a baseline analysis against which changes

KEY CONCEPTS

- **It is better to have a general and approximate understanding of the range of health issues that may be affected by climate change rather than having a very detailed understanding of only some specific risks.**

- **Vulnerability and adaptation assessments should not be abstract assessments of potential risks in the distant future. Instead, they should be grounded in current health realities and aim to improve health now and increase resilience to a changing climate.**

- **Health adaptation measures should be identified and prioritized. This stage requires the leadership of health policymakers and practitioners who are most directly involved in implementation.**

- **It is important to prioritize the interventions that should bring the greatest**

This chapter draws heavily on the WHO publication *Protecting Health from Climate Change: Vulnerability and Adaptation Assessment*. We thank all those who contributed to the process of developing that guidance, particularly Peter Berry, Carlos Corvalan, Elena Villalobos-Prats, Marilyn Aparicio, Hamed Bakir, Christovam Barcellos, Badrakh Burmaajav, Jill Ceitlin, Edith Clarke, Nitish Dogra, Winfred Austin Greaves, Andrej M Grjibovski, Guy Hutton, Iqbal Kabir, Vladimir Kendrovski, George Luber, Bettina Menne, Lucrecia Navarro, Piseth Raingsey Prak, Mazouzi Raja, Ainash Sharshenova, and Ciro Ugarte. We also express our appreciation to the US Environmental Protection Agency, Health Canada, and the government of Costa Rica for their support to this work.

in disease risk and protective measures can be monitored, provide the opportunity for building capacity, and strengthen the case for investment in health protection.

What Health Issues Should a Vulnerability and Adaptation Assessment Cover?

As a general guide, it is usually better to have a general and approximate understanding of the range of health issues that may be affected by climate change rather than having a very detailed understanding of only some specific risks. The best approach is therefore usually to scope the various mechanisms through which climate change may affect health risks before focusing on those that are indicated to be the most important in terms of current and likely future health burden, as well as the degree to which they are amenable to preventative interventions.

The experience to date across a range of countries and settings suggests the following broad categories of health risks to consider:

- *The direct physical effects of extreme heat and thermal stress.* Increased average temperatures over recent decades have translated into higher frequency and intensity of heat waves, exacerbating cardiovascular and respiratory diseases and heat-related mortality. There is high confidence that the warming trend will continue in the future and is a significant risk that large areas of the world may be unsafe for outdoor physical activity before the end of the century.

- *Climate change-related alterations in the frequency, intensity, and duration of other extreme weather events (e.g., floods, droughts, and windstorms).* Each year, these events affect millions of people, damage critical public health infrastructure, and cause billions of dollars of economic losses. The frequency and intensity of some types of extreme weather event are expected to increase over coming decades as a consequence of climate change (IPCC 2013), suggesting that the associated health impacts could increase without additional prevention actions.

- *Infectious diseases transmitted by water, food, vectors, or zoonotic reservoirs.* Higher temperatures tend to accelerate microbial growth and survival and can alter the distribution and abundance of disease vectors, such as the mosquitoes that transmit malaria and dengue fever. Changing precipitation patterns and more extreme rainfall events can reduce the amount of water available for hygiene purposes, cause contamination of water sources through flooding, and affect the ecology and behavior of vectors.

- *Air quality.* Higher temperatures tend to increase ozone levels, particularly in and around urban areas, while warmer conditions and increased levels of carbon dioxide in the atmosphere can favor the release of airborne allergens. Higher temperatures and reduced precipitation can cause desertification and lead to wildfires and dust storms, all of which affect respiratory health.

- *Nutrition and food security.* Higher temperatures and changes in precipitation can decrease agricultural production and therefore the quality and quantity of available food. Food shortages tend to increase food prices, putting the poorest populations at particular risk. This can exacerbate existing levels of nutrition, in turn associated with much higher susceptibility to diseases such as diarrhea, malaria, and acute respiratory infections.

- *Indirect effects through climate-induced economic dislocation and environmental decline.* The cumulative effects of climate change, including long-term trends, for example, those associated with sea level rise or desertification, may undermine economic growth and drive migration, placing pressure on health and other protection systems and potentially heightening tensions and the risk of conflict.

In addition to these major categories of risks, it is important to keep an open mind to health risks that may not be the most important in global terms but may be particularly important for particular populations or in certain settings. For example, the foodborne illness ciguatera is caused by eating certain reef fish contaminated with toxins originally produced by dinoflagellates living in tropical and subtropical waters and is associated with meteorological conditions that may be affected by climate change. While not a major health burden in global terms, it is a significant risk to the lives and livelihoods or those specific populations dependent on reef fishing (Llewellyn 2010).

CLINICAL CORRELATES 12.1   CLIMATE CHANGE, MIGRATIONS, AND REFUGEE HEALTH NEEDS

Environmental change has the potential to displace massive numbers of people. The Office of the UN High Commissioner for Refugees estimates the current number of forcibly displaced people to be more than 43 million ("Resources for Speakers" n.d.). Forced migration results from lack of resources such as food and water or violence that occurs as a result of resource scarcity and civil unrest. Caring for the health needs of this many displaced individuals is a daunting task, and as environmental change continues to occur, forecasts are that the number of refugees will increase.

Experts predict that changing weather patterns are likely to make many human-inhabited regions of the world uninhabitable in the next fifty years. Geographical regions at risk include low-lying coastal settlements, farm regions dependent on rivers fed by snowmelt and glacier melt, subhumid and arid regions, and humid areas in Southeast Asia vulnerable to changes in monsoon patterns (Sachs 2007).

The health issues of refugees are complex and range from chronic diseases, to infectious communicable diseases, to malnutrition and mental illness. One strategy to help mitigate these needs would be to implement electronic medical records systems within refugee camps. Using data gathered from health visits, policymakers could make evidence-based decisions in regard to disease surveillance, as well as the allocation of resources, thus increasing the efficiency of care.

Climate change is likely to make many regions of the world uninhabitable over the next fifty years. Managing the needs of refugee health will require massive amounts of resources. Information technology may increase efficiency of health care delivery and resource allocation.

What Other Nonclimate Factors Should Be Considered?

While adverse health effects of climate variability and change will be felt by all countries and populations, effects will be very strongly mediated by social and environmental determinants that are not directly related to climate change. Consideration of these factors is therefore an essential dimension of any vulnerability and adaptation assessment. There is a wide range of determining factors that will be more or less specific to different health issues, but among the most important that cut across all health risks are geography, poverty, age, and gender.

The physical location in which populations are situated is a major determinant of their exposure to meteorological hazards and their vulnerability. For example, populations living in tropical megacities are likely to be at particular risk of suffering health impacts of extreme heat as the effects of long-term climate change and short-term weather variation combine with the urban heat island effect and elevated levels of air pollution.

Socioeconomic status and, particularly, poverty are among the most important determinants within and between populations. The poorest countries suffer the burdens of climate-sensitive health outcomes such as undernutrition, vector-borne diseases, and diarrhea that are orders of magnitude greater than those in the richer nations. Even within the same country, burdens of these diseases are typically several times greater among the poorest compared to the richest populations (World Health Organization 2009a). Such differences are also important within more developed countries. For example, those living in poorer-quality housing with poorer insulation are likely to suffer more from the health effects of hot and cold extremes. Taking account of such differences within vulnerability and adaptation assessments provides an opportunity to advance health equity.

Individual characteristics, particularly age and gender, are also important determinants. Some of the clearest examples include the generally higher susceptibility of young children to climate-sensitive diseases such as malaria, diarrhea, and asthma and the increased vulnerability of older people to health effects of thermal extremes. Gender is also critically important and is determined by both biological differences and social norms, with classic examples being much higher mortality rates of women than men in the Bangladesh floods of the 1970s, as women were less likely to have learned to swim or to leave the house to seek safety in the absence of a male family member. It is not the case, however, that one sex is always more vulnerable than the other. For example, evidence from some countries shows that the rate of suicides in the aftermath of droughts is particularly high among male rural farmers, which may be due to the psychological effects of men being unable to fulfill their traditional role in providing economically for the household. Initiatives to build health resilience to extreme weather events should therefore pay particular attention to mental health in this population group (World Health Organization 2009b).

CLINICAL CORRELATES 12.2   HOSPITAL PREPAREDNESS AND VULNERABILITY ASSESSMENT

Climate change and associated effects of extreme weather events, poor air quality, vector-borne diseases, and disruptions in the supply of food and water are likely to increase demand for health care services. Hospitals must therefore undertake an evaluation of their vulnerability and their ability to respond to increasing short- and long-term needs. Comprehensive tools exist for such analysis, such as the American Hospital Association's Hazard Vulnerability Analysis tool (http://www.ashe.org).

Assessments must be tailored to address specific geographical climate-related risks. For example, All Children's Hospital in Florida recognized the severe hurricane risk of the geographical area when planning the design of its 2010 building (Brands et al. 2013). It rallied stakeholders and, using evidence from the breakdown in hospital services during Hurricane Katrina, sought to design a completely self-sufficient hospital that could function at full capacity for one month. They developed an analysis tool to identify potential risks and identified core needs that included (1) generating power, (2) protecting the structural integrity of the building and safeguarding electrical and mechanical equipment, (3) ensuring backup systems for air temperature control, water supply, plumbing, and sewage disposal, (4) storing essential supplies with which to operate the hospital for one month, and (5) creating a fail-proof transportation system to and from the hospital to ensure delivery of supplies and evacuation of patients. Hospitals throughout the United States need to undergo self-assessment and have alternative plans to function in a limited resource setting. Health care providers are essential stakeholders and should be involved in all stages of assessment and planning.

Hospitals should perform vulnerability assessments to adequately prepare for increases in health care needs in emergency situations.

Vulnerability and Adaptation Assessment

Framing and Scoping the Assessment

There is no set rule for the scope of a vulnerability and adaptation assessment; this will be a function of the mandate for the assessment (e.g., whether it is called for by a national ministry of health, a city authority, or as an academic research project) and the time and resources available to the project team.

In order for an assessment that meets its goals, however, it is critically important to be clear from the outset on issues such as the geographical regions to be considered, the health outcomes to be considered, and the specific questions to be addressed. This in turn will determine the kinds of expertise that need to be included within the project team, the range of stakeholders needed, and the strategy for communicating the results of the assessment.

For example, in several countries, national ministries of health have commissioned health vulnerability and adaptation assessments with the objective of ensuring that both the formal health system and the wider range of health-determining sectors (such as water or energy supply) have an objective assessment of the scale and nature of climate risks to health and guidance on potential responses. The assessment is generally used to both define the responsibilities of the health sector and contribute the health perspective to cross-government action to address climate change.

To meet this need, health ministries have therefore set up a core steering committee of the concerned operational sectors and experts on health and climate change, which have established a wider expert group covering the main health issues that are considered to be of interest (e.g., heat stress, nutrition, vector-borne disease, waterborne disease, air quality, and occupational health), identifying individuals or establishing subgroups to look at each of these sets of risks (figure 12.1). This larger project team is then responsible for carrying out the risk assessment, analysis, and reporting

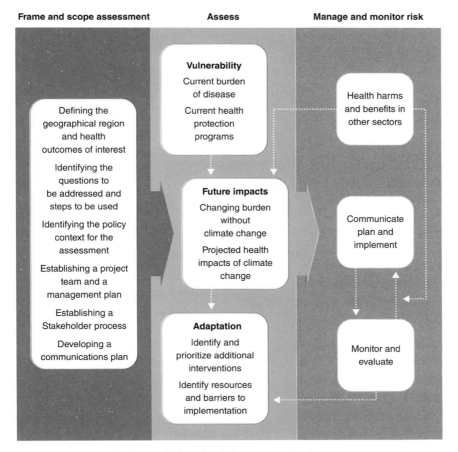

Figure 12.1   Steps in Conducting a Health Vulnerability and Adaptation Assessment
Source: WHO (2013).

under a common structure and directing the outcomes of the assessment to institutions or stakeholder groups that are expected to act on them (e.g., in addressing the potential effects of climate change on waterborne disease risks, specific recommendations may be made to disease surveillance services, and to water and sanitation providers).

Understanding the Current Situation

Vulnerability and adaptation assessments should not be abstract assessments of potential risks in the distant future; instead they should be grounded in current health realities and aim to improve health now, as well as increasing resilience to a changing climate. The starting point for the assessment is therefore the health situation as it currently stands. This is typically addressed through documentation of recent data on the main climate risk factors for health in the context of other drivers (e.g., frequency of heat waves or floods), current health impacts (e.g., the number of deaths or hospitalizations from extreme events, or morbidity or mortality from climate-sensitive diseases), and the capacity of health systems to manage these risks (e.g., the coverage of surveillance and response systems for infectious diseases, and known weaknesses in these systems).

This step should identify populations and regions with particular vulnerability to health effects associated with weather, current climate variability, and recent climate change. Some of the most important relationships are shown in table 12.1.

In addition to identifying particularly vulnerable population groups, it is often useful to do spatial risk mapping of areas at highest risk. For

Table 12.1   Vulnerability to Climate-Sensitive Health Outcomes by Subpopulation

Groups with Increased Vulnerability	Climate-Related Vulnerabilities
Infants and children	Heat stress, ozone air pollution, waterborne and food-borne illnesses, vector-borne diseases, malnutrition
Pregnant women	Heat stress, extreme weather events, waterborne and food-borne illnesses, vector-borne diseases
Elderly people and people with chronic medical conditions	Heat stress, air pollution, extreme weather events, waterborne and food-borne illnesses, vector-borne diseases
Impoverished and low socioeconomic status	Heat stress, extreme weather events, air pollution, vector-borne infectious diseases, waterborne and food-borne diseases
Outdoor workers	Heat stress, air pollution, vector-borne infectious diseases, ultraviolet light exposure

Source: Adapted from Balbus and Malina (2009).

example, populations living in low-lying plains are particularly susceptible to flooding following extreme rainfall, both through exposure of their own homes and also of critical infrastructure and services, such as health facilities.

Analyses of the relationships of health outcomes and their determinants to weather and climate patterns (sensitivity analyses) are essential to vulnerability and adaptation assessments. Such analyses usually assess the relationships between specific health data and weather variables, such as temperature, precipitation, relative humidity, and extreme weather events and patterns. These are typically assessed through time series analysis (e.g., quantitative analysis of the degree to which daily or weekly variations in temperature are associated with mortality rates) or spatial correlation (e.g., analyzing the degree to which spatial variations in temperature and precipitation determine distributions of vector-borne diseases such as malaria or dengue). Health data are generally available from ministries of health and weather data from national meteorological and hydrological services. However, the level of detail of the analysis and the robustness of the conclusions depend on the quality of the underlying data. It is often very difficult to obtain data that are reliable, of high spatial and temporal resolution, and covering the same time period and location for health, meteorology, and other determinants. Careful analysis and judgment is therefore required both to conduct and interpret sensitivity analysis. Caution is necessary when interpreting correlations based on low-resolution data or making inferences outside the location or data range in which the original analysis was conducted. As for the rest of the assessment, the aim is not to carry out a perfect analysis but to provide the most useful possible information for decision making. The ultimate judgment on the robustness or otherwise of the analysis should rest with those responsible for acting on it.

The final component of understanding the current situation with regard to climate-sensitive disease risks is an assessment of the capacity of existing health systems to manage these challenges. As climate change acts mainly through exacerbating existing current health problems rather than creating entirely novel ones, a wide range of policies and programs already exists to address the main relevant diseases. However, the continued high burden of health issues such as malnutrition, malaria, and diarrhea in many countries demonstrates that control programs are not currently adequate to address the current burden of climate-sensitive diseases. Even in the richest countries, shocks such as extreme weather events or disease epidemics can often overwhelm health services, at least temporarily. It is therefore critically important to review the capacity of the health sector in the wide sense—including not only the ministry of health, nongovernmental organizations, and private sector health actors but also other relevant actors such as emergency services, water and sanitation service providers, and local authorities. Representatives from all relevant organizations and institutions should be consulted to find out what is working well, what could be improved, and the capacity of the programs to address possible increases in the incidence or changes in the geographical range of the health outcomes of concern.

To assess the capacity and performance of current programs, the following kinds of questions are relevant (WHO 2013):

- What is the management structure for the program? This information is necessary to identify constraints and opportunities for modifying the program.

- What human and financial resources are available? Cataloguing these assets is important when planning additional policies and programs.

- How effective is the program in controlling the current health burden? Less-than-optimal effectiveness may be the result of limited human and financial resources, limited laboratory and material supplies, limited coordination among partners, administrative inefficiencies, and other factors. Addressing this question should include evaluations of overall effectiveness, particularly of programs serving vulnerable populations and regions.

- How robust are core health system functions (such as human resource planning, disease surveillance, and emergency preparedness and response) to extreme weather events? This is important for identifying existing gaps that may be exacerbated by a more variable climate.

- How might proposed changes to the program in the next five to ten years affect its ability to address relevant climate-sensitive health outcomes?

Many metrics can be used to measure the effectiveness of these programs, including trends in reductions in the number of injuries, illnesses, or deaths; coverage of appropriate geographical regions and vulnerable groups; and the extent to which planned changes are likely to increase the ability of the program or activity to further reduce current health burdens.

Health system capacity needs to be assessed not just as a static property. Resilience to climate change requires more than just well-resourced and well-organized health systems but also flexibility and adaptive management to take account of evolving challenges to health due to climate change and rapid changes in other determinants. Today few health policies and programs are tailored to take into consideration weather conditions and seasonal trends, current climate variability, and recent climate change. Most, such as surveillance and disease control programs, were designed assuming a stable climate. Furthermore, the institutions that administer these policies and programs may have structures that enhance or restrict their flexibility to integrate new information and respond to new conditions. Assessment of health system capacity should therefore look explicitly at the degree to which these systems can respond to a rapidly changing disease landscape.

CLINICAL CORRELATES 12.3   FOOD SECURITY AND VULNERABILITY PREPAREDNESS

Climate change is anticipated to have far-reaching impacts on food production and certain aspects of food quality (Batisti and Naylor 2009). Currently one-third of children in developing countries are malnourished by anthropometric standards. It is essential to use an evidence-based approach to understand why current systems are failing as researchers and policymakers attempt to stabilize food security. Central America has the highest prevalence of stunting (23 percent) and the lowest rates of improvement over the past twenty-five years, while nearby South America has lower levels of stunting and the highest rates of improvement despite economic stagnation in both regions (Bryce et al. 2008). A recent *Lancet* series analyzes how and why nutrition programs fail and reports that some failures can be traced to a lack of political commitment, while others can be traced to failure to support programs that have evidence-based results (Bryce et al. 2008). What public health professionals and clinicians can learn from this is that malnutrition is knowable and treatable and that with proper programs, we have the tools to address the issue. Clinicians must serve as spokespersons in their local political arena to advocate for evidence-based nutrition programs.

Evidence-based approaches should be used to assess and address the health impacts of food security among vulnerable populations.

Understanding Future Impacts on Health

The next stage is to consider how changing climate conditions may be expected to alter the incidence and geographical range of climate-sensitive health outcomes. Over the extended time periods that characterize climate change, other important health determinants will also be altering significantly, which may act against, reinforce, or otherwise interact with climate effects. These interactions will vary in both their importance and predictability.

For example, climate scientists have comparatively high confidence that climate change will continue to increase the frequency and intensity of extreme high temperatures in summer. There is also a long-term trend toward urbanization, and aging populations in most of the world. Taken together, there is a clear indication that the expanding megacities should strengthen early warning, preparedness, and response for the health effects of heat waves, with a particular focus on older populations, who tend to be the most vulnerable. In contrast, climate models indicate a general tendency toward increased variation in rainfall, but there is much less consistency in projections of changing patterns of floods or droughts for particular regions or localities. Local factors such as land use, flood defenses, and the quality of infrastructure also exert a strong effect on whether changes in precipitation are translated into dangerous floods or drought. This is not to say that events that are uncertain should be ignored; on the contrary, decision makers in the health and related sectors will instead need to ensure sufficient spare capacity, or flexibility, to be able to cope with the range of possible future conditions.

Either quantitative or qualitative methods, or a combination of the two, may be used to assess future risks depending on available data and the nature of the issue. Quantitative approaches are generally more useful in terms of data and analytical requirements and may be more appropriate when the causal pathway between the climate factors and health outcomes is simpler and better understood. For example, some assessments have combined information on projected changes in the distribution of daily temperatures from climate models; the observed relationship between the variations in daily temperature and daily mortality rates of different age groups; and from time series studies, with projected changes in the age distribution of populations over the coming few decades, in order to project the potential impact of climate change on heat-attributable mortality in specific cities.

The advantages of this method are that it can take into account both the size of the underlying burden of disease and the size of the proportional change. It can also be used to produce an aggregate estimate of the effect of climate change across a wide range of impact pathways and provide some indication of the relative importance of different health impacts (e.g., whether changes in flood frequency may be more or less of a health problem than increasing vector-borne disease).

In other cases, qualitative methods may be preferable, either because of lack of data on which to base a quantitative assessment or because the causal chain between climate and the health outcomes is more diverse and complex. For example, qualitative methods were used to identify the range of health determinants and exposures sensitive to climate change and imagine the possible kinds of future health impacts that could develop over the coming twenty years in Tashkent, Uzbekistan (WHO 2013). In addition to the projected changes in climate, the exercise identified trends in key determinants, including increased proportions of the population under age fourteen and over fifty-five, migratory pressures into urban areas, and increased traffic volume and industrial and commercial activity. These are expected to lead to:

- Increased emissions of greenhouse gases and particulates and higher levels of ground-level ozone, contributing to climate change and lowering local air quality with associated increases in respiratory and cardiac disease

- Greater production of solid waste and higher demands on water and solid waste infrastructure, compromising the quality and quantity of the water supply, with associated risks of water-borne disease

- Reductions in agricultural land under production, lowering capacity to produce local foods, particularly fruits, vegetables, and grains that sustain a healthy diet

- Warmer summer temperatures increasing energy demand for air-conditioning

Even without a full quantitative analysis, this exercise helped local planners understand the specific pressures that climate change may place on the health systems and the need for both general protection measures such as the planned rollout of universal health insurance and more specific interventions, such as monitoring and management of air quality.

One aspect that is particularly important to consider in assessing future risks is the time period of the assessment. In practice, there is usually a trade-off between the kinds of information that are available from climate models (which are better at predicting interdecadal trends rather than year-to-year variation), projections of socioeconomic determinants (which tend to be much more accurate in the short rather than the long term), and the time horizon of policymakers, which is rarely beyond a few years into the future. Despite these constraints, the assessment should aim as far as possible to cover the period over which decisions will take effect. For example, if one goal of the assessment is to determine the siting and standards for health care infrastructure, then it is appropriate to consider climate risks over the likely lifetime of the buildings (i.e., several decades). In contrast, when considering issues such as the deployment of vector control interventions, where control programs can be adjusted relatively quickly, a shorter time period may be appropriate.

Identifying and Prioritizing Health Adaptation Measures

This part of the assessment discusses how to identify changes to current policies and programs in order to address the risks that have been identified in the earlier stages of the assessment. This stage in particular requires the leadership of health policymakers and practitioners who are most directly involved in implementation.

As for all of the assessment, adaptation measures for climate change need to be placed in a wider context. It is important to recognize that some of the most important measures that will protect health from climate change are general and include poverty alleviation and greater and more equitable access to all preventative and curative health services. At the same time, climate change poses new challenges, and alters the nature of existing ones. For example, increasing temperatures lead not only to more frequent heat waves but to extremes that are beyond the range of historical experience for particular locations, such as the European heat wave of 2003 (Beniston and Diaz 2004; Stott, Stone, and Allen 2004). It is therefore necessary to build forward-looking control programs that are also flexible in the face of changing conditions. The added value of a vulnerability and adaptation assessment is that it provides direction on the specific changes that need to be made to cope with climate risks.

The diversity of links between climate and health presents a challenge in identifying adaptation options. In contrast to individual diseases or other specific threats, addressing the health risks of climate change requires a range of interventions; there is no vaccine for the health impacts of climate change. It can therefore be helpful to structure the different areas in which action is needed to respond to this challenge. For example, African ministries of health and of environment have together identified and endorsed a set of functions that need to be strengthened in order to increase health resilience. These effectively serve as the headings under which specific adaptation measures can be identified. While there is no specific and definitive approach, in recent years, a range of policy processes and experience from pilot projects have started to converge on a similar set of headings. Figure 12.2 shows a set of proposed areas of intervention, based on this emerging experience.

These broad headings can help to ensure that the response is sufficiently comprehensive. Under each heading, however, it is necessary to identify more specific actions to take. The best approach may be to begin by generating a list of all potential choices without regard to technical feasibility, cost, or other limiting criteria (Ebi and Burton 2008). This theoretical range of choice (White 1961) includes currently implemented interventions, new or untried interventions, and other interventions that are theoretically possible.

The next step is to evaluate the identified policies and programs to determine which measures are practical for a particular situation within existing technological, financial, and human capital constraints. This step generates a list of policies and programs from which policymakers and

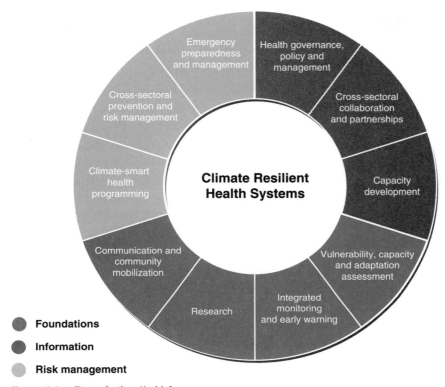

Figure 12.2 Climate Resilient Health Systems

Source: US Global Change Research Program. Available at http://www.globalchange.gov/

decision makers can choose. Criteria that can be used to determine which choices are practical include the following:

- *Technical feasibility.* Is the choice technically viable and available? For example, although a possible program to address potential changes in the geographical range of malaria is vaccination, this option is not currently available.

- *Operationally feasibility.* Does the health system have an adequate workforce, sustainable financial resources, service delivery mechanisms, and technical knowledge and capacity to deliver the interventions or programs?

- *Degree of effectiveness.* How effective is the proposed policy or program in reducing the incidence of the adverse health outcome? For example, not all malaria prophylactics are effective in all regions because of the development of drug resistance.

- *Economic efficiency.* How costly is the policy or program in relation to the expected benefits, and who would be expected to bear the cost?

+ *Environmental, social, and legal acceptability.* Does the proposed policy or program have environmental consequences that are unacceptable, contravene current regulations, or likely to conflict with the laws and social customs of the affected population?

Because resources are always limited, it is important to prioritize interventions that should bring the greatest benefits to health and health equity. This needs to involve relevant stakeholders and typically involve at least consideration, and ideally analysis, of the significance of the health issue being addressed, benefits and effectiveness, costs, and feasibility. Costs should be compared not only relative to current program expenditures, but against the costs of inaction: the health damages and costs to health services that can be expected if no action is taken. It is often possible to identify "no-regrets" interventions: those that will bring health benefits regardless of the specific climate scenario that eventually occurs in a location.

Finally, it is important to recognize that climate change adaptation and greenhouse gas mitigation policies implemented in other sectors can also present risks or opportunities for health. In many countries, for example, increased water stress, partly attributable to climate change, is stimulating greater use of treated wastewater in the agriculture sector, presenting risks of chemical and biological contamination in agricultural produce. In Jordan, one of the main components of its national health adaptation strategy and plan is to manage the potential human health risks arising from these exposures. In contrast, many policies for reducing greenhouse gas emissions, such as transitioning to cleaner energy sources to generate electricity, or more sustainable modes of transport, present opportunities for major health gains (Haines, McMichael et al. 2009). In these cases, the task of health actors is to assess the health implications of these policies and ensure that the health implications are appropriately valued in the decision-making process, that is, promoting choices that will bring the greatest health, as well as environmental benefits.

Integration, Implementation, and Iteration

The main purpose of the vulnerability and adaptation process is to identify effective adaptation options to protect health. However, these will rarely be stand-alone interventions; instead they will constitute the health component of the broader effort to address climate change risks across different sectors and at the same time serve to ensure climate resilience in health programming. It is therefore very important that both the development of such assessments and any implementation of the resulting recommendations are fully integrated into these broader processes.

Many countries have developed overall strategies and established intersectoral policy mechanisms for adaptation to climate change. The way in which these are translated into programs varies among countries. For example, the least developed countries have developed national adaptation programs of action (NAPAs) to meet the most urgent and immediate needs for adaptation, with support through the UN Framework Convention on Climate Change. While these are important, they address only some of the challenges posed by climate change, and in most cases the coverage of health challenges and proposed health interventions has been relatively weak (Manga et al. 2010). There is an important opportunity to improve this situation through national adaptation plans now being developed under the UNFCCC. These move on from the more immediate and project-based approach of the NAPAs, taking a longer-term view, and aim to mainstream climate change risks into the programs of the various affected sectors. Ministries of health are now working with their counterparts from ministries of the environment to develop the health components of national adaptation plans, in many cases with the support and guidance of WHO (2013). In this context, a high-quality vulnerability and adaptation assessment for health serves the crucial role of providing comprehensive, relevant, and evidence-based guidance on the risks and the interventions that should be addressed within the national adaptation plans.

The assessments also serve an equivalent function in programming for health and health-determining sectors. Most countries have strategic health plans for five or more years into the future, and in this case, assessments inform the mainstreaming of climate risks into health planning. In Nepal, for example, the government is developing a national strategy and plan of action on health adaptation to climate change, at the same time bringing together their various policies on water, sanitation and hygiene into a One-WASH policy. They have commissioned a health vulnerability and adaptation assessment to describe the full range of expected health risks, while at the same time having a particular focus on the challenges that climate change is expected to present to health through the water and sanitation pathway, including drying of water sources, disruption of water and sanitation infrastructure, and resulting risks of diarrheal disease. The assessment is therefore the cornerstone of both the overall health response and a means to identify specific interventions, such as climate-resilient water safety plans, that should help ensure Nepal's continued progress in reducing the burden of diarrheal disease, despite the new challenges of climate change. Integration into these processes also helps to mobilize resources from multiple sources, including funds for climate change adaptation, core health programs, and investment in health-determining sectors such as water and sanitation or food and nutrition security. This mutual alignment also reduces duplication and improves efficiency.

One particular feature of the health response to climate change is the need to iteratively revise and develop the assessment over time. The links between climate and health are very real, but they are also complex, subject to considerable uncertainty and alteration as other modulating factors change. Climate change and health is also a relatively new and fast-moving field, with improving methods and expanding experiences. Vulnerability and adaptation assessments should therefore be periodically revisited, in line with the policy cycle—for example, being updated in time to inform each revision of a national adaptation plan or health strategy. Monitoring and evaluation are critical to this iterative approach, requiring the identification and long-term measurement of indicators that allow tracking of hazards, risk factors, adaptation measures, and eventual health outcomes and that their relationships be reassessed over time (English, Sinclair et al. 2009).

CLINICAL CORRELATES 12.4   "NO REGRETS" FOR SMALL-SCALE FARMING

Expansion of small-scale farming is one way to bring resilience into the agricultural sector. Industrial farming is an energy-intense way to provide nutrition because growers rely on external inputs such as water, light, and pesticides to suit the needs of the crops. These crops are often transported long distances to reach consumers. Small-scale farmers tend to sow crops that grow naturally in the local environment and therefore require less energy-intense external inputs. Industrial farms also tend to grow few crop varieties, thus limiting the nutritional variation in our diets and the biodiversity of the foods we consume. Small-scale farming does the opposite: it incorporates resilience into its design by maintaining a genetically diverse seed bank. For example, Seeds of Change, an organization based in Santa Fe, New Mexico, grows over a thousand varieties of food plants on land originally farmed by the indigenous Tewa people. The organization explicitly propagates unusual varieties in order to maintain genetic diversity in the seed bank and preserve the ability to select specific seeds for seasonal propagation that are best adapted to climate conditions at a given time.

Thus, small-scale farming decreases demand for water, fuel, and agrochemicals and safeguards the future of our food supply by maintaining seed diversity. Indirect benefits of small-scale farming include strengthening of the local economy, as well as improving access to fresh and healthy food sources. This is an example of a "no-regrets" strategy that would bring health and environmental benefits irrespective of how the climate changes in the future.

Small-scale farming is an example of a no-regrets initiative that has a positive impact on health in the present while at the same time builds resilience for the future.

Conclusion

All vulnerability and adaptation assessments share a common goal: to better understand current and future health risks from climate variability and climate change and to guide policies and programs to ensure that public health is protected. Beyond that commonality, all assessments are different, shaped by the nature of the climate hazard and the resulting health risks in diverse locations, the varying socioeconomic circumstances of the exposed populations, and the differing capacity of systems to protect their health.

For this reason, guidance on vulnerability and adaptation assessments outlines the main steps of a process to be followed rather than a highly directive and specific set of instructions or checklists. Health vulnerability and adaptation assessments are also in their infancy, and the greatest progress that is being made in this field is through learning by doing as they are carried out across a diverse range of settings. Despite this, lessons are already beginning to emerge from both the methodological development and the early experiences of their application.

First, connection to stakeholders and their ownership of the process is critical. The best assessments are carried out under the direction of and in consultation with the decision makers who will be expected to use the results. This ensures that the assessment stays relevant, facilitates access to data and expertise, and provides constant feedback on the type and standard of evidence that will be sufficient to influence decisions. Stakeholders are much more likely to act on the results of an assessment if they have participated in its production rather than having it delivered to them after it has been completed.

Second, data and information are essential. For this reason, many countries are selecting disease surveillance as the top-priority intervention in their national adaptation plans for health. Strengthening disease surveillance systems and connecting them to meteorological and other environmental information can meet the immediate need of targeting control measures, allow the development of early warning systems, and lay the foundation for the sustained monitoring that will track long-term success as well as improve future vulnerability and adaptation assessments.

Third, the link to active programs to support implementation is vitally important. Assessments are least useful when they are stand-alone academic exercises and most useful when designed from the outset as a component of an overall program that can mobilize resources to carry out interventions and establish monitoring systems to track success.

The risks of climate change provide an opportunity and a challenge to the health sector to demonstrate leadership in protecting vulnerable populations, through its own actions and its collaboration with others. Vulnerability and adaptation assessments are a fundamental contribution to that task.

DISCUSSION QUESTIONS

1. List the broad categories of climate-related health risks that are important to consider, as well as the important nonclimate factors. Of these, which do you think are most applicable to your community? Your region? Your country?

2. What should the starting point for a vulnerability and adaptation assessment be? What are the ways in which this information can be accessed and documented?

3. It is important to recognize that climate change adaptation and greenhouse gas mitigation policies implemented in other sectors can also present with risks and opportunities for health. Find and discuss an instance in which this might occur and offer a possible solution.

KEY TERM

Health vulnerability and adaptation assessment: Allows countries to assess which populations are most vulnerable to different kinds of health effects, identify weaknesses in the systems that should protect them, and specify interventions to respond.

References

Balbus, J. M., and C. Malina. 2009. "Identifying Vulnerable Subpopulations for Climate Change Health Effects in the United States." *Journal of Occupational and Environmental Medicine* 51(1):33–37.

Batisti, D. S., and R. L. Naylor. 2009. "Historical Warnings of Future Food Insecurity with Unprecedented Seasonal Heat." *Science* 323:240–44.

Beniston, M., and H. F. Diaz. 2004. "The 2003 Heat Wave as an Example of Summers in a Greenhouse Climate? Observations and Climate Model Simulations for Basel, Switzerland." *Global and Planetary Change* 44(1–4):3–81.

Brands, C. B., R. H. Hernandez, A. Stenberg, G. Carnes, J. Ellen, M. Epstein, and T. Strouse. 2013. "Complete Self-Sufficiency Planning: Designing and Building Disaster-Ready Hospitals." *Southern Medical Journal* 106(1):63–68.

Bryce, J., D. Coitinho, I. Darnton-Hill, D. Pelletier, and P. Pinstrup-Andersen. 2008. "Maternal and Child Undernutrition: Effective Action at National Level." *Lancet* 371:510–26.

Ebi, K., and I. Burton 2008. "Identifying Practical Adaptation Options: An Approach to Address Climate Change-Related Health Risks." *Environmental Science and Policy* 11:359–69.

English, P. B., A. H. Sinclair, Z. Ross, H. Anderson, V. Boothe, C. Davis, K. Ebi, et al. 2009. "Environmental Health Indicators of Climate Change for the United States: Findings from the State Environmental Health Indicator Collaborative." *Environmental Health Perspectives* 117:1673–81.

Haines, A., A. J. McMichael, K. R. Smith, I. Roberts, J. Woodcock, A. Markandya, B. G. Armstrong, et al. 2009. "Public Health Benefits of Strategies to Reduce Greenhouse-Gas Emissions: Overview and Implications for Policy Makers." *Lancet* 37:2104–14.

Intergovernmental Panel on Climate Change. 2013. *Working Group I Contribution to the Fifth Assessment Report of the Intergovernmental Panel on Climate Change: Climate Change 2013: The Physical Science Basis: Summary for Policymakers.* Geneva: IPCC Secretariat.

Llewellyn, L. E. 2010. "Revisiting the Association between Sea Surface Temperature and the Epidemiology of Fish Poisoning in the South Pacific: Reassessing the Link between Ciguatera and Climate Change." *Toxicon* 56:691–97.

Manga, L., M. Bagayoko, T. Meredith, and M. Neira. 2010. "Overview of Health Considerations within National Adaptation Programs of Action for Climate Change in Least Developed Countries and Small Island States." World Health Organization. http://www.who.int/phe/Health_in_NAPAs_final.pdf

McMichael, A., R. Woodruff, P. Whetton, K. J. Hennessy, N. Nicholls, and S. Hales. 2003. *Human Health and Climate Change in Oceania: A Risk Assessment.* Canberra, Commonwealth of Australia.

"Resources for Speakers on Global Issues: Refugees." n.d. http://www.un.org/en/globalissues/briefingpapers/refugees/index.shtml

Sachs, J. 2007. "Climate Change Refugees." *Scientific American* 296 (May 20).

Stott, P. A., D. A. Stone, and M. R. Allen. 2004. "Human Contribution to the European Heatwave of 2003." *Nature* 432:610–14.

White, G. F. 1961. "The Choice of Use in Resource Management." *Natural Resources Journal* 1(1):23–40.

World Health Organization. 2009a. *Gender, Climate Change and Health.* Geneva: World Health Organization.

World Health Organization. 2009b. *Protecting Health from Climate Change: Connecting Science, Policy and People.* Geneva: World Health Organization.

World Health Organization. 2013. *Protecting Health from Climate Change: Vulnerability and Adaptation Assessment.* Geneva: World Health Organization.

World Meteorological Organization/World Health Organization. 2012. *Atlas of Health and Climate.* Geneva: World Meteorological Organization.

CHAPTER 13

CLIMATE CHANGE HEALTH IMPACT PROJECTIONS

Looking into the Future

Jeremy Hess

The potential adverse health impacts of climate change have been a topic of discussion ever since Arrhrenius (1896) broached the question of whether the Earth would warm as a result of fossil fuel combustion in 1896. Yet up through 1991, when Longstreth penned the first modern commentary on the topic in the health literature, the concerns were qualitative, as our understanding of the relationships between atmospheric processes and human health impacts was too limited to quantify likely impacts and was primarily expressed in the form of cautionary narratives rather than testable propositions. Our ability to conceptually model the possible impacts still far outpaced our ability to model the impacts mathematically.

During the 1990s, the field of environmental health made significant progress toward quantifying the likely health impacts of environmental changes at a range of scales. In its broadest sense, this process is termed *health impact assessment* (also *health risk assessment*), and the first consensus statement regarding how such estimates should be made was published in 1999 (European Centre for Health Policy 1999). Generally such assessments are aimed at clarifying and, where possible, improving the health impacts of decisions made outside the health sector using a mix of quantitative and qualitative methods (Lock 2000), though the methods have continued to evolve in recent years.

The methodological advances that helped advance the science of health impact assessments spurred hopes that similar methods might be used to quantify climate

KEY CONCEPTS

- **Climate change health impact projections are modeled, scenario-based estimates of the risks of adverse health impacts associated with climatic change.**

- **As models, health impact projections are simplifications of real-world processes.**

- **Climate change health impact projections are not predictions but projections—estimates of likely impacts associated with a stipulated set of conditions, typically scenarios of greenhouse gas emissions.**

- **Climate change health impact projections are similar to other modeling efforts in environmental health, including health impact assessment, which use scenarios and known exposure-outcome associations to project human health impacts.**

KEY CONCEPTS (*CONTINUED*)

- Health impact projections use retrospectively derived exposure-outcome associations from epidemiological studies. Some associations are better studied than others.

- Some exposure-outcome pathways are relatively direct (e.g., heat and heat-related illness) while others are less so (e.g., rainfall patterns, forage abundance, rodent population size, and the zoonosis hantavirus pulmonary syndrome). Generally more direct pathways are easier to model.

- It is important to be clear what projected health impacts of climate change are being compared to, whether adaptation has been included, and how.

- Climate change health impact projection science is relatively young and is likely to grow and change significantly in coming decades.

change health impacts. At the same time, while many public health experts felt that the most severe climate change health impacts were still likely decades away, there was growing concern that they would become the dominant global health challenge of the twenty-first century (Chan 2007). Practitioners also expressed a need for **projections** that could be used in comparative risk assessments (Campbell-Lendrum and Woodruff 2006), wherein estimates of health impacts attributable to various exposures can be compared across settings to help prioritize policies and other public health interventions.

Early on it was not clear that epidemiology was yet up to the task. In 2001, McMichael outlined three challenges for epidemiology in relation to climate change: retrospective analyses of associations between climate-sensitive environmental exposures and health outcomes, surveillance for current public health impacts highly likely to be attributable to climate change, and scenario-based health risk assessments of projected climate change health impacts. He was careful to note the interplay between the first priority, retrospective analyses to derive exposure-outcome associations, and the third, health impact projection, as projections are predicated on the ability to quantify these relationships. He also noted that the third task, conducting scenario-based health risk assessments, was perhaps the least familiar of the three.

In the years that followed, the number of papers devoted to each steadily increased, and several health impact projections were published, notably a global projection done by McMichael and colleagues at the World Health Organization (McMichael, Campbell-Lendrum et al. 2004). The requirements for pursuing climate change health impact projections—topical fluency, access to global circulation model outputs to use as exposure data, access to relevant exposure-outcome associations, and fluency with the modeling and mapping approaches required to produce projections—are now relatively common in many public health settings. It appears that the field is likely poised on the edge of a significant expansion in projection efforts, fueled partly out of a recognized need to perform quantitative risk assessment and partly out of the increasingly available skills and inputs.

Despite this, there are no guides to conducting climate change health impact projections and no expert consensus on the approaches that should be used, how to address various methodological considerations, how to uniformly express disease burdens, and whether and how to include adaptation into the projections. This chapter is an introduction to these issues and a modest attempt to begin filling that gap. After a conceptual overview of climate change health impact projections and related topics, I review the different approaches that have been used, consider important concerns identified to date, and consider frontiers in conducting and using climate change health impact projections.

A Conceptual Overview of Climate Change Health Impact Projections

At base, a climate change health impact projection is a modeled, scenario-based estimate of the risks of adverse health impacts associated with climatic change. While not all climate change health impacts will necessarily be adverse, salutary changes are of less concern in preparedness and planning efforts, and adverse impacts tend to be the focus of health impact projection studies. Climate change health impact projections may focus on determinants of adverse health impacts (the distribution of exposures that serve as risk factors in the causal pathway) or extend the analysis to the outcomes themselves (Confalonieri and Menne 2007); either way, they aim to quantify components of the causal pathway linking environmental variables and human health impacts on a population basis. The process is outlined in figure 13.1.

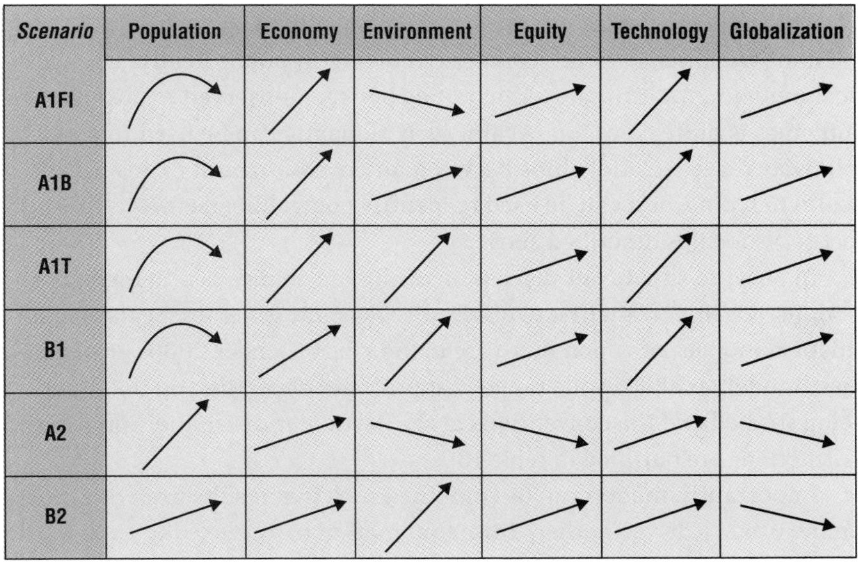

Scenario	Population	Economy	Environment	Equity	Technology	Globalization
A1FI						
A1B						
A1T						
B1						
A2						
B2						

Figure 13.1   The General Approach to Climate Change Health Impact Projection

The remainder of this section is devoted to unpacking the definition to gain additional insights into the process, starting with the fundamental nature of the approach: modeling.

Modeling

Models are representations that "[mimic] relevant features of the situation being studied" (Bender 2000, 1). Models, particularly mathematical models that use equations to represent either theoretical dynamics or observations, are central to scientific inquiry. They allow for characterization of systems and their components and for exploration of system behavior as various parameters are manipulated, including experimentation that may not be feasible for practical or ethical reasons.

Models are fundamental tools in studying climate change and its potential impacts. In particular, global circulation models (GCMs), complex mathematical models of the Earth's atmosphere and oceans that include many atmospheric and terrestrial layers divided up into thousands of three-dimensional gridded spaces, are used to study the likely environmental impacts of shifts in greenhouse gas emissions, such as changes in temperature, precipitation, and sea level. These changes can be used as health-relevant exposures themselves if there is a direct relationship between the exposure and health outcomes (e.g., ambient temperature and heat-related illness). They can also be used to generate indirect estimates of how health-relevant exposures may shift (e.g., warming, combined with changes in precipitation, can result in prolonged drought with potentially significant consequences for food supply and thus nutritional outcomes in certain regions).

Models of a different sort are also fundamental to public health. Modeling done by climate scientists is relatively rare in public health, but statistical modeling to estimate associations between observed exposures and outcomes is quite common. Again, such modeling can be used to describe relatively direct relationships between an environmental exposure and a health outcome, or it can be used to identify controlling factors in the indirect relationships described above.

In order to situate our discussion of climate change health impact projections, it is important first to briefly discuss some general aspects of mathematical models, of which there are many kinds (Bender 2000). In general, these models exhibit a wide range of approaches depending on the situation being studied and the conventions of the particular discipline. Some major distinctions are outlined in table 13.1.

Importantly, models can be combined such that results from one model can be used to drive another. This combination can be used to expand the scope (i.e., the range of factors modeled) or scale (i.e., spatial and temporal

Table 13.1   Some Simple Binary Classifications of Mathematical Models

Linear: Employ Linear Equations Exclusively	Nonlinear: Employ Nonlinear Equations or a Mix of the Two
Static (also equilibrium): Time invariant	Dynamic: Include an element of time
Discrete: Treat objects in the model separately	Continuous: Describe collective behavior of objects in model
Deterministic: Outputs depend entirely on prior conditions	Probabilistic: Include randomness using probability distributions
Deductive: Based on theory	Inductive: Based on empirical observations

dimensions) of the effort. In this sense climate change health impact projections are combination models, as they all include GCM projections of data from possible climate futures and modeled estimates of associations between environmental exposures and health outcomes.

While models can be powerful tools, they are by nature subject to a number of limitations, all of which ultimately undermine their validity to some degree. Perhaps most important, models are based either on historical observations or theory (though some theoretical models incorporate significant empirical elements). In the first case, models based on historical observations by definition cannot account for observations outside the historical data set on which they are based and thus are fundamentally inadequate for predicting, hedging against, and taking advantage of extreme and rare events (e.g., the "turkey problem"; Taleb 2012). In the second, theoretical models are relatively untested and therefore may not describe the systems under study as well as users would like. Another significant limitation to models is that as simplifications, they may misrepresent system behaviors deriving from factors that are not included among the model's components. While to an extent this concern can be addressed through sensitivity testing, there are fundamental uncertainties involved in modeling that are inherently difficult to characterize fully.

We move next to issues related to generating the GCM outputs used in health impact projections, then to considerations of exposure-outcome association modeling, after which we finally return to the topic of modeling climate-sensitive health impacts.

Modeling Climate Change Health Impacts

The Role of GCM Projections

In the climate change literature, the word *projections* has a very specific meaning. The Intergovernmental Panel on Climate Change (IPCC) defines *climate change projections* as the "response of the climate system to emission or concentration scenarios of greenhouse gases and aerosols, or radiative forcing scenarios, often based upon simulations by climate models" (Baede et al. 2007). Elaborating on this, the IPCC notes that "climate projections are distinguished from climate predictions in order to emphasise that climate projections depend upon the emission/concentration/radiative forcing scenario used, which are based on assumptions . . . that may or may not be realised, and are therefore subject to substantial uncertainty" (Baede et al. 2007). Predictions, in contrast, are attempts to generate best estimates of future states, usually starting with current conditions. Weather forecasts, for instance, are near- and medium-term predictions of the weather for a specified location. Predictions or forecasts are not dependent on scenarios (put differently, the scenarios used in predictions are invariant from present conditions apart from the mechanics of the processes being used in the prediction; the underlying drivers remain unchanged).

The Role of Scenarios

As the above paragraph makes clear, projections are based on **scenarios**, which are essentially alternate images or storylines for future states that include details relevant to the processes being projected. The scenarios used to project global climate change have been determined by the IPCC, which first released scenarios (named IS92) in 1992; in 1996, these scenarios were revisited with an updated knowledge base, and the IPCC Special Report on Emissions Scenarios (IPCC SRES) was published in 2000 (Nakicenovic and Swart 2000). As noted in the SRES Summary for Policymakers:

> Future greenhouse gas (GHG) emissions are the product of very complex dynamic systems, determined by driving forces such as demographic development, socio-economic development, and technological change. Their future evolution is highly uncertain. Scenarios are alternative images of how the future might unfold and are an appropriate tool with which to analyse how driving forces may influence future emission outcomes and to assess the associated uncertainties. (Intergovernmental Panel on Climate Change 2000, 4)

The SRES scenarios encapsulated storylines for global development and cooperation regarding climate change mitigation. They were categorized using a taxonomy and nomenclature, with scenario families being the largest class and the four families named A1, A2, B1, B2; scenario families were subdivided into groups, with group members having "similar demographic, societal, economic and technical-change storylines" (Baede et al. 2007).

The scenarios were representations of various development trajectories and were divided based on the degree of economic versus environmental focus (A scenario family versus B scenario family) and global versus regional development (1 scenario family versus 2 scenario family). From each group, one scenario was considered illustrative, or representative of the general storyline; these scenarios (the A1B, A2, B1, B2 scenarios from the SRES) were most commonly used in projection studies. The SRES scenarios were used to generate projections for the IPCC's Third and Fourth Assessment Reports.

More recently, the scenarios were updated again prior to the Fifth Assessment Report and reoriented to focus primarily on the radiative forcings (energy imbalances) driving climate change. The new scenarios are referred to as representative concentration pathways, and there are four: RCP8.5, RCP6, RCP4.5, and RCP2.6. The numbers identifying each of the RCPs refer to the magnitude of the energy imbalance (measured in watts per square meter[2]) in the scenario in the year 2100; the RCPs roughly correspond with year 2100 atmospheric carbon dioxide concentrations of about 490 parts per million (ppm), 650 ppm, 850 ppm, and 1,370 ppm, respectively (van Vuuren et al. 2011). In addition to quantifying forcing, the RCPs also quantify rates of emissions and concentrations of each of the major greenhouse gas concentrations. Data for each of the scenarios, which are meant to minimize duplication of modelers' efforts and facilitate interdisciplinary science, include baseline and historical emissions data and projected emissions and concentration data going forward to 2100, subdivided into cells measuring half a degree of latitude and longitude (Wayne 2013). The RCP scenarios are freely available for download.

Of note, the RCPs are being used to develop new, related pathways for global socioeconomic development, termed the shared socioeconomic pathways (SSPs), that can be used alongside the RCPs in impact research (O'Neill et al. 2014). (For additional information on the SSPs and their relevance to health impacts projections, see Ebi et al. 2014.)

It is important to note that the scenarios used to project climate change health impacts were in fact devised to provide inputs into GCMs, which then project changes in the climate. These scenarios, particularly the RCP scenarios, are entirely silent in regard to changes over time in the many factors and social systems known to affect population health, commonly called as the social determinants of health (Marmot and Wilkinson 2009), though the SSPs are expected to fill this gap. Unless explicitly stated, in projections using the RCPs, these factors have typically not been addressed in projections of climate change health impacts, and if they are addressed, it is typically through models of the pathway between climate-related exposure and health outcome.

Characterization of Projected Exposures

The exposures of interest in climate change health impact projections are taken from GCM projections. There are a host of issues related to model outputs that are relevant for generating estimates of these exposures, from which GCMs or ensemble GCM outputs are used, whether outputs are scaled down from their original relatively coarse resolution to a finer resolution more applicable for health impacts modeling and what downscaling approaches are used. The issues attending these questions are complex and have been reviewed extensively in the literature. A thorough discussion is beyond the scope of this chapter but Carbone (2014) has conducted an excellent recent review.

Another issue that deserves more attention here is the question of how exposures are quantified for health impact modeling once these other concerns have been addressed. Most climate change health impact projections to date have used what is commonly termed the delta method, which refers to the exposure that is being projected and how it was derived. Gosling, McGregor, and Lowe (2009) refer to the application of the delta method to projection of health impacts from changes in temperature associated with climate change, highlighting that the exposure is a change in mean temperature:

> A mean climate warming [is applied] to the observed present-day climate to create a temperature projection time series that can be applied to the observed present temperature-mortality relationship. The degree of climate warming is calculated as the difference between the future period and present period mean temperatures, as estimated by climate models, to give a temperature anomaly. (Gosling et al. 2009, 32)

The term *delta method* was coined by Déqué (2007), and a thorough analysis of many studies using the delta method was done by Gosling McGregor, and Paldy in 2007. Gosling and colleagues developed a modified delta method in which projected changes in both mean temperature and temperature variability are included in the exposure of future populations and demonstrated that the combination of these two shifts is likely to result in greater heat-related mortality compared with projections of increased mean temperature alone.

The exposure-outcome associations used in the delta method (and modified approaches) are modeled inputs, commonly developed from retrospective analyses using various regression techniques (Bender 2009). Poisson regression models, used to generate estimates of relative risks associated with various exposures (Frome and Checkoway 1985), are particularly common in environmental health, though a number of other approaches may be more appropriate depending on the nature of the exposure and the outcome and the stipulated relationship between the two. For example, the approaches used to study the relationship between temperature and associated health outcomes include descriptive, case control, case only, case crossover, time series, spatial, synoptic, and others (Huang et al. 2011). Basu and Samet (2002) have suggested that case crossover and time series are the most appropriate designs for studying heat-health relationships because of the short duration of the exposure and the brief lag between exposure and outcome.

Choosing and Quantifying Exposure-Outcome Associations

These projections focus on various path-dependent factors known or hypothesized to affect the potential for human health impacts from climate change. A wide array of health impacts are known to be climate sensitive, ranging from injuries like blunt and penetrating trauma commonly experienced in extreme weather events, to many vector-borne and zoonotic diseases, to food-borne and waterborne illnesses, to depression and other mental health concerns (Frumkin et al. 2008). In many cases, the pathways leading from environmental conditions to human exposure to actual morbidity and mortality are remarkably complex (Portier et al. 2010). Consequently, the easiest pathways to model are the ones that are most direct (i.e., the shortest and least complex causal pathways) and the most consistent across populations. Cholera's sensitivity to weather and climate variability is well established, for instance, but the impacts of these varying exposures are mediated by a wide range of factors from governance to socioeconomic status to season to climatic variability and tend to vary markedly by setting (Murray, McBean, and Bhatt 2012).

Other considerations are important as well, such as how well exposures can be characterized in both the retrospective analyses and the GCM projections. For instance, levels of airborne pollutants such as particulate matter can be measured at monitoring stations, and these measurements can serve as proxies for population-level exposure to the same species at a larger spatial scale with some degree of confidence (Miller et al. 2007). Similarly, temperature measured at one location is frequently used as a proxy for temperature exposure across a larger area (Green et al. 2010). In both cases, the assumption of scalability can facilitate health impact projection, though it is important to recognize that this simplification can come at a cost.

Assumptions regarding extrapolation of exposure may mask significant variability in actual exposures at the individual level, obscuring dynamics that may be significant for public health action (see, for example, Jerrett et al. 2005 for a discussion related to particulate air pollution, and Harlan et al. 2013 for a discussion related to heat.)

Despite this concern, acute heat illness serves as a good example of a direct and relatively consistent pathway, wherein the environmental condition of ambient warmth (e.g., maximum daily temperature) can be clearly correlated with a population health outcome (e.g., the incidence of emergency department visits for acute heat illnesses such as heat exhaustion and heat stroke). As populations can be acclimatized to different baseline levels of heat exposure, the relationship is not always consistent across different settings, though the overall relationship between temperature and heat illness tends to be similar even if specifics vary within a certain range (Ye et al. 2012). For this reason, heat-related health impacts are thus far the most commonly projected climate change health impact (Huang et al. 2011).

CLINICAL CORRELATES 13.1 PROJECTING HEALTH IMPACTS OF EXTREME WEATHER EVENTS

The ways through which extreme weather events affect human health are complex, interrelated, and context dependent. Therefore, creating accurate models to predict impacts of future events is difficult, a fact that may hinder robust disaster preparedness among medical service agencies. In the direct wake of extreme weather, the need for medical services to treat injury increases. Secondary impacts, including human displacement, infectious disease, and loss of shelter and clean water, soon follow. However, the extent to which a particular event may affect an area depends on many factors that include ecosystem characteristics, health infrastructure, demographics, and the wealth of that region ("A Bad Climate for Development" 2009). As models to predict impact of extreme weather events improve, the medical community must take these risks to life and longevity seriously and prepare accordingly.

Medical service agencies are an essential component of adaptive management and must prepare with imperfect information for climate change effects.

Comparisons and the Counterfactual

Climate change health impact projections commonly take a few different forms depending on what changes are projected into the future and, by implication, what referent is used in comparison. By definition, investigators include projected future climatic conditions in their models, but otherwise there is no consistent guidance regarding whether investigators should also project shifts in population demographics and sensitivity to the exposures being analyzed. For instance, since we can be most confident about the validity of recently observed relationships, should we restrict projections to recently derived exposure-outcome associations and apply them to present-day populations without attempting to include adaptation? Or since we are often projecting far into the future, should we project population differences in resilience (ability to resist the deforming impact of an exposure) when trying to determine health impacts?

These questions refer to counterfactuals, or hypothetical explorations of what might have happened if initial conditions had been as stipulated (Balke and Pearl 2011). Ultimately the individual investigator will be responsible for answering these questions, though the research community may come together to generate a consensus regarding these and other pressing questions (e.g., using the delphi method; Adler and Ziglio 1996) regarding climate change health impact projection methods.

When considering these issues, it is also important to note that many exposure-outcome associations used in climate change health impact projections are expressions of relative risk, for example, relative risk of mortality associated with one temperature relative to another during a specific period of time, or relative risk of mortality associated with an extreme weather event compared with mortality risk during a nonevent baseline period. In these instances, the counterfactual is a population without the exposure of interest. However, in climate change health impact projections, this assumption generally does not hold, as the exposure develops over a sufficiently long period that other, significant changes in the population, many of which may affect the exposure-outcome association, will have occurred.

This is an important limitation of static models, which project impacts at a particular point in time without allowing for dynamic consideration of important feedbacks. For instance, socioeconomic development is known to be a major driver of population health status, and vice versa. Climate change is expected to have adverse impacts on population health status and thus to impede development over time, but it is not clear whether it might be more strategic to invest in development generally or mitigate climate change to protect health in low- and middle-income countries. Preliminary work using dynamic modeling techniques suggests that investment in development is likely to have a higher return in the short and medium terms, though climate change mitigation will have a more significant impact on population health several decades hence (Tol, Ebi, and Yohe 2007).

Merging Data Streams in the Climate Change Health Impact Model

As noted, several approaches have been used to project health impacts associated with climate change, all of which use GCM outputs to generate estimates of future exposures. The approach used to link these outputs with health outputs must accommodate the nature of climate change health impacts, which are expected to be not only significant but also "nonlinear, region specific, and time dependent" (Chan et al. 1999, 330). Ideally, the projection modeling effort would accommodate these dynamics.

To date, however, the approach used to project health effects appears to have depended more on the usual approach in the investigator's discipline than on some of these other considerations. For instance, economists have tended to use economic models that estimate costs associated with climate change health impacts; in these models, which are typically inductive, nonlinear, continuous, and deterministic and can be dynamic or static, use health impacts as part of an overall estimating equation of damages to a local or world economy (Bosello, Roson, and Tol 2006).

Climate Change Health Impact Projections in the Health Literature

Because we are particularly interested in projections of specific health impacts, most of which have been done by public health scientists, I focus on this subset of climate change health impact projections. Perhaps twenty such projections have been published, and the number is growing rapidly. Many have focused on heat and associated impacts (Huang et al. 2011; Voorhees et al. 2011; Li, Horton, and Kinney 2013), though some have focused on air quality and respiratory disease (Gosling et al. 2009; Tagaris et al. 2009; Sheffield et al. 2011; Chang, Hao, and Sarnat 2014), some on heat and air quality (Knowlton et al. 2008), and a few on diarrheal disease (Kolstad and Johansson 2011), nutrition (Lloyd, Kovats, and Chalabi 2011), and infectious diseases (Slater and Michael 2012; Zhang et al. 2012; Ogden et al. 2014). A handful of studies have used projections not only for the purpose of generating estimates of disease burdens but as a means to the end of exploring uncertainty resulting from methodological choices and data constraints and thereby to clarify further research priorities (Kolstad and Johansson 2011; Wu et al. 2014).

While approaches have varied, generally these investigators used linear, deterministic, static models calibrated to a particular future point in time to generate their estimates. Their models are empirical, in the sense that they involve higher-order abstractions from observed relationships that are simplified using general equations and assumptions regarding the future scenarios being projected. They all use some form of the delta method, though differences between future and present-day temperature are not necessarily the exposures that are projected; sometimes temperature shifts are used to drive air quality changes, and sometimes other exposures, such as changes in relative humidity, drive other ecological changes relevant to health, such as the relative abundance of ticks that can transmit Lyme disease (Ogden et al. 2014).

Investigators modeling climate change health impacts must answer a number of questions in the course of their modeling efforts, including:

- What are the model's scope and scale?
- What populations will be included? Will the analysis be stratified?
- What exposure factors will be included in the response function?
- How will impacts be expressed?
- Will the model include adaptation? If so, how?
- How will uncertainty be considered and assessed?

To date, analysts have taken a wide range of approaches to these considerations. This has limited the comparability of results, even for the same general exposures and health outcomes (Huang et al. 2011). Clarification of best practices regarding health impact projections, stratified by exposure and health outcome, will be an important next step in the evolution of climate change health impact projections science.

Work that better clarifies the relationships between environmental exposures and health impacts, McMichael's first task, will also be important to improving the utility of climate change health impact projections. Recent work has identified this as one of the primary sources of uncertainty in health impact projections (Kolstad and Johansson 2011; Wu et al. 2014). Because of the complexity of many exposure-outcome pathways, their diversity across settings, and our incomplete understanding of the specific dynamics in many cases, many pathways are oversimplifications. The equations used to summarize observed relationships, particularly in areas that are not well studied, are subject to confounding and other potential sources of bias and should be viewed as such. Moreover, unless the underlying pathways have been extensively researched, it is important to note that the relationships described in exposure-outcome pathways may not always be explicitly causal. Determining causality in environmental health is a difficult task that often requires various forms of evidence, including observational and experimental studies, and satisfies evidentiary criteria that can help distinguish correlation from causation (Hill 1965). In some cases, the exposure-outcome associations modeled in climate change health impact projections are, strictly speaking, correlations that are strongly suspected to represent causal relationships, an important caveat to keep in mind.

Characterization of Risk

Risk characterization is important because it funnels into risk communication, policymaking, and intervention prioritization. Climate change health impact projections have employed several approaches to characterizing risk and expressing its magnitude relative to other public health threats. Many studies express outcomes in terms of an increase in counts per unit time, for example, the number of excess deaths per day from a given exposure anticipated in a given setting at a given point in time assuming a particular emissions scenario. Some of these risk estimates are stratified, often by age or other demographic factors.

Some studies also characterize relative risks, for example, in comparison with population risk in some baseline period or in some other referent population. Some studies also explicitly link their risk estimates, for example, excess cases of acute asthma exacerbations due to elevated ozone concentrations that require a visit to the emergency department, to metrics such as disability adjusted life years (DALYs) that allow for comparative risk assessment (Longfield et al. 2013). Several investigators have recommended that DALYs are the appropriate metric for climate change health impact projections for this reason (Zhang, Bi, and Hiller 2007; Xun et al. 2009). One challenge with using DALYs, however, is that valuation metrics have not been assigned to all of the outcomes that may be of interest; another is that valuation is context dependent and heavily influenced by per capita incomes and other contextual factors. Despite these issues, the comparability that use of DALYs allows can confer significant advantage on studies that are able to employ this metric from a policymaking perspective.

Frontiers in Climate Change Health Impact Projection

While the future is fraught with uncertainty, we can speculate about potential innovations in the science of climate change health impact projections. Several developments are likely.

First, we are likely to see a continued expansion of climate change health impacts modeling as the techniques become more familiar, expertise in the public health community develops, and there is demand for such modeled impacts among a broader range of stakeholders. Related to this, it is likely that models will be integrated into planning efforts in certain jurisdictions in order to guide adaptation planning and that these models will be continuously updated using principles of adaptive management (Ebi 2011a, 2011b; Hess, McDowell, and Luber 2012), a framework that uses regularly updated models to facilitate management of complex systems subject with multiple stakeholders (Holling 1978; National Research Council 2004). Using climate change health impact projections in this way is likely to become more common as models become more adept at projecting medium-term impacts and can be revised as surveillance evidence accumulates.

Second, the range of projected health impacts is likely to broaden as we learn more about historical relationships between weather, climate variability, climate change, and health. This increased breadth will likely include health impacts that have not been projected previously, for example, nutritional impacts associated with drought and with ocean acidification, to name two relevant exposures, as well as projections of health impacts specific to new regions. We may also be able to project impacts related to weather extremes and to events with conditional probabilities, for example, failure of a sewage treatment plant in the setting of an extreme precipitation event or power outage during a severe heat wave.

Third, our projections will likely become more refined as we continue to deepen our understanding of factors affecting the central relationships we project. As we learn more about factors that amplify or blunt certain exposures, for example, how neighborhood microclimates may affect ambient temperatures at a granular level, and about factors that modify the effects of exposure in susceptible populations, such as air-conditioning prevalence and electricity prices, we will be able to make more refined projections that take these factors into account.

Fourth, we will likely see incorporation of alternative modeling techniques to characterize health impacts. These techniques may include approaches that accommodate dynamic factors and feedbacks within the systems being modeled or allow for more realistic characterization of novel scenarios through the development of virtual worlds populated with agents operating based on various predetermined principles. Incorporating novel approaches such as these will likely make it even more difficult to compare health impacts across studies, but will also likely improve the ability to approximate some relationships of interest.

Finally, as public health invests more heavily in climate change health impact projections and they are used more widely, it is likely that there will be additional efforts to clarify best practices regarding modeling choices. Such efforts are already underway in regard to modeling of the health cobenefits of climate change mitigation activities (Remais et al. 2014). Accommodating the wide range of exposures, health outcomes, and spatial and temporal scales at which projections are done will be challenging, but systematically addressing several central modeling issues could significantly clarify research priorities and improve the applicability of projections.

CLINICAL CORRELATES 13.2 CLINICAL PRACTICE AND ADAPTIVE MANAGEMENT

Clinicians are important stakeholders in adaptation planning and projective assessment. They are in a unique position to see the impacts of climate-sensitive diseases on a case-by-case basis and see in real time the outcomes of health-related climate mitigation policies. Therefore, clinicians must play an active role in surveillance, as well as in generating feedback to the health policy process. One application of this model is the detection and treatment of climate-sensitive infectious diseases. For example, Lyme disease, a tick-borne infection, is expanding its range due to changing environmental and climatic patterns. Clinicians practicing within known and newly expanding Lyme regions may choose to change their practice of testing and treating. Overtreatment results in misuse of antibiotics, whereas undertreatment can lead to disease complications. Local prevalence of Lyme is often unknown, and there are no currently accepted guidelines for when to treat suspected cases. Therefore, clinicians must feed back into the adaptive management system to provide public health and policymakers with data to support or refute wide-scale practice recommendations.

Clinicians are stakeholders in adaptation planning and must respond in an active way by analyzing their management practices and feeding this information back to the level of policymaking institutions.

Conclusion

In a relatively brief period, the public health community has moved from being limited to qualitative risk assessments of the health impacts of climate change to being able to quantify some likely impacts. These projections are made using global circulation models, emissions scenarios, and models linking environmental exposures and health impacts. To date, most projections made by public health scientists have used the delta method to project a relatively narrow set of impacts at fixed points in the future, and many have ignored complex issues related to adaptation and dynamic feedbacks in the systems being modeled. Those that have incorporated adaptation have used widely varying methods. Nevertheless, the projections to date have given us some sense of the order of magnitude of health impacts we might expect from climate change, and such modeling efforts are becoming more and more common, a trend that is likely to continue. In the future, it is likely that such modeling efforts will become more refined and will be applied to a wider range of settings and a broader suite of health impacts. An expert consensus regarding best practices may emerge.

DISCUSSION QUESTIONS

1. What three tasks did McMichael identify for the field of epidemiology in its effort to characterize the health impacts of climate change?

2. What is the difference between a prediction and a projection?

3. Why do we use models to project health impacts of climate change?

4. What are the main differences between the different types of scenarios that have been used to project climate change in global circulation models?

5. Name at least five different data streams that need to be merged to project climate change health impacts.

6. What factors can affect the validity of a climate change health impact projection?

7. What issues should one consider before applying climate change health impacts projected for one region to another geographical area?

8. List some of the ways in which risk is characterized and quantified in climate change health impact projections.

9. At the end of the chapter several frontiers in climate change health impact projection science are listed. Try to find an example of a recent study that illustrates how one or more of these frontiers has been pushed since this book was published.

KEY TERMS

Models: Models are representations that "[mimic] relevant features of the situation being studied" (Bender 2000).

Projections: Defined by the Intergovernmental Panel on Climate Change as the "response of the climate system to emission or concentration scenarios of greenhouse gases and aerosols, or radiative forcing scenarios, often based upon simulations by climate models" (Baede et al. 2007).

Scenarios: Alternate images or storylines for future states that include details relevant to the processes being projected.

References

Adler, M., and E. Ziglio 1996. *Gazing into the Oracle: The Delphi Method and Its Application to Social Policy and Public Health.* London: Jessica Kingsley.

Arrhenius, S. 1896. "On the Influence of Carbonic Acid in the Air upon the Temperature of the Ground." *Philosophical Magazine* 41:266.

"A Bad Climate for Development." 2009. *Economist,* September 17.

Baede, A., P. van der Linden, and A. Verbruggen. 2007. "Annex II: Glossary." *In Climate Change 2007: Synthesis Report,* edited by R. Pauchari and A. Reisinger, 76–99. Geneva: Intergovernmental Panel on Climate Change.

Balke, A., and J. Pearl 2011. "Probabilistic Evaluation of Counterfactual Queries." University of California, Department of Statistics Papers. http://escholarship .org/uc/item/6vh9k0cf

Basu, R., and J. M. Samet. 2002. "Relation between Elevated Ambient Temperature and Mortality: A Review of the Epidemiologic Evidence." *Epidemiologic Reviews* 24:190–202.

Bender, E. A. 2000. *An Introduction to Mathematical Modeling.* New York: Dover.

Bender, R. 2009. "Introduction to the Use of Regression Models in Epidemiology." *Methods in Molecular Biology* 471:179–95. doi:10.1007/1978–1001–59745–59416–59742_59749

Bosello, F., R. Roson, and R. Tol. 2006. "Economy-Wide Estimates of the Implications of Climate Change: Human Health." *Ecological Economics* 58:579–91.

Campbell-Lendrum, D., and R. Woodruff. 2006. "Comparative Risk Assessment of the Burden of Disease from Climate Change." *Environmental Health Perspectives* 114:1935–41.

Carbone, G. J. 2014. "Managing Climate Change Scenarios for Societal Impact Studies." *Physical Geography* 35:22–49.

Chan, M. 2007. "Climate Change and Health: Preparing for Unprecedented Challenges." Paper presented at the 2007 David E. Barmes Global Health Lecture, Bethesda, MD.

Chan, N. Y., K. L. Ebi, F. Smith, T. F. Wilson, and A. E. Smith. 1999. "An Integrated Assessment Framework for Climate Change and infectious Diseases." *Environmental Health Perspectives* 107:329–37.

Chang, H. H., H. Hao, and S. E. Sarnat. 2014. "A Statistical Modeling Framework for Projecting Future Ambient Ozone and Its Health Impact due to Climate Change." *Atmospheric Environment* 89:290–97.

Confalonieri, U., and B. Menne. 2007. "Human Health." In *Climate Change 2007: Impacts, Adaptation and Vulnerability. Contribution of Working Group II to the Fourth Assessment Report of the Intergovernmental Panel on Climate Change,* edited by M. L. Parry, O. F. Canziani, J. P. Palutikof, P. J. Van der Linden, and C. E. Hanson, 391–431. Cambridge: Cambridge University Press.

Déqué, M. 2007. "Frequency of Precipitation and Temperature Extremes over France in an Anthropogenic Scenario: Model Results and Statistical Correction according to Observed Values." *Global and Planetary Change* 57(1):16–26.

Ebi, K. 2011a. "Adaptive Management to the Health Risks of Climate Change." In *Climate Change Adaptation in Developed Nations*, edited by J. Ford and L. Berrang-Ford, 924–30. New York: Springer.

Ebi, K. 2011b. "Climate Change and Health Risks: Assessing and Responding to Them through 'Adaptive Management.'" *Health Affairs* 30:924–30.

Ebi, K. L., T. Kram, D. P. van Vuuren, B. C. O'Neill, and E. Kriegler. 2014. "A New Toolkit for Developing Scenarios for Climate Change Research and Policy Analysis." *Environment: Science and Policy for Sustainable Development* 56(2):6–16.

European Centre for Health Policy. 1999. "Health Impact Assessment: Main Concepts and Suggested Approach." Gothenburg consensus paper. Brussels: WHO Regional Office for Europe.

Frome, E. L., and H. Checkoway.1985. "Use of Poisson Regression Models in Estimating Incidence Rates and Ratios." *American Journal of Epidemiology* 121:309–23.

Frumkin, H., J. Hess, G. Luber, J. Malilay, and M. McGehin. 2008. "Climate Change: The Public Health Response." *American Journal of Public Health* 98:435–45.

Gosling, S., G. McGregor, and J. A. Lowe.2009. "Climate Change and Heat-Related Mortality in Six Cities Part 2: Climate Model Evaluation and Projected Impacts from Changes in the Mean and Variability of Temperature with Climate Change." *International Journal of Biometeorology* 53(1):31–51.

Gosling, S. N., G. R. McGregor, and A. Paldy. 2007. "Climate Change and Heat-Related Mortality in Six Cities Part 1: Model Construction and Validation." *International Journal of Biometeorology* 51:525–40.

Green, R. S., R. Basu, B. Malig, R. Broadwin, J. J. Kim, and B. Ostro. 2010. "The Effect of Temperature on Hospital Admissions in Nine California Counties." *International Journal of Public Health* 55:113–21.

Harlan, S. L., J. H. Declet-Barreto, W. L. Stefanov, and D. B. Petitti. 2013. "Neighborhood Effects on Heat Deaths: Social and Environmental Predictors of Vulnerability in Maricopa County, Arizona." *Environmental Health Perspectives* 121(2):197.

Hess, J., J. McDowell, and G. Luber. 2012. "Integrating Climate Change Adaptation into Public Health Practice: Using Adaptive Management to Increase Adaptive Capacity and Build Resilience." *Environmental Health Perspectives* 120:171–79.

Hill, A. B. 1965. "The Environment and Disease: Association or Causation?" *Proceedings of the Royal Society of Medicine* 58:295.

Holling, C. 1978. *Adaptive Environmental Assessment and Management*. New York: Wiley.

Huang, C., A. G. Barnett, X. Wang, P. Vaneckova, G. FitzGerald, and S. Tong. 2011. "Projecting Future Heat-Related Mortality under Climate Change Scenarios: A Systematic Review." *Environmental Health Perspectives* 119:1681–90.

Intergovernmental Panel on Climate Change 2000. *Intergovernmental Panel on Climate Change: Special Report on Emissions Scenarios: Summary for Policymakers*. Cambridge: Cambridge University Press.

Jerrett, M., A. Arain, P. Kanaroglou, B. Beckerman, D. Potoglou, T. Sahsuvaroglu, J. Morrison, and C. Glovis. 2005. "A Review and Evaluation of Intraurban Air

Pollution Exposure Models." *Journal of Exposure Science and Environmental Epidemiology* 15:185–204.

Knowlton, K., C. Hogrefe, B. Lynn, C. Rosenzweig, J. Rosenthal, and P. L. Kinney. 2008. "Impacts of Heat and Ozone on Mortality Risk in the New York City Metropolitan Region under a Changing Climate." In *Seasonal Forecasts: Climatic Change and Human Health,* edited by M. C. Thomson, C. Madeleine, R. Garcia-Herrera, and M. Beniston, 143–60. New York: Springer.

Kolstad, E. W., and K. A. Johansson. 2011. "Uncertainties Associated with Quantifying Climate Change Impacts on Human Health: A Case Study for Diarrhea." *Environmental Health Perspectives* 119:299–305.

Li, T., R. M. Horton, and P. L. Kinney. 2013. "Projections of Seasonal Patterns in Temperature-Related Deaths for Manhattan, New York." *Nature Climate Change* 3:717–21.

Lloyd, S. J., R. S. Kovats, and Z. Chalabi. 2011. "Climate Change, Crop Yields, and Undernutrition: Development of a Model to Quantify the Impact of Climate Scenarios on Child Undernutrition." *Environmental Health Perspectives* 119(12):1817.

Lock, K. 2000. "Health Impact Assessment." *British Medical Journal* 320(7246):395.

Longfield, K., B. Smith, R. Gray, L. Ngamkitpaiboon, and N. Vielot. 2013. "Putting Health Metrics into Practice: Using the Disability-Adjusted Life Year for Strategic Decision Making." *BMC Public Health* 13(Supp. 2):S2.

Longstreth, J. 1991. "Anticipated Public Health Consequences of Global Climate Change." *Environmental Health Perspectives* 96:139–44.

Marmot, M., and R. Wilkinson 2009. *Social Determinants of Health.* New York: Oxford University Press.

McMichael, A. J. 2001. "Global Environmental Change as 'Risk Factor': Can Epidemiology Cope?" *American Journal of Public Health* 91:1172–74.

McMichael, A., D. Campbell-Lendrum, S. Kovats, S. Edwards, P. Wilkinson, T. Wilson, R. Nicholls, et al. 2004. "Global Climate Change." In *Comparative Quantification of Health Risks,* edited by M. Ezzati, A. Lopez, A. Rodgers, and C. Murray. Geneva: World Health Organization.

Miller, K. A., D. S. Siscovick, L. Sheppard, K. Shepherd, J. H. Sullivan, G. L. Anderson, and J. D. Kaufman. 2007. "Long-Term Exposure to Air Pollution and Incidence of Cardiovascular Events in Women." *New England Journal of Medicine* 356:447–58.

Murray, V., G. McBean, and M. Bhatt. 2012. "Case Studies." In *Managing the Risks of Extreme Events and Disasters to Advance Climate Change Adaptation: A Special Report of Working Groups I and II of the Intergovernmental Panel on Climate Change (IPCC),* edited by C. Field, V. Barros, T. Stocker, D. Qin, D. J. Dokken, K. L. Ebi, M. D. Mastrandrea, et al., 487–542. Cambridge: Cambridge University Press.

Nakicenovic, N., and R. Swart, eds. 2000. *Intergovernmental Panel on Climate Change Special Report on Emissions Scenarios.* Cambridge: Cambridge University Press.

National Research Council. 2004. *Adaptive Management for Water Resources Project Planning.* Washington, DC: National Academies Press.

O'Neill, B., E. Kriegler, K. Riahi, K. L. Ebi, S. Hallegatte, T. R. Carter, R. Mathur, and D. P. van Vuuren. 2014. "A New Scenario Framework for Climate Change Research: The Concept of Shared Socioeconomic Pathways." *Climatic Change* 122:387–400.

Ogden, N. H., M. Radojević, X. Wu, V. R. Duvvuri, P. A. Leighton, and J. Wu. 2014. "Estimated Effects of Projected Climate Change on the Basic Reproductive Number of the Lyme Disease Vector *Ixodes scapularis.*" *Environmental Health Perspectives* 122:631–38

Portier, C., K. Thigpen-Tart, S. R. Carter, C. H. Dilworth, A. E. Grambsch, J. Gohlke, J. Hess, et al. 2010. *A Human Health Perspective on Climate Change.* Raleigh, NC: Research Triangle Park, Environmental Health Perspectives, National Institute of Environmental Health Sciences.

Remais, J. V., J. J. Hess, K. L. Ebi, A. Markandya, J. M. Balbus, P. Wilkinson, A. Haines, and Z. Chalabi. 2014. "Estimating the Health Effects of Greenhouse Gas Mitigation Strategies: Addressing Parametric, Model, and Valuation Challenges." *Environmental Health Perspectives.* 122:447–55. doi:10.1289/ehp.1306744.

Sheffield, P. E., K. Knowlton, J. L. Carr, and P. L. Kinney. 2011. "Modeling of Regional Climate Change Effects on Ground-Level Ozone and Childhood Asthma." *American Journal of Preventive Medicine* 41:251–57.

Slater, H., and E. Michael. 2012. "Predicting the Current and Future Potential Distributions of Lymphatic filariasis in Africa Using Maximum Entropy Ecological Niche Modelling." *PLoS One* 7(2):e32202.

Tagaris, E., K. J. Liao, A. J. DeLucia, L. Deck, P. Amar, and A. G. Russell. 2009. "Potential Impact of Climate Change on Air Pollution–Related Human Health Effects." *Environmental Science and Technology* 43):4979–88.

Taleb, N. N. 2012. *Antifragile: Things That Gain from Disorder.* New York: Random House Digital.

Tol, R., K. Ebi, and G. Yohe. 2007. "Infectious Disease, Development, and Climate Change: A Scenario Analysis." *Environment and Development Economics* 12:687–706.

van Vuuren, D., J. Edmonds, M. Kainuma, K. Riahi, and J. Weyant 2011. "A Special Issue on the RCPs." *Climatic Change* 109:1–4.

Voorhees, A. S., N. Fann, C. Fulcher, P. Dolwick, B. Hubbell, B. Bierwagen, and P. Morefield. 2011. "Climate Change-Related Temperature Impacts on Warm Season Heat Mortality: A Proof-of-Concept Methodology Using BenMAP." *Environmental Science and Technology* 45:1450–57.

Wayne, G. 2013. *The Beginner's Guide to Representative Concentration Pathways.* Skeptical Science.org.

Wu, J., Y. Zhou, Y. Gao, J. S. Fu, B. A. Johnson, C. Huang, Y.-M. Kim, and Y. Liu. 2014. "Estimation and Uncertainty Analysis of Impacts of Future Heat Waves on Mortality in the Eastern United States." *Environmental Health Perspectives* 122(1):10.

Xun, W., A. Khan, E. Michael, and P. Vineis. 2009. "Climate Change Epidemiology: Methodological Challenges." *International Journal of Public Health* 55:85–96.

Ye, X., R. Wolff, W. Yu, P. Vaneckova, X. Pan, and S. Tong. 2012. "Ambient Temperature and Morbidity: A Review of Epidemiological Evidence." *Environmental Health Perspectives* 120(1):19–28.

Zhang, Y., P. Bi,, and J. E. Hiller. 2007. "Climate Change and Disability-Adjusted Life Years." *Journal of Environmental Health* 70(3):32–36.

Zhang, Y., P. Bi, Y. Sun, and J. E. Hiller. 2012. "Projected Years Lost due to Disabilities (YLDs) for Bacillary Dysentery Related to Increased Temperature in Temperate and Subtropical Cities of China." *Journal of Environmental Monitoring* 14:510–16.

CHAPTER 14

COMMUNITY-BASED SENTINEL SURVEILLANCE AS AN INNOVATIVE TOOL TO MEASURE THE HEALTH EFFECTS OF CLIMATE CHANGE IN REMOTE ALASKA

David Driscoll

How do you measure and reduce the health effects of climate change in culturally diverse communities spread across an area as wide as the distance between California and Georgia? Suppose this vast region is served by few, if any, roads, medical facilities, or communications infrastructure. Add blizzards, floods, and forest fires, and you have the conundrum facing researchers at the Institute for Circumpolar Health Studies (ICHS) at the University of Alaska in 2010. In Alaska, and the circumpolar north, air travel is the only viable transport option to rural and isolated communities and is both expensive and vulnerable to inclement weather conditions. These characteristics make research costly, difficult to schedule, and time-consuming.

Public health research is sorely needed in Alaska and other regions of the circumpolar north as climate change continues to alter the environmental conditions, and therefore the health, of the people who live there. Changes to Arctic sea ice, water temperature, permafrost, plant and animal diversity and harvesting availability, storms and seasonal precipitation, and temperatures are all points of vulnerability for Alaskans and other residents of the circumpolar north. The impact of these drastic and ongoing changes on the health of people living in this region has yet to be definitively assessed. Here we describe the health effects of climate change in the circumpolar north in the context of a study by the University of Alaska's ICHS to assess the well-being of affected populations, work with

KEY CONCEPTS

- Because climate change poses myriad intertwined threats to the health of residents of Alaska, and other areas of the circumpolar north, mixed-method designs are required to understand the complex climatological, cultural, and locational context of this region's public health.

- Training members of the lay public to participate in the collection of environmental observations and health status reporting garners active engagement in climate change surveillance, creating community buy-in for long-term adaptation strategies.

- Sentinel surveillance using repeated household surveys that ask participants to report both health and environmental observations is a low-expense, high-yield method of study that complements community-based efforts to design plans for adaptation to climate change.

participant community members to promote understanding of the relationship between environment and health, and move forward with community-based adaptations to the new climate reality. The methodology employed was crafted to answer the specific challenges present in public health research in the circumpolar north and respond to the particular vulnerabilities that communities in the region face. The findings assisted local, state, tribal, and federal governments in identifying priority areas for adaptation investment and determining how to develop actions and policies to promote adaptation to climate change.

The Public Health Context: Sentinel Surveillance and Community-Based Research in Public Health

Sentinel Surveillance

Public health agencies rely on a mix of data to monitor disease and such contributing factors as environmental, economic, and sociocultural characteristics. In areas with widespread access to robust health care systems, clinical data are usually collected in the course of health service delivery. In this way, clinically based sentinel surveillance systems allow public health scientists and policymakers to identify health trends.

Challenges to Clinically Based Surveillance Systems

The conduct of clinically based surveillance systems in rural and remote communities is limited by the availability of secondary data. This limitation is directly associated with the paucity of health care facilities from which reliable health data can be regularly collected. For example, 75 percent of Alaskan communities are not connected to a road that leads to a hospital (DeGross 2001). In addition, clinics in small communities that lack a resident physician or nurse practitioner may not be required to report health data the way larger facilities and hospitals must. Therefore clinically based reporting is not a viable way to gather health data in small communities.

A second challenge to clinically based reporting is that it is inherently biased to reflect health care uptake patterns. Patients who cannot and do not seek health care due to geographic, economic, or social barriers are likely to differ from the people on whom hospital or clinic data are routinely reported. Due to these distinctions, clinical data do not adequately represent the public health of many populations. For example, a resident of rural Alaska experiencing a health incident may not be noted in clinically based aggregate health data unless the severity of the health condition warrants that the patient be moved by medevac to a hub with a hospital, where data collection is more regular.

In addition, data reported by health care facilities may not contain the nuance and context that can be provided by other means of reporting, specifically a repeated self-report survey.

Survey-based public health surveillance emerged in response to these inadequacies of clinically based reporting. In bypassing the health system, surveys collect patient-level data for a sample representative of the entire population of interest. The National Health and Nutrition Survey and the Behavioral Risk Factor Surveillance System are two examples of large survey-based surveillance systems. These large-scale, repeated surveys ask participants to self-report on a variety of structured health outcomes and behaviors.

One way to hybridize these methods is to conduct ongoing and systematic collection of observations by lay observers using a structured surveillance instrument with the goal of maximizing stakeholder participation.

Occurring outside the health care venue, **community-based sentinel surveillance** systems allow researchers to collect extensive contextual data. An engaged study population given many open-ended questions within the survey instrument enables researchers located in far-off hub locations to collect nuanced contextual data in addition to quantifiable data. The use of sentinel sites for a community-based household survey allows viable data to be collected across a large geographical area with a widely dispersed population. Surveys maximize the use of limited resources when travel to each hard-to-reach study site would be prohibitive. In a research environment where study sites are hundreds of miles from research institutions, community-based household surveys are a particularly useful data collection tool.

Studies Employing This Methodology

Recently the public health and social science research communities have turned to participant communities to give shape to research methods and goals. A major producer of work on climate change adaptation in rural populations of the circumpolar north is J. D. Ford, who has worked with and studied Canadian Aboriginal populations intensively. McClymont and Myers (2012) designed community-based participatory research by northern communities with a focus on building capacity for decision making at the community level and promoting health-related adaptation plans. Harper, Edge, et al. (2012) also endorsed using a community-based, transdisciplinary approach to climate health impact research. Bell (2013) concluded that further research into the effects of climate change on health needs to integrate the classical health research "disease focus" with social science focus on socioeconomic and human system factors. Furgal, a consulting stakeholder in the design of this study, has done further work in his home nation that brought together Canadian Aboriginal community members, government representatives, and researchers to work on the assessment of community vulnerabilities and the implementation of viable adaptation measures (Furgal and Seguin 2006). Finally, the Alaska Native Tribal Health Consortium (Brubaker et al. 2011) has conducted detailed analysis of location-specific climate change impacts in northern Alaska.

This chapter describes how a team from the ICHS employed a similar model to the national surveys described above to track local environmental events and their perceived health impacts in rural and remote communities in Alaska. Researchers elaborated on these models by adding an open-ended comment section to each question, which provided qualitative and contextual data with which to inform and refine the quantitative survey data.

This study differs from previous literature in a few ways. The ICHS study covered multiple sites in three different regions of the state, each with its own distinct ecological profile and therefore with a diversity of climate vulnerabilities and adaptation needs. This complements intensive studies of single-location case studies, such as those conducted by the Alaska Native Tribal Health Consortium. Furthermore, the ICHS study involves the ongoing, systematic collection of surveillance data over the course of multiple years. In addition, our blend of public health and social science methods allowed us to optimize our survey instrument to engage community members in both data collection and the long-term study outcomes of community adaptation. Because our survey instrument allowed subjects to report both health status and observed climactic changes, we are positioned to draw conclusions about the impact of climate change on public health in the circumpolar north.

CLINICAL CORRELATES 14.1 ALASKAN NATIVES, NUTRITIONAL HEALTH, AND CLIMATE CHANGE

Alaskan native communities continue to face negative climate-related changes to their nutritional health. According to historians, "Drastic and disastrous shifts in diet can be traced to the Canadian government's forced settlement of these nomadic peoples in the years following World War II" (Lougheed 2010). Separation from ancestral ways of living and the introduction of modern food practices into Alaska resulted in decreased reliance on healthy traditional food sources. Today only 10 to 35 percent of adult dietary energy is derived from traditional foods, and a recent survey showed that nearly 70 percent of Inuit preschoolers live in food-insecure households.

Nutritional deprivation manifests as obesity and diabetes in these populations, secondary to consumption of energy-rich, nutrition-poor food. Fresh food is extremely expensive secondary to transportation costs. Traditional foods may seem like a good alternative, but these foods have been associated with high levels of persistent organic pollutants and heavy metals and could carry long-term deleterious health risks. In addition, climate change has altered the natural environment such that hunting is made more complicated by thinning ice and shifts in the availability of healthy fish populations. According to James Ford, a geographer at McGill University, "In many cases we're seeing young people who aren't going hunting because it's too dangerous. They don't have the knowledge, they don't have the skills, and they don't have the equipment" (Lougheed 2010, 390).

Traditional Alaskan native food sources have become threatened, and modern diseases such as obesity, diabetes and malnutrition are on the rise.

Climate and Health in the Far North

What Is the Arctic? What Is the Circumpolar North?

The Arctic Circle is the parallel of latitude that runs 66°33′44″ north of the equator.

North of the Arctic Circle, the sun is visible at midnight on at least one day of the year (the summer solstice) and is below the horizon at noon on at least one day of the year (the winter solstice). The term **circumpolar north** refers to that region within and bordering the Arctic Circle in which human residents share common challenges associated with life in the far north and includes all of Alaska and portions of Russia, Northern Europe, Greenland and Canada (Armstrong, Rogers, and Rowley 1978).

Why study the circumpolar north in relation to climate change? This area has experienced some of the greatest regional warming on Earth since the 1970s (Huntington and Weller 2004). Temperatures in the interior of Alaska have risen over 3°C (7°F) since 1950, and the ambient air temperature in the circumpolar north could increase another 5°C (9°F) during this century (Larsen et al. 2008). This warming trend will have substantial impacts on the health of the region's 13.1 million residents (World Health Organization 2003; "Population Distribution" 2009). Some of the current environmental changes to the region's defining characteristics include the following (Hinzman et al. 2005; McBeath 2003):

• Reduction of **sea ice** (frozen seawater that may float on the ocean surface or be attached to coasts or the seafloor)

- Thawing **permafrost** (a layer of soil below the ground surface that remains frozen throughout the year for at least two or more sequential years)

- Increased precipitation

- Decreased duration of snow cover

- Increase in extreme weather event intensity and impact

- Changes in seasonal patterns

Vulnerability in the Circumpolar North

Although the circumpolar north encompasses several nations and dozens of languages, residents of the region share three significant vulnerabilities to climate change: limited built infrastructure, reliance on a subsistence lifestyle, and limited access to information.

Built Infrastructure

Roads, bridges, ports, rail lines, and similar public works are noticeable by their absence throughout much of Alaska and the circumpolar north. The paucity of built infrastructure in northern latitudes can increase the likelihood of adverse health outcomes from environmental changes associated with climate change. For example, because many Alaskan communities are unreachable by any road system, emergency evacuation must occur by other means. This puts children, people with disabilities, and the elderly at greater risk because of the discomfort, difficulty, and danger of traveling long distances by boat, four-wheeler, or airplane. Extreme weather events of increasing strength and frequency also threaten supply lines by making it potentially impossible for supply barges to reach villages during the narrow seasonal window when they can safely pass to shore. Rural Alaska, like other circumpolar places, is increasingly reliant on supplies of food, fuel, and medicine, so an interruption in the supply of essential materials could be catastrophic (Berner and Furgal 2005).

Subsistence

In urban centers, an empty freezer is solvable with a quick trip to the store and is vulnerable only to the availability of cash. An empty freezer indicates something more harrowing in the circumpolar north, a high-priority threat to food security. Getting food to remote locations can be logistically impossible, so subsistence users store up many kinds of fish, game, and wild flora through the long Alaskan winter. For generations, subsistence users have hunted on ice sheets whose permanent features made sea mammal hunting a reliably fruitful prospect and relied on detailed knowledge of the land and seasons to put food on the table. Now, thinning ice has made subsistence much more high risk and low yield (Brubaker, Bell, and Rolin 2009).

On top of new dangers inherent in subsistence activities, changes in animal migration patterns threaten the availability of wild food harvests, including sea mammals, fish, fowl, and berries. Traditional food storage and preservation are also vulnerable to climate change. Permanent underground caverns have acted as freezers for generations, but rising temperatures are causing these to thaw, which threatens food safety (Brubaker, Bell, and Rolin 2009). Warmer summers also shorten the window during which harvested meat can be preserved by drying. Warming coastal water temperatures are a primary vulnerability for subsistence and recreational shellfish harvesters. Warmer temperatures encourage algal blooms that cause high concentrations of toxins in local seafoods, resulting in the sometimes fatal **paralytic shellfish poisoning (PSP)**. (The toxins are produced by a species of dinoflagellate called *Alexandrium tamarense*, and it accumulates in filter-feeder bivalves when warm water hosts red tide algal blooms.) Symptoms of PSP range in severity from limb numbness to nausea to full respiratory failure (Centers for Disease Control and Prevention 2011).

Information

Many communities in the circumpolar north are isolated in terms of geography and access to local information. Very-high-frequency (VHF) radio connects many Alaskan communities to each other, but those signals are usually relayed through a hub station in a larger village hundreds of miles away. The circumpolar north is so vast, sparsely populated, and dangerous that there is a paucity of accurate, up-to-the-minute climate event data that could make a profound difference in the public's health as climactic change progresses. In addition, few data collection mechanisms are in place for air or water quality warnings, severe weather event warnings, or algae bloom warnings to be disseminated in a timely manner. With an improved information dissemination system, the direction of sudden storms could be more accurately predicted and air and water quality warnings quickly acted on, and shellfish from at-risk waters avoided.

Residents of the circumpolar north living in isolated communities face climate changes greater than those at middle and lower latitudes. Populations that practice subsistence, often in remote communities, as well as those who already face a variety of health and socioeconomic challenges, will be most vulnerable to the health effects of climate change (Parkinson and Butler 2005). While some health outcomes are easily assessed, like exposure to extreme heat or storms, others follow more complicated pathways and make assessment more challenging. Potential health effects in the region include the following:

Direct Effects

- Increase in hyperthermia, particularly among the elderly and very young
- Injuries, deaths, and illnesses resulting from storms and floods
- Increase in subsistence-practice–related injuries and deaths

Indirect Effects

- Changes in availability of subsistence foods, resulting in increased reliance on expensive, nontraditional, and potentially less healthy food options, with an attendant increase in obesity, diabetes, hunger, and heart disease.
- Damage to water sources and infrastructure due to erosion and subsidence
- Increase in respiratory ailments from changes in allergens and air pollution from increased wildfire activity
- Encroachment of wildlife-borne, waterborne and vector-borne diseases (Parkinson and Butler 2005)
- Mental health concerns and loss of community identity (Willox et al. 2012)

Practically all descriptions of Alaska include a declaration of the state's size, and yet it cannot be understated. Across this massive expanse of land are some of the most varied terrains on the planet and more coastline than the contiguous United States combined. Well over half the state's population resides in its major urban centers of Fairbanks and Anchorage, but 25 percent of all Alaskans and 46 percent of Alaska Native residents live in communities of fewer than one thousand people. Only thirteen state roads connect urban centers, and nearly one-quarter of the state's population live in towns and villages that are reachable only by boat or aircraft (US Census Bureau 2013).

There are enormous differences in lifestyles and living conditions between Alaska's metropolitan areas and its smallest rural communities, not the least of which is reliance on **subsistence** hunting, fishing, and gathering, that is, the customary and traditional uses of wild resources for direct personal or family consumption as food, shelter, fuel, clothing, tools or transportation. The livelihood and well-being of nonurban Alaskans is exceptionally vulnerable to climate change because of the particularly close relationship residents have with their environment (Bureau of Land Management 2008).

Public Health in Alaska

Alaska's health care system is multitiered and expansive, intersecting many private, nonprofit, and governmental structures whose responsibilities have shifted over time. The Indian Health Service (IHS) and Alaska Native Tribal Healthcare Consortium (ANTHC) work together to run hundreds of care centers across Alaska. Itinerant public health nurses and regular **medevac** services (medical evacuation usually by aircraft, from small communities to hub sites with increased access to health care) are a bigger part of rural Alaska's medical care experience than are a locally based hospital or doctor. As in many other rural areas, primary care providers are in short supply. There are over sixty **Health Professional Shortage Areas (HPSAs)** and medically underserved areas (MUAs) in Alaska, representing nearly two-thirds of the state's territory (Department of Health and Human Services 2013). Primary care HPSAs are based on a physician-to-population ratio of 1:3,500. In other words, when there are 3,500 or more people per primary care physician, an area is eligible to be designated as a primary care HPSA. A network of public health centers and offices in twenty- communities and regular visits by public health nurses bring care to approximately 280 additional small communities and villages (Bertolli et al. 2008). Community health aides (CHAs) deliver basic medical and emergency help in isolated Alaska communities. While nearly all villages have a clinic, many are staffed by village health aides, and patients must be flown to a hub location before receiving advanced medical attention. Health care, and therefore health data reporting, are made sparse by the unique challenges presented by the region.

Participation in public health surveillance systems for rural and specifically indigenous populations is low across America, but especially difficult in Alaska. For example, there are almost no available trend data on asthma prevalence for Alaska Natives (Gessner and Neeno 2005). Any effort to track the health effects of climate change faces the challenge presented by this paucity of available secondary health data (Ford, Vanderbilt, and Berrang-Ford 2012).

Alaska's Distinct Ecoregions

The Arctic is climatologically diverse, with at least three distinct regions (figure 14.1). The northwest region has a cool to cold climate; the average high temperature in July is 58°F, and the average high temperature in January is 5°F. Average precipitation is low—only nine inches of rain and forty-seven inches of snow annually. These predominantly coastal villages are particularly vulnerable to storms and erosion. Navigation of these waters is blocked by sea ice most of the year, and very few villages are connected

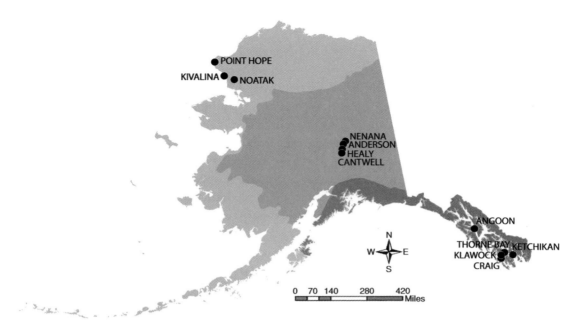

Figure 14.1   Climatological Regions in Alaska

to roads. The predominant Alaska Native groups in this region are Inupiaq to the north, Yup'ik to the west, and Aleutian to the southwest. In 2010, the villages of Point Hope, Kivalina, and Noatak had 1,562 residents, over 90 percent of whom were Alaska Native. Arctic tundra characterizes the northwestern section of the state; short plants and spongy earth are underlaid by permafrost and covered with snow most months of the year.

The tundra gives way to mountain ranges that border the interior, where temperatures regularly reach over 85°F in the summer and plummet to -50°F in the winter. The average annual precipitation is generally low, just exceeding twelve inches. Population centers in this region concentrate around the highways. The predominant Alaska Native groups in this region are culturally distinct Athabaskan tribes. In 2010, Healy, Anderson, and Cantwell had 1,486 residents, of whom approximately 30 percent are of Alaska Native ancestry.

The southeast region of the state contains a temperate rain forest and dramatic fjords where cliffs plunge into the sea. It has a cool, moist climate with an average annual rainfall in the region that exceeds 150 inches and an annual average snowfall exceeding 36 inches. The average high temperature in July is 65°F, and the average high temperature in January is 39°F. Many communities in the region are unconnected to any road system and are accessible only by sea and air. The predominant Alaska Native groups in this region are Tlingit, Tsimshian, and Haida. In 2010, Ketchikan and

Angoon had 8,509 residents. The racial makeup of Ketchikan was approximately 60 percent white, and 25 percent Alaska Native while Angoon was roughly 75 percent Alaska Native and 10.5 percent white.

CLINICAL CORRELATES 14.2 BARRIERS TO HEALTH CARE IN ALASKA

Health care in Alaska is made difficult by the enormous geography, the dispersion of human settlements, and a shortage of health care providers. Alaska Natives face these barriers in addition to poor baseline community health. Alaska Natives die at higher rates than other Americans from tuberculosis (500 percent higher), alcoholism (519 percent higher), diabetes (195 percent higher), unintentional injuries (149 percent higher), homicide (92 percent higher), and suicide (72 percent higher) (Indian Health Service n.d.). The reality of health care in Alaska is that travel to major medical centers requires medevac in the majority of cases, which is subject to weather and fuel availability. Primary care facilities are scarce.

In the era of climate change, with less predictable weather and rising fuel prices, transportation may become exponentially more difficult, and Alaska Native communities may become more isolated from health resources. Telemedicine has emerged as an interesting option to deal with transportation and provider barriers. A recent initiative through the Indian Health Service has advanced ophthalmic and diabetic care. Populations at risk of diabetic retinopathy (leading cause of blindness among diabetics) can receive annual eye exams from a technician. and images can be forwarded to specialists in the continental United States for recommendations. In addition, local primary care doctors can consult in real time with subspecialists (Carroll, Culle, and Kokesh 2011). Connecting vulnerable Alaskan communities to health care must use a multifaceted approach that could include telemedicine.

Alaska natives suffer disproportionate morbidity and mortality from preventable and treatable diseases. Telemedicine may be a means to overcome barriers to health care for Alaska natives.

What We Did and Why

This section describes how we crafted our study, the reasons for actions we took, some of the specific the challenges we faced, and what we did to overcome them.

Figure 14.2 provides an outline of how we designed our multidisciplinary approach.

In September 2010, the ICHS at the University of Alaska initiated a two-year study to promote informed planning for community-based adaptation to climate change in Alaska. The initial study surveillance goals were aligned with the Centers for Disease Control's Building Resilience against Climate

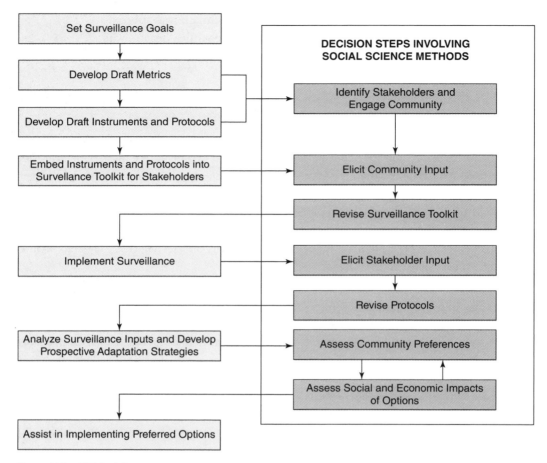

Figure 14.2   ICHS Study Design

Effects (BRACE) goals developed by its National Center for Environmental Health (NCEH). The study was conducted with support from the CDC and in partnership with ANTHC and Alaska Community Services (ACS).

The Study Approach

Step 1: Find Out What We Need to Know about Climate Change and Health in Alaska

Researchers pulled together a team of national and international experts, including many of the researchers mentioned earlier, as well as local stakeholders to assess the impacts of climate change on vulnerable populations within each of the three regions of the state.

Justification: By soliciting the input and participation of a wide scope of stakeholders, researchers were able to draw on a range of perspectives and expertise to assess the vulnerability of each unique region, ensure the survey would take on a final shape that its intended audience would be receptive to and find easy to complete, and form or strengthen working relationships with community member networks.

Based on a literature review and the colloquium's vulnerability assessment, the ICHS identified several areas of interest in measuring the health effects of climate change in three ecologically distinct regions of Alaska. From these areas of interest, five surveillance elements and several attendant observations were outlined for each.

Step 2: Decide Whether to Use a Survey

The colloquium input led researchers to craft a survey that covered the main concerns across the state, which ran along similar lines of those in other climate change vulnerability research. It was determined that a structured survey instrument would be most appropriate for the collection of these data because it could best answer the challenges of conducting research in the region.

Justification: Compared to long-term, on-site research or repeated site visits to communities, surveys require relatively few financial resources. Recall that all of the communities in question are far from urban centers, and most are accessible only by boat or airplane. Traveling researchers would have run up against not only the expense but also the risk of traveling so far by those means. The weather in the remote circumpolar north often requires travel plans to be rescheduled, which presents additional delays and barriers to successful and efficient completion of research.

In addition, direct participation by engaged lay observers detailed descriptions of environmental challenges specific to each region, as well as insight into a variety of health outcomes and risk factors that would not be identified quickly, if at all, by any passive surveillance systems available in Alaska at the time.

Step 3: Test the Survey

Once the survey was designed to ICHS researchers' satisfaction, colloquium stakeholders were called back to evaluate the instrument and provide feedback about how effective they thought it would be in the field. Pretesting of the draft instrument with community representatives found some questions too long and detailed. Researchers revised the surveillance tool kit to streamline survey questions, making them easier to read and understand. This shaped the survey instrument into something scientifically viable, as well as easy and rewarding to participate in. The final study instrument and protocol were implemented with repeated submissions of structured observations of the same metrics over the course of twelve months beginning in spring 2011.

Justification: Having a colloquium of scientific and lay community leaders evaluate the study helped shape the survey instrument into a useful research tool. It is important to note that engaged and informed community residents are necessary for the successful implementation of such a sentinel surveillance system. For that reason, it is very important that participants find questions relatable to priorities in their own lives. Embracing the reflexive process of revision brought important insights to the research team regarding content, language, and cultural barriers.

Step 4: Solicit Respondents

Our response was to implement surveillance with awareness and good faith. In the first month of the study, we spent several days in each study community meeting with participants in one-on-one and group settings to discuss the study objectives and protocols and to provide training in completing and returning the surveys. We were well aware of the experiences that indigenous people have had with researchers, including climate change research. Sensitive to the issue of participant authorship and conscious of our responsibility as researchers to those taking time to help, a twenty-dollar gift certificate or store credit incentive was provided to each participant on receipt of their monthly survey.

Justification: By flying out to the villages and spending time face-to-face with participants, researchers were able to create individual and community buy-in that resulted in high response rates and kept surveys coming in over the year.

By working closely with stakeholders in a reflexive and responsive way, researchers were able to create a comprehensive research instrument that garnered significant participant interest and provided data on a broad expanse of subjects. The distinctive blend of social science and public health approaches helped this study overcome some of the challenges that face community-based surveillance research.

Step 5: Assess Vulnerabilities

We were aware of the broad vulnerabilities common to the circumpolar north. However, the goal of this study was to identify the vulnerabilities most significant to each community's particular stakeholders and then work within the communities to create strategies for adaptation.

Community Vulnerability Self-Assessments

A **vulnerability assessment** evaluates susceptibility to potential threats and identifies corrective actions that can reduce or mitigate the risk of serious consequences from adverse phenomena. It is an essential aspect of any undertaking to adapt to or mitigate negative health outcomes. This important precursor to action allows researchers to understand the context of their research question, identify challenges and resources, and build a baseline of understanding to inform conclusions and advisory outcomes. The vulnerability assessment is what glues a study's findings to the real world—how it becomes applicable research that can make a difference.

Following collection and analysis of the data from each study community project, investigators visited each site to present their findings and engage the communities in creating their own vulnerability assessment. Participants worked with researchers to map their community and identify features that might be vulnerable to climate change, such as water and food sources, rivers, and coastlines. Through informal discussion, study participants voiced their agreement or disagreement with the surveillance findings. Participants also discussed causal associations between the primary environmental effects and health outcomes they observed and recorded in the surveillance data, and helped craft prospective adaptation strategies to mitigate those causal associations. By bringing lay observers' attention to their environment in conjunction with health concerns, researchers were able to aid participants in crafting a vulnerability assessment for their own communities on the way to creating the adaptation plan. The adaptation plans that emerged were thereby both community oriented and data driven.

Northwest

Residents of the Northwest focused on vulnerabilities to food security, including accidental injury during harvesting due to melting sea ice. Other food security vulnerabilities included changes to migratory routes of animals relied on for subsistence meats. Caribou harvesters described changes in migration routes and an increase in predators like polar bears and wolves. Unexpectedly intense storms and temperature trends that weaken ice or flood trails exacerbate these vulnerabilities. Residents also prioritized health issues associated with air and water quality, predominantly related to increased particulate loads due to upstream erosion, unusual warmth and low precipitation.

At the time of the presentations, Kivalina's water system was shut down due to large loads of particulates from upstream erosion, and Noatak's airport was closed due to erosion from the Noatak River, which runs next to it.

Interior

Residents of Interior Alaska were concerned about a broad scope of air quality issues, including growing allergen levels and increased forest fire smoke.

Residents were also concerned about water quality as melting permafrost and erosion result in heavy loads of particulate in water sources, as in the Northwest. Residents noted that increasing population might add additional stress to these vulnerabilities

Southeast

Residents of the Southeast were concerned about the significant food security threat presented by PSP. There was also concern for air quality, although their worry was an increase in black mold in the community. Injuries resulting from frost-heave damage to infrastructure and difficulty in accessing health care were particularly noted by some participants in this region. During a visit to the study site community of Angoon, researchers found that the community's resident physician had quit, leaving Angoon without formal medical care, let alone a mechanism for reporting health data to concerned agencies.

Self-Assessment Priorities Statewide

In the Northwest and Southeast, water security ranked first in community concerns about the health effects of climate change, and it ranked first as the most frequent concern across all three regions. Second across the state was food security, which was of preeminent concern in the Interior and ranked second in concern in the Northwest and third in the Southeast. Respiratory concerns came in third overall, followed by cold-related injuries and PSP.

Community evaluation of researchers' findings helped bring participants' attention to community-specific vulnerabilities to climate change. Informal discussion between researchers and participants encouraged feedback and idea synthesis and resulted in a framework responsive to the particular needs of each region. It also led to enthusiasm among participants for further participation in designing and executing emergent adaptation plans.

A community-based approach to sentinel surveillance systems has been used effectively to study the health effects of climate change in the circumpolar north.

Findings, Reporting Back to the Community, and Adaptation Plans

With analysis completed, researchers returned to each of the eight communities and presented their findings. Following the community engagement model, participants were invited to comment, critique, and discuss with researchers, as well as brainstorm about appropriate community adaptations. Adaptations were judged by both their prospective impact and ease of implementation. Thus, community members and researchers focused on information delivery as a broad-reaching means by which to help community members mitigate existing concerns and vulnerabilities while laying groundwork of success by setting achievable goals within adaptation plans.

Findings by Region

Residents of southeastern Alaska had three top health priorities they considered linked to environmental conditions:

- *Unintentional injury:* Caused by or related to extreme weather events were of concern
- *Food security:* High levels of algae-related toxin in local shellfish when water temperatures rise, and the resulting high-risk of PSP
- *Indoor and outdoor air quality:* Increased allergies and mold prevalence

PSP was an expected vulnerability in the Southeast, though unintentional injury was less expected. Researchers and participants concluded the greatest community need was for more information about all vulnerability points and that local adaptation to the top community concerns would be best promoted with alerts disseminated by all local media. This included monthly electronic mailings (the *Alaska Climate and Health Bulletin*), links to time-sensitive and Web-based materials such as the Allergy Advisor or NOAA Weather Alerts, as well as updates using text messages. Local radio and print media were included as well in an effort to increase region-wide awareness of imminent severe weather and of warm water temperatures that could result in PSP cases.

Residents of the Interior region described a host of prospective causal associations to health phenomena:

- *Respiratory ailments:* Asthma and allergies associated with wind-blown dust in the spring, increasing pollen levels in fall, and smoke from forest fires in summer
- *Water security:* Eroding riverbeds caused by melting permafrost clog water infrastructure unable to handle high sediment loads

Though complaints from the region were unique, the proposed adaptation measures mirrored those promoted in Southeast. Erosion can be linked to disintegrations in both water and air quality, and erosion is often caused or exacerbated by extreme weather. An effective, if not perfect, adaptation technique would be to alert residents to impending extreme weather using all available local media, while simultaneously beginning work on mitigating erosion.

The following issues arose in the Northwest:

- *Food security:* Unexpectedly intense storms and temperature trends weaken ice and exacerbate vulnerability to food insecurity.

- *Air quality:* Erosion exacerbated by storms lowers air quality.

- *Water quality:* Upriver erosion was a concern.

Again, customized, timely information and alerts were determined to be the best way to initiate adaptation mechanisms in the region. Residents of both villages recommended that adaptation strategies include better erosion control. They also recommended that health education materials be developed and disseminated in each community.

The research team particularly recommended efforts to disseminate data on air and water quality from existing monitoring efforts to community members as a cost-effective and necessary first step toward climate change adaptation. At the very least, these should include warnings related to particulates from smoke and pollen and perhaps include information related to monitoring for PSP outbreaks in the Southeast region. Additional adaptation strategies commonly mentioned by our participants include better access to quality health care for unintentional injuries and other common outcomes, water systems and other infrastructure that remain safer and efficient despite growing erosion and other aspects of severe weather events, and more information on the availability of alternative foods in light of reductions in traditional subsistence food sources.

CLINICAL CORRELATES 14.3 ALASKA: FOOD SECURITY, HUMAN HEALTH, AND THE AQUATIC ENVIRONMENT

Rising carbon dioxide (CO_2) concentrations in the atmosphere have direct impacts on the world's oceans, leading to changes that affect human settlements that rely on the ocean for their livelihood. Rising CO_2 levels result in ocean acidification, changes to the density structure of the upper ocean, alterations in the upwelling of winds and changes in the timing, and volume of freshwater runoff into coastal marine waters (Bindoff et al. 2007). Such changes result in higher levels of toxic as well as nontoxic algae that are relevant to human health, particularly that of Alaskans. Based on 2010 reports, fifty-three thousand individuals are employed by the seafood industry, and Alaska Native populations rely directly on seafood as a primary source of nutrition ("Alaska Economic Performance Report" 2010). Harmful algae blooms produce toxins that accumulate in marine species and when consumed cause toxic syndromes such as amnesic, paralytic, neurotoxic, and diarrheic shellfish poisoning. Indirect effects from nontoxic blooms include reductions in the dissolved oxygen concentration of oceans and reductions in biodiversity, which together alter the aquatic ecosystem and affect fishing and food gathering in Alaskan communities.

Elevated CO_2 levels in the atmosphere change ocean dynamics and affect the health and livelihoods of thousands of Alaskans.

Conclusion

Researchers concluded that a community-based sentinel surveillance system is a helpful way to measure the health effects of climate change in a rural region with a paucity of primary health care centers.

Weaving together public health and social science methods from the very beginning of the study was immensely beneficial. The deliberate process of developing first metrics, then an instrument, and finally a data collection tool in a colloquium setting brought to the study additional expertise from both content-area experts and residents of rural and isolated villages in Alaska. This improved the quality of the surveillance tool for use in a region of the country with few secondary data sources. This process should prove effective in other regions of the nation and across the circumpolar north as well.

Using the surveillance tool to collect community-based, sentinel surveillance data is an effective means to assess the nature and extent of health effects of climate change on communities located across Alaska. The inclusion of open-ended response fields created an instrument far more flexible than many large-scale, self-reporting surveys, which served two purposes. It permitted community members to explain their answers and therefore provide nuance to the quantitative data. It also engaged community members more directly with the survey, allowing them to make their own observations and submit them to rigorous analysis. This further engaged them in the research process and in the actions to be taken on its completion.

Third, the presentation of the sentinel surveillance data contributed to productive discussions of the prospective causal relationships between environmental events and the health outcomes described. For example, an explicit recognition of the association between unusual weather events and unintentional injuries provided insights into such mediating factors as unsafe ice or building conditions, which were obvious to participants but might not have been otherwise identified by project investigators. These discussions tended to be quite far reaching, with the scope of prospective adaptation strategies encompassing local policies and built infrastructure.

The adaptation strategies that resulted from this process are both locally determined and data driven. This combination of factors would seem auspicious for the successful conduct of one or more of these adaptation strategies at the circumpolar regional level.

DISCUSSION QUESTIONS

1. What are the strengths and weaknesses of community-based adaptation planning?

2. How can researchers best use limited resources to assess the connection between environmental and health phenomena?

3. What are some of the major challenges facing residents of the circumpolar north as a result of climate change?

KEY TERMS

Circumpolar north: The region within and bordering the Arctic Circle in which human residents share common challenges associated with life in the far north; includes all of Alaska and portions of Russia, Northern Europe, Greenland and Canada.

Community-based sentinel surveillance: Ongoing and systematic collection of observations by lay observers using a structured surveillance instrument with the goal of maximizing stakeholder participation.

Health Professional Shortage Area (HPSA): A US federal government designation that may refer to a geographic area, a specific population group, or a facility with a shortage of health professionals.

Medevac: Medical evacuation aircraft that fly patients from small communities to hub locations where medical resources are available.

Paralytic shellfish poisoning (PSP): A potentially fatal toxin that attacks the nervous system, caused by *Alexandrium tamarense*, a species of dinoflagellate. PSP accumulates in filter-feeder bivalves when warm water hosts red tide algal blooms. Symptoms range in severity from numbness to nausea to full respiratory failure.

Permafrost: A layer of soil below the ground surface that remains frozen throughout the year for at least two or more sequential years.

Sea ice: Frozen seawater that floats on the ocean surface or is attached to coasts or the sea floor.

Sentinel surveillance: Health care facilities report data to public health agencies regularly through review of patient data collected in the course of service delivery. In this way, facility-based sentinel surveillance systems allow clinicians and policymakers to identify health trends.

Subsistence: The customary and traditional use of wild resources for direct personal or family consumption as food, shelter, fuel, clothing, tools, or transportation.

Vulnerability assessment: Evaluation of susceptibility to potential threats and identification of corrective actions that can reduce or mitigate the risk of serious consequences from adverse phenomena.

References

Alaska Economic Performance Report. 2010. Department of Commerce, Community and Economic Development. http://commerce.alaska.gov/dnn/Portals/6/pub/2010_Alaska_Economic_Performance_Report.pdf

Armstrong, T. E., G. W. Rogers, and G. R. Rowley. 1978. *The Circumpolar North: A Political and Economic Geography of the Arctic and Sub-Arctic.* London: Methuen.

Bell, E. J. 2013. "Climate Change and Health Research: Has It Served Rural Communities?" *Rural Remote Health* 13:2343. http://www.ncbi.nlm.nih.gov/pubmed/23398298

Berner, J., and C. Furgal. 2005. "Arctic Climate Impact Assessment." In *Impacts of a Warming Arctic*, 863–906. Cambridge: Cambridge University Press.

Bertolli, J., A. Roussel, J. Harris, D. Lentine, J. Gable, R. Fichtner, J. Kauffman, M. Landen, and R. Bryan. 2008. "Surveillance of Infectious Diseases among American Indians and Alaska Natives." *Journal of Health Disparities Research and Practice* 2:121–44. http://digitalscholarship.unlv.edu/cgi/viewcontent.cgi?article=1096&context=jhdrp

Bindoff, N. L., J. Willebrand, V. Artale, A. Cazenave, J. Gregory, S. Gulev, K. Hanawa, et al. 2007. "Observations: Oceanic Climate Change and Sea Level." In *Climate Change 2007: The Physical Science Basis Contribution of Working Group I to the Fourth Assessment Report of the Intergovernmental Panel on Climate Change*, edited by S. Solomon, D. Qin, M. Manning, Z. Chen, M. Marquis, K. B. Avery, M. Tignor, and H. L. Miller, 385–432. Cambridge: Cambridge University Press.

Brubaker, M. Y., J. N. Bell, J. E. Berner, and J. A. Warren. 2011. "Climate Change Health Assessment: A Novel Approach for Alaska Native Communities." *International Journal of Circumpolar Health* 70:266–73. http://www.ncbi.nlm.nih.gov/pubmed/21703129

Brubaker, M., J. Bell, and A. Rolin. 2009. *Climate Change Effects on Traditional Inupiaq Food Cellars Center for Climate and Health. ANTHC.* CCH bulletin 1. 2009. http://www4.nau.edu/tribalclimatechange/tribes/docs/tribes_InupiaqFoodCellars.pdf

Bureau of Land Management. U.S. Department of the Interior. 2008. "Subsistence." http://www.blm.gov/ak/st/en/prog/subsistence.html

Carroll, M., T. Culle, and J. Kokesh. 2011. "Innovation in Indian Healthcare: Using Health Information Technology to Achieve Health Equity for American Indian and Alaska Native Populations." *Perspectives in Health Information Management* 8:1d.

Centers for Disease Control and Prevention. 2011. "Paralytic Shellfish Poisoning—Southeast Alaska May-June 2011." http://www.cdc.gov/mmwr/preview/mmwrhtml/mm6045a3.htm

DeGross, D. 2001. "Healthcare in Alaska." Alaska Center for Rural Health. http://www.healthcareersinalaska.info/images/uploads/Article_-_Health_Care_in_Alaska_-_DeGross.pdf

Department of Health and Human Services, Health Resources and Services and Administration. 2013. "Find Shortage Areas: MUA/P by State and Country." http://muafind.hrsa.gov/index.aspx

Ford, J. D., W. Vanderbilt, and L. Berrang-Ford. 2012. "Authorship in IPCC 565 AR5 and Its Implications for Content: Climate Change and Indigenous Populations in WGII." *Climate Change* 113:201–13. http://link.springer.com/article/10.1007%2Fs10584–011–0350-z

Furgal, C., and J. Seguin. 2006. "Climate Change, Health, and Vulnerability in Canadian Northern Aboriginal Communities." *Environmental Health Perspectives* 114:1964–70. http://www.ncbi.nlm.nih.gov/pmc/articles/PMC1764172/

Gessner, B. D., and T. Neeno. 2005. "Trends in Asthma Prevalence, Hospitalization Risk, and Inhaled Corticosteroid Use among Alaska Native and Nonnative Medicaid Recipients Younger Than 20 Years." *Annals of Allergy, Asthma and Immunology* 94:372–79. http://www.sciencedirect.com/science/article/pii/S1081120610609908

Harper, S. L., V. L. Edge, C. A. Willox, and Rigolet Inuit Community Government. 2012. "Changing Climate, Changing Health, Changing Stories' Profile: Using an EcoHealth Approach to Explore Impacts of Climate Change on Inuit Health." *Ecohealth* 9(1):89–101. http://www.ncbi.nlm.nih.gov/pubmed/22526749

Hinzman, L., N. D. Neil, W. Bettez, B. F. Robert, S. Chapin, M. B. Dyurgerov, C. L. Fastie, et al. 2005. "Evidence and Implications of Recent Climate Change in Northern Alaska and Other Arctic Regions." *Climatic Change* 72:251–98. http://www.imedea.uibcsic.es/master/cambioglobal/Modulo_3_03/Summary%20changes%20and%20climate%20in%20the%20Arctic.pdf

Huntington, H., and G. Weller. 2004. "Arctic Climate Impact Assessment." In *Impacts of a Warming Arctic*, 15–18. Cambridge: Cambridge University Press.

Indian Health Service. n.d. *IHS Fact Sheets: Indian Health Disparities.* http://info.ihs.gov/Disparities.asp

Larsen, P. H., S. Goldsmith, O. Smith, M. L. Wilson, K. Strzepek, P. Chinowsky, and B. Saylor. 2008. "Estimating Future Costs for Alaska Public Infrastructure at Risk from Climate Change." *Global Environmental Change.* http://www .climatechange.Alaska.gov/aag/docs/O97F18069.pdf

Lougheed, T. 2010. "Food Security: The Changing Landscape of Arctic Traditional Food." *Environmental Health Perspectives* 118(9):386–93.

McBeath, J. 2003. "Institutional Responses to Climate Change: The Case of the Alaska Transportation System." http://link.springer.com/content /pdf/10.1023%2FA%3A1025840627213.pdf

McClymont, P., and E. Myers. 2012. "Community-Based Participatory Process: Climate Change and Health Adaptation Program for Northern First Nations and Inuit in Canada." *International Journal of Circumpolar Health* 71:1–8. http://www.ncbi.nlm.nih.gov/pubmed/22584509

Parkinson, A. J., and J. C. Butler. 2005. "Potential Impacts of Climate Change on Infectious Diseases in the Arctic." *International Journal of Circumpolar Health* 64:478–86. http://www.ncbi.nlm.nih.gov/pubmed/16440610

"Population Distribution." 2009. University of the Arctic International Secretariat.

US Census Bureau. 2013. "Quick Facts." http://quickfacts.census.gov/qfd /states/02000.html

Willox, A C., S. L. Harper, J. D. Ford, K. Landman, K. Houled, V. L. Edge, and Rigolet Inuit Community Government. 2012. "From This Place and of This Place: Climate Change, Sense of Place, and Health in Nunatsiavut, Canada." *Social Science and Medicine* 75:538–47. http://www.ncbi.nlm.nih.gov/pubmed/22595069

World Health Organization. 2003. "Climate Change and Human Health: Risks and Responses." World Health Organization. http://www.who.int/globalchange /publications/climchange.pdf

PROTECTING ENVIRONMENTAL JUSTICE COMMUNITIES FROM THE DETRIMENTAL IMPACTS OF CLIMATE CHANGE

Cecilia Martinez, Nicky Sheats

The problems posed by environmental risks to the health and livelihoods of communities across the globe are daunting. Even as we develop more sophisticated scientific methods for understanding their scope and magnitude, our efforts are seemingly unable to keep pace with the increasing range and complexity of environmental hazards that are emerging. Our society is now confronting what is arguably the most significant human-induced environmental problem in history: climate change. After decades of examination, deliberation, and debate, the scientific community has come to a consensus that anthropogenic climate change is in fact occurring and that the potential impacts on human settlements are as substantial as they are wide-ranging (IPCC 2007, 2014). Research and policy strategies for climate mitigation are critical. But as essential as greenhouse gas reduction is to the future of our global environment, equally as important is the need to build protections for communities against the damaging impacts already underway. The era of climate change has caused researchers, civil society organizations, and governments across the globe to focus on research and strategies that will reduce the harmful societal impacts caused by this global threat.

A global assessment coordinated by the World Health Organization (WHO 2011), taking into account only a subset of the possible health impacts, found that between 1970 and 2004, over 140,000 excess deaths annually could be attributed to the changing climate. Approximately 600,000 deaths occurred worldwide as a result of

KEY CONCEPTS

- **This chapter examines how environmental justice research can be integrated into climate change and public health analyses and planning, and seeks to illustrate how climate resiliency research and planning can more effectively address environmental justice concerns and issues of inequality.**

- **The fundamental problem of vulnerability in environmental justice is that communities live with already existing physical and social challenges, which are compounded by climate change events.**

- **Several investigations have found that communities of color and low-income communities are already disproportionately exposed to airborne pollutants. Given these existing disproportionate exposures, the prospect of increased levels of air pollution due to climate change is particularly**

KEY CONCEPTS (CONTINUED)

troubling to environmental justice communities.

- If overall temperatures and the frequency of heat waves increase as predicted, the future health and viability of vulnerable environmental justice communities must be addressed.

- In order to make communities resilient to extreme weather events, community-level adaptation plans should be created that address the specific issues identified in this chapter.

- Changes to, and loss of, biodiversity due to climate change are affecting Indigenous communities' ability to lead a subsistence existence and also negatively affects cultural practices as well.

- It is critical that more research and resources, and more responsive methods, be developed to assess and mitigate the public health impacts of climate change on environmental justice communities.

weather-related natural disasters in the 1990s (95 percent of which were from poor countries). Moreover, climate-sensitive diseases are among the largest global killers (WHO 2005). In the 1980s and 1990s, almost 1.3 million people lost their lives due to climate and weather events, and another 3.3 billion lives were affected in some manner (WHO 2005). Moreover, between 2030 and 2050, climate change is expected to cause 250,000 additional deaths per year globally, with the direct costs to health projected to be $2 to $4 billion annually (WHO 2014). More recently the "super" typhoon that struck the Philippines on November 8, 2013, was recorded as the fourth most intense tropical cyclone in history with the preliminary impacts of a death toll at 8,000, damages of $12 billion, 4 million displaced people, 500,000 destroyed homes and nearly 9.8 million affected people (UN News Centre 2014). Climate change and human health is already a problem of crisis proportions in many parts of the world.

The range of climate impacts include an increase in the intensity and incidence of heat waves; increased incidence and severity of weather events such as hurricanes, droughts and tornadoes; an increase in air pollutant effects as emissions interact with changing weather patterns; an increased risk of allergens-related disease; and expansion or changing paths for the transmission of pathogens (IPCC 2014). Issues of mental and social distress exacerbated by displacement have also been identified as potential effects arising from a changing climate (Albrecht et al. 2007). The climate and human health research concludes there is a range of both direct and indirect climate impacts. Direct effects include deaths and injuries that are caused by an event itself. Indirect or secondary effects are those that can result from, or are mediated by changes in ecological systems and existing social and economic conditions.

The problem of social and economic inequalities present among countries at the global level has been the subject of intense negotiations at international forums, and it is generally understood that developing countries have lesser capacities to adapt or be resilient to climate impacts (Confalonieri et al. 2008). In the United States, the important question of how climate change impacts are distributed across communities in the context of historical environmental inequalities should also be of concern in climate assessment and planning. Many communities are already experiencing the effects of climate-related events, including drought in the Midwest and Southwest, floods along the Mississippi River, and early and severe snowstorms on the East Coast (Zaffos 2011). In 2011 alone, an estimated 1,270 tornadoes were responsible for 544 deaths and $25 billion in damages (Zaffos 2011). Hurricane Katrina caused an estimated 1,833 deaths and displaced more than 1 million people (Blanchard 2008; Plyer 2014). On October 29, 2012, Superstorm Sandy hit the northeastern seaboard of the United States, the Greater Antilles, the Bahamas, and eastern Canada. Reminiscent of Katrina, the effects of Superstorm Sandy unleashed a range of environmental impacts from trauma and injury to toxic exposure to the physical displacement of residents. Sandy's total economic toll is estimated at over $20 billion in infrastructure damage and losses including over 650,000 houses and 300,000 businesses damaged or destroyed (Burritt and Sullivan 2012; National Oceanic and Atmospheric Administration 2015). Communities already affected by sea level changes and extreme weather events demonstrate that analyses of unequal impacts associated with climate-related events are crucial.

It is evident that environmental change now stands to exacerbate the risks to public health in many significant ways. Still, research and planning in this area are relatively new. In 1990, Congress established the US Global Change Research Program to conduct national assessments of the potential impacts of climate change, but it was not until 1997 that the process earnestly began to include public health (Patz et al. 2000). In 2007, the National Research Council (NRC; 2007) conducted a review of the US Climate Change Science Program and concluded that a knowledge gap existed and that "efforts to understand climate change impacts on society, to analyze mitigation and adaptation strategies, and to study regional impacts are 'relatively immature'" (Ebi et al. 2009, 589). These conclusions underscore the fact that historically less research and fewer resources have been directed to climate adaptation and public health compared to other topics such as energy, economics, agriculture, and biodiversity. Similarly, referring to the outcomes of the UN Conference of Parties 15 (COP 15) negotiations in 2012, Rosenzweig and Wilbanks (2010) conclude that "it has taken about 35 years for scientists to bring the global climate change issue to the attention of the world's people and their leaders . . . however interdisciplinary work on impacts, adaptation, and vulnerability is still critically needed to advance the development of the solution phase" (103).

On the policy side, President Obama issued executive order 13514, Federal Leadership in Environmental and Energy Performance, which established the Interagency Climate Change Adaptation Task Force (2011) with making recommendations on how federal policies, programs, and planning can prepare the nation for the impacts of climate change (Interagency Climate Change Adaptation Task Force, 2011). In one of its first reports, the task force reiterated the call for adaptation planning and stated, "While Federal agencies have made progress in helping communities build resilience to climate change impacts, much more can be done, particularly for vulnerable populations. Within communities, some populations—such as children, elderly and low-income citizens—are more vulnerable to climate impacts due to higher sensitivity to health threats. Tribal nations are also disproportionately affected by climate change because of their strong dependence on natural resources for economic development, subsistence, social cohesion, and culture" (10).

It is the issue of **vulnerability** that is of special concern to the **environmental justice (EJ) community**. While climate adaptation and **resiliency** has now achieved a priority position on the nation's policy and research agendas, it is our contention that research on the problem of social and environmental inequality in climate change remains relatively immature. Clearly the impacts experienced by communities in the United States are different from those of the global South. However, the nation is by no means immune to the problem of inequality within its borders; in some cases, the impacts on EJ communities, low-income communities—Indigenous communities and communities of color—have reached crisis conditions.

This chapter offers an introduction to the importance of rooting climate and public health research in an examination of inequality in our society. Using an EJ framework, we discuss several important climate change-related impacts that disproportionately affect EJ communities and demonstrate why incorporating a structural approach is required.

CLINICAL CORRELATES 15.1 HOSPITAL ACCESS, VULNERABLE POPULATIONS, AND SUPERSTORM SANDY

The closing of Bellevue hospital in New York City in the wake of Superstorm Sandy highlights the need to intensify resources in environmental justice communities. Bellevue Hospital is the largest public hospital in the city, with 828 inpatient beds and multiple clinics that handle nearly 500,000 outpatient and 145,000 emergency visits per year. More than 80 percent of Bellevue patients are medically underserved. ("Bellevue Hospital Center" 2015). When Superstorm Sandy hit New York City on the evening of October 29, 2012, it caused power outage throughout the hospital and severe flooding, which ultimately forced the hospital to evacuate all patients and close its doors (Uppal et al. 2013).

To make matters worse for patients, the hospital remained closed for three months after the storm. The effect that this closure had on the city's most vulnerable populations is unknown. Those who relied on Bellevue for intensive outpatient care and those requiring hospitalization would have had to travel outside their neighborhood on unreliable postdisaster public transportation to seek care from other already severely overcrowded hospitals. In retrospect, many aspects of Bellevue's design were not prepared for a storm surge, despite its location along the water (Teperman 2013). This incident highlights the need to intensify resources in environmental justice communities, which have historically experienced low investment or disinvestment that makes them vulnerable to natural disasters.

Hospitals serving environmental justice communities require more state, local, and federal funding in order to prepare for natural disasters.

Climate Resiliency and Environmental Justice

Even with our best science, precise predictions about how and to what extent climate change will affect different communities are extremely difficult. We do know that environmental changes are occurring and that their impacts on people and communities do not occur in isolation; they are also determined to a great extent by existing social, political, economic, and environmental conditions (Intergovernmental Panel on Climate Change 2014). Acknowledgment of these uncertainties and complexities in the science of climate change has resulted in the development of a policy and planning framework built on the concept of resiliency. The priority of climate resiliency planning is to enhance the capacity of communities to prepare for and protect against impacts associated with climate-related events. Moreover, absent full and complete predictive knowledge about the scope and magnitude of these occurrences and their impacts, climate resiliency also focuses on increasing community capacity for effective and timely recovery (O'Brien et al. 2004; Smit and Wandel 2006).

A crucial component of climate resiliency planning therefore must include assessments of existing unequal environmental conditions and capacities to both withstand and recover from environmental threats. The climate and public health literature has largely defined differential impacts among individuals and communities as variations in vulnerability. The vulnerabilities associated with climate change are a function of the direct effects of climate-related events and ecosystem trends and the capacity of people and communities to be resilient when these events occur. In disaster management, *vulnerability* is defined as the "diminished capacity to anticipate, cope with, resist and recover from the impact of hazards" (International Federation of Red Cross and Red Crescent Societies n.d.). Climate resiliency therefore is interdisciplinary in nature and draws significantly from the fields of planning, public health and disaster management.

Two general questions frame an analysis of vulnerability: What is the scope and intensity of the threat, and What are the factors that create the condition of vulnerability? These two questions are also critically important in the EJ field.

An important methodological problem is that vulnerability can be conceptualized in different and sometimes competing ways. As O'Brien et al. (2004) suggest, there are two general frameworks of vulnerability in climate change research, each with significantly different methodological approaches to resiliency research and planning. The first is defined as an end point approach, whereby vulnerability is essentially viewed as the impacts that result from the added effects of climate change influences. This approach uses predictions presented by climate modeling, and from these predictions projects potential impacts on individuals with existing health predispositions. Community vulnerabilities are understood as the aggregate of individual vulnerabilities, which leads to an individualized-based risk framework. An example of this approach is demonstrated by the Centers for Disease Control and Prevention's (CDC) Building Resilience against Climate Effects (BRACE) framework (2012) which defines the following steps to climate change planning:

Step 1. Forecast climate impacts and assess vulnerabilities.

Step 2. Project the additional burden of health outcomes.

Step 3. Assess public health interventions for suitable interventions for the impacts of greatest concern.

Step 4. Develop and implement a climate and health adaptation plan.

Step 5. Evaluate impacts of the plan and its implementation.

In this approach, existing health conditions are the baseline for assessment, and climate-related impacts are measured as the additional risks to the baseline presented by climate events. While this approach certainly has some analytical merit, it does not easily integrate issues of existing inequality and therefore from an EJ perspective can be viewed as useful but also as containing a significant risk of being incomplete.

A second vulnerability framework that more easily incorporates EJ concerns is identified by O'Brien et al. (2004) as the "starting point" approach. Environmental and social processes are included in this approach, which requires diagnoses of "inherent social and economic processes of marginalization and inequalities as the causes of climate vulnerability" (5). The authors conclude that if "the underlying causes and contexts of vulnerability are not taken into account, there is a danger of underestimating the magnitude (large), scope (social and environmental) and urgency (high) of climate change" (12). In this approach, vulnerability addresses climate risks in the context of institutional inequalities, which are determined by political and economic factors.

The starting point approach corresponds to an EJ framework for understanding climate change and incorporates the structural or institutional issues that contribute to the existing unequal distribution of risk. Climate impacts should not be divorced from the legacy of pollution and environmental harms already experienced by communities. To exclude or discount these processes in climate resiliency planning and research at a minimum presents incomplete analysis of vulnerability and, more significant, may reinforce and maintain patterns of inequality. Understanding the social geography of vulnerability in climate and public health is as essential as understanding pathways of exposure. As Cutter (2006) notes, "The underlying dimensions of a place, including its social institutions, construct and define risks . . . Hazards and risks, then, are more than just the probability of occurrence of an extreme event. They include the underlying factors that contribute to risks in the first place" (11).

Most climate change planning efforts focus on the additional health effects caused by climate change and identification of affected populations without addressing the underlying dimensions of place that Cutter articulated. In an EJ or starting point approach, existing environmental, social, and political stressors that create the condition of vulnerability are addressed, thus presenting a more accurate understanding of the full scope of climate change and its impacts on vulnerable communities. From an EJ perspective, the fundamental problem of vulnerability is that communities live with existing physical and social challenges, which are compounded by climate change events. The challenges of building equitable climate-resilient communities emanates from the fact that vulnerability is determined by both individual-based and structural-based risk factors. As the research and practice of resilient communities continues to advance, EJ is critical to a full examination of the challenges and opportunities for an equitable climate resilient future. Fortunately, a significant body of research on environmental inequality and its causes has been developed over the past thirty years, including studies examining how and to what extent race, poverty, and institutional structures and practices are determinant factors in creating such conditions.

An EJ structural-based approach to public health planning and implementation is critical for building climate resiliency that does not reinforce historical inequality. Therefore, public health research and planning on climate-related vulnerability could greatly benefit from the work in this area. In the next sections, we examine how EJ research can be integrated into climate change and public health analyses and planning. It should be noted that this is an introduction into the issues associated with this integrative framework. As such, the examples cited are briefly outlined as a summary. Our goal is to illustrate how climate resiliency research and planning can more effectively address EJ concerns and issues of inequality

Cumulative Impacts, Environmental Justice, and Climate Change

A disproportionate number of polluting facilities are often located in EJ communities, and the issue of **cumulative impacts** focuses on how to address the problem of multiple pollutants emitted by multiple facilities (Morello-Frosch et al. 2011; California EPA 2010; Bullard et al. 2007; Mohai and Saha 2007). The current system of environmental protection does not effectively regulate the dangerous mixture of multiple toxins that often occurs in EJ neighborhoods, partly because it attempts to control pollution by establishing individual standards for each pollutant that do not account for their cumulative concentrations or effects (California EPA 2010; National Environmental Justice Advisory Council 2004; Environmental Protection Agency 2003). Another important aspect of cumulative impacts is social vulnerabilities that all too frequently exist in communities of color and low-income communities. These vulnerabilities include a lack of access to fresh food, a lack of planned open space, poor public infrastructure, health disparities, racial discrimination, poverty and crime (Morello-Frosch et al. 2011). When these social vulnerabilities are combined with pollution from multiple facilities, conditions are created that are conducive to the production of detrimental health impacts. The issue of cumulative impacts has multiple impacts and interactions. It includes the interaction of multiple pollutants as well as the interaction of multiple social vulnerabilities. It also encompasses the interaction of pollution with social vulnerabilities and the detrimental health impacts produced by all of the aforementioned. Cumulative impacts can be a difficult issue to understand and address because its different aspects are so intertwined.

For example, health disparities can both contribute to and be a result of cumulative impacts.

Multiple polluting facilities that overburden communities with pollution may contribute to health disparities that consistently plague Indigenous communities, communities of color, and low-income communities in the United States (National Center for Health Statistics 2013; Morello-Frosch et al. 2011; Adler and Rehkopf 2008; Waldron 2007; Dressler, Oths, and Gravlee 2005; Spalter-Roth Rowenthal, and Rubio 2005; Mensah et al. 2005). EJ research has investigated these disproportionate or unequal exposures to pollution, which can include a range of hazards from poor air quality to brownfields and toxic waste siting to unequal regulatory enforcement (Cutter 2006; Agyeman, Bullard, and Evans 2003; Mohai, Pellow, and Timmons 2009; Pearsall and Pearce 2010; Bullard and Wright 2009; Tsosie 2007). The EJ research and advocacy community has had a long-standing call for addressing the methodological shortcomings (Brulle and Pellow 2005; Corburn 2002) in both our legal system and in conventional research that have addressed pollutants individually and not accounted for their cumulative effects. A 2004 National Environmental Justice Advisory Council (NEJAC) report emphasized the need to address the inequity of public health research through the development and implementation of a cumulative risk and impacts assessment framework. NEJAC also called for place-based assessments and the inclusion of the effects of psychosocial and physical factors, as well as environmental factors, that may compound health risks for individuals in a community. A cumulative impacts framework or policy would focus on addressing the aggregation, and possible synergy, of risks and impacts from multiple pollutants emitted by multiple sources. It would also seek to account for social vulnerabilities.

A high level of cumulative impacts can also make EJ communities especially vulnerable to several detrimental impacts of climate change. For example, communities with a significant number of polluting facilities can be at higher risk of toxic contamination left behind by receding storm surge waters. This risk may be more widespread in low-income communities where the risk of flooding can be intensified due to poor infrastructure that includes an inadequate drainage system. When cumulative impacts are combined with existing health disparities that include a relative lack of access to quality health care (Little-Blanton and Hoffman 2005; Spalter-Roth et al. 2005; Williams and Rucker 2000), EJ communities may also become especially vulnerable to climate change–related heat stress, increases in air pollution and elevations in the risk of vector borne disease.

Because communities with a high level of cumulative impacts will be more vulnerable to climate change, they will be in need of community-level resiliency plans. Since cumulative impacts may result in detrimental health impacts and contribute to the creation of health disparities, these communities also need a coherent cumulative impacts strategy that at the very least will reduce their levels of pollution and ideally address other aspects of cumulative impacts (Morello-Frosch et al. 2011; California EPA 2010; NEJAC 2004). It is important to understand that an effective cumulative impacts strategy or public policy will not only make communities healthier in general; it will also make them more resilient to the detrimental impacts of climate change and should be part of adaptation planning.

When recovering from what is perhaps the best-known detrimental impact of climate change, an increased number of extreme weather events, care should be taken that the problem of cumulative impacts in EJ communities is not perpetuated or exacerbated. This can be accomplished in part by taking three steps during poststorm reconstruction: (1) determine if the structure being rebuilt will emit significant amounts of pollution; (2) determine if the structure is being rebuilt in an EJ community with a high level of cumulative impacts due in part to multiple sources of pollution; and (3) not rebuild a structure that emits significant amounts of pollution in an EJ community suffering from high levels of cumulative impacts until existing pollution is reduced, or at least a strategy is in place to do so.

Air Quality, Environmental Justice, and Climate Change

While the full extent of climate change impacts on air quality is yet to be known, an extensive body of research on the effects of air pollution on human health has been conducted. Major pollutants of concern include ozone, particulate matter, sulfur dioxide, nitrogen oxides, and volatile organic compounds due to their health impacts (Tagaris et al. 2010; Ebi and McGregor 2008). Particulate matter and ozone are air pollutants of priority concern (Caiazzo et al. 2013; Tagaris et al. 2010). A recent MIT study concluded that in 2005, particulate matter contributed to a staggering 200,000 premature deaths and estimated 10,000 early mortalities were ozone related (Caiazzo et al. 2013). The investigation focused on fine particulate matter, or PM2.5, airborne particles less than 2.5 microns in diameter. These very small particles are considered more harmful to health than larger particles because they can penetrate deep into the lungs (Pope and Dockery 2006; Brunkreef and Holgate 2002). In addition to early mortality, fine particulate matter has been linked to a wide range of problems including respiratory disorders, cardiovascular disease, and lung cancer (Pope and Dockery 2006; Jarrett et al. 2005; Pope et al. 2004; Dockery et al. 1993). Ozone is also associated with emergency room visits for respiratory problems, diminished lung function, and asthma (Tagaris et al. 2009, 2010; Ebi and McGregor 2008; Knowlton et al. 2004; Kinney 1999).

In the context of a changing climate, important research topics include how the concentration, transport, dispersion, and deposition of air pollutants are and will be affected (Ebi and McGregor 2008). Research indicates that climate change directly affects local air quality by altering chemical reaction rates, as well as affecting the transport, dispersion, and deposition of air pollutants. These direct effects of climate change increase the burden of illness and mortality across different communities and regions (Ebi and McGregor 2008). For example, studies estimate that air pollution-related deaths will increase in approximately two-thirds of the states due to changes in climate (Tagaris et al. 2009, 2010). It is projected that fine particulate matter will affect premature mortality rates in the Great Lakes area and northeast, while the southern states are expected to experience a greater incidence of ozone related deaths and other health effects (Tagaris et al. 2009, 2010). There are also indications that climate change will increase ozone concentrations in Los Angeles, Houston, Chicago, New York, and Atlanta and may cause more violations of the daily 8-hour average ozone air quality health standard in Los Angeles, New York and Houston (Tagaris et al. 2010). It has been estimated that climate change–induced increases in particulate matter concentrations will cause four thousand additional premature deaths per year and elevations in ozone concentrations will account for another three hundred early mortalities (Tagaris et al. 2009, 2010). Projections concerning climate change and particulate matter are thought to be less certain than those involving climate change and ozone (Ebi and McGregor 2008).

Several climate-related issues could exacerbate problems already affected by fine particulate matter and ozone, which are less severe than premature mortality. For example, increased carbon dioxide levels can result in longer growing seasons for ragweed and other aeroallergens, which could cause an increase in allergic reactions and asthma episodes (Luber et al. 2014). Ozone can exacerbate allergic conditions (Ebi and McGregor 2008), and both ozone and particulate matter have been connected to reduced lung function (Knowlton et al. 2004; Brunekreef et al. 1997) and asthma (Tagaris et al. 2009, 2010; Knowlton et al. 2004; Kinney 1999; Schwartz et al. 1993; Pope 1989). Although these conditions are a concern to a wide range of populations, asthma is also an EJ issue since it disproportionately affects children of color (Akinbami et al. 2014; Environmental Protection Agency n.d.). It should be noted that the studies cited here that linked particulate matter to asthma (Schwartz et al. 1993 and Pope 1989) investigated particles less than 10 microns in diameter and not fine particulate matter.

From an EJ framework, the ultimate question is what impact climate change will have on the distributional burden of illness and mortality due to air pollution among different communities across the nation (Ebi and McGregor 2008). Several investigations have found that communities of color and low-income communities are already disproportionately exposed to airborne pollutants (California EPA 2010; Ash et al. 2009; Pastor et al. 2005; Pastor, Sadd, and Morello-Frosch 2004; Houston, et al. 2004; Jarrett et al. 2001; Wernette and Nieves 1992). Given these existing disproportionate exposures, the prospect of increased levels of air pollution due to climate change is particularly troubling for EJ communities. This is one reason that some EJ advocates and researchers maintain that climate change policy should address greenhouse gas toxic copollutants, such as particulate matter and its precursors, as well as greenhouse gases (Boyce and Pastor 2012; Environmental Justice and Science Initiative 2010; Kaswan 2008; Sheats et al. 2008). By doing so, such a policy orientation would at least partially incorporate a cumulative impacts framework, which encompasses existing disproportionate pollution burdens. If climate change policy does not address preexisting pollution inequalities it runs the risk of reinforcing them.

CLINICAL CORRELATES 15.2 ASTHMA DISPARITIES AND ENVIRONMENTAL HEALTH

The Centers for Disease Control and Prevention report that asthma prevalence increased from 7.3 percent in 2001 to 8.4 percent in 2010, thus affecting 25.7 million individuals annually (Akinbami et al. 2012). Deteriorating air quality due to climate change is a concerning threat to children in environmental justice communities. Clinicians, regulators, public health officials, and housing authorities must come together to address this large and vulnerable population.

Deteriorating air quality threatens to increase rates of respiratory illness, especially in children and among those in environmental justice communities.

Heat Waves, Environmental Justice, and Climate Change

The impacts of climate on weather patterns, and particularly the incidence of high-temperature degree-days or heat waves, is an area of substantial research (National Aeronautics and Space Administration 2010). According to the Centers for Disease Control there were approximately eight thousand premature deaths in the United States between 1979 and 1999 due to heat-related stress (EPA 2008), and the number of deaths associated with a July 1995 Chicago heat wave was estimated to be as high as seven hundred (Cooney 2011; Whitman et al. 1997). People with preexisting illnesses such as cardiovascular, respiratory and cerebrovascular disease are especially vulnerable to heat-related stress (Basu 2009). The incidence of these illnesses is not uniform across socioeconomic status, however. A number of studies have found that race and socioeconomic status are important variables in contributing to the vulnerability to heat stress for a variety of reasons (Cooney 2011; Uejio et al. 2011; Balbus and Molina 2009; Basu 2009; Harlan et al. 2006; O'Neill, Zanobetti, and Schwartz 2003; Curriero et al. 2002; Klinenberg 2003; Whitman et al., 1997; Greenberg et al. 1983). The impact of temperature increases and heat waves will continue to be a public health problem and one of the primary predicted effects of climate change (Uejio et al. 2011; O'Neill et al. 2003; Curriero et al. 2002). While large urban centers are not the only communities vulnerable to heat-induced health risks, they have been identified as particularly susceptible to this problem (Ueijio et al. 2011) and are places where large numbers of people live in in a physical infrastructure that exacerbates the effects of high degree temperatures. The research indicates that the incidence of extreme heat in urban areas will continue to be an important public health problem because of the **urban heat island (UHI)** effect.

The UHI effect refers to the higher thermal storage capacity of the urban environment, which, in combination with a relatively high concentration of heat sources, contributes to an increase in temperatures relative to surrounding areas. The UHI effect results in both elevated surface and air temperatures. Surfaces, including roofs, roads, and sidewalks, absorb heat that can result in surface temperatures up to 18 to 27 degrees Fahrenheit (F.) higher than surrounding areas during the daytime, and 9 to 18 degrees F. higher during nighttime (Environmental Protection Agency 2008). Heat absorption by city surfaces also contribute to elevated urban air temperatures that can range from 2 to 10 degrees F. higher than in neighboring rural and suburban areas (EPA 2008; Berdahl and Bertz 1997). Importantly, higher daytime temperatures result in absorption of heat, which radiates at night, thereby raising nighttime temperatures. These nighttime temperature increases can be even more problematic than daytime heat and have been linked to increased deaths, particularly among the elderly and the socially isolated (Environmental Protection Agency 2008).

UHIs are also associated with elevated emissions of air pollutants and greenhouse gases due to the increased use of energy required to meet the added demand for cooling buildings during periods of high temperatures. It is estimated that the UHI effect can be responsible for as much as 5 to

10 percent of peak electricity demand (Hewitt, Mackres, and Shickman 2014; Akbari 2005). Increased electricity needed for cooling increases the need for additional generating capacity, and peak-load generating units are brought online quickly to meet this demand. However, these units are generally the least efficient and increase emissions of pollutants. Due to this chain of events, a rise in demand due to climate change–related temperature elevations would have implications for heat-related air quality conditions experienced by urban populations. This is an EJ issue since so many people of color and low-income Americans live in cities.

While the research on the racial determinants of the distribution of heat-related morbidity and mortality is relatively small, a few studies have found that further investigation in this area is well warranted. For example, there are indications that blacks (Uejio et al. 2011; Basu 2009; O'Neill et al. 2003; Curriero et al. 2002; Klinenberg 2003; Whitman et al. 1997; Greenberg et al. 1983), people of low and moderate income (Balbus and Molina 2009; Basu 2009; Harlan et al. 2006; O'Neil et al. 2003; Curriero et al. 2002; Klinenberg 2003) as well as Latinos (Uejio et al. 2011; Harlan et al. 2006) are particularly vulnerable to heat stress. Research has found income disparities to be an important variable of heat stress vulnerability due to higher exposure rates (Harlan et al. 2006) and limited material resources (Balbus and Molina 2009; Harlan et al. 2006; Klinenberg, 2003; Greenberg et al. 1983) and social capital (Harlan et al. 2006; Klinenberg 2003) for coping. For example, in New York City, a strong correlation between income and the use of air-conditioning, an obvious mechanism to combat high temperatures, was found to have implications for low-income communities (New York City Department of Health and Mental Hygiene 2007). Inadequate access to air-conditioning may also be a factor in the disproportionate risk of mortality due to heat stress faced by blacks (O'Neill, Zanobetti, and Schwartz 2005).

Another contributing factor to heat stress is the problem of social isolation and inadequate neighborhood infrastructures (O'Neill, Zanobetti, and Schwartz 2003; Klinenberg 2003). Disparities in physical and social capital investment and the creation of historically poor neighborhoods should be taken into account in estimating differences in vulnerability (Williams and Collins 2001; Committee on Public Health Strategies to Improve Health 2011). The effects of past racial segregation practices also means that people of color are more likely than whites to live in poor-quality housing, which pose a greater risk of exposure to conditions that can contribute to heat and other health risks such as indoor allergens (Committee on Public Health Strategies to Improve Health 2011). This inequality is evident in that approximately 40 to 45 percent of black,

Latino, and native individuals live in poor neighborhoods (Braverman, Egerter, and Mockenhaupt 2011; National Environmental Justice Advisory Council 2004).

The physical, economic, and social infrastructures are important variables in climate resiliency because they can and do affect the capacity for sustaining strong social networks. Klinenberg (2003) examined an African American Chicago neighborhood that had a high mortality rate during the city's 1995 heat wave and concluded that poor infrastructure helped to create conditions that foster social isolation among its residents. The legacy of historic discriminatory practices such as redlining, the unequal effects of public infrastructure investments such as the engineering of highway systems through neighborhoods of color, and the disparities in the siting of NIMBY industries have created a pattern of unequal neighborhood capacities. Where people live and the condition of their neighborhoods is not only a consequence of the private real estate market. It is a product of unequal public housing subsidies and urban development programs as well. The infrastructure of today's cities was built with massive public and private investments and guided by planning models and public decisions that reproduced and reinforced segregation and inequality. Public health must now contend with the environmental and EJ impacts of this historical inequality (Braverman et al. 2011)

The higher heat mortality risk experienced by blacks may in part be due to living in disproportionate numbers in older and substandard housing (Jacobs 2011) that may increase heat exposure and constrain heat mitigation efforts (Uejio et al. 2011). Racial discrimination could play a role in confining relatively more blacks to this substandard housing. Several studies also produced evidence that Latinos living in Phoenix may be more vulnerable to heat stress. One investigation found more heat distress calls were made from neighborhoods with higher proportions of Latinos (and blacks, the linguistically isolated, and renters) (Uejio et al. 2011), and another determined that poor Latino neighborhoods experienced elevated levels of heat stress exposure (Harlan et al. 2006).

If overall temperatures and the frequency of heat waves increase as predicted, the future health and viability of vulnerable EJ communities must be addressed. We have suggested that heat stress vulnerability of these communities is linked to societal problems such as the negative impacts of urban redevelopment, socioeconomic inequality, discrimination, and the urban heat island effect. To address community heat stress vulnerability in the context of these challenging issues, EJ advocates, urban planners, and health professionals will surely have to work closely together.

Extreme Weather Events and Environmental Justice

An increased number of extreme weather events, particularly storms, may be among the most noticeable and well-known climate change–related impacts, and there are many EJ aspects connected to these highly destructive occurrences. Katrina, Sandy, and other disasters have shown that race and class affect evacuation from, impacts caused by, and response to extreme storms (Fair Share Housing Center et al. 2014; Enterprise Community Partners 2013; Furman Center and Moelis Institute 2013; Cutter et al. 2010; Bullard and Wright 2009; National Fair Housing Alliance 2006; Pastor et al. 2006). Bullard and Wright (2009) also remind us that existing inequalities affect impacts from and response to extreme storms. This discussion focuses primarily on Katrina and Sandy due to their destructive force and since they are the most recent US disasters that have galvanized societal interest.

Evacuation

New Orleans residents left stranded during Katrina were disproportionately of color and low income (Pastor et al. 2006), and there are various factors that might explain this phenomenon. For example, blacks in New Orleans relied more on public transit than whites and thus may have had a more difficult time fleeing the city (Pastor et al. 2006). In addition, government warnings regarding storms may not be as effective for people of color for several reasons. One is that that blacks and Latinos may rely more on the use of meetings or social networks to obtain information than other populations. Another is a higher level of distrust of government that may exist among some segments of EJ communities (Pastor et al. 2006).

Low-income residents may face a lack of resources that leaves them with no way to leave and no-where to go if they could leave (Pastor et al. 2006).

Impacts

For both Katrina and Sandy there is evidence that environmental justice communities suffered more damage than other communities (Enterprise Community Partners 2013; Logan 2006; Pastor et al. 2006). Residents of these neighborhoods may have suffered disproportionately in other ways also, for example, poststorm psychological ailments may be more prevalent in these communities (Enterprise Community Partners 2013; Pastor et al. 2006).

It is not clear why EJ communities suffer disproportionately from these storm-related impacts, but several reasonable explanations have ben offered. It could be that due to a lack of resources and racial discrimination, low-income communities and communities of color are more likely to be built on low ground and therefore are more prone to flooding (Bullard and Wright 2009; Logan 2006; Pastor et al. 2006). A higher percentage of residents of these communities may also live in sub-par housing (Jacobs 2011) that is more damage prone (Uejio et al. 2011). A higher incidence of psychological problems could possibly be because of color, and low-income people feel they have less control over their lives than do other storm survivors (Pastor et al. 2006).

Recovery

Low-income and of color residents may have more difficulty recovering from extreme storms for a number of reasons, including limited income, intensification of existing poverty, limited savings, limited insurance, barriers to communication, communities overburdened with pollution, health disparities, and racial discrimination (Bullard and Wright 2009; Pastor et al. 2006). It is probably easy for most people to understand how a limited income or poverty can make it more difficult to recover from an extreme storm, but it may be more difficult to comprehend, and perhaps accept, why being of color would also inhibit recovery. However, at least one report found that recovery from Katrina was slower for blacks relative to whites even at similar income levels (Bullard and Wright 2009). One reason this could be true is racial discrimination, especially discrimination related to housing and insurance. Housing discrimination can make it even more difficult for people of color to find housing in a market that has been reduced by the destructive force of an extreme weather event (Bullard and Wright 2009; National Fair Housing Alliance 2006). This may be one reason that a smaller percentage of blacks displaced by Katrina returned than displaced whites (Bullard and Wright 2009). Difficulty obtaining loans and satisfactory insurance can also reduce the resources available for residents of color to rebuild homes and businesses destroyed by an extreme weather event (Bullard and Wright 2009; Pastor et al. 2006). Businesses of color rooted in their own communities may also find it more difficult to recover because their of color clientele may suffer disproportionately high rates of both temporary and permanent displacement (Bullard and Wright 2009).

There is some evidence from both Katrina and Sandy that low-income residents and residents of color have found it more difficult than white residents to access poststorm governmental services (Fair Share Housing et al. 2014; Bullard and Wright 2009). One reason is that that the Federal Emergency Management Association services tend to focus on homeowners rather than renters and a higher percentage of renters than homeowners tend to be low-income and of color (Samara 2014; Furman Center and

Moelis Institute 2013). After Katrina, one reason that low-income residents may have found it more difficult to find housing, besides the basic problem of limited resources, was that a significant amount of public housing was destroyed or closed and not quickly rebuilt or reopened (Bullard and Wright 2009; Logan 2006; National Fair Housing Alliance 2006). There is some fear that this public housing will not be fully replaced (Bullard and Wright 2009).

Language can present barriers to both the emergency response to (Pastor et al. 2006) and recovery from (Fair Share Housing Center et al. 2014) severe storms, especially for the portion of the EJ population for which English is not their first language. This is particularly true if the government does not ensure that recovery information is fully and correctly translated into other languages besides English (Fair Share Housing Center et al. 2014; Pastor et al. 2006).

In order to make communities resilient to extreme weather events, community-level resiliency plans should be created that address the specific issues identified in this section of the chapter. These plans should be made and implemented by a partnership that involves community groups and EJ organizations that are provided with a sufficient amount of resources to allow them to be full partners (Pastor et al. 2006).

Indigenous Rights and Climate Change

There are approximately 565 federally recognized tribes within the United States, and numerous others whose recognition was either terminated or never acknowledged by the US governmental process. The history of American Indian tribes and Indigenous peoples is unique and underscores how the complexities and intersectionalities of social and economic policies contribute to disproportionate climate change impacts. Indigenous history is also crucial in understanding the range of historical accumulation of societal stressors that are the background to human-induced climate change.

The Indigenous experience is one of being the object of forced assimilationist and removal policies. Many tribal communities were relocated to entirely different regions or their rights to homeland areas were severely diminished. Duran and Duran (1995) explain that experiences of these types of societal-induced external stressors has resulted in a "soul wound" that continues in the community fabric from one generation to another. In fact, governmental policies and programs were explicitly designed to "kill the Indian, save the man." ("Kill the Indian, Save the Man" was the signature phrase of General Richard H. Pratt, who founded and developed Indian boarding schools in the United States in order to culturally assimilate American Indians.)

The concept of historical trauma is used to explain the generational consequences of traumatic experience. It is defined as a "cumulative trauma over both the life span and across generations that results from massive cataclysmic events" (Yellow Horse 1999, 111). King, Smith, and Gracey (2009) note, "Indigenous health is widely understood to also be affected by a range of cultural factors, including racism, along with various Indigenous-specific factors, such as loss of language and connection to the land, environmental deprivation, and spiritual, emotional, and mental disconnectedness. The definition of indigeneity is, therefore, inherently social, and includes major elements of cultural identity. Being isolated from aspects of this identity is widely understood to have a negative effect on Indigenous health" (77).

The result is that the scope and range of environmentally mediated climate change impacts on Indigenous peoples can be of a different character from other rural and urban populations. In part, this is also due to the fact that tribes in the United States have a unique political status as sovereign governments. In addition, tribes and tribal communities have retained cultural, linguistic, and livelihood practices such as hunting, fishing, and gathering that are very closely tied to nature and the environment. Therefore, cultural practices of Indigenous communities are strongly rooted in place, and the quality of life is dependent on the quality of that environment. Environmental changes that affect the quality and character of place can have significant intrusive implications.

Lynn et al. (2013) note that "American Indians and Alaska Natives face unique and disproportionate challenges from climate change that are not yet widely understood in academic or policy arenas" (546). Moreover, the reality is that "tribal access to resources is strongly influenced by the legal and regulatory relationship that tribes have with the federal government; and . . . tribes have a unique and multi-faceted relationship with places, ecological processes and species" (546; see also Reo and Parker 2013). Functionally, Indigenous peoples historically and contemporarily depend on the ecosystem for food, medicine, ceremonies, and other cultural practices (Whyte 2013). Their cultural frameworks are not oriented toward a commodification of the environment as a system of ecoservices. Rather, they view the environment as a source of livelihood and believe that plants and animals are spiritual in nature, which creates an entirely different ethic and practice in relationship to nature. For example, Lynn et al. (2013), explain that "water is held sacred by many Indigenous peoples, and considered by some to be a traditional food. In combination with other stressors, climate change may affect tribes' relationships with traditional foods, including access, availability, harvesting strategies and ability to store, process and use foods in traditional ways" (546). For Indigenous peoples, climate change portends not only to affect the physical character of the ecosystem and its processes. In so doing, it also affects how Indigenous communities will be able to continue to sustain longstanding cultural practices that are rooted in an understanding and knowledge of place.

The effects of climate change are already at a critical stage in many Indigenous communities. For example, in Alaska, rising sea levels, increased flooding, and melting permafrost are resulting in forced relocation and new disease. There is coastal erosion due to loss of protective sea ice, which is threatening Alaskan village infrastructures, water supplies, and health and safety systems (Cochran et al. 2013). For tribes in the Pacific Northwest and First Nations in Canada, salmon is a fundamental cultural and food resource, but quantitative and qualitative changes in the species are having consequences on Indigenous livelihoods (Jacob, McDaniels, and Hinch 2010). In the Southwest, there are droughts and changing river flows. The National Climate Assessment points out that the "Southwest's 182 federally recognized tribes and communities in its U.S.-Mexico border region share particularly high vulnerabilities to climate changes such as high temperatures, drought, and severe storms" (Garfin et al. 2014, 465). In the Great Lakes region, the growing range of wild rice, an Indigenous staple for Ojibwe communities, has been altered due to warming winters and changing water levels (Minnesota Department of Natural Resources 2008).

Reminiscent of past experiences, Indigenous peoples in the United States are now being forced to relocate their entire communities, as the environmental conditions attributable to a changing climate can no longer sustain their human settlements. The melting permafrost and ice in Alaska sea ice is contributing to intensive flooding and erosion. In 2009, the US Army Corps of Engineers identified 178 Alaskan communities that are threatened by erosion and 26 that are priority action communities. The Village of Kivalina, already being forced to relocate because of flooding, filed suit in federal court arguing that five oil companies, fourteen electric utilities, and the country's largest coal company were responsible (Barringer 2008). The total cost for relocation has been estimated at $400 million. Though the plaintiffs were unsuccessful in their suit, the issues facing Indigenous peoples in the Arctic as well as the Gulf Coast illustrate that climate change will compound the historical stresses that have been a part of community life.

Juxtapositioned with these real and potential risks is the fact that there are Indigenous communities that are currently with no electricity or potable water systems. Infrastructure systems in Indian Country are sorely in need of development and maintenance. In addition to the basic systems of electricity and water, other infrastructure needs such as housing, economic development, and health care continue to be a challenge for Indigenous communities. The National Congress of American Indians (NCAI) (n.d.) points out that 40 percent of on-reservation housing is considered substandard (compared to 6 percent outside Indian Country), and nearly one-third of homes on reservations are overcrowded. In addition, fewer than half of the homes on reservations are connected to public sewer systems, and 16 percent lack indoor plumbing. The NCAI also reports that 50 percent of Native homes are without phone service.

Climate vulnerability for Indigenous peoples is integrally connected to cultural rights. Changes in the ecosystem fundamentally alter the capacity for communities to continue to maintain their livelihoods and their spiritual and ceremonial practices. Moreover, the information and knowledge systems that are the underpinning of adaptive capacities are also at risk. The experiential and traditional knowledge of Indigenous peoples has developed over generations and adapted to the local culture and environment. It is transmitted orally from generation to generation (Ellen, Parkes, and Bicker 2000) and is the culmination of living in specific environments. More and more, traditional Indigenous knowledge is acknowledged by Western science and is being incorporated into the bank of climate change information and data because it is recognized that it offers intricate and sophisticated information about the environment. Thus, traditional Indigenous knowledge has gained legitimacy in the Western scientific community for its contribution to a fuller understanding of a range of environmental changes including climate change (Doyle, Redsteer, and Eggers 2013; Weinhold 2010b; Cochran and Geller 2002; Ellen et al. 2000).

While traditional knowledge can contribute to the wider understanding of climate change, because this knowledge has developed based on a preclimate change reality, it is also endangered. As climate change affects ecosystems, the extant knowledge base of Indigenous peoples is also threatened, and traditional knowledge will need to adapt to this changing condition. Weinhold (2010b) explains that "for some Native Americans, traditional knowledge developed over millennia of living on specific lands has been rendered almost meaningless, with many tribes evicted from the ecosystems they historically occupied and confined to reservations, sometimes on harsh, unproductive land" (A65).

Climate change resiliency efforts in Indigenous communities therefore must incorporate the myriad of historical, legal, and cultural complexities. Resiliency will require, as Whyte (2013) notes, the need to engage and contest hardships due to historical public and private actions, such as cultural discrimination and disrespect for treaty rights; and "how to pursue comprehensive aims at robust living like building cohesive societies, vibrant

cultures, strong subsistence and commercial economies and peaceful relations with a range of non-tribal neighbors from small towns to nation states
to the United Nations" (518).

CLINICAL CORRELATES 15.3 AMERICAN INDIAN AND ALASKA NATIVE HEALTH ISSUES

Native Americans comprise 564 federally recognized tribes and constitute roughly 1 percent of the US population. Their unique cultural and historical backgrounds as well as their current means of livelihood make them a particularly vulnerable group to environmental change (Weinhold 2010a). Important current health-related disparities include the following:

- In 2006, American Indian and Alaska Natives (AI/AN) had an infant death rate 48 percent greater than whites.

- In 2009 AI/AN adults more often lived in inadequate and unhealthy housing compared to white householders.

- In 2009, the percentage of AI/AN adults living in poverty was larger than any other US racial or ethnic group.

At the same time, AI/ANs have maintained a whole range of cultural practices that are highly effective in addressing health issues. Unfortunately, these practices have been marginalized by the conventional health care system. For example, Alaska natives derive 80 percent of their sustenance from the natural surroundings (Weinhold 2010a). Because of their ties to the land, these communities have been some of the first to experience the impacts of climate change and continue to be vocal and active proponents of addressing environmental changes. The domestic health community has a duty to address such blatant health disparities. In addition, we can appreciate and learn from both traditional AI/AN and western science about how to adapt during times of environmental strife.

American Indian and Alaska Native populations are sentinel observers of climate change and are particularly vulnerable to changes because of historical policies and practices, which have contributed to a range of community health issues and because of their reliance on local environments.

Summary and Recommendations

Summary

In the introduction to this chapter we highlighted the need to determine
if there are unequal climate change impacts on communities across our

nation. The knowledge and experience of EJ researchers and advocates should lead climate change researchers in general to have a heightened concern that communities of color and low-income communities in particular are especially vulnerable to the detrimental impacts of climate change. However, we have argued that the standard approach that many researchers use to engage climate change resiliency issues, while having merit, also contains a structural problem that does not facilitate the sufficient incorporation of EJ concerns.

The chapter also explores several specific issues that we feel should be an important part of the discussion surrounding climate change and protecting EJ communities. The first is cumulative impacts. A disproportionate number of polluting sources and social vulnerabilities combine to produce detrimental cumulative environmental and health impacts in EJ communities. These cumulative impacts and the conditions that combine to create them can also make EJ communities particularly vulnerable to the detrimental impacts of climate change.

The effect that climate change will have on air quality is another important EJ issue. It has been projected that climate change will cause additional premature deaths by resulting in higher fine particulate matter and ozone concentrations in some areas of the country. This is especially problematic for EJ communities because many of them already suffer from disproportionately high levels of air pollution.

Some investigations have yielded evidence that blacks, Latinos, and low-income Americans are particularly vulnerable to heat stress. Many factors may contribute to this vulnerability, including a lack of resources, social isolation, racial discrimination, and the heat island effect.

Race and low income can detrimentally affect issues related to extreme weather events, including evacuation, impacts, response, and recovery. Factors that might cause extreme weather events to disproportionately affect EJ communities are a lack of financial resources, including insurance; racial discrimination and disparities; communication barriers that can include language; and high amounts of neighborhood pollution.

Changes to, and loss of, biodiversity due to climate change are affecting Indigenous communities' ability to lead a subsistence existence and also negatively affects cultural practices as well. Some Indigenous communities have had to relocate due to climate change impacts. Indigenous communities contain a significant amount of traditional knowledge that is being recognized by mainstream science as important to the understanding of ecosystem operations. For Indigenous communities, resiliency will mean using both traditional and mainstream knowledge to cope with the historical trauma caused by destructive acts such as forced removal, forced assimilation, and cultural discrimination, as well as the effect of climate change on culture and subsistence lifestyles.

To address climate change–related EJ issues identified in this chapter we offer the following recommendations.

Recommendations

Community-level climate change resiliency plans should be prepared for as many EJ communities as possible. Two important issues related to these plans that need to be highlighted are:

+ "Community level" is not meant to refer to a municipal government. The geographic scope of these plans should coincide with neighborhoods within municipalities and not with the municipalities themselves.

+ Community residents, local community groups, and EJ organizations should play an integral role in creating and implementing these community-level resiliency plans. This type of community involvement would require that residents, community groups, and EJ organizations have access to sufficient resources to allow them to be equal partners with government in the development and implementation of these plans.

Public policy and community-level resiliency plans should address cumulative impacts.

If rebuilding is necessary after an extreme weather event, a cumulative impacts policy should be in place before a polluting facility is reconstructed in an EJ community that already has a high level of pollution.

Climate change mitigation policy should address toxic greenhouse gas copollutants, such as particulate matter and its precursors, as well as greenhouse gases. Special attention should be devoted to copollutants that affect EJ communities with high levels of cumulative impacts.

Community-level resiliency policy should address greenhouse gas copollutants that adversely affect local residents.

Public policy and community-level resiliency plans for indigenous communities should address, in addition to other more commonly discussed issues, historical trauma and climate change impacts on subsistence living and cultural practices.

Public policy and community-level resiliency plans should address evacuation, impacts, and recovery connected to extreme weather events and the factors that cause these events to have a disproportionate impact on EJ communities. Factors that should be addressed include:

- Racial discrimination, particularly those types that may pose the greatest impediments to resiliency efforts such as housing and insurance discrimination. Actions should be taken in an effort to ensure that these types of discrimination no longer exist or are at least minimized.

- The gap in procuring government resources after an extreme weather event that appears to exist between residents of EJ communities and other communities.

Conclusion

It is crucial that more research and resources, and more responsive methods, be developed to assess and mitigate the public health impacts of climate change on EJ communities. Clearly many aspects of the current system inadequately address their needs. These disparities are the result of the difference in adaptation and disaster preparedness, as well as capacities to withstand and recover from the physical and social impacts of climate change–related issues. Effective public health planning can both lessen and make communities more resilient to the negative effects of climate change–related environmental impacts. With the projected increase in the occurrence of climate change–related environmental impacts, it is critical to address the environmental and health disparities they produce.

Campbell-Lendruma, Corvalána, and Neiraa (2007), state, "Adaptation to climate change is essentially a matter of basic public health protection. . . . Ultimately, however, the public health community needs to go beyond reacting to a changing climate. A true preventive strategy needs to ensure the maintenance and development of healthy environments from local to global levels" (235–36). EJ communities should not be burdened with more climate change–related impacts than any other communities and all communities should be protected from these impacts. We have already offered a set of more specific recommendations but more generally in order to reduce climate change–related vulnerabilities and increase climate change–related resiliency in EJ communities our society needs to:

- Address the root causes of vulnerability, such as poverty, racial discrimination, ineffective governance and planning, and unequal and inadequate access to resources and livelihoods. To reiterate, we must address:

  o Racial bias and discrimination

  o Economic inequality

  o Unequal political power and access

  o Indigenous rights

- ◆   Reduce the impact of the climate change threat itself (through mitigation, prediction, and warning and preparedness)

- ◆   Build the capacity of EJ communities to withstand climate change related threats

Mitigating climate change and ensuring that EJ communities are resilient to the inevitable detrimental impacts of climate change are obligations our society must meet.

DISCUSSION QUESTIONS

1.   What are environmental justice communities, and what are some of the reasons these communities are vulnerable to climate change?

2.   Explain the concept of cumulative impacts, and list the ways in which these impacts may make environmental justice communities particularly vulnerable to climate change.

3.   Discuss the ways in which indigenous populations, such as American Indians and Alaska Natives, face unique and disproportionate challenges from climate change.

KEY TERMS

Cumulative impacts: The effect of multiple pollutants emitted by multiple Sources and their interaction with each other and social vulnerabilities.

Environmental justice (EJ) communities: Indigenous communities, communities of color and low-income communities.

Environmental justice: The Environmental Protection Agency defines environmental justice as the fair treatment and meaningful involvement of all people regardless of race, color, national origin, or income, with respect to the development, implementation, and enforcement of environmental laws, regulations, and policies

Resiliency: Focuses on increasing community capacity for an effective and timely recovery; used interchangeably with *adaptation.*

Urban heat island (UHI) effect: Refers to the higher thermal storage capacity of the urban environment, which in combination with a relatively high concentration of heat sources, contributes to an increase in temperatures relative to surrounding areas.

Vulnerability: In disaster management, defined as the "diminished capacity to anticipate, cope with, resist and recovery from the impact of hazards" (International Federation of the Red Cross and Red Crescent Societies, n.d.).

References

Adler, N. E., and D. H Rehkopf. 2008. "US Disparities in Health: Descriptions, Causes, and Mechanisms." *Annual Review of Public Health* 29:235–52.

Agyeman J., R. Bullard, and B. Evans, eds. 2003. *Just Sustainabilities: Development in an Unequal World.* Cambridge, MA: MIT Press.

Akbari, H. 2005. *Energy Saving Potential and Air Quality Benefits of Urban Heat Island.* Berkeley, CA: Lawrence Berkeley National Laboratory.

Akinbami, L., J. Moorman, A. Simon, and K. Schoendorf. 2014. "Trends in Racial Disparities for Asthma Outcomes among Children 0 to 17 Years, 2001–2010." *Journal of Allergy and Clinical Immunology* 134:547–53. http://www.aaaai.org /about-the-aaaai/newsroom/news-releases/Black-children-were-twice -as-likely-to-have-asthma.aspx

Akinbami, L. J., J. E. Moorman, C. Bailey, H. Zahran, M. King, C. Johnson, and X. Liu. 2012. "Trends in Asthma Prevalence, Health Care Use and Mortality in the United States, 2001–2010." NCHS data brief 94.

Albrecht, G., G. Sartore, L. Connor, N. Higginbotham, S. Freeman, B. Kelly, and, G. Pollard. 2007. "Solastalgia: The Distress Caused by Environmental Change." *Australasian Psychiatry* 15 (S1):S95–S98. doi:10.1080/10398560701701288

Ash, M., J. Boyce, G. Chang, J. Scoggins, and M. Pastor. 2009. *Justice in the Air: Tracking Toxic Pollution from America's Industries and Companies to Our States, Cities, and Neighborhoods.* Amherst, MA: Political Economy Research Institute.

Balbus, J., and C. Molina. 2009. "Identifying Vulnerable Subpopulations for Climate Change Health Effects in the United States." *Journal of Occupational and Environmental Medicine* 51(1):33–57.

Barringer, F. 2008. "Flooded Village Files Suit, Citing Corporate Link to Climate Change." *New York Times*, February 27. http://www.nytimes.com/2008/02/27 /us/27alaska.html?_r=0

Basu, R. 2009. "High Ambient Temperature and Mortality: A Review of Epidemiologic Studies from 2001 to 2008." *Environmental Health* 8(1):40.

"Bellevue Hospital Center." 2015. Wikipedia. http://en.wikipedia.org/wiki /Bellevue_Hospital_Center

Berdahl, P., and S. Bertz. 1997. "Preliminary Survey of the Solar Reflectance of Cool Roofing Materials." *Energy and Buildings* 25:149–58.

Blanchard, W. 2008. "Deadliest U.S Disaster: Top Fifty." Washington, DC: Federal Emergency Management Agency.

Boyce, J. K., and M. Pastor. 2012. *Cooling the Planet, Clearing the Air: Climate Policy, Carbon Pricing, and Co-Benefits.* Portland, OR: Economics for Equity and Environment.

Braverman, P. A., S. A. Egerter, and R. E. Mockenhaupt. 2011. "Broadening the Focus: The Need to Address the Social Determinants of Health." *American Journal of Preventive Medicine* 40:S4-S18.

Brulle, R. J., and D. N Pellow, eds. 2005. *Power, Justice, and the Environment.* Cambridge, MA: MIT Press.

Brunekreef, B., and S. T. Holgate. 2002. "Air Pollution and Health." *Lancet* 360 (9341):133–42.

Brunekreef, B., N. A. Janssen, J. de Hartog, H. Harssema, M. Knape, and P. van Vliet. 1997. "Air Pollution from Truck Traffic and Lung Function in Children Living near Motorways." *Epidemiology* 8:298–303.

Bullard, R. D., P. Mohai, R. Saha, and B. Wright. 2007. *Toxic Wastes and Race at Twenty: 1987–2007.* Cleveland, OH: United Church of Christ.

Bullard, R. D., and B. Wright, eds. 2009. *Race and Environmental Justice after Hurricane Katrina: Struggles to Reclaim, Rebuild and Revitalize New Orleans and the Gulf Coast.* Boulder, CO: Westview Press.

Burritt, C., and B. K. Sullivan. 2012. "Hurricane Sandy Threatens $20 Billion in Economic Damage." Bloomberg Business. October 30. http://www.bloomberg .com/news/2012–10–29/hurricane-sandy-threatens-20-billion-in-u-s -economic-damage.html

Caiazzo, F., A. Ashok, I. A. Waitz, S.H.L. Yim, and S.R.H. Barret. 2013. "Air Pollution and Early Deaths in the United States. Part 1: Quantifying the Impact of Major Sectors in 2005." *Atmospheric Environment* 79:198–208.

California Environmental Protection Agency. 2010. *Cumulative Impacts: Building a Scientific Foundation.* Sacramento, CA: Office of Environmental Health Hazard Assessment. http://oehha.ca.gov/ej/pdf/CIReport123110.pdf

Campbell-Lendruma, D., C. Corvalána, and M. Neiraa. 2007. "Global Climate Change: Implications for International Public Health Policy." *Bulletin of the World Health Organization* 85:161–244. http://www.who.int/bulletin /volumes/85/3/06–039503/en/

Centers for Disease Control and Prevention. 2012. "CDC Policy on Climate Change and Public Health." http://www.cdc.gov/climateandhealth/policy.htm

Cochran, P. L., and A. L Geller. 2002. "The Melting Ice Cellar: What Native Traditional Knowledge Is Teaching Us about Global Warming and Environmental Change." *American Journal of Public Health* 92(9):1404–1409.

Cochran, P., O. H. Hutingtom, C. Pungowiyi, S. Tom, F. S. Chapin III, H. P. Huntington, N. G. Maynard, and S. F. Trainor. 2013. "Indigenous Frameworks for Observing and Responding to Climate Change in Alaska." *Climatic Change* 120:557–67.

Committee on Public Health Strategies to Improve Health. 2011. *For the Public's Health: Revitalizing Law and Policy to Meet New Challenges.* Washington DC: National Academies Press.

Confalonieri, U., B. Menne, R. Akhtar, K. Ebi, M. Hauengue, R. Kovats, B. Revich, et al. 2008. "Human Health." In *Climate Change, 2007: Synthesis Report. Contribution of Working Groups I, II and III to the Fourth Assessment Report of the Intergovernmental Panel on Climate Change*, edited by Core Writing Team, R. K. Pachauri, and A. Reisinger. Geneva: Intergovernmental Panel on Climate Change. http://www.ipcc.ch/pdf/assessment-report/ar4/wg2/ar4-wg2-chapter8.pdf

Cooney, C. M. 2011. "Preparing a People: Climate Change and Public Health." *Environmental Health Perspectives* 119:a166-a171.

Corburn, J. 2002. "Environmental Justice, Local Knowledge and Risk: The Discourse of a Community-Based Cumulative Exposure Assessment." *Environmental Management* 29:451–66.

Curriero, F. C., K. S. Heiner, J. M. Samet, S. L. Zeger, L. Strug, and J. A. Patz. 2002. "Temperature and Mortality in Eleven Cities of the Eastern United States." *American Journal of Epidemiology* 155(1):80–87.

Cutter, S. 2006. *Hazards, Vulnerability and Environmental Justice.* New York: Earthscan.

Cutter, S. L., E. T. Emrich, J. T. Mitchell, B. J. Boruff, M. Gall, M. C. Schmidtlein, C. G. Burton, and G. Melton. 2010. "The Long Road Home: Race, Class, and Recovery from Hurricane Katrina." *Environment: Science and Policy for Sustainable Development* 48(2):8–20. doi:10.3200/ENVT.48.2.8–20

Dockery, D. W., C. A. Pope, X. Xiping, J. D. Spengler, J. H. Ware, M. E. Fay, B. G. Ferris, and F. E. Speizer. 1993. "An Association between Air Pollution and Mortality in Six U.S. Cities." *New England Journal of Medicine* 329:1753–59.

Doyle, J. T., M. H. Redsteer, and M. J. Eggers. 2013. "Exploring Effects of Climate Change on Northern Plains American Indian Health." *Climate Change* 120(3):643–55. doi: 10.1007/s10584–013–0799-z

Dressler, W. W., K. S. Oths, and C. C. Gravlee. 2005. "Race and Ethnicity in Public Health Research: Models to Explain Health Disparities." *Annual Review of Anthropology* 34:231–52.

Duran, E., and B. Duran. 1995. *Native American Postcolonial Psychology.* Albany: State University of New York Press.

Ebi, K. L., J. Balbus, P. L. Kinney, E. Lipp, D. Mills, M. S. O'Neill, and M. L. Wilson. 2009. "U.S. Funding Insufficient to Address the Human Health Impacts of and Public Health Responses to Climate Variability and Change." *Environmental Health Perspectives* 117:857–62.

Ebi, K., and G. McGregor. 2008. "Climate Change, Tropospheric Ozone and Particulate Matter, and Health Impacts." *Environmental Health Perspectives* 116:1449–55.

Ellen, R. P., P. Parkes, and A. Bicker, eds. 2000. *Indigenous Environmental Knowledge and Its Transformations: Critical Anthropological Perspectives.* Amsterdam: Gordon and Breach Publishing Group.

Enterprise Community Partners. 2013. "Hurricane Sandy: Housing Needs One Year Later." Research brief, October. Columbia, MD.

Environmental Justice and Science Initiative. 2010. "Letter on EPA Authority to Regulate Greenhouse Gases and Climate Change Co-Pollutant Policy." June 8, 2010.

Environmental Protection Agency. n.d. *Children's Environmental Health Disparities: Black and African American Children and Asthma.* Washington, DC: US Environmental Protection Agency. http://www.epa.gov/epahome /sciencenb/asthma/HD_AA_Asthma.pdf

Environmental Protection Agency. 2003. *Framework for Cumulative Risk Assessment.* Washington, DC: US Environmental Protection Agency.

Environmental Protection Agency. 2008. *Reducing Urban Heat Islands: Compendium of Strategies.* Washington, DC: US Environmental Protection Agency. http://www.epa.gov/heatisld/resources/compendium.htm

Fair Share Housing Center, Housing and Community Development Network of New Jersey, Latino Action Network, and NAACP New Jersey State Conference. 2014. *The State of Sandy Recovery.* Cherry Hill, NJ: Fair Share Housing Center.

Furman Center and Moelis Institute for Affordable Housing Policy. 2013. *Sandy's Effects on Housing in New York City.* New York: Furman Center.

Garfin, G., G. Franco, H. Blanco, A. Comrie, P. Gonzalez, T. Piechota, R. Smyth, and R. Waskom. 2014. "Southwest." In *Climate Change Impacts in the United States: The Third National Climate Assessment,* edited by J. M. Melillo, T. C. Richmond, and G. W. Yohe, 462–86. US Global Change Research Program. doi:10.7930/J08G8HMN

Greenberg, J. H., J. Bromberg, C. M. Reed, T. L. Gustafson, and R. A. Beauchamp. 1983. "The Epidemiology of Heat Related Deaths, Texas—1950, 1970–79, and 1980." *American Journal of Public Health* 73:805–807.

Harlan, S. L., A. J. Brazel, L. Prashad, W. L. Stefanov, and L. Larsen. 2006. "Neighborhood Microclimates and Vulnerability to Heat Stress." *Social Science and Medicine* 63:2847–63.

Hewitt, V., E. Mackres, and K. Shickman. 2014. *Cool Policies for Cool Cities: Best Practices for Mitigating Urban Heat Islands in North American Cities.* Washington, DC: American Council for an Energy Efficient Economy.

Houston, D., J. Wu, P. Ong, and A. Winer. 2004. "Structural Disparities of Urban Traffic in Southern California: Implications for Vehicle Related Air Pollution Exposure in Minority and High Poverty Neighborhoods." *Journal of Urban Affairs* 26:565–92.

Interagency Climate Change Adaptation Task Force. 2011. *Federal Actions for a Climate Resilient Nation: Progress Report of the Interagency Climate Adaptation Task Force.* Washington, DC: Interagency Climate Change Adaptation Task Force

International Federation of Red Cross and Red Crescent Societies. n.d. "What Is Vulnerability?" International Federation of Red Cross and Red Crescent Societies. http://www.ifrc.org/en/what-we-do/disaster-management/about-disasters/what-is-a-disaster/what-is-vulnerability/

Intergovernmental Panel on Climate Change. 2007. *Climate Change, 2007: Synthesis Report. Contribution of Working Groups I, II and III to the Fourth Assessment Report of the Intergovernmental Panel on Climate Change,* edited by M. L. Parry, O. F. Canziani, J. P. Palutikof, P. J. van der Linden, and C. E. Hanson. Geneva, Switzerland: Intergovernmental Panel on Climate Change. http://www.ipcc.ch/report/ar4/

Intergovernmental Panel on Climate Change. 2014. *Fifth Assessment Report: Climate Change 2013.* Geneva: Intergovernmental Panel on Climate Change." http://www.ipcc.ch/report/ar5/

Jacob, C., T. McDaniels, and S. Hinch. 2010. "Indigenous Culture and Adaptation to Climate Change: Sockeye Salmon and the St'at'ime People." *Mitigation and Adaptation Strategies for Global Change* 15:859–76.

Jacobs, D. E. 2011. "Environmental Health Disparities in Housing." *American Journal of Public Health* 101:S115–22.

Jarrett, M., R. T. Burnett, P. Kanaroglou, J. Eyles, N. Finkelstein, C. Giovis, and J. R. Brook. 2001. "A GIS–Environmental Justice Analysis of Particulate Air Pollution in Hamilton, Canada." *Environment and Planning A* 33:955–73.

Jarrett, M., R. T. Burnett, R. Ma, C. A. Pope, D. Krewski, K. B. Newbold, G. Thurston, et al. 2005. "Spatial Analysis of Air Pollution and Mortality in Los Angeles." *Epidemiology* 16:727–36.

Kaswan, A. 2008. "Environmental Justice and Domestic Climate Change Policy." *Environmental Law Reporter* 38:10287–345.

King, M., A. Smith, and M. Gracey. 2009. "Indigenous Health Part 2: The Underlying Cause of the Health Gap." *Lancet* 374:75–85.

Kinney, P. L. 1999. "The Pulmonary Effects of Outdoor Ozone and Particle Air Pollution." *Seminars in Respiratory and Critical Care Medicine* 20:601–607.

Klinenberg, E. 2003. *Heat Wave: A Social Autopsy of Disaster.* Chicago: University of Chicago Press.

Knowlton, K., J. Rosenthal, C. Hogrefe, B. Lynn, S. Gaffin, R. Goldberg, C. Rosenzweig, et al. 2004. "Assessing Ozone-Related Health Impacts under a Changing Climate." *Environmental Health Perspectives* 112:1557–63.

Little-Blanton, M., and C. Hoffman. 2005. "The Role Of Health Insurance Coverage in Reducing Racial/Ethnic Disparities in Health Care." *Health Affairs* 24:398–408.

Logan, J. R. 2006. *The Impact of Katrina: Race and Class in Storm-Damaged Neighborhoods.* Providence, RI: Brown University.

Luber, G., K. Knowlton, J. Balbus, H. Frumkin, M. Hayden, J. Hess, M. McGeehin, et al. 2014. "Human Health." In *Climate Change Impacts in the United States: The Third National Climate Assessment*, edited by J. M. Melillo, T. C. Richmond, and G .W. Yohe, 220–56. Washington, DC: US Global Change Research Program.

Lynn, K., J. Daigle, J. Hoffman, F. Lake, N. Michelle, D. Ranco, C. Viles, et al. 2013. "The Impacts of Climate Change on Tribal Traditional Foods." *Climatic Change* 120:545–56.

Mensah, G. A., A. H. Mokdad, E. S. Ford, K. J. Greenlund, and J. B. Croft. 2005. "State of Disparities in Cardiovascular Health in the United States." *Circulation* 111:1233–41.

Minnesota Department of Natural Resources. 2008. "Natural Wild Rice in Minnesota." St. Paul: Minnesota Department of Natural Resources. http://files.dnr.state.mn.us/fish_wildlife/wildlife/shallowlakes/natural-wild-rice-in-minnesota.pdf

Mohai, P., D. Pellow, and R. Timmons. 2009. "Environmental Justice." *Annual Review of Environment and Resources* 34:405–30.

Mohai, P., and R. Saha. 2007. "Racial Inequality in the Distribution of Hazardous Waste: A National-Level Reassessment." *Social Problems* 54:343–70.

Morello-Frosch, R., M. Zuk, M. Jarrett, B. Shamasunder, and A. D. Kyle. 2011. "Understanding the Cumulative Impacts of Inequalities in Environmental Health: Implications for Policy." *Health Affairs* 30:879–87.

Murphy, J. S., and M. T. Sandel. 2011. "Asthma and Social Justice: How to Get Remediation Done." *American Journal of Preventive Medicine* 41(2S1):S57–58.

National Aeronautics and Space Administration. 2010. "Urban Heat Islands." http://earthobservatory.nasa.gov/IOTD/view.php?id=4770

National Center for Health Statistics. 2013. *Health, United States, 2012: With Special Feature on Emergency Care.* Hyattsville, MD: National Center for Health Statistics.

National Congress of American Indians. n.d. "Housing and Infrastructure." National Congress of American Indians. http://www.ncai.org/policy-issues /economic-development-commerce/housing-infrastructure

National Environmental Justice Advisory Council, Cumulative Risks/Impacts Work Group. 2004. *Ensuring Risk Reduction in Communities with Multiple Stressors: Environmental Justice and Cumulative Risks/Impacts.* Washington, DC: US Environmental Protection Agency.

National Fair Housing Alliance. 2006. *Still No Home for the Holidays: A Report on the State of Housing and Housing Discrimination in the Gulf Coast Region.* Washington, DC: National Fair Housing Alliance.

National Oceanic and Atmospheric Administration. 2015. "Sandy's Legacy: Improved Storm Surge Prediction Tools." http://www.regions.noaa.gov/north-atlantic /highlights/sandys-legacy-improved-storm-surge-prediction-tools/

National Research Council. 2007. *Evaluating Progress of the US Climate Change Science Program: Methods and Preliminary Results.* Washington, DC: National Academies Press.

New York City Department of Health and Mental Hygiene. 2007. "Air Conditioner in Home by High-Risk (DPHO) Neighborhood, 2007 (Unadjusted for Age)." http://goo.gl/4sVv9k

O'Brien, K., S. Eriksen, A. Schjolden, and L. Nygaard. 2004. *What's in a Word? Conflicting Interpretations of Vulnerability in Climate Change Research.* Oslo, Norway: Center for International Climate and Environmental Research.

O'Neill, M. S., A. Zanobetti, and J. Schwartz. 2003. "Modifiers of the Temperature and Mortality Association in Seven US Cities." *American Journal of Epidemiology* 157:74–1082.

O'Neill, M. S., A. Zanobetti, and J. Schwartz. 2005. "Disparities by Race in Heat-Related Mortality in Four US Cities: The Role of Air Conditioning Prevalence." *Journal of Urban Health* 82:191–97.

Pastor, M., R. D. Bullard, J. K. Boyce, A. Fothergill, R. Morello-Frosch, and B. Wright. 2006. *In the Wake of the Storm: Environment, Disaster, and Race after Katrina.* New York: Russell Sage Foundation.

Pastor, M., R. Morello-Frosch, and J. L. Sadd. 2005. "The Air Is Always Cleaner on the Other Side: Race, Space, and Ambient Air Toxics Exposures in California." *Journal of Urban Affairs* 27:127–48. doi:10.1111/j.0735–2166.2005.00228.x

Pastor, M., Jr., J. L. Sadd, and R. Morello-Frosch. 2004. "Waiting to Inhale: The Demographics of Toxic Air Release Facilities in 21st-Century California." *Social Science Quarterly* 85:420–40. doi:10.1111/j.0038–4941.2004.08502010.x

Patz, J. A., M. A. McGeehin, S. M. Bernard, K. L. Ebi, P. L. Epstein, A. Grambsch, D. J. Gubler, et al. 2000. "The Potential Health Impacts of Climate Variability and Change for the United States: Executive Summary of the Report of the Health Sector of the U.S. National Assessment." *Environmental Health Perspectives* 108:367–76.

Pearsall, H., and J. Pearce. 2010. "Urban Sustainability and Environmental Justice: Evaluating the Linkages in Planning/Policy Discourse." *Local Environment* 15:569–80.

Plyer, A. 2014. "Facts for Features: Katrina Impact. Data Center." http://www.datacenterresearch.org/data-resources/katrina/facts-for-impact/

Pope, A. 1989. "Respiratory Disease Associated with Community Air Pollution and a Steel Mill, Utah Valley." *American Journal of Public Health* 79:623–28.

Pope, C., R. T. Burnett, G. D. Thurston, M. J. Thun, E. E. Calle, D. Krewski, and J. Godleski. 2004. "Cardiovascular Mortality and Long-Term Exposure to Particulate Air Pollution, Epidemiological Evidence of General Pathophysiological Pathways of Disease." *Circulation* 109:71–77.

Pope, C. A., and D. W. Dockery. 2006. "Health Effects of Fine Particulate Air Pollution: Lines That Connect." *Journal of the Air and Waste Management Association* 56:709–42.

Reo, N. J., and A. Parker. 2013. "Rethinking Colonialism to Prepare for the Impacts of Rapid Environmental Change." In *Climate Change and Indigenous Peoples in the United States*, edited by J. K. Maldonado, C. Benedict, and T. Pandya, 163–74. New York: Springer.

Rosenzweig, C., and T. Wilbanks. 2010. "The State of Climate Change Vulnerability, Impacts, and Adaptation Research: Strengthening Knowledge Base and Community." *Climatic Change* 100 (May):103–106. doi:10.1007/s10584–010–9826–5

Samara, T. R. 2014. *Rise Of the Renter Nation: Solutions to the Housing Affordability Crisis.* Brooklyn, NY: Homes for All Campaign of the Right to the City Alliance.

Schwartz, J., D. Slater, T. V. Larson, W. E. Pierson, and J. Q. Koenig. 1993. "Particulate Air Pollution and Emergency Room Visits for Asthma in Seattle." *American Review of Respiratory Disease* 147:826–31.

Sheats, N., T. Onyenaka, S. Gupta, V. Caffee, T. Carrington, K. Gaddy, and P. Montague. 2008. *An Environmental Justice Climate Change Policy for New Jersey.* Trenton: New Jersey Environmental Justice Alliance and Center for the Urban Environment.

Smit, B., and J. Wandel. 2006. "Adaptation, Adaptive Capacity and Vulnerability." *Global Environmental Change* 16:282–92.

Spalter-Roth, R., T. A. Rowenthal, and M. Rubio. 2005. *Race, Ethnicity, and the Health of Americans.* Sydney S. Spivack Program in Applied Social Research and Social Policy. http://www2.asanet.org/centennial/race_ethnicity_health.pdf

Tagaris, K., L. Kuo-Jen, A. J. DeLucia, L. Deck, P. Amar, and A. G. Russell. 2010. "Sensitivity of Air Pollution–Induced Premature Mortality to Precursor Emissions under the Influence of Climate Change." *International Journal of Environmental Research and Public Health* 7:2222–37.

Targaris, E., K. J. Liao, A. J. Delucia, L. Deck, P. Amar, and A. G. Russell. 2009. "Potential Impact of Climate Change on Air Pollution-Related Human Health Effects." *Environment Science and Technology* 43:4979–88.

Teperman S. 2013. "Hurricane Sandy and the Greater New York Health Care System." *Journal of Trauma and Acute Care Surgery* 74:1401–10.

Tsosie, R. A. 2007. "Indigenous People and Environmental Justice: The Impact of Climate Change." *University of Colorado Law Review* 78:1625.

Uejio, C. K., O. V. Wilhelmi, J. S. Golden, D. M. Mills, S. P. Gulino, and J. P. Samenow. 2011. "Intra-Urban Societal Vulnerability to Extreme Heat: The Role of heat Exposure and the Built Environment, Socioeconomics, and Neighborhood Stability." *Health and Place* 17:498–507.

United Nations News Centre. 2014. "One Year after Devastating Storm, UN Says Philippines 'Well on Road to Recovery.'" http://www.un.org/apps/news/story .asp?NewsID=49281#.VL09-ScXU3U

Uppal, A., L. Evans, N. Chitkara, P. Patrawalla, M. A. Mooney, D. Addrizzo-Harris, E. Leibert, et al. 2013. "In Search of the Silver Lining: The Impact of Superstorm Sandy on Bellevue Hospital." *Annals of the American Thoracic Society* 10:135–42.

US Army Corps of Engineers. 2009. *Alaska Baseline Erosion Assessment.* US Army Corps of Engineers. Alaska District.

Waldron, H. 2007. *Trends in Mortality Differentials and Life Expectancy for Male Social Security-Covered Workers, by average Relative Earnings.* Washington, DC: US Social Security Administration, Office of Research, Evaluation and Statistics.

Weinhold, B. 2010a. "Climate Change and Health: A Native American Perspective." *Environmental Health Perspectives* 118(2):A64–65.

Weinhold, B. 2010b. "Health Disparities: Climate Change and Health: A Native American Perspective." *Environmental Health Perspectives* 118:a64-a65. http:// dx.doi.org/10.1289/ehp.118-a64

Wernette, D. R., and L. A. Nieves. 1992. "Breaking Polluted Air." *EPA Journal* 18:16.

Whitman, S., G. Good, E. R. Donoghue, N. Benbow, S. Wenyuan, and S. Mou. 1997. "Mortality in Chicago Attributed to the July 1995 Heat Wave." *American Journal of Public Health* 87:1515–18.

Whyte, K. P. 2013. "Justice Forward: Tribes, Climate Adaptation and Responsibility." *Climatic Change* 120:517–530. doi:10.1007/s10584–013–0743–2

Williams, D. R., and C. Collins. 2001. "Racial Residential Segregation: A Fundamental Cause of Racial Disparities in Health." *Public Health Report* 226:404–16.

Williams, D. R., and T. D. Rucker. 2000. "Understanding and Addressing Racial Disparities in Health Care." *Health Care Financing Review* 21(4):75–90.

World Health Organization. 2005. "Climate Change and Human Health." Fact sheet. http://www.who.int/globalchange/news/fsclimandhealth/en/

World Health Organization. 2011. "The Social Dimensions of Climate Change, Discussion Draft." Geneva: World Health Organization.

World Health Organization. 2014. "Climate Change and Health." Fact sheet 266. http://www.who.int/mediacentre/factsheets/fs266/en/

Yellow Horse, M. 1999. "Oyate Ptayela: Rebuilding the Lakota Nation through Addressing Historical Trauma among Lakota Parents." In *Voices of First Nations People*, edited by H. Weaver, 109–26. Binghamton, NY: Haworth Press.

Zaffos, J. 2011. "Extreme Measures: The Push to make Climate Research Relevant." *Daily Climate*, November 2. http://wwwp.dailyclimate.org/tdc-newsroom/2011/11/weather-extremes

CHAPTER 16

CLIMATE CHANGE COMMUNICATION

Stuart Capstick, Adam Corner, Nick Pidgeon

A central concern for many social scientists working in climate change research is the promotion of effective **public engagement** with the personal, social, and political dimensions of climate change. Two of the main arguments for doing so are that in democratic societies, people should be involved in important decision-making processes in this area, and that closer personal engagement leads to attitudes and behaviors that can make a constructive contribution to addressing climate change (Höppner and Whitmarsh 2011; Oskamp 1995). From these basic premises there has now developed a substantial literature that has sought to set the conditions for **pro-environmental behavior** change (such as reducing energy consumption or switching from driving a car to cycling) and to develop **climate change communication** in ways that make the topic more comprehensible and personally relevant (Moser 2010; Steg and Vlek 2009). This is a critical task and a demanding one, entailing as it does the communication of a global problem that is at once more abstract and less salient than many other social issues and yet also has the potential to lead to more serious and long-term implications than many of the previous challenges that humanity has faced (Moser 2010). Public health professionals have themselves made the case for a concerted effort to communicate about climate change, and this chapter aims to discuss some of the key considerations that are of relevance to doing so.

The question of how to effectively communicate the health risks of climate change can be posed from several perspectives. In the first instance, the effects of climate change on human populations can to a large extent be viewed as a public health issue, as has been outlined

KEY CONCEPTS

- **Public health professionals have made the case for a concerted effort to communicate about climate change; the effects of environmental changes will be experienced by people predominantly through impacts on health and well-being.**

- **It is highly problematic to assume that public skepticism or lack of engagement about climate change derives principally from a lack of information or education on climate change.**

- **There is a strong evidence base that the ways in which we understand and respond to climate change is intimately connected with our values and worldviews.**

- **The language of uncertainty, so central to scientists' vocabulary, is typically unfamiliar to members of the public and may generate the impression that the science of climate change is less well understood than it actually is. It has been argued that the communication about climate**

KEY CONCEPTS (*CONTINUED*)

change should be reframed away from uncertainty and reoriented towards risk.

- Nisbet (2009) suggests that communication about climate change that connects to health that which are already familiar and seen as important (such as heat-stroke and asthma) can make the issue seem more personally relevant.

- A number of researchers have also suggested that the strategy of using tailored and targeted health communication can also be applied to communicating climate change. Tailored approaches to communication are premised on the notion that specific messages should be devised that resonate with particular audiences.

- Health practitioners are in a distinctive position with respect to being able to convey messages. As Frumkin and McMichael (2008) have noted, the health sector has an opportunity to demonstrate leadership on climate change because health professionals are seen as having moral authority, professional prestige, and a reputation for science-based analysis.

elsewhere in this book. That is, the effects of environmental changes will be experienced by people predominantly through impacts on our health and well-being. On this view of the problem, climate change becomes an additional, albeit important, driver of public health policy, and communicating effectively about climate-related health risks is important for this reason. A subtly different view of the overlap between climate change and its impacts on public health, however, is to ask whether the more familiar and well-understood territory of health might be a useful way of conveying information about climate change. That is, might the relationships between health and climate change lead to communication approaches that foster public engagement with both?

A large and growing body of research has shown that climate change communication requires careful consideration, in part because of the complex nature of the topic itself, but also because there are many elements of individual and social psychology which affect the ways in which climate change is conceptualized and messages about it are received. In this chapter we first discuss research which has examined public understanding of climate change, as a basis for thinking about some of the principles which can be applied to ensure sound communication. We next examine some of the approaches which have been used to communicate about specific climate impacts, with a particular focus on heat events and flood risk. We then move on to consider some of the targeted research which has looked at ways of structuring communication about climate change from a health perspective.

When there are so many other challenges facing health care providers, why take on the problem of climate change as well? Writing in the *British Medical Journal* in 2013, Costello, Montgomery, and Watts of the Institute for Global Health argue that the implications of climate change for public health are "profoundly worrying" and that health practitioners "need to shout from the rooftops that climate change is a health problem." They argue that those working in health cannot escape a responsibility for reducing carbon emissions any more than they can for alleviating poverty or reducing tobacco use. Writing in the

CLINICAL CORRELATES 16.1 PHYSICIAN ATTITUDES ON CLIMATE CHANGE

A 2014 survey of National Medical Association physicians shows the following attitudes (Sarfaty et al. 2014):

- Over 97 percent believe that climate change is happening and 62 percent believe that this change is mostly or entirely caused by human activities.

- Approximately 88 percent of participants believe that climate change is directly related to patient care and that it has caused harm in their communities over the past decade.

- Most physicians agree that climate change is currently affecting their patients' health due to severe weather (88 percent), increases in severity of chronic disease. (88 percent), increased allergic symptoms (80 percent) and heat-related morbidity (75 percent).

- Most physicians believe that certain groups of people, specifically the young, the old, and those with chronic diseases, are affected more than others.

A large majority (78 percent) of physicians think that their personal and professional actions can contribute to effective action on climate change. This survey indicates that most physicians are aware of the impacts of climate change on health. Further work is needed to address how to involve and educate more health care providers who may be in a position to respond to the needs of patients who are subject to the effects of climate change.

Recent surveys indicate that most physicians are aware of the impacts of climate change on health.

Lancet's series on Health and Climate Change in 2009, Mike Gill and Robin Stott are of the view that there is no group better placed than health professionals to spell out the importance of acting on climate change. They argue that health practitioners have an important story to tell about the links between climate change and health and possess the public trust needed that will help this to be heard, adding: "We must be innovative and imaginative in how we amplify the voice of health practitioners, and disseminate the message, its significance to us all, and its urgency, by using all our existing networks."

Public Understanding of Climate Change and Principles of Climate Change Communication

As with communication in other domains, an understanding of audience characteristics and prior beliefs can be critical, as these may strongly influence how new messages about climate change are interpreted.

Climate change is now a topic that is almost universally recognized by people, at least in developed nations (and increasingly, worldwide (Brechin and Bhandari 2011; BBC World Service Trust 2010; Pidgeon 2012). The meanings attached to the idea of climate change often vary immensely, however, leading to the many disagreements and disputes about climate change with which many of us are now familiar (Hulme 2009).

The notion of climate change or global warming has been in the public domain since at least the late 1980s. Research into public understanding at this time emphasized the common misconceptions held by people, especially a confusion between weather and climate, and a conflation between climate change and the (largely unrelated) environmental problem of stratospheric ozone depletion (Kempton 1991, 1997; Bostrom et al. 1994). There is evidence that these misconceptions have diminished over time, but that new ones have formed in their place—in particular, a widespread tendency to overemphasize the role of natural climate change while underplaying the importance of anthropogenic emissions (Reynolds et al. 2010; Gallup 2012). More generally, research has shown that people's immediate associations with climate change often relate to imagery such as of melting ice or heat—but also that climate change is associated for some with alarmist imagery (such as concerning disaster or apocalyptic notions) or, conversely, with a skeptical viewpoint, for example, that climate change constitutes a conspiracy theory (Lorenzoni et al. 2006; Smith and Leiserowitz 2012).

Over the past quarter century, levels of concern about climate change have tended to rise and fall within the United States and worldwide: figure 16.1 shows the proportion of the US public who report they personally worry about global warming (Gallup 2013; see also Capstick et al. 2015) reaching a peak in the year 2000 and then fluctuating to the present time. The decline in public concern about climate change that occurred recently has been variously attributed to economic circumstances (Scruggs and Benegal 2012), cyclical patterns in public attention (Ratter, Philipp, and von Storch 2012), and the activities of opinion-forming elites (Brulle, Carmichael, and Jenkins 2012).

Whatever the reasons behind the declines in public concern in the Untied States and elsewhere in, there has been a continuing sense of unease among many involved in communicating climate change that **climate change skepticism** among the public has proven so difficult to address, despite the solid evidence base for the reality, severity, and human contribution to climate change (IPCC 2013) and near unanimity among scientists about the basic tenets of climate science (Anderegg et al. 2010). A number of studies in different parts of the developed world have now outlined the characteristics of public skepticism about climate change, as well as their

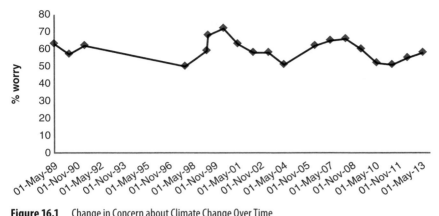

Figure 16.1   Change in Concern about Climate Change Over Time

Note: The percentage of respondents responding that they worry "a great deal" or "a fair amount" about global warming over the time period.

Source: Data from Gallup polling (US data).

foundations in personal and political outlook (Capstick and Pidgeon 2014a; Whitmarsh 2011; Poortinga et al. 2011; McCright and Dunlap 2011; Smith and Leiserowitz 2012; Hobson and Niemeyer 2013; Engels et al. 2013).

More generally, it has been established that people's perspectives on climate change are determined by a range of demographic, psychological, and cultural factors. Women express higher levels of overall concern about climate change than do men (McCright 2010; Brody et al. 2008; O'Connor, Bord, and Fisher 1999). Levels of concern also vary with age: some research has viewed this in terms of an inverse linear relationship (Semenza, Ploubidis, and George 2011; Kellstedt, Zahran, and Vedlitz 2008), although others have suggested that those in the youngest and oldest age groups are less concerned overall than are middle-aged people (Upham et al. 2009; Capstick, Pidgeon, and Whitehead 2013). Studies also suggest that ethnicity plays a role in determining climate change attitudes; for example, Leiserowitz and Akerlof (2010) find that Hispanics and African Americans often supported a range of action on climate change at higher levels than did whites. Other US studies have also noted that nonwhite research participants tend to be more concerned about climate change (Malka, Krosnick, and Langer 2009; Wood and Vedlitz 2007).

A growing body of research has demonstrated that people's values and political ideology are particularly important influences on their perspectives on climate change and how communication about it is received (Kahan 2010). Particularly in the United States, climate change has become an increasingly politicized and partisan issue (McCright and Dunlap 2011) with longitudinal survey data showing an ever-widening gap between

Democrat and Republican positions on the issue (Dunlap and McCright 2008). One study suggested that the lowest levels of belief in climate change are found among those who affiliate with the Tea Party, with only around a third (34 percent) of these study participants accepting the basic reality of climate change, compared to 78 percent of Democrats (Leiserowitz et al. 2011).

In a related manner, a growing body of research has suggested that people's **cultural worldviews** underpin the ways in which they understand climate change (Bellamy and Hulme 2011; Kahan, Jenkins-Smith, and Braman 2011; Kahan et al. 2012; Capstick and Pidgeon 2014a, 2014b; Leiserowitz 2006; Leiserowitz et al. 2010; Steg and Sievers 2000; Thompson and Rayner 1998; Thompson, 2003; West, Bailey, and Winter 2010). For people holding a worldview in which collective organization and shared problem solving are seen as desirable attributes for society (described as "egalitarians"), climate change tends to be seen as something of importance and a matter for personal concern. This is argued to be a direct consequence of the fact that responses to climate change tend to be portrayed in ways that align with egalitarian intuitions, requiring as they do participation by all and constraints on economic activity. By contrast, a cultural worldview that emphasizes freedom to act autonomously with few restrictions on personal choices (as is the case for "individualists") is incommensurate with the large-scale social dilemma of climate change; consequently those holding this worldview tend to downplay the importance or even reality of climate change.

A related strand of literature has applied social psychological insights into the different types of **values** that people typically hold and how these tend to be related to their attitudes toward climate change. A value is usually defined as a "guiding principle in the life of a person" (Schwartz 1992). Over several decades, and through research conducted in over sixty countries, there is now a huge body of evidence that shows that certain values and beliefs tend to go together, while others tend to be opposed to each other. There are two broad categories of values, which are known as "self-enhancing' (or "extrinsic") and "self-transcending" (or "intrinsic"). People who identify strongly with "self-enhancing" or "extrinsic" values (e.g., materialism, personal ambition) tend not to identify strongly with "self-transcending" or "intrinsicy" values (e.g., benevolence, respect for the environment). There are some important practical implications to this research with respect to people's likely degree of engagement with climate change. People who hold self-transcendent values (especially pro-environmental values and high levels of altruism) are more likely to engage in sustainable behavior (Stern 2000), show higher concern about environmental risks like climate change (Slimak and Dietz 2006), are more likely to perform specific actions such as recycling (Dunlap, Grieneeks, and Rokeach 1983) and are more likely to support climate mitigation policies (Nilsson, von Borgstede, and Biel 2004).

Importantly for climate change communication, preexisting values and worldviews not only influence prior beliefs but also act as a perceptual filter for new information. In an experimental setting where study participants were presented with information about climate change from a putative expert on the subject, people offered different appraisals of whether they saw this expert as trustworthy and knowledgeable, depending on the extent to which their own preconceptions matched those of the expert (Kahan et al., 2011). This finding, the study authors argued, relates to people's propensity to seek out information that is congenial to their preexisting outlook on life (Schulz-Hardt et al. 2000). Corner, Whitmarsh, and Xenias (2012) have also highlighted people's tendency to interpret information about climate change according to preexisting beliefs, finding that study participants who already hold skeptical views about climate change are more likely to appraise information within a skeptical news article (one that casts doubt on climate change) as being convincing and reliable than would nonskeptics; conversely, nonskeptics were more inclined to react favorably towards nonskeptical information. In research that examined people's interpretations of the unusually cold weather experienced across Europe in late 2009 and 2010, Capstick and Pidgeon (2014b) found that those already holding skeptical viewpoints tended to interpret these events as evidence against climate change, whereas those who were more accepting of the reality and importance of climate change tended to see the cold weather as a form of evidence supporting its existence.

There have been mixed findings concerning the extent to which connections are made by people between climate change and human health. Leiserowitz (2007) makes the point that not a single respondent out of a US survey sample of 673 adults made an unprompted association between climate change and health impacts in work carried out in the United States in 2002 and 2003. A study by Akerlof et al. (2010) did find widespread public acceptance of, and concern about, health risks from climate change, however: in 2008 and 2009, just over half the respondents in this national US survey agreed that climate change would cause more disease epidemics over the next twenty years, with around a third of respondents also of the opinion that people in the United States "are being harmed now" by climate change. However, the authors of this study also stressed there had been little spontaneous association made by people between climate change and human health risks (rather, they agreed in response to specific survey items).

Qualitative work carried out in Canada in 2010 and 2011 found that health effects were mentioned by most participants when they were asked about global environmental change, although the most prominent categories of response obtained related to air pollution and problems from ultraviolet radiation. These authors also noted that people's reference to health risks in the context of climate change were not contextualized to personal or community health or understood in any detail (Cardwell and Elliott 2013).

As a consequence of the limited connections made by people between human health and climate change, the studies noted draw the conclusion that communication be developed that seeks to affirm such links. Both the Akerlof et al. (2010) and Leiserowitz (2007) studies recommended developing public health communication designed specifically to increase the salience of health risks from climate change. Cardwell and Elliott (2013) took this a stage further and argued for a reframing of climate impacts from an environmental issue to a public health issue in order to increase public engagement with climate change. This, they argue, would be achieved via a public health framing because this could underscore the personal relevance of climate change to individuals. Likewise, Petrovic, Madrigano, and Zaval (2014) propose that a reemphasis on the health benefits of reducing fossil fuel use has the potential to be more compelling than an emphasis on climate change mitigation, particularly for those of a conservative political orientation. We return to these arguments in some more detail below.

With respect to the communication of climate change in more general terms, a number of studies have examined how this can be done most appropriately and effectively. One of the first points to emphasize here, made repeatedly over the years, but nonetheless often overlooked, is that it is highly problematic to assume that public skepticism or lack of engagement derives principally from a lack of information or education on climate change. Certainly research suggests that recognition of important facts, such as the high level of scientific consensus about the human causation of climate change, can exert a critical influence on attitudes (Lewandowsky, Gignac, and Vaughan 2013). However, it is now clear that what has come to be termed the **information deficit model** of climate change communication, assuming that there is a "deficit" of knowledge that requires addressing, is inadequate to promote meaningful engagement with this topic (Moser and Dilling 2011).

Because there is now a strong evidence base that the ways in which we understand and respond to climate change is intimately connected with our values and worldviews, a number of researchers and campaigners have suggested that climate change communication needs to be designed in such a way as to emphasize certain values over others.

One of the key publications to address this line of argument is Crompton's (2010) *Common Cause* handbook (available at http://valuesandframes.org/; see also Crompton 2011). Crompton argues that for bigger-than-self problems such as climate change, which require shared efforts to address, communication should affirm self-transcendent values that focus on, for example, closeness to family and friends and commitment to the wider community because these are more likely to foster a durable and deeper sense of engagement. This would seem to be congruent with approaches that have been used in community health promotion (Hatcher, Allensworth, and Butterfoss 2010) whereby the needs and interdependencies of groups are emphasized, as well as with the importance of social capital and community resilience for health (Poortinga 2012). However, this is a type of different message from that often used to encourage action on climate change, where economic incentives or self-interest are often invoked—for example, where people may be encouraged to act on climate change to save money (as the US Environmental Protection Agency suggests: http://www.epa.gov/climatechange/wycd/).

Messages emphasizing economic incentives may work in the short term or for isolated behaviors. However, the argument of Crompton and others is that in the long term, encouraging people to act out of self-interest, for what is essentially a common interest problem, is counterproductive (see also Thøgersen and Cromptom 2009). Recent experimental evidence would seem to bear this out. One recent study found that people at a gas station were more likely to get their tires checked when they were shown a message about the environmental benefits of correctly inflated tires, rather than the money they might save (Bolderdijk et al. 2013). Another paper found that when car sharing was described as a money-saving rather than proenvironmental activity, participants were less likely to engage in subsequent proenvironmental behaviors such as recycling (Evans et al. 2013).

A related area that is important to consider is the careful use of images and language. Images are powerful communication tools, but they have proven to be something of a sticking point for climate change communicators. This is because for most audiences in industrialized nations, climate change is something vague, abstract, and very difficult to visualize. Several studies (Manzo 2010; O'Neill and Nicholson-Cole 2009) have presented evidence that typically "environmentalist" images of melting ice caps and polar bears can produce strong emotional reactions in some people, but may also produce a feeling of powerlessness, as these sorts of images do not relate easily to people's lives. Manzo (2010) draws attention to the commonly used image in climate change communications of vulnerable people (often children) from developing countries against a ravaged landscape. This type of image, Manzo argues, exemplifies the paradoxes and pitfalls of certain types of climate change communication: while images of famine and desolation may make climate change seem important, they can simultaneously lead to participants' feeling unable to do anything about the problem.

A recent analysis (O'Neill et al. 2013) of a wide range of images used to visualize climate change likewise found that some images (e.g., of climate impacts, such as cracked ground) made the issue more salient in participants' minds, but at the same time tended to undermine self-efficacy (the sense that one can do anything about the problem). Other images, such as portrayals of energy futures (e.g., electric cars or ecohouses) were more successful in engendering a feeling of empowerment to act. None of the images these researchers investigated, however, provoked both of these types of responses, suggesting that visualizing climate change is a critical area for future inquiry and illustrating that there are no guaranteed ways of bringing about public engagement using visual representations.

A further challenge for climate change communicators is selecting the language and terminology for describing climate change and its effects. For a start, although the terms *climate change* and *global warming* are often used interchangeably (although in the United States *global warming* is more common, and in the United Kingdom *climate change* tends to dominate), even this seemingly superficial distinction is problematic. Research has identified systematic differences in the way that people interpret the terms *climate change* and *global warming*, with *global warming* perceived as more emotionally engaging than *climate change* (Whitmarsh 2009). Republicans have also been found to be more likely to endorse the reality of *climate change* than *global warming* (Schuldt, Konrath, and Schwarz 2011).

The language of **uncertainty**, so central to scientists' vocabulary, is typically unfamiliar to members of the public and may generate the impression that the science of climate change is less well understood than it actually is (Budescu, Broomell, and Por 2009; Corbett and Durfee 2004). The everyday meaning of uncertainty is negative, and it is commonly equated with ignorance (Shome and Marx 2009). In addition, when people with initially different views about the seriousness and reality of climate change are presented with conflicting or uncertain information about climate change, they are likely to assimilate the information in different ways (Corner, Whitmarsh, and Xenia 2012) and may even polarize in their views, becoming even more convinced of their initial views than they were previously (Kahan et al. 2011). Behavioral scientists have drawn attention to the ways in which people process uncertain information in the context of climate change, in many cases concluding that the risks associated with it are not of a kind that tend to promote concern or action (Patt and Weber 2014).

As Weber (2006) points out, the abstract nature of climate change, and the sense that climate risks are often presented as occurring in the future and in probabilistic terms, are factors that are unlikely to evoke a strong emotional response.

It has been argued that communication about climate change should be reframed away from "uncertainty" and oriented toward "**risk**," a concept that most people are more familiar with (Pidgeon and Fischhoff 2011). Framing climate change as being about risk (rather than a set of uncertain predictions about the future) turns the problem into something that most people are used to dealing with. Risk is the language of the insurance, health, and national security sectors. Pidgeon and Fischhoff suggest that the more the risks of climate change can be brought to life through vivid mental models' (e.g., practical examples of the risks of sea level rise), the more likely it is that people will respond to climate risks in a proactive way.

In addition to paying attention to the particular types of language and imagery used to communicate climate change, some researchers have stressed the need to think in broader terms about the types of **narratives** used to give meaning to climate change. As Westerhoff and Robinson (2013) note, narratives in this sense are not judged on the basis of their relative truth, but on the quality, relevance, and meaning that they bring to a particular audience. For example, instead of providing people with information that is abstract, complex, and irrelevant to daily life, we might consider presenting information in ways that connect climate change to personal experiences and concerns. Westerhoff and Robinson suggest that through the use of everyday language familiar to one's audience and portraying positive messages of local agency and empowerment, people are more likely to be engaged with the subject of climate change.

Work by the Climate Outreach Information Network (COIN) (Corner and van Eck 2014) has also suggested a number of ways in which the often complex, and perhaps unappealing, messages from the Intergovernmental Panel on Climate Change (IPCC) could be made more engaging and inspiring. One of the recommendations of this research was that rather than rely solely on facts to communicate, there is an urgent need to human stories to be told about climate change, that are able to bring climate change to life. COIN has assembled a number of such stories through its Moving Stories project, focusing on people who have been displaced or migrated in the context of climate change, in order to give a human voice to an issue more usually confined to academia and the development sector (Randall, Salsbury, and White 2014). As the authors of the Moving Stories report outline, while the experiences of people affected by climate change are often traumatic, they can also be powerful and inspiring.

A rather different way in which narratives have often been used with respect to climate change is in the conveying of apocalyptic futures. Movies such as *The Day after Tomorrow* and *The Age of Stupid* present to us a vision of a world devastated by our inaction on climate change. The deliberate use of these types of messages by climate change communicators is controversial, however. Some research suggests that the fear-inducing messages often contained in such movies, whereby the prospect of dire futures from environmental destruction is emphasized, can prompt action among the public (Howell 2011; Lowe et al. 2006) and for environmentalists (Veldman, 2012). Other researchers have, however, argued that such messages instead lead to disengagement and can bring about apocalypse fatigue with respect to climate change (Nordhaus and Shellenberger 2009).

A recent US study (Feinberg and Willer 2010) found that apocalyptic messages about climate change affected different people in different ways. For those who believe in a just world—that bad things don't, by and large, happen to good people—messages that ended in dire consequences actually increased their skepticism about climate change. The researchers suggested that the conflict between the negative impacts of climate change and their belief in a just world led to the message being ignored and was used as evidence that climate change was not occurring.

The use of appeals based on fear or guilt has a long history in the health behavior domain, and research has shown the potential for fear-based messages to change attitudes or verbal expressions of concern (Witte and Allen 2000). However, the impact of fear appeals is context and audience specific (Das, de Wit, and Stroebe 2003; Hoog, Stroebe, and de Wit 2005). While fear of a negative outcome (e.g., lung cancer) *can* be an effective way of promoting behavioral changes (e.g., giving up smoking), the link between the threat and the behavior must be personal and direct; furthermore, the recipient of the message must perceive an efficacious way of mitigating the threat through their behavior (Witte and Allen 2000). Typically, though, climate change is perceived as neither a direct nor a personal threat, and so deliberate attempts to instill fear or guilt in people carry a considerable risk of backfiring. At the very least, simply invoking fear without pointing to a means of attenuating it is unlikely to be an effective communication strategy (O'Neill and Nicholson-Cole 2009).

Some of the key insights that we consider above are applied and developed in *Connecting On Climate: A Guide to Effective Climate Change Communication*, developed by the Center for Research on Environmental Decisions at Columbia University and ecoAmerica (available at connecting-onclimate.org; see also Markowitz, Hodge, and Harp 2014). This accessible guide outlines ten principles designed to help engage audiences in a positive

Table 16.1   Ten Principles of Climate Change Communication

Communication Principle	Examples of Practical Considerations
1. Put yourself in your audience's shoes.	Consider who your audience trusts and respects. Can any of these individuals help deliver climate change communication?
2. Channel the power of groups.	Which of the values of your audience's existing groups align with climate solutions?
3. Emphasize solutions and benefits.	Highlight the local, personal, and wider benefits of climate solutions, including improving health.
4. Bring climate impacts close to home.	Help people identify the locally and personally relevant impacts of climate change.
5. Connect climate change to issues that matter to your audience.	Draw attention to the connections between climate change and health, such as risks from heat-related illness.
6. Use images and stories to make climate change real.	Use images that depict people or households rather than landscapes or bar charts.
7. Make climate science meaningful.	Incorporate real-life comparisons to help contextualize information, and connect any statistics used to authoritative messengers.
8. Acknowledge uncertainty, but show what you know.	Use short, simple statements to show that the vast majority of scientists believe climate change is real and human caused.
9. Approach skepticism carefully.	Consider emphasizing solutions to climate change (principle 3) rather than countering with facts and figures.
10. Make behavior change easy.	Illustrate positive actions that other people are taking in the audience's community.

Source: Adapted from Markowitz et al. (2014).

manner with the concepts and challenges of climate changes. These include the recommendations that effective climate communication should be tailored to people's values and priorities, use images and stories that inspire and empower people, and apply proven strategies that help enable behavior change. Each of the principles developed for the guide is summarized in table 16.1, together with practical examples provided by its authors to help communicators achieve these aims.

Communicating the Impacts of Climate Change

Of the many consequences of climate change that are projected to affect people across the world, some of the most frightening and immediately visible are those arising from extreme weather events. There are important concerns for health professionals arising from the need to communicate effectively around extreme events such as flooding and heat waves, and we consider these in some detail in this chapter. There is also a sense, however, in which the experience of extreme weather, whether encountered directly or vicariously through acquaintances or the news media, may act to raise the prominence of climate change in ways that have been difficult to achieve so far.

Typically the more **psychological distance** associated with climate change—that is, the more climate change is seen as temporally, socially, or geographically removed from one's own life or as being scientifically uncertain—the less concern people express about the issue (Spence, Poortinga, and Pidgeon 2012). By contrast, because of the importance of direct, personal experience for climate risk perceptions (Weber 2010), as well as the salience of a perceived association between weather and climate (Smith and Joffe 2013), there is substantial research interest in how people's encounters with and interpretations of weather affect their views on climate change. This is particularly the case because weather events in the future are increasingly likely to be outside of the normal everyday range of experience (Rahmstorf and Coumou 2011).

Experience and interpretation of extreme weather may act as a strong signal or focusing event (Renn 2011; November, Penelas, and Viot 2009) whereby future climatic events are made more imaginable. Research in the United Kingdom by Spence et al. (2011) and Capstick et al. (2013) has suggested that in cases where people directly experienced flooding, this was associated with higher levels of concern about climate change and willingness to act to help address it. More recently in the United States, Rudman, McLean, and Bunzl (2013) found that the experiences of Hurricanes Irene and Sandy led to greater concern about, and acceptance of, the reality of climate change.

Structuring communication that emphasizes the consequences of climate change with reference to such events is complex, however. First, the connections between extreme weather events and climate change are not straightforward, and the links between individual events and climate change are scientifically difficult to establish (at least at the time at which they occur). In addition, and as Marshall (2014) cautions, there is a high risk of ill-designed messaging around extreme weather events backfiring, potentially leading to the reinforcement of existing cultural divides or promoting a backlash against communicators (e.g., if it appears the message is being conveyed by environmentalists: "I told you so"). Nevertheless, Marshall suggests that because extreme weather events are real, local, and immediate and because they relate to personal experience and real-life stories that can generate empathy, such events can offer the prospect of helping to communicate about climate change in new, powerful, and convincing ways.

As well as drawing on the experience and consequences of extreme weather in this manner, health professionals may also be concerned to communicate directly about the problems directly arising from such events.

One of the principal health concerns arising from climate change in many parts of the world is the additional risks to vulnerable populations arising from heat events (see chapter 2). The elderly and those with chronic illnesses are among those most susceptible to health problems and increased mortality from periods of intense heat (Kovats and Hajat 2008; Semenza et al. 1996, 1999) and so are among those most at risk from the consequences of climate change (McGeehin and Mirabelli 2001).

Commonly provided advice from health authorities designed to reduce the risks from heat events includes measures such as the avoidance of alcohol, reduction in physical activity, and regular hydration (Hajat, O'Connor, and Kosatsky 2010). However, it has been argued that the passive dissemination of such advice (e.g., through websites) is unlikely to be effective given that high-risk groups include those who are socially isolated or may have a disability with a cognitive or behavioral component (Kovats and Ebi 2006). Moreover, even if health warnings are received by people, elements of individual risk perception may impede preventive responses. Lane et al. (2013), for example, found that although most elderly people and caregivers in their research understood the dangers of heat and the importance of age as a risk factor, nevertheless this was seen primarily as an issue for "other people" (see also Sheridan 2007).

Guidance provided by Health Canada (2011, http://www.hc-sc.gc.ca /ewh-semt/pubs/climat/index-eng.php) on communicating health risks from extreme heat emphasizes several key factors that should be taken into account by practitioners, including selection of appropriate means of communication, planning communication in advance of the summer months, and the careful incorporation of a series of evidence-based messages. Health Canada's guidance suggests that successful communication should target heat-vulnerable individuals either directly or through social networks. For example, supporting organizations such as community outreach programs and residential homes may be involved in measures to promote awareness of health issues around heat events and in the development of heat response plans. The US Environmental Protection Agency has itself developed fact sheets tailored to older people and their caregivers providing advice on ways of reducing risks from excessive heat (http://www.epa.gov/research /aging/factsheets/itdhpfehe-rd.html).

Wolf et al. (2010) suggest that a successful communication strategy for preventing heat morbidity should include provision of advice to a population in general, in combination with tailored messages for those over the age of seventy-five. These authors sound a note of caution, however, concerning potential problems in tailoring advice to older people, recommending that practitioners be particularly aware of the substantial importance the elderly place on a sense of independence, which can lead to reluctance to seek help during heat events (see also Kosatsky et al. 2009). Similarly, while social networks are often emphasized as an important influence that can help to prevent and respond to health risks in general among the elderly, a number of authors have pointed out that these networks may at times exert a detrimental influence in the context of heat events. This is because a person's social network may at times provide (perhaps unwarranted) reassurance or otherwise play down the risks arising from heat stress (Abrahamson et al. 2009; Sampson et al. 2013; Wolf et al. 2010). Wolf et al. (2010) emphasize the potential for formal and informal institutions to challenge assumptions that often circulate within social groups about the ability of older people to use "common sense" to cope with heat events without the provision of additional support. In providing health advice in the context of heat events, Sampson et al. (2013) suggest that it is important furthermore for health practitioners to be aware of the importance of cultural and economic factors that can influence susceptibility to heat. For example, individuals may hold the view that having previously lived in a warmer climate lowers a person's vulnerability to heat events or may be constrained by economic circumstances leading to unwillingness to use air-conditioning (see also Toloo et al. 2013).

As with increased risk of extreme heat events from climate change, there is projected to be greater incidence and severity of flooding in future as a result of a warming climate system (Hirabayashi et al. 2013; Milly, Dunne, and Delworth 2002). Dangers to health from increased flooding include injuries and death as a direct results of the physical impacts of floods, as well as the potential for increased fecal-oral transmission of disease in flood conditions (Ahern et al. 2005). The impacts of flooding may occur over an extended period of time, with additional stresses placed on people's mental health as those affected try to recover routines, relationships, and property that have been disrupted (UK Health Protection Agency 2011; Stanke et al. 2012).

Effective communication with respect to flood risk can entail intensive efforts directed toward enhancing citizen preparedness. Lichterman (2000), for example, outlines several community-based programs in which people are trained in preparing their home and family to cope with disaster events (including preparation of emergency kits and developing evacuation plans), as well as receiving training in advanced medical aid and disaster mental health. O'Sullivan et al. (2012) argue that such preparedness can contribute to high levels of resilience against flood events.

A recent review by Parker and Tapsell (2009) looked at several European studies that considered communication around flood risks and people's responses to such information. These authors caution that while there has been much attention to how official flood warnings have operated through formal agencies, in practice people tend to seek out information about flood risk in a variety of ways, including though personal observation of environmental cues (such as water levels) and obtaining informal warnings through social networks. Nevertheless, Parker and Tapsell (2009) offer a series of recommendations for creating effective communication around flooding. These include the use of learning-by-doing activities within local communities and the setting up of informal communication networks in local communities by which arrangements can be made to help the elderly and infirm in an emergency. Parker and Tapsell also stress that individuals and communities should feel ownership of flood warning and self-protection systems. Although information provision from government agencies is important, this can nevertheless be associated with the message that responsibility for protection ultimately rests with the authorities. Perhaps controversially, Parker and Tapsell also suggest that flood risk communication works best when this creates a lack of certainty in people's minds, causing them to question their environment and their safety within it.

Careful consideration of the objectives and frameworks of communication around flood risk is advocated by Demeritt and Nobert (2014). These authors suggest that there has to date been a variety of conflicting advice about what information should be transmitted, the ways this should occur, and to whom information should be made available. They argue that there have been four broad approaches used to communicate flood risk (and risk more generally), which differ according to basic aims and practice. First, a risk message model aims to inform people about flood risk in as direct a manner as possible. While the appeal of such a model is in a straightforward imperative for citizens to be provided with information and for authorities to be transparent in their dealings, this model may be criticized for being premised on the notion that "experts" possess superior knowledge of risk, which they then convey to the ignorant. A related model of risk communication, but one with more practical objectives, is the risk instrument model. Here again, there is presumed to be a largely didactic flow of information— the assumption being that overcoming a lack of knowledge will be sufficient to reduce risk. Here, a desirable outcome in risk communication is taken to be that which leads to appropriate responses. From this perspective, a communicator may be motivated, for example, to generate fear or otherwise tap into negative emotions so as to motivate preparedness. Two further models discussed by Demeritt and Nobert are the risk dialogue model and the risk government model. In the first of these, the communication of risk is no longer seen as a one-way process, but is based on an exchange of information as part of processes of public participation; in the latter, public participation in risk management is again seen as integral, to the extent that such approaches arguably constitute a strategy for transferring responsibility onto individuals (in much the same ways in which much health communication emphasizes individual responsibility for leading healthier lifestyles).

In summary, these four models of flood risk communication illustrate that identification of best practice in the communication of climate impacts—whether around heat events, flooding, or other consequences of climate change—should not be considered solely a technical matter, but one bound up with more value-laden questions about the reasons for communicating and assumptions about what constitutes appropriate forms of communication. As such, although questions of what works in communicating climate change are essential to ask, it is also important for health professionals to be clear in advance what they are attempting to achieve from doing so. Does the impetus for communication arise from a concern that climate change directly contributes to increased health risks, and so demands a response from health professionals in specific circumstances? Alternatively, might health professionals who are aware of the importance of climate change feel moved to speak out on the subject and apply their knowledge and expertise to effect positive change? There are, moreover, a number of instances where there are strong synergies between acting to mitigate the causes of climate change and the promotion of public health.

In the final section of this chapter, we turn to research and guidance that has approached the communication of climate change from a public health perspective. There are a number of advantages to this approach, which has been used as both a practical means of effecting engagement with climate change and a way of tackling the wider social issues underpinning both environmental and health issues.

CLINICAL CORRELATES 16.2 COMMUNICATING HEALTH BENEFITS OF CLIMATE-CONSCIOUS LIVING

Clinicians can communicate the benefits of climate-conscious living as a win-win situation for patients:

- Choosing to walk or cycle as a means of transportation in urban areas can reduce the burden of heart disease, diabetes, obesity, some cancers, and depression (Ganten, Haines, and Souhami 2010).

- Reducing consumption of animal products limits cattle-related methane gas production and may decreases risks of ischemic heart disease and colon cancer (Roberts 2010).

- Consuming fewer animal products addresses world hunger as feeding grain to animals forces up world grain prices and is an inefficient use of food energy (Roberts 2008).

- Advocating for improved coal burning technology would result in reductions of greenhouse gas emissions as well a reduce rates of respiratory infections and asthma exacerbations caused by fine particulate matter in the ambient air.

Initiating conversations about the health benefits of living in an environmentally conscious way is one method for improving health as well as improving environmental literacy.

Communicating Climate Change through a Focus on Health

As early as 1993, Edward Maibach and his colleagues explored the overlap between public perceptions of climate change and its health impacts, as well as lessons from the public health sector for climate change communicators (Maibach 1993; see also Maibach, Roser-Renouf, and Leiserowitz 2008). The potential advantages of using a public health **frame** have since been stressed by a number of authors in recent years (we use the term *frame* or *framing* here to refer to the selection or emphasis of particular meanings within communication; see Scheufele 1999). Nisbet (2009) argues that the public health implications of climate change represent a powerful interpretive resource in this regard. He suggests that communication about climate change that connects to health problems that are already familiar and seen as important (such as heat stroke and asthma) can make the issue seem more personally relevant. Nisbet suggests that a public health frame also has the potential to make climate change seem more relevant at a local level by replacing distant imagery such as is typically used in climate change communication (e.g., remote Arctic regions) with more socially proximate neighborhoods and localities.

Several research studies have also examined the consequences of climate change communication that emphasizes public health. Maibach et al. (2010) found that portraying climate change in ways that encourage people to consider its health contexts—particularly, in terms of affirming the health benefits from taking action on climate change—offers an engaging frame of reference able to make climate change seem more personally significant and relevant to people. As well as pointing toward the advantage of using a health framing, these findings are consistent with other work from both health and climate change communication research that emphasizing a "gain" frame (emphasizing the benefits of action rather than the negative consequences of not acting) produces more positive attitudes toward taking action on climate change (Spence and Pidgeon 2010; Rothman et al. 2006).

In related research, Myers et al. (2012) tested different messages about climate change framed either as an environmental, public health, or national security risk. Messages were tested across each of six attitudinal groups termed the "Six Americas" (an approach we discuss in more detail later), encompassing those who were particularly concerned about climate change, as well as those who were dismissive or doubtful about the subject. Across all groups, the public health frame elicited the most positive responses. Myers et al. conclude from this work that a public health framing of climate change has the potential to inspire hope in the context of discussion around climate change, which the researchers describe as more consistent with support for taking action on climate change. This is a promising finding for both climate change communication and health practitioners, as it would seem to suggest that an emphasis on health has the potential to appeal directly to different audiences who might otherwise see the problem very differently. As Maibach et al. (2011) note, a public health frame thus offers the prospect of shifting the climate change debate from one based on environmental values, to one based on public health values, which are more widely held regardless of ideology and political outlook. A note of caution should be sounded here, however, as some separate research has found that the outcomes of health messages in the climate change domain may depend on a person's political orientation. Petrovic et al. (2014) found that an emphasis on health (stressing that fossil fuel burning leads to air pollution harmful to human health) was more likely to lead to attitude change among conservatives than a comparable emphasis on climate impacts. The reverse effect was obtained for liberals, however, who were more responsive to a framing emphasizing the climate change consequences of fossil fuel use than they were to one emphasizing health consequences from air pollution.

Research in the United Kingdom has also suggested that presenting information about climate change in the context of health can be an effective means of engaging people who vote conservative (those toward the right of the political spectrum) who are otherwise among those least engaged with the topic. Mocker (2012) showed research participants two versions of a video where an actor gave a speech on low-carbon transport. Both videos discussed transport problems and the need for electrification and increased use of public transport, cycling, and walking. Whereas one version of the video framed these issues around economic and nationalistic concerns, the other video discussed the issues in the context of the dangers and benefits for community health. The results of this study suggested that of these two versions, incorporating an emphasis on community health prompted a greater feeling of empowerment and personal motivation to act on climate change.

As well as stressing the advantages of applying a health frame to promote engagement with climate change, health practitioners have also emphasized the cobenefits that acting on health can bring for climate change, and vice versa. A number of authors have noted that a variety of major public health issues share common roots with climate change. As Maibach et al. (2011) note succinctly, "Global warming offers America an opportunity to make choices that are healthier for us, and for our climate" (19). Ganten, Haines, and Souhami (2010) argue that reducing the use of private cars in urban areas, with an associated increasing walking and cycling, could reduce the burden of heart disease, diabetes, some cancers, and depression, as well as contributing to emissions reduction. Webb and Egger (2013) similarly suggest that interventions designed to reduce greenhouse gas emissions might also have public health benefits in the area of tackling obesity (see also Edwards and Roberts 2009). McMichael et al. (2009) argue that well-judged mitigation policies also have the advantage of bringing health gains, with benefits accrued from moving away from air-polluting energy generation, choosing transport methods that encourage physical activity and social contact, and changing carbon-intensive food choices. These authors indeed suggest that pursuing such approaches presents the opportunity for the revitalization of health promotion strategies. Haines, Campbell-Lendrum, and Corvalán (2006) have stressed that mitigation of climate change through reduction in the use of fossil fuels can also lead to health benefits by reducing air pollution. Because of these cobenefits, and others, Maibach et al. (2011) argue that health practitioners should reinforce the point that taking action can result in a win-win situation.

It has been also been suggested that the insights generated from many years of developing health communication approaches be applied to climate change communication. One simple but powerful use of a health communication approach is given by Maibach et al. (2011) in the context of many people's reluctance to accept the widespread agreement of climate science experts regarding the reality and human causation of climate change (Anderegg et al. 2010; Intergovernmental Panel on Climate Change 2013). These authors suggest that a health care analogy can be useful in helping people understand that we often consider it wise to act when there is widespread agreement on a subject, even if this is not unanimous. The example they give is that if 95 percent of the world's leading pediatricians were to agree that a child was seriously ill, most parents would likely act on their advice rather than on that of the 5 percent who disagree.

More generally, Frumkin and McMichael (2008) and Maibach et al. (2008) have drawn attention to the use of **social marketing** in promoting health behaviors, and the potential for its extension to encourage appropriate responses to climate change at the personal and collective level. McKenzie-Mohr (2013) has developed in some detail the use of social marketing to foster sustainable behaviors, based on a pragmatic five-stage approach. The steps that McKenzie-Mohr recommends practitioners adopt for encouraging pro-environmental behavior are the selection of specific behaviors to be changed or promoted; identification of the barriers and benefits of behavior change; development of appropriate strategies; piloting of the strategy; and broad-scale implementation and evaluation (see www.cbsm.com). While there is now an evidence base that social marketing techniques for behavior change can be successful (Gordon et al. 2006), some authors have cautioned that as a strategy for climate change engagement, this can be limiting. Corner and Randall (2011) argue that we cannot sell climate change in the same way commercial goods are sold and that motivating a proportional response to climate change (bringing about more than small-scale and piecemeal behavior change) requires engaging people at a deeper level than is possible with social marketing.

A number of researchers have also suggested that the strategy of using tailored and targeted health communication can also be applied to communicating climate change. Tailored approaches to communication are premised on the notion that specific messages should be devised that resonate with particular audiences, an approach that has been adopted to promote specific health behaviors (Noar et al. 2011) and in social marketing approaches (McKenzie-Mohr 2000).

Probably the most prominent research program to have developed such a **segmentation** approach in the area of climate change has been the Yale Project on Climate Change Communication (see http://environment .yale.edu/climate-communication/). In a series of publications and reports, the case has been made that climate change is perceived differently across each of six attitudinal groups, termed "Global Warming's Six Americas" (see Leiserowitz et al. 2013; Maibach et al. 2011; Leiserowitz and Smith 2010). As a consequence of these different yet coherent ways of understanding climate change, it is argued that public education and engagement strategies are most likely to be successful where these are tailored to these target audiences (Maibach et al. 2011). Specific strategies for engaging those who are already concerned about climate change include providing information about what kind of actions can be taken to limit climate change; for those who are least concerned about climate change (or may dispute its existence), information relating to how climate scientists know that climate change is real or caused by humans is more relevant (Roser-Renouf et al. 2014).

Bostrom, Böhm, and O'Connor (2013) also argue that targeting and tailoring climate change communication makes sense, based on a wider literature supporting such an approach from health risk communication, although these authors caution that to date, direct evidence of the effectiveness of tailoring climate change communication remains elusive. Other researchers have adopted a variety of alternative approaches to dividing up publics in such a way as to customize communication to particular groups (Agyeman et al. 2007; Featherstone et al. 2009; Rose, Dade, and Scott, 2007).

As well as giving consideration to audience characteristics and the structure of communication, it is worth bearing in mind that health practitioners are themselves in a distinctive position with respect to being able to convey messages. As Frumkin and McMichael (2008) have noted, the health sector has an opportunity to demonstrate leadership on climate change because health professionals are seen as having moral authority, professional prestige, and a reputation for science-based analysis. Because of their special position, these authors argue that health professionals are well placed to motivate people toward appropriate personal actions and collective decisions and to provide guidance to industry and policymakers. Indeed, health professionals may be able to exert political influence in the area of climate change mitigation through being clear about the substantial public health benefits that such policies can also bring. As Bloomberg and Aggarwala (2008) point out, "Even a politician who is convinced that global warming is a scientific fraud, or who refuses to work to save the world unless every other nation does so first, cannot ignore proposals that will directly improve the health of his or her constituents" (421).

CLINICAL CORRELATES 16.3 CLINICIAN RESPONSIBILITIES REGARDING THE HEALTH IMPACTS OF CLIMATE CHANGE

Evidence shows that global climate change is currently having profound impacts on human health and will continue to do so in the future (Climate Change 2013). Physicians have the expertise to understand these health effects and the professional responsibility to patients and to society to be advocates of improved health on a global scale. Thus, some argue that it is within the professional domain of clinicians to educate themselves and patients of the health effects of climate change and engage on an organizational level to reduce greenhouse gas emissions (Abelsohn 2013).

Clinicians are in a unique position to educate their patients and the public about the health impacts of climate change.

Conclusion

The communication of climate change can be approached in a number of ways, with a range of decisions required as to how language, imagery, narratives, emotional content, and values are portrayed. Now that we have reached a point where the impacts of climate change are manifesting for people across the world, this might represent the chance to draw attention to climate change being a current and local issue, although careful consideration is needed concerning how to do so appropriately and in ways that do not alienate audiences. Moreover, there is a need to communicate about the risks inherent in climate impacts themselves. The structuring of communication in ways that emphasize the linkages between climate change and health offers a unique opportunity to engage people with the issue of climate change. Health professionals are uniquely placed to be able to present these messages to the public and decision makers. Their position in society and ability to understand and represent science-based issues makes them well-placed to support efforts to address and communicate about climate change.

DISCUSSION QUESTIONS

1. What role do values, worldviews, and political beliefs play in determining how messages about climate change are received?

2. What are the best ways to communicate risk and uncertainty?

3. How can communicators overcome the psychological distance of climate change?

4. Why might it be advantageous to stress issues of public health when communicating about climate change?

KEY TERMS

Climate change communication: Material designed to inform, persuade, or engage about climate change; may be delivered face-to-face or using a variety of media.

Climate change skepticism: The holding of doubts about the physical reality, human causation, or importance of climate change, and/or concerning the ability of human action to effectively address it.

Cultural worldview: A preference for a particular type of social control and organization; for example, egalitarians emphasize equal status and collective problem-solving whereas individualists emphasize personal autonomy and economic freedom.

Frames, framing: The selection and emphasis of particular meanings in communication; for example, a public health frame in climate change communication stresses the relevance of public health to climate change.

Information deficit model: A common or default assumption in communication, that the audience requires education, information, or facts in order to be engaged with a topic.

Narratives: Stories and meaning making in communication, for example, through relating climate change to people's real-life experiences.

Pro-environmental behavior: Personal action that contributes to addressing climate change, such as reducing energy use in the home.

Psychological distance: The perception of being disconnected from an issue such as climate change; psychological distance has four dimensions: temporal (distance in time), social (distance between oneself and others), spatial (geographical distance), and uncertainty (how certain it is that an event will happen).

Public engagement: The extent to which people are cognitively, affectively (emotionally), and behaviorally connected with a problem such as climate change.

Risk: The potential for consequences where something of value is at stake and outcomes are uncertain.

Segmentation: The use of statistical techniques to group a population according to common characteristics.

Social marketing: The application of principles from commercial marketing for socially desirable ends.

Uncertainty: The probability that a statement is (in)valid. The IPCC uses shorthand statements (such as "very likely") to equate to numerical probabilities (e.g., "very likely" corresponds to "percent above 90 percent probability").

Values: In the psychology literature, a guiding principle in the life of a person.

References

Abelsohn, A. 2013. "Should Family Physicians and Family Medicine Organizations Pay Attention?" *Canadian Family Physician* 59:462–66.

Abrahamson, V., J. Wolf, I. Lorenzoni, B. Fenn, R. S. Kovats, P. Wilkinson, and R. Raine. 2009. "Perceptions of Heatwave Risks to Health: Interview-Based Study of Older People in London and Norwich, UK." *Journal of Public Health* 31(1):19–126.

Agyeman, J., B. Doppelt, K. Lynn, and H. Hatic. 2007. "The Climate-Justice Link: Communicating Risk with Low-Income and Minority Audiences." In *Creating a Climate for Change*, edited by S. Moser and L. Dilling, 119–38. Cambridge: Cambridge University Press.

Ahern, M., R. Kovats, P. Wilkinson, R. Few, and F. Matthies. 2005. "Global Health Impacts of Floods: Epidemiologic Evidence." *Epidemiologic Reviews* 27(1):36–46.

Akerlof, K., R. DeBono, P. Berry, A. Leiserowitz, C. Roser-Renouf, K. L. Clarke, A. Rogaeva, et al. 2010. "Public Perceptions of Climate Change as a Human Health Risk: Surveys of the United States, Canada and Malta." *International Journal of Environmental Research and Public Health* 7:2559–2606.

Anderegg, W., J. Prall, J. Harold, and S. Schneider. 2010. "Expert Credibility in Climate Change." *Proceedings of the National Academy of Sciences* 107:12107–12109.

BBC World Service Trust. 2010. *Africa Talks Climate Change: The Public Understanding of Climate Change in Ten Countries.* London: BBC World Services Trust. www.africatalksclimate.com

Bellamy, R., and M. Hulme. 2011. "Beyond the Tipping Point: Understanding Perceptions of Abrupt Climate Change and Their Implications." *Weather, Climate and Society* 3(1):48–60.

Bloomberg, M., and R. Aggarwala. 2008. "Think Locally, Act Globally: How Curbing Global Warming Emissions Can Improve Local Public Health." *American Journal of Preventive Medicine* 35:414–23.

Bolderdijk, J., L. Steg, E. Geller, P. Lehman, and T. Postmes. 2013. "Comparing the Effectiveness of Monetary versus Moral Motives in Environmental Campaigning." *Nature Climate Change* 3:413–46.

Bostrom, A., G. Böhm, and R. O'Connor. 2013. "Targeting and Tailoring Climate Change Communications." *Wiley Interdisciplinary Reviews: Climate Change* 4:447–55.

Bostrom, A., M. Granger-Morgan, B. Fischhoff, and D. Read. 1994. "What Do People Know About Global Climate Change?" *Risk Analysis* 14:959–70.

Brechin, S., and M. Bhandari. 2011. "Perceptions of Climate Change Worldwide." *Climate Change* 2:871–85.

Brody, S., S. Zahran, A. Vedlitz, and H. Grover. 2008. "Examining the Relationship between Physical Vulnerability and Public Perceptions of Global Climate Change in the United States." *Environment and Behavior* 40:72–95.

Brulle, R., J. Carmichael, and J. Jenkins. 2012. "Shifting Public Opinion on Climate Change: An Empirical Assessment of Factors Influencing Concern over Climate Change in the US, 2002–2010." *Climatic Change* 114:169–88.

Budescu, D., S. Broomell, and H. Por. 2009. "Improving Communication of Uncertainty in the Reports of the Intergovernmental Panel on Climate Change." *Psychological Science* 20:299–308.

Capstick, S., N. Pidgeon, and M. Whitehead 2013. *Public Perceptions of Climate Change in Wales: Summary Findings of a Survey of the Welsh Public Conducted during November and December 2012.* Cardiff: Climate Change Consortium of Wales,

Capstick, S., and N. Pidgeon. 2014a. "What *Is* Climate Change Skepticism? Examination of the Concept Using a Mixed Methods Study of the UK Public." *Global Environmental Change* 24:389–401.

Capstick, S., and N. Pidgeon. 2014b. "Public Perception of Cold Weather as Evidence for and against Climate Change." *Climatic Change* 122:695–708.

Capstick, S., L. Whitmarsh, W. Poortinga, N. Pidgeon, and P. Upham. 2015. "International Trends in Public Perceptions of Climate Change over the Past Quarter Century." *Wiley Interdisciplinary Reviews Climate Change* 6(1):35–61.

Cardwell, F., and S. Elliott. 2013. "Making the Links: Do We Connect Climate Change with Health? A Qualitative Case Study from Canada." *BMC Public Health* 13(1):208.

Climate Change. 2013. "The Physical Science Basis: Fifth Assessment Report of the Intergovernmental Panel on Climate Change." http://www.climatechange2013.org

Corbett, J., and J. Durfee. 2004. "Testing Public (Un)Certainty of Science Media Representations of Global Warming." *Science Communication* 2:129–51.

Corner, A., and A. Randall. 2011. "Selling Climate Change? The Limitations of Social Marketing as a Strategy for Climate Change Public Engagement." *Global Environmental Change* 21:1005–14.

Corner, A., and C. van Eck. 2014. *Science and Stories: Bringing the IPCC to life.* Oxford: Climate Outreach Information Network.

Corner, A., L. Whitmarsh, and D. Xenias. 2012. "Uncertainty, Skepticism and Attitudes towards Climate Change: Biased Assimilation and Attitude Polarisation." *Climatic Change* 114:463–78.

Costello, A., H. Montgomery, and N. Watts. 2013. "Climate Change: The Challenge for Healthcare Professionals." *British Medical Journal* 347:f6060.

Crompton, T. 2010. *Common Cause: The Case for Working with Our Cultural Values.* UK: World Wildlife Fund. www.valuesandframes.org

Crompton, T. 2011. "Finding Cultural Values That Can Transform the Climate Change Debate." *Solutions* 2(4):56–63.

Das, E., J. de Wit, and W. Stroebe. 2003. "Fear Appeals Motivate Acceptance of Action Recommendations: Evidence for a Positive Bias in the Processing of Persuasive Messages." *Personality and Social Psychology Bulletin* 29:650–64.

Demeritt, D., and S. Nobert. 2014. "Models of Best Practice in Flood Risk Communication and Management." *Environmental Hazards* 13:313–28.

Dunlap, R. E., J. K. Grieneeks, and M. Rokeach. 1983. "Human Values and Pro-Environmental Behavior." In *Energy and Material Resources: Attitudes, Values, and Public Policy,* edited by W. Conn, 145–68. Boulder, CO: Westview.

Dunlap, R., and A. McCright. 2008. "A Widening Gap: Republican and Democratic Views on Climate Change." *Environment: Science and Policy for Sustainable Development* 50(5):26–35.

Edwards, P., and I. Roberts. 2009. "Population Adiposity and Climate Change." *International Journal of Epidemiology* 38:1137–40.

Engels, A., O. Hüther, M. Schäfer, and H. Held. 2013. "Public Climate-Change Skepticism, Energy Preferences and Political Participation." *Global Environmental Change* 23:1018–27.

Evans, L., G. Maio, A. Corner, C. Hodgetts, S. Ahmed, and U. Hahn. 2013. "Self-Interest and Pro-Environmental Behaviour." *Nature Climate Change* 3:122–25.

Featherstone, H., E. Weitkamp, K. Ling, and F. Burnet. 2009. "Defining Issue-Based Publics for Public Engagement: Climate Change as a Case Study." *Public Understanding of Science* 18:214–28.

Feinberg, M., and R. Willer. 2010. "Apocalypse Soon? Dire Messages Reduce Belief in Global Warming by Contradicting Just-World Beliefs." *Psychological Science* 22(1):34–38.

Frumkin, H., and A. McMichael. 2008. "Climate Change and Public Health: Thinking, Communicating, Acting." *American Journal of Preventive Medicine* 35:403–10.

Gallup. 2012. "In U.S., Global Warming Views Steady Despite Warm Winter." http://www.gallup.com/poll/153608/Global-Warming-Views-Steady-Despite -Warm-Winter.aspx

Gallup. 2013. "Americans' Concerns about Global Warming on the Rise." Gallup Online. http://www.gallup.com/poll/161645/americans-concerns-global -warmingrise.aspx

Ganten, D., A. Haines, and R. Souhami. 2010. "Health Co-Benefits of Policies to Tackle Climate Change." *Lance* 376:1802–1804.

Gill, M., and R. Stott. 2009. "Health Professionals Must Act to Tackle Climate Change." *Lancet* 374(9706):1953–55.

Gordon, R., L. McDermott, M. Stead, and K. Angus. 2006. "The Effectiveness of Social Marketing Interventions for Health Improvement: What's the Evidence?" *Public Health* 120:1133–39.

Haines, A., R., D. Campbell-Lendrum, and C. Corvalán. 2006. "Climate Change and Human Health: Impacts, Vulnerability and Public Health." *Public Health* 120:585–96.

Hajat, S., M. O'Connor, and T. Kosatsky. 2010. "Health Effects of Hot Weather: From Awareness of Risk Factors to Effective Health Protection." *Lancet* 375:856–63.

Hatcher, M., D. Allensworth, and F. Butterfoss. 2010. "Promoting Community Health." In *Health Promotion Programs: From Theory to Practice*, edited by C. Fertman and D. Allensworth. San Francisco: Jossey-Bass.

Hirabayashi, Y., R. Mahendran, S. Koirala, L. Konoshima, D. Yamazaki, S. Watanabe, H. Kim, and S. Kanae. 2013. "Global Flood Risk under Climate Change." *Nature Climate Change* 3:816–21.

Hobson, K., and S. Niemeyer. 2013. "'What Sceptics Believe': The Effects of Information and Deliberation on Climate Change Skepticism." *Public Understanding of Science* 22:396–412.

Hoog, N., W. Stroebe, and J. de Wit. 2005. "The Impact of Fear Appeals on Processing and Acceptance of Action Recommendations." *Personality and Social Psychology Bulletin* 31:24–33.

Höppner, C., and L. Whitmarsh. 2011. "Public Engagement in Climate Action: Policy and Public Expectations." In *Engaging the Public with Climate Change: Communication and Behaviour Change*, edited by L. Whitmarsh, S. O'Neill, and I. Lorenzoni, 47–65. London: Earthscan.

Howell, R. A. 2011. "Lights, Camera . . . Action? Altered Attitudes and Behaviour in Response to the Climate Change Film *The Age of Stupid*." *Global Environmental Change* 21:177–87.

Hulme, M. 2009. *Why We Disagree about Climate Change*. Cambridge: Cambridge University Press.

Intergovernmental Panel on Climate Change. 2013. "Summary for Policymakers." In *Climate Change 2013: The Physical Science Basis. Contribution of Working Group I to the Fifth Assessment Report of the Intergovernmental Panel on Climate Change*, edited by T. Stocker, D. Qin, G.-K. Plattner, M. Tignor, S. Allen, J. Boschung, A. Nauels, et al. Cambridge: Cambridge University Press.

Kahan, D. 2010. "Fixing the Communications Failure." *Nature* 463:296–97.

Kahan, D., H. Jenkins-Smith, and D. Braman. 2011. "Cultural Cognition of Scientific Consensus." *Journal of Risk Research* 14:147–74.

Kahan, D., E. Peters, M. Wittlin, P. Slovic, L. Ouellette, D. Braman, and G. Mandel. 2012. "The Polarizing Impact of Science Literacy and Numeracy on Perceived Climate Change Risks." *Nature Climate Change* 2:732–35.

Kellstedt, P., S. Zahran, and A. Vedlitz. 2008. "Personal Efficacy, the Information Environment, and Attitudes toward Global Warming and Climate Change in the United States." *Risk Analysis* 28:113–26.

Kempton, W. 1991. "Lay Perspectives on Global Climate Change." *Global Environmental Change* 1:183–208.

Kempton, W. 1997. "How the Public Views Climate Change." *Environment* 39(9):12–21.

Kosatsky, T., J. Dufresne, L. Richard, A. Renouf, N. Giannetti, J. Bourbeau, M. Julien, J. Braidy, and C. Sauve. 2009. "Heat Awareness and Response among Montreal Residents with Chronic Cardiac and Pulmonary Disease." *Canadian Journal of Public Health* 100:237–40.

Kovats, R., and K. Ebi. 2006. "Heatwaves and Public Health in Europe." *European Journal of Public Health* 16:592–99.

Kovats, R., and S. Hajat. 2008. "Heat Stress and Public Health: A Critical Review." *Annual Review of Public Health* 29:41–55.

Lane, K., K. Wheeler, K. Charles-Guzman, M. Ahmed, M. Blum, K. Gregory, G. Nathan, N. Clark, and T. Matte. 2013. "Extreme Heat Awareness and Protective Behaviors in New York City." *Journal of Urban Health* 91:403–14.

Leiserowitz, A. 2006. "Climate Change Risk Perception and Policy Preferences: The Role of Affect, Imagery, and Values." *Climatic Change* 7:45–72.

Leiserowitz, A. 2007. "Communicating the Risks of Global Warming: American Risk Perceptions, Affective Images, and Interpretive Communities." In *Creating a Climate for Change*, edited by S. Moser and L. Dilling, 45–72. Cambridge: Cambridge University Press.

Leiserowitz, A., and K. Akerlof. 2010. *Race, Ethnicity and Public Responses to Climate Change.* New Haven, CT: Yale Project on Climate Change. http://environment.yale.edu/uploads/RaceEthnicity2010.pdf

Leiserowitz, A., E. Maibach, C. Roser-Renouf, G. Feinberg, and P. Howe. 2013. *Global Warming's Six Americas, September 2012.* New Haven, CT: Yale Project on Climate Change Communication. http://environment.yale.edu/climate/publications/Six-Americas-September-2012

Leiserowitz, A., E. Maibach, C. Roser-Renouf, and J. Hmielowski. 2011. *Politics and Global Warming: Democrats, Republicans, Independents, and the Tea Party.* New Haven, CT: Yale Project on Climate Change Communication. http://environment.yale.edu/climate/files/PoliticsGlobalWarming2011.pdf

Leiserowitz, A., E. Maibach, C. Roser-Renouf, N. Smith, and E. Dawson. 2010. *Climate Change, Public Opinion and the Loss of Trust.* New Haven, CT. http://environment.yale.edu/climate/publications/climategate-public-opinion-and-the-loss-of-trust

Leiserowitz, A., and N. Smith. 2010. *Knowledge of Climate Change across Global Warming's Six Americas.* New Haven, CT: Yale Project on Climate Change Communication. http://environment.yale.edu/climate-communication/files/Knowledge_Across_Six_Americas.pdf

Lewandowsky, S., G. Gignac, and S. Vaughan. 2013. "The Pivotal Role of Perceived Scientific Consensus in Acceptance of Science." *Nature Climate Change* 3:399–404.

Lichterman, J. 2000. "'A Community as Resource' Strategy for Disaster Response." *Public Health Reports* 115(2–3):262–65.

Lorenzoni, I., A. Leiserowitz, M. Doria, W. Poortinga, and N. Pidgeon. 2006. "Cross National Comparisons of Image Associations with `Global Warming' and `Climate Change' among Laypeople in the United States of America and Great Britain." *Journal of Risk Research* 9:265–81.

Lowe, T., K. Brown, S. Dessai, M. Doria de França, M. K. Hayne, and K. Vincent. 2006. "Does Tomorrow Ever Come? Disaster Narrative and Public Perceptions of Climate Change." *Public Understanding of Science* 15:435–57.

Maibach, E. 1993. "Social Marketing for the Environment: Using Information Campaigns to Promote Environmental Awareness and Behavior Change." *Health Promotion International* 8:209–24.

Maibach, E., P. Baldwin, K. Akerlof, G. Diao, and M. Nisbet. 2010. "Reframing Climate Change as a Public Health Issue: An Exploratory Study of Public Reactions." *BMC Public Health* 10(1):299.

Maibach, E., A. Leiserowitz, C. Roser-Renouf, and C. Mertz. 2011. "Identifying Like-Minded Audiences for Global Warming Public Engagement Campaigns: An Audience Segmentation Analysis and Tool Development." *PLoS One* 6(3):e17571.

Maibach, E., C. Roser-Renouf, and A. Leiserowitz. 2008. "Communication and Marketing as Climate Change–Intervention Assets: A Public Health Perspective." *American Journal of Preventive Medicine* 35:488–500.

Malka, A., J. Krosnick, and G. Langer. 2009. "The Association of Knowledge with Concern about Global Warming: Trusted Information Sources Shape Public Thinking." *Risk Analysis* 29:633–47.

Manzo, K. 2010. "Beyond Polar Bears? Re-Envisioning Climate Change." *Meteorological Applications* 17:196–208.

Markowitz, E., C. Hodge, and G. Harp. 2014. *Connecting on Climate: A Guide to Effective Climate Change Communication.* New York and Washington, DC: Center for Research on Environmental Decisions and ecoAmerica. www.connectingonclimate.org

Marshall, G. 2014. *After the Floods: Communicating Climate Change around Extreme Weather.* Oxford: Climate Outreach Information Network.

McCright, A. 2010. "The Effects of Gender on Climate Change Knowledge and Concern in the American Public." *Population and Environment* 32(1):66–87.

McCright, A., and T. Dunlap. 2011. "The Politicization of Climate Change and Polarization in the American Public's Views of Global Warming, 2001–2010." *Sociological Quarterly* 52:155–94.

McGeehin, M., and M. Mirabelli. 2001. "The Potential Impacts of Climate Variability and Change on Temperature-Related Morbidity and Mortality in the United States." *Environmental Health Perspectives* 109(Suppl. 2):185.

McKenzie-Mohr, D. 2000. "Promoting Sustainable Behavior: An Introduction to Community-Based Social Marketing." *Journal of Social Issues* 56:543–54.

McKenzie-Mohr, D. 2013. *Fostering Sustainable Behavior: An Introduction to Community-Based Social Marketing.* Gabriolo Island, BC: New Society Publishers.

McMichael, A., M. Neira, R. Bertollini, D. Campbell-Lendrum, and S. Hales. 2009. "Climate Change: A Time of Need and Opportunity for the Health Sector." *Lancet* 374:2123–25.

Milly, P., R., K. Dunne, and T. Delworth. 2002. "Increasing Risk of Great Floods in a Changing Climate." *Nature* 415:514–17.

Mocker, V. 2012. "'Blue Valuing Green': Are Intrinsic Value Frames Better Than Economic Arguments to Communicate Climate Change and Transport Policies to Conservative Audiences?" Master's thesis, Oxford University.

Moser, S. 2010. "Communicating Climate Change: History, Challenges, Process and Future Directions." *WIREs Climate Change* 1:31–53.

Moser, S., and L. Dilling. 2011. "Communicating Climate Change: "Closing the Science-Action Gap." In *Oxford Handbook of Climate Change and Society,* edited by R. Norgaard, D. Schlosberg, and J. Dryzek, 161–74. New York: Oxford University Press.

Myers, T. A., M. C. Nisbet, E. W. Maibach, and A. A. Leiserowitz. 2012. "A Public Health Frame Arouses Hopeful Emotions about Climate Change." *Climatic Change* 113:1105–12.

Nilsson, A. C., von Borgstede, and A. Biel. 2004. "Willingness to Accept Climate Change Strategies: The Effect of Values and Norms." *Journal of Environmental Psychology* 24:267–77.

Nisbet, M. 2009. "Communicating Climate Change: Why Frames Matter for Public Engagement." *Environment: Science and Policy for Sustainable Development* 51(2):12–23.

Noar, S., N. Harrington, S. Van Stee, and R. Aldrich. 2011. "Tailored Health Communication to Change Lifestyle Behaviors." *American Journal of Lifestyle Medicine* 5:112–22.

Nordhaus, T., and M. Shellenberger. 2009. "Apocalypse Fatigue: Losing the Public on Climate Change." *Yale Environment blog.* http://e360.yale.edu/feature /apocalypse_fatigue_losing_the_public_on_climate_change/2210/

November, V., M. Penelas, and P. Viot. 2009. "When Flood Risk Transforms a Territory: The Lully Effect." *Geography* 94:189–97.

O'Connor, R., R. Bord, and A. Fisher. 1999. "Risk Perceptions, General Environmental Beliefs, and Willingness to Address Climate Change." *Risk Analysis* 19:461–71.

O'Neill, S., M. Boykoff, S. Niemeyer, and S. Day. 2013. "On the Use of Imagery for Climate Change engagement." *Global Environmental Change* 23:413–21.

O'Neill, S., and S. Nicholson-Cole. 2009. "'Fear Won't Do It': Promoting Positive Engagement with Climate Change through Visual and iconic Representations." *Science Communication* 30:355–79.

O'Sullivan, J., R. Bradford, M. Bonaiuto, S. De Dominicis, P. Rotko, J. Aaltonen, K. Waylen, and S. Langan. 2012. "Enhancing Flood Resilience through Improved Risk Communications." *Natural Hazards and Earth System Sciences* 12:2271–82.

Oskamp S. 1995. "Applying Social Psychology to Avoid Ecological Disaster." *Journal of Social Issue* 51:217–39.

Parker, D., S., and S. Tapsell. 2009. "Understanding and Enhancing the Public's Behavioural Response to Flood Warning Information." *Meteorological Applications* 16:103–14.

Patt, A. G., and E. U. Weber. 2014. "Perceptions and Communication Strategies for the Many Uncertainties Relevant for Climate Policy." *Climate Change* 5:219–32.

Petrovic, N., J. Madrigano, and L. Zaval. 2014. "Motivating Mitigation: When Health Matters More Than Climate Change." *Climatic Change* 126:245–54.

Pidgeon, N. 2012. "Public Understanding of, and Attitudes to, Climate Change: UK and International Perspectives and Policy." *Climate Policy* 12(suppl. 1):S85-S106.

Pidgeon, N., and B. Fischhoff. 2011. "The Role of Social and Decision Sciences in Communicating Uncertain Climate Risks." *Nature Climate Change* 1(1):35–41.

Poortinga, W. 2012. "Community Resilience and Health: The Role of Bonding, Bridging, and Linking Aspects of Social Capital." *Health and Place* 18:286–95.

Poortinga, W., A. Spence, L. Whitmarsh, S. Capstick, and N. Pidgeon. 2011. "Uncertain Climate: An Investigation of Public Skepticism about Anthropogenic Climate Change." *Global Environmental Change* 21:1015–24.

Rahmstorf, S., and D. Coumou. 2011. "Increase of Extreme Events in a Warming World." *Proceedings of the National Academy of Sciences* 108:17905–17909.

Randall, A., J. Salsbury, and Z. White. 2014. *Moving Stories: The Voices of People Who Move in the Context of Environmental Change.* Oxford: Climate Outreach Information Network. www.climateoutreach.org.uk/portfolio-item /moving-stories-climate-and-migration/

Ratter, B., K. Philipp, and H. von Storch. 2012. "Between Hype and Decline: Recent Trends in Public Perception of Climate Change." *Environmental Science and Policy* 18:3–8.

Renn, O. 2011. "The Social Amplification/Attenuation of Risk Framework: Application to Climate Change." *Climate Change* 2:154–69.

Reynolds, T., A. Bostrom, D. Read, and M. Morgan. 2010. "Now What Do People Know about Global Climate Change? Survey Studies of Educated Laypeople." *Risk Analysis* 30:1520–38.

Roberts, I. 2008. "The Economics of Tackling Climate Change." *British Medical Journal* 336:165–66.

Roberts I. 2010. "Doctors and Climate Change." *Lancet* 76:1801–1802.

Rose, C., P. Dade, and J. Scott. 2007. *Research into Motivating Prospectors, Settlers and Pioneers to Change Behaviours That Affect Climate Emissions.* Campaign Strategy. http://www.campaignstrategy.org/articles/behaviourchange_climate.pdf

Roser-Renouf, C., N. Stenhouse, J. Rolfe-Redding, E. Maibach, and A. Leiserowitz. 2014. "Engaging Diverse Audiences with Climate Change: Message Strategies for Global Warming's Six Americas." In *The Routledge Handbook of Environment and Communication,* edited by A. Hanson and R. Cox. London: Routledge.

Rothman, A., R. Bartels, J. Wlaschin, and P. Salovey. 2006. "The Strategic Use of Gain and loss-Framed Messages to Promote Healthy Behaviour: How Theory Can Inform Practice." *Journal of Communication* 56:202–20.

Rudman, L., M. McLean, and M. Bunzl. 2013. "When Truth Is Personally Inconvenient, Attitudes Change: The Impact of Extreme Weather on Implicit Support for Green Politicians and Explicit Climate Change Beliefs." *Psychological Science* 24:2290–96.

Sampson, N., C. Gronlund, M. Buxton, L. Catalano, J. White-Newsome, K. Conlon, M. O'Neill, S. McCormick, and E. Parker. 2013. "Staying Cool in a Changing Climate: Reaching Vulnerable Populations during Heat Events." *Global Environmental Change* 23:475–84.

Sarfaty, M., M. Mitchell, B. Bloodhart, C. Berg, and E. Maibach. 2014. "National Medical Association Physician Survey." George Mason University Center for Climate Change Communication. http://climatechangecommunication.org

Scheufele, D. 1999. "Framing as a Theory of Media Effects." *Journal of Communication* 4:103–22.

Schuldt, J., S. Konrath, and N. Schwarz. 2011. "'Global Warming' or 'Climate Change'? Whether the Planet Is Warming Depends on Question Wording." *Public Opinion Quarterly* 75:115–24.

Schulz-Hardt, S., D. Frey, C. Luthgens, and S. Moscovici. 2000. "Biased Information Search in Group Decision Making." *Journal of Personality and Social Psychology* 78:655–69.

Schwartz, S. 1992. "Universals in the Content and Structure of Values: Theoretical Advances and Empirical Tests in 20 Countries." *Advances in Experimental Social Psychology* 25:1–65.

Scruggs, L., and S. Benegal. 2012. "Declining Public Concern about Climate Change: Can We Blame the Great Recession?" *Global Environmental Change* 22:505–15.

Semenza, J., J. McCullough, D. Flanders, M. McGeehin, and J. Lumpkin. 1999. "Excess Hospital Admissions during the 1995 Heat Wave in Chicago." *American Journal of Preventive Medicine* 16:269–77.

Semenza, J., G. Ploubidis, and L. George. 2011. "Climate Change and Climate Variability: Personal Motivation for Adaptation and Mitigation." *Environmental Health* 10(1):46.

Semenza, J., C. Rubin, K. Falter, J. Selanikio, W. Flanders, H. Howe, and J. Wilhelm. 1996. "Heat-Related Deaths during the July 1995 Heat Wave in Chicago." *New England Journal of Medicine* 335(2):84–90.

Sheridan, S. C. 2007. "A Survey of Public Perception and Response to Heat Warnings across Four North American Cities: An Evaluation of Municipal Effectiveness." *International Journal of Biometeorology* 52:3–15.

Shome, D., and S. Marx. 2009. *The Psychology of Climate Change Communication: A Guide for Scientists, Journalists, Educators, Political Aides and the Interested Public.* New York: Centre for Research on Environmental Decisions.

Slimak, M., and T. Dietz. 2006. "Personal, and Ecological Risk Perception." *Risk Analysis* 26:1689–1705.

Smith, N., and H. Joffe. 2013. "How the Public Engages with Global Warming: A Social Representations Approach." *Public Understanding of Science* 22(1):16–32.

Smith, N., and A. Leiserowitz. 2012. "The Rise of Global Warming Skepticism: Exploring Affective Image Associations in the United States over Time." *Risk Analysis* 32:1021–32.

Spence, A., and N. Pidgeon. 2010. "Framing and Communicating Climate Change: The Effects of Distance and Outcome Frame Manipulations." *Global Environmental Change* 20:656–67.

Spence, A., W. Poortinga, C. Butler, and N. Pidgeon. 2011. "Perceptions of Climate Change and Willingness to Save Energy Related to flood Experience." *Nature Climate Change* 1:46–49.

Spence, A., W. Poortinga, and N. Pidgeon. 2012. "The Psychological Distance of Climate Change." *Risk Analysis* 32:957–72.

Stanke, C., V. Murray, R. Amlôt, J. Nurse, and R. Williams. 2012. "The Effects of Flooding on Mental Health: Outcomes and Recommendations from a Review of the Literature." *PLoS Currents* 4.

Steg, L., and I. Sievers. 2000. "Cultural Theory and Individual Perceptions of Environmental Risks." *Environment and Behavior* 32:250–269.

Steg, L., and C. Vlek. 2009. "Encouraging Pro-Environmental Behaviour: An Integrative Review and Research Agenda." *Journal of Environmental Psychology* 29:309–17.

Stern, P. C. 2000. "New Environmental Theories: Toward a Coherent Theory of Environmentally Significant Behavior." *Journal of Social Issues* 56:407–24.

Thøgersen, J., and T. Crompton. 2009. "Simple and Painless? The Limitations of Spillover in Environmental Campaigning." *Journal of Consumer Policy* 32:141–63.

Thompson, M. 2003. "Cultural Theory, Climate Change and Clumsiness." *Economic and Political Weekly* 38:5107–12.

Thompson, M., and S. Rayner. 1998. Risk and Governance Part I: The Discourses of Climate Change." *Government and Opposition* 33:139–66.

Toloo, G., G. FitzGerald, P. Aitken, K. Verrall, and S. Tong. 2013. "Evaluating the Effectiveness of Heat Warning Systems: Systematic Review of Epidemiological Evidence." *International Journal of Public Health* 58:667–81.

UK Health Protection Agency. 2011. *The Effects of Flooding on Mental Health.* http://www.hpa.org.uk/webc/HPAwebFile/HPAweb_C/1317131767423

Upham, P., L. Whitmarsh, W. Poortinga, K. Purdam, A. Darnton, C. McLachlan, and P. Devine-Wright. 2009. *Public Attitudes to Environmental Change: A Selective Review of Theory and Practice: A Research Synthesis for the Living with Environmental Change Programme, Research Councils UK.* Swindon: Economic and Social Research Council/Living with Environmental Change Programme.

Veldman, R. G. 2012. "Narrating the Environmental Apocalypse: How Imagining the End Facilitates Moral Reasoning among Environmental Activists." *Ethics and the Environment* 17(1):1–23.

Webb, G. J., and G. Egger. 2013. "Obesity and Climate Change Can We Link the Two and Can We Deal with Both Together?" *American Journal of Lifestyle Medicine* 8:200–204.

Weber, E. U. 2006. "Experience-Based and Description-Based Perceptions of Long-Term Risk: Why Global Warming Does Not Scare Us (Yet)." *Climatic Change* 77:103–20.

Weber, E. U. 2010. "What Shapes Perceptions of Climate Change?" *Climate Change* 1:332–42.

West, J., I. Bailey, and M. Winter. 2010. "Renewable Energy Policy and Public Perceptions of Renewable Energy: A Cultural Theory Approach." *Energy Policy* 38:5739–48.

Westerhoff, L., and J. Robinson. 2013. *The Meanings of Climate Change: Exploring Narrative and Social Practice in the Quest for Transformation."* https://circle.ubc.ca/handle/2429/44563

Whitmarsh, L. 2009. "What's in a Name? Commonalities and Differences in Public Understanding of 'Climate Change' and 'Global Warming.'" *Public Understanding of Science* 18:401–20.

Whitmarsh, L. 2011. "Skepticism and Uncertainty about Climate Change: Dimensions, Determinants and Change over Time." *Global Environmental Change* 21:690–700.

Witte, K., and M. Allen. 2000. "A Meta-Analysis of Fear Appeals: Implications for Effective Public Health Campaigns." *Health Education and Behavior* 27:591–615.

Wolf, J., W. N. Adger, I. Lorenzoni, V. Abrahamson, and R. Raine. 2010. "Social Capital, Individual Responses to Heat Waves and Climate Change Adaptation: An Empirical Study of Two UK Cities." *Global Environmental Change* 20:44–52.

Wood, B., and A. Vedlitz. 2007. "Issue Definition, Information Processing, and the Politics of Global Warming." *American Journal of Political Science* 51:552–68.

PART 4

TAKING ACTION
Adaptation, Mitigation, and Governance

CHAPTER 17

INTERNATIONAL PERSPECTIVE ON CLIMATE CHANGE ADAPTATION

Kristie L. Ebi

Climate change is altering the mean and variability of temperature, precipitation, and other weather variables, and sea level rise is increasing the regions at risk of storm surges, saltwater intrusion into freshwater, and inundation (IPCC 2012). Impacts are already evident in many sectors and regions, with some species extinction, childhood mortality, and changing landscapes already attributed to climate change (IPCC 2014). Changing weather patterns are often not the only driver of impacts, but can exacerbate other stresses to significantly increase risks. These stresses are and will be unevenly distributed, with low- and middle-income countries at higher risk. Growing understanding of the breadth and depth of these multiple stresses means that climate change has moved from being simply a pollution problem to an issue of global development and equity.

Adaptation and **mitigation** are the main policy approaches to manage the risks of climate change. The Intergovernmental Panel on Climate Change (IPCC 2012) defines *adaptation* as: "in human systems, the process of adjustment to actual or expected climate and its effects, in order to moderate harm or exploit beneficial opportunities. In natural systems, the process of adjustment to actual climate and its effects; human intervention may facilitate adjustment to expected climate."

The importance of adaptation has increased over the past twenty years with the breadth and depth of scientific understanding that the planet is committed to additional warming over the next few decades no matter the success or failure of mitigation activities (IPCC 2014; van Vuuren et al. 2011). Implementing a wide range of adaptation policies

KEY CONCEPTS

- Adaptation is one of the two main policy approaches for managing the risks of climate change. The framing of adaptation has changed over time, leading to a more nuanced understanding of the strategies, policies, and measures needed to increase resilience to the health risks of current and future climate variability and change.

- The health risks of climate change are a function of three factors: hazards created by climate change, such as changes in temperature, precipitation, and extreme weather and climate events, and the consequences for natural systems that have relevance for human health; who or what (region) is exposed to those hazards; and the vulnerability of exposed individuals and communities.

- Understanding the effectiveness of current health system policies

KEY CONCEPTS (*CONTINUED*)

and programs is a first step in understanding what modifications are needed to address the risks of a changing climate.

- Many current health adaptation options focus on improving health system functions. While these are critically important, they will only be sufficient to protect population health as the climate continues to change if they explicitly incorporate projected climate variability and change. Adaptive risk management is needed.

- The costs of health adaptation may be significant over coming decades. The costs of adaptation later in the century will depend on the extent and speed with which greenhouse gas emissions can be reduced in the short term.

and measures is critical in the short term if human and natural systems are to successfully prepare for and cope with the changes built into the climate system, although it will not be possible to prevent all impacts. It is not just the changing weather patterns themselves that need to be adapted to, but also the consequences of those changing patterns, such as increases in the geographical range of insects and other disease vectors leading to the possible spread of infectious diseases into new regions. Over the longer term, the magnitude and pattern of climate change impacts will depend on the mix of adaptation and mitigation, with rapid and successful reductions in greenhouse gas emissions decreasing how much adaptation will be needed later this century (Smith et al. 2014; van Vuuren et al. 2011). Slower and less comprehensive mitigation will increase the likelihood of crossing thresholds that could result in dangerous impacts to human and natural systems (Haines et al. 2014).

Historical Perspective

National and international organizations began seriously considering the possible consequences for human and natural systems of increasing greenhouse gas emissions in the 1970s. For example, in 1970, MIT convened a Study of Critical Environmental Problems (1970), focusing on environmental problems whose large, prevalent, and cumulative effects on ecological systems would have worldwide significance. The primary concerns were the effects of pollution on humans through changes in climate, ocean ecology, and large terrestrial ecosystems. Climatic effects included increasing carbon dioxide (CO_2) content of the atmosphere, particle concentration in the atmosphere, and emissions from subsonic and supersonic aircraft contaminating the troposphere and stratosphere. These topics, discussions, and conclusions highlight important historical perspectives that carry forward to today: climate change is an environmental pollutant, with consequences possibly felt in the future, and reducing greenhouse gas emissions through mitigation is the key activity to avoid negative consequences.

This perspective is understandable in the context of other environmental concerns starting in the 1960s. The publication of *Silent Spring* by Rachel Carson (1962) about the environmental hazards of pesticides, particularly on birds, helped launch the contemporary environmental movement. The 1970s and 1980s saw new environmental issues arise, including stratospheric ozone and acid rain. Stratospheric ozone depletion went from an unknown issue in early 1970 to a multilateral environmental agreement in 1985 and an international treaty (Montreal Protocol on Substances the Deplete the Ozone Layer) in 1987 that led to successful reduction of the emissions of ozone-depleting chemicals (United Nations 2009). Throughout the 1970s and 1980s, there was ongoing scientific and policy debate about the effects of sulfur deposition (acid rain) on ecosystem resources in the United States, resulting in the US Congress passing the Acid Deposition Act 1980, establishing an eighteen-year assessment and research program that successfully reduced the relevant emissions (Lackey and Blair 1997; Likens and Bormann 1974).

Lessons from these and similar environmental problems include that an agent (pesticides, chemicals that deplete ozone, sulfur compounds) can harm the environment; reducing the agent was relatively easy and successful after overcoming initial resistance; and reduction led to improvements in the impacts of concern. In short, humans can create environmental problems, and they can resolve these on fairly short timescales once there is the political commitment to do so. Ozone-depleting agents and sulfur are typically short-lived compared with carbon dioxide. Furthermore, alternatives or substitutes were often readily available. For these problems, a key first step in managing the problem was risk identification (identifying which agents of concern led to adverse impacts), followed by the scientific determination of a level of exposure that would result in "acceptable" risk (where *acceptable* was defined by regulators), usually in terms of risk to human health (Bernard and Ebi 2001). This approach and its successes informed efforts to understand the impacts of and strategies to control climate change.

The framing under this approach is that impacts are directly related to emissions and the way to manage impacts is to reduce greenhouse gas emissions. Mitigation is the primary policy task. That perspective is reflected in the language in the UN Framework Convention on Climate Change (UNFCCC) and activities since its negotiation, underscoring the original intention that the treaty should focus on reducing the source of climate change (e.g., mitigation) rather than on adapting to the changes (Schipper 2006), even though the inherent inertia in the climate system means the Earth is committed to decades of climate change no matter the success of mitigation (e.g., there is a climate change commitment) (IPCC 2014; van Vuuren et al. 2011). Adaptive capacity in the convention was considered to be an indicator of the extent to which societies could tolerate changes in climate, not a policy objective. Climate change policy during the 1990s and early 2000s was characterized by this tension between mitigation and adaptation. Increasing scientific understanding, and increasing impacts of climate change, moved this discourse to how to most effectively promote adaptation and mitigation locally, nationally, and internationally, taking into consideration their interactions and trade-offs.

Climate change is moving from being considered primarily a pollution problem to a much more complex and nuanced worldwide challenge involving questions not just about the costs of strategies, policies, and measures to control, prepare for, respond to, and recover from impacts, but also about sustainable development, equity, and social justice. As scientific understanding of climate change and its impacts has increased, so has the social construction of what impacts are unacceptable. The Framework Convention specified three criteria for what it termed dangerous anthropogenic interference with the climate system (United Nations 1992): time for ecosystems to adapt naturally, food production not to be threatened, and economic development enabled in a sustainable matter. However, these are not quantifiable criteria that can be measured and monitored (Burton, Chandani, and Dickinson 2011). Furthermore, while these criteria are clearly important, they are not the only possible impacts of climate change that could have large-scale consequences. For example, there are growing concerns about a wide range of other consequences that could be considered dangerous, including the availability of sufficient quantities of safe water in some regions; the impacts of changing patterns of extreme weather and climate events; changes in the geographical range and incidence of climate-sensitive health outcomes; melting of large ice sheets in Greenland, the Arctic, and Antarctica; sea level rise; and the acidification of the oceans (Smith et al. 2009).

The Copenhagen Accord states the international scientific consensus that a global mean surface temperature increase of 2°C above preindustrial levels is the upper limit of what human societies could adapt to and that anything above that concentration would be dangerous (United Nations 2009). However, this is more a political than a scientific consensus. From the perspective of the health sector, it basically says that morbidity and mortality due to less than a 2°C increase in global mean surface temperature is acceptable; this is at variance with the principles of public health. Research indicates the impacts associated with a 2°C increase are greater than previously indicated, suggesting that 2°C may represent the threshold between dangerous and extremely dangerous (Anderson and Bows 2011). Pledges for greenhouse gas emission reductions put forward since the Copenhagen Accord lead to a 50:50 chance of a peak global temperature increase of at least 3°C above preindustrial levels, with some estimates as large as 3.9°C (Parry 2010). The magnitude and extent of future climate change is an important context for adaptation.

Framework for Adaptation

Research over the past thirty years on the impacts of climate change has led to a more nuanced framework of how climate change could affect human and natural systems. The magnitude and extent of possible risks of climate change depend on the interaction of (IPCC 2012):

+ Changes in temperature, precipitation, and other weather variables and in sea level rise and ocean acidification

+ Human and natural systems exposed to these changes, including people and their livelihoods, infrastructure, economic, social, or cultural assets, environmental services, and resources

+ Vulnerability of these systems, where vulnerability is defined as the propensity or predisposition to be affected

Figure 17.1 illustrates this framework. The figure shows the three components of risk, highlighting that realized risk (e.g. impacts) can influence

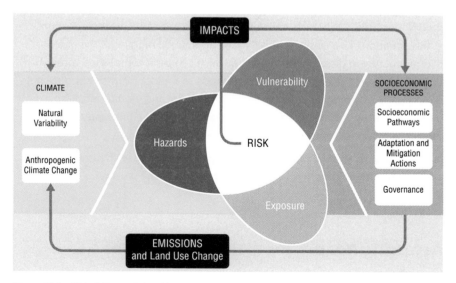

Figure 17.1   Risk of Climate-Related Impacts

Source: IPCC (2014). Reproduced with permission from the IPCC Fifth Assessment.

subsequent development, including through risk management and climate change adaptation, and that development is a driver of anthropogenic climate change. Using this framework, adaptation is understood to increase resilience by decreasing hazards, exposures, or vulnerability.

An important issue this framing does not incorporate is the iterative nature of adaptation (Ebi 2011; Hess, McDowell, and Luber 2012). Health policymakers and decision makers are generally concerned with managing risks over short timescales, often the next five to ten years. Because climate will continue to change for decades to centuries, adaptation needs to simultaneously consider the short term of importance for current decisions, as well as how climate change over longer timescales could affect the robustness of these decisions, in an iterative cycle of assessment, implementation, monitoring, and evaluation (National Research Council 2009). It is important to consider whether choices made today are likely to be resilient under new and different weather patterns, how easily these choices could be modified to adjust to changing situations, and what the consequences might be for population health.

CLINICAL CORRELATES 17.1 THE ROLE OF INDUSTRIALIZED NATIONS IN ADDRESSING THE UNEQUAL DISTRIBUTION OF CLIMATE-SENSITIVE ILLNESS

The United Nations estimates that the cost of treating climate-related health problems in the near future will be on the order of billions and most of these costs will be borne by geographical areas of the world that do not have the infrastructure or financial reservoirs to respond appropriately (United Nations 1992). What role can the medical community of wealthier nations play in addressing this situation? The World Health Organization (n.d.) highlights the need to strengthen health infrastructure in developing countries, which can be accomplished through outreach education of health workers, investment in methods to rapidly diagnose and treat climate-sensitive illness, and investment in technology for surveillance and monitoring. Perhaps most important is that we must promote an attitude among the medical community that the global health crisis is relevant to everyone and that solutions are possible.

Industrialized nations can and should play a role in helping to mitigate the impacts of climate change–related health effects in resource-poor regions of the world.

Assessing Adaptation Needs and Options

Health systems have more than a century of experience with implementing policies and measures to reduce the burden of climate-related health outcomes. However, current programs were typically not designed to account for changes in the incidence, seasonality, and geographical range of these outcomes in a changing climate. Adaptation assessments are designed to identify opportunities to modify current and design new strategies, policies, and measures to increase the capacity of health systems to prepare for, cope with, respond to, and recover from the impacts of climate variability and change (WHO 2013). Adaptation assessments can be conducted at any scale, from local to national.

Adaptation assessments share similar features across sectors (Preston, Yuen, and Westaway 2011). Basic aims include identifying high-priority health outcomes and vulnerable populations; modifications to current and planned programs to address the additional risks of climate change; and opportunities for new policies and measures to reduce burdens of climate-sensitive health outcomes. In most cases, an adaptation assessment builds on the results of a vulnerability assessment (Lindgren and Gustafson 2001). This process is intended to characterize the existing situation, including factors that increase or decrease vulnerability, such as population characteristics, disease burdens, functioning of health care systems, and effectiveness of programs to control the burden of health outcomes. Assuming a vulnerability assessment identified how the current burden of climate-related health outcomes could change with climate change over specific temporal and spatial scales, the main steps in conducting an adaptation assessment include these (Ebi et al. 2013; WHO 2013):

- Evaluating the effectiveness of policies and measures to reduce the current burden of climate-sensitive health outcomes

- Identifying adaptation options to manage the health risks of current and projected climate change

- Evaluating and prioritizing adaptation options

- Identifying human and financial resources needs and options to overcome possible barriers, constraints, and limits to implementation

- Developing monitoring and evaluation programs to facilitate continued effectiveness of policies and measures in a changing climate

In the United States, the Centers for Disease Control and Prevention developed the BRACE framework (Building Resilience Against Climate Effects) to facilitate risk management of the health risks of climate change, including using modeling to project risks, engaging all relevant stakeholders, and regularly updating models and risk management plans as new information becomes available (Marinucci et al. 2014).

Identifying, prioritizing, and implementing strategies, policies, and measures to address the health risks of climate change must be based on an evaluation of the strengths and weaknesses of current policies and measures to address current climate variability and recent climate change (Ebi 2009; Frumkin et al. 2008; Jackson and Shields 2008). A first step in adaptation may be to enhance these programs to address current climate variability (Ebi 2011; Hess et al. 2012). Determining where populations are affected by current climate variability can facilitate identifying the additional policies and measures needed now. At the same time, implementing options that address only current vulnerabilities may not be sufficient to protect against health risks from future and possibly more severe climate change (Ebi 2011; Hess et al. 2012; Smith et al. 2014).

Because a health ministry, nongovernmental organization, and others may have individual or joint responsibility for programs designed to manage climate-relevant health outcomes, representatives from all relevant organizations and institutions should be consulted to determine what is working well, what could be improved, and the capacity of the policies and measures to address possible increases in incidence or changes in the geographical range of the health outcome of concern (Lim et al. 2005). The increase in extreme weather and climate events means that organizations and agencies responsible for disaster risk management are important partners.

Awareness, motivation for action (at political, institutional, societal, and individual levels), human and financial resources, and institutional capacity are essential for any response to climate change (Ebi et al. 2013). Thus, national and local policymaking processes, institutions, and resources influence the choices of which policies and measures to implement to address the current and future health risks of climate change (Bowen and Ebi 2015). These should be explicitly considered when conducting an adaptation assessment.

There is a significant need to evaluate the effectiveness of adaptation options to increase resilience to climate change (Bouzid, Hooper, and Hunter 2013; Hutton and Menne 2014). Studies also need to conduct economic evaluations of the costs and benefits of adaptation options. The challenge is establishing frameworks and indicators for measuring costs and effectiveness over the short time period of a project when the goal is to facilitate individuals and societies preparing for and coping with climate change over decades and longer.

The number of national health vulnerability and adaptation assessments is growing. For example, an assessment for the Solomon Islands used a qualitative, participatory process to estimate the likelihood and consequences of health risks of climate change and to identify potential adaptation policies and measures to reduce and manage risks (Spickett and Katscherian 2014). Vector-borne and respiratory diseases were considered to be extreme risks. Adaptation actions were categorized as legislative or regulatory (e.g., regulate and enforce disease notification procedures), public education and communication, surveillance and monitoring (e.g., improving capacity, including laboratory capacity), ecosystem intervention (e.g., integrated vector management), infrastructure development (e.g., strengthening networks across sectors), technology or engineering (e.g., modify building design), health intervention (e.g., training health professionals), and research and information (e.g., develop **early warning systems**).

Unfortunately, few low- and middle-income countries have undertaken comprehensive health adaptation assessments. For example, an analysis in Fiji of the extent to which the health risks of climate change are accounted for in climate change policies found minor incorporation into the Fiji National Climate Change Policy and the corresponding National Climate Change Adaptation Strategy, as well as the Public Health Act (Morrow and Bowen 2014). Efforts are underway to increase the capacity of low- and middle-income countries to undertake vulnerability and adaptation assessments and implement options to reduce current and projected risks (Neira et al. 2014).

CLINICAL CORRELATES 17.2 E-HEALTH AND TRANSLATIONAL ADAPTIVE MANAGEMENT

Using emerging mobile technologies to crowd-source health information is a recent innovation that has the potential to create benefits in communities vulnerable to climate change. Traditionally, public health assessment systems have tended to rely on remote "experts" to create health maps and identify health issues within a community. Crowd-sourcing in the context of public health is a way of amassing information from the local community in order to build a larger picture and gain fresh insight into a situation. The Voices of Youth Maps Initiative in Haiti is an example of its use in disaster management. In Haiti, coordinators educate youth to identify environmental situations that create the potential for infectious disease spread. They are then taught how to use global positioning system and mobile technology to report infectious threats. Armed with smart phones, youth are empowered to serve as advocates for their community and are better able to protect themselves and others while at the same time creating viable and meaningful information about their communities.

The health sector can continue to work with this concept as an adaptive strategy for climate change. For example, communities can be educated to identify outbreaks of diarrheal diseases in their neighborhood, contaminated water sources, urban areas with high levels of heat vulnerability, and more. Projects such as these build social resilience while improving efficiency of resource use. Clinicians working in these areas can play a vital role in educating their patients to identify and document risks.

Community investment and education are crucial factors for building resilience to the myriad impacts of climate change.

National Adaptation Programmes of Action and National Adaptation Plans

All countries that are signatories to the UNFCCC are required to submit regular national reports covering their greenhouse gas emissions, climate change vulnerabilities, and adaptation and mitigation options to manage risks. Non-Annex I countries (a negotiated list of developing countries; http://unfccc.int/parties_and_observers/parties/non_annex_i/items/2833 .php) submit National Communications (see http://unfccc.int/national _reports/non-annex_i_natcom/items/2979.php). Nearly all developing countries have submitted one, with many working on their third. In addition, least developed countries (LDCs) developed National Adaptation Programmes of Action (NAPAs) to identify their most "urgent and immediate adaptation needs." These were submitted to the UNFCCC for possible funding from the Least Developed Country Fund. Urgent needs were defined as those for which further delay in implementation would increase vulnerability to climate change or increase adaptation costs at a later stage ("Least Developed" 2012). Generally staff within ministries of the environment conducted the assessments, focusing on current or near-term impacts and consulting the relevant sectors to verify information. Despite the near lack of involvement of ministries of health in developing the NAPAs, health is prioritized in most of them. For example, among the Pacific island LDCs, Kiribati, Tuvalu, and Vanuatu ranked vector- and waterborne diseases as priority climate change risks to address in the short term. Unfortunately, limited adaptation funding has focused on the health concerns identified in the NAPAs.

Under the Cancun Adaptation Framework (United Nations 2010), a process was established to enable LDCs to formulate and implement National Adaptation Plans (NAPs) that build on the NAPAs, but shift the focus toward identifying medium- and long-term adaptation needs, and toward identifying strategies and policies to address these needs (http://unfccc.int/adaptation/items/5852.php). Other countries have begun or are beginning to use this modality in their adaptation assessments.

There is often a misperception that developed countries are taking the lead on adaptation because low- and middle-income countries are most at risk from climate change and have considerable human and financial resource constraints for implementing adaptation options. In fact, the UNFCCC has been funding adaptation projects under various funds since the late 1990s. For example, the Global Environment Facility funded three large regional adaptation projects in the Caribbean in the late 1990s and early 2000s: Pacific Islands Climate Change Assistance Programme, 1997–2002, with $4 million; Caribbean Planning for Adaptation to Global Climate Change, 1998–2002, with $6.7 million; and Mainstreaming Adaptation to Climate Change in the

Caribbean, 2004–2007, with $5.3 million (Nurse and Moore 2005). There has been similar funding in other highly vulnerable countries and regions. Lessons learned from the considerable expertise and experience gained in low- and middle-income countries on developing and implementing adaptation policies and measure could be helpful for all countries.

CLINICAL CORRELATES 17.3 STRATEGIES TO ADDRESS WATERBORNE DISEASES

Diarrheal diseases are the second leading cause of death in children under age five, killing more than two thousand per day, more than AIDS, malaria, and measles combined (Centers for Disease Control and Prevention 2013). Reports show that 88 percent of cases are attributed to unsafe water conditions and poor hygiene (Black, Morris, and Bryce 2003). Projections are that climate change is likely to exacerbate water stress in many vulnerable areas, likely intensifying this problem (UN 2012). Experts estimate that every $1 invested in prevention yields an average return of $25.50 in terms of the cost of resources needed to treat illness (Tindyebwa 2004). Adaptive options to address this issue as laid out by the Centers for Disease Control and Prevention (2013) include:

- Governments and ministries of health can:
  - Provide rotavirus vaccination
  - Invest in safe drinking water, hygiene, and sanitation infrastructure
  - Support clear and targeted health promotion and behavioral change programs
- Nongovernmental and aid organizations can:
  - Increase the adoption of proven measures against diarrhea such as rotavirus vaccination, breastfeeding, oral rehydration therapy, and household and community systems for treating and storing water
- Health care facilities can:
  - Ensure availability of adequate medical supplies such as oral rehydration solution
  - Improve training programs for health workers and educate them on the proper treatment of diarrhea
  - Ensure that facilities for handwashing, provision of safe water, and proper disposal of human waste are provided at all health care facilities
  - Encourage appropriate antibiotic use
- Communities can:
  - Discourage or eliminate open defecation
  - Construct basic sanitation facilities

Combating diarrheal illness requires buy-in from multiple stakeholders and is a global, climate-sensitive issue for which adaptive management is essential.

Adaptation Options

There are many schemes for categorizing adaptation options, including from the perspective of actors and their responsibilities (Ebi 2009); from the perspective of the types of actions (e.g., legislative, technical, educational, and behavioral/cultural; McMichael et al. 2001); and from the perspective of the main health system functions, such as monitoring health status and diagnosing and investigating health problems (Frumkin et al. 2008). Because these categorizations focus on options by health outcome, they may not be as effective to address the major concerns of this century, including food and water security and extreme weather and climate events. For example, climate change can affect food security not just through malnutrition but also through impacts on diarrheal diseases and malaria (World Bank 2008). Promoting food security requires considering the interactions of a range of issues that often cross departmental structures within ministries of health and other responsible ministries.

To reinforce the iterative nature of adaptation, strategies, policies, and measures to adapt to the health impacts of climate change can be categorized as incremental, transitional, and transformational actions (O'Brien et al. 2012). Incremental adaptation occurs when information on the risks of climate change is integrated into policies and measures without changing underlying assumptions. This includes improving health system services for climate-relevant health outcomes without necessarily considering the possible impacts of climate change. Transitional adaptation occurs with changes in underlying assumptions, including shifts in attitudes and perceptions. This includes vulnerability mapping, early warning systems, and other measures when they explicitly incorporate climate change. Transformation occurs with changes in social and other structures that mediate the construction of risk (Kates, Travis, and Wilbanks 2012). While there is considerable interest in transformational adaptation, examples do not yet exist.

Incremental Adaptation: Improving Health System Functions

Most health adaptation is focusing on improving health system functions, such as surveillance and interpretation of data related to the impacts of climate change, outbreak investigation and response, regulations, education, enhancing partnerships, and conducting research (Frumkin et al. 2008; Semenza and Menne 2009). Enhancing current programs is critical because the baseline health status of a population may be the most important predictor of health impacts in a changing climate and of the costs of adaptation and inaction (Pandey 2010). Reducing background rates of disease and injury can improve population resilience and minimize poor health outcomes from climate change. The design and implementation of incremental policy changes should be grounded in an understanding of the adequacy of existing policies and measures and how their effectiveness could change under different scenarios of climate and socioeconomic change.

Surveillance is the core activity for identifying the incidence and distribution of climate-relevant diseases and the factors responsible (Last 2001). Surveillance programs are designed to keep local, regional, national, and global public health departments and ministries of health informed about the health status of the populations they serve and the real and potential problems they face (Wilson and Anker 2005). Surveillance involves systematically collecting data, including on risk factors and potential exposures that affect the incidence and distribution of a disease, and interpreting and distributing information to all relevant actors (including health system decision makers, health care providers, and others) so that informed decisions can be taken.

Modifying or expanding current surveillance programs may be recommended in areas where changing weather patterns may increase the incidence or facilitate the spread of infectious diseases. For example, because the risk of salmonella may increase with warmer ambient temperatures that favor the growth and spread of the bacteria (Kovats et al. 2004), enhancing current salmonella control programs and improving measures to encourage adherence to proper food-handling guidelines can lower current and future disease burdens.

Table 17.1 provides examples of health system activities in Europe focused on the potential impacts of climate change on infectious diseases.

Transitional Adaptation

Transitional adaptation moves beyond focusing on reducing the current adaptation deficit to explicitly incorporating climate change into the design of programs and measures, including how these options could increase population health resilience to climate change and how climate change could alter the effectiveness of the options. Indicators of community functioning and connectedness are relevant because communities with high levels of social capital tend to be more successful in disseminating health and related messages, providing support to those in need (Ebi and Semenza 2008).

Among the adaptation options being used or considered that are transitional when they incorporate climate change are these:

- **Vulnerability mapping**
- **Early warning systems**
- **E-health**

Table 17.1   Examples of Health System Activities in Europe to Address Infectious Disease Risks under Climate Change

Indicator-based surveillance: collection, (trend) analysis, and interpretation of data	Routine data analysis from mandatory notification (e.g., the 49 infectious diseases and conditions notifiable at the EU level)
	Pharmacy-based monitoring of prescription and nonprescription drug sale or health-related data preceding diagnosis
	Sentinel surveillance (collection and analysis of high quality and accurate data at a geographic location; e.g., tick-borne encephalitis, Lyme borreliosis)
	Vector surveillance (monitor distribution of vectors (e.g., *Aedes albopictus*)
	Real-time surveillance (instantaneous data collection with dynamic and sequential data analysis, e.g., hospital admissions or dead bird surveillance)
	Mortality from infectious diseases (monitor cause-specific deaths from infectious diseases based on medical records, autopsy reports, death certificates)
	Syndromic surveillance (e.g., monitor emergency room admissions for symptoms indicative of infectious diseases)
Event-based epidemic intelligence; early identification of infectious disease threats	Screening of (international) news media and other sources
	Case reports (e.g., clinician-based reporting)
	Science watch (e.g., screening scientific reports for discoveries and new findings)
	Interdisciplinary reporting on infectious disease threats (e.g., from agriculture, industry, environment

Source: Adapted from Semenza and Menne (2009).

Vulnerability Mapping

Mapping the locations of populations particularly vulnerable to current climate variability and future climate change is increasingly being used in adaptation planning, spurred by the availability and use of geospatial data and remote-sensing capabilities. Better understanding of where suscepti-ble populations are located can help target adaptation activities, focusing services on the most sensitive and effectively using scarce health system resources. To enhance such mapping efforts, it would be beneficial to include indicators of the capacity of communities to cope with current and future changes in weather patterns.

For example, the European Centre for Disease Prevention and Control implemented the European Environment and Epidemiology (E3) Network (http://E3geoportal.ecdc.europa.eu/) that links environmental, remotely sensed, demographic, epidemiological, and other data sets for integrated analysis of environmental conditions related to infectious disease threats (Semenza et al. 2013). The network is facilitating identifying short-term events associated with environmental conditions that can improve and accelerate early warning and response activities and facilitate identify-ing long-term trends that will build the evidence base for strategic health system policies and measures. The E3 network was used to identify the environmental profile of cases of locally acquired malaria (*Plasmodium vivax*) from 2009 to 2012 in Greece, to guide malaria control efforts in affected regions and in nonaffected regions whose characteristics suggested possible malaria transmission (Sudre et al. 2013). A model was developed to predict the suitability of areas of persistent malaria transmission; it included variables such as day- and nighttime land surface temperature, vegetation seasonal variations, altitude, land cover, and demographic indicators. Regions of concern were those with low elevation, elevated temperatures, and intensive year-round irrigated agriculture with complex cultivation patterns. Based on this, recommendations were made of where to implement spraying and other malaria control measures. This model could be used to determine what the consequences for malaria transmission might be of higher surface temperatures and changes in seasonal vegetation with climate change.

Vulnerability mapping carried out in other sectors of the projected impacts of climate change, such as flooding zones (e.g., Hirabayashi et al. 2013) can be helpful input for health systems to increase resilience to (in this case) more extreme precipitation and flooding events.

Early Warning Systems

Disaster risk management has become more urgent with increases in the frequency and intensity of many extreme weather and climate events (IPCC 2012). An effective management option is an early warning system coupled with improved fine-scale understanding of where human and natural systems are particularly vulnerable. Early warning systems are being increasingly implemented in health and other sectors as skill in seasonal forecasting has increased and with increased sophistication in using these forecasts to warn populations of impeding risks and how to most effectively prepare and respond. Effective early warning systems take into consideration the range of factors that can drive risk and are most effective when developed in collaboration with end users (Lowe, Ebi, and Forsberg 2011).

Much of the focus in the health sector has been on heat wave early warning systems. Components of effective early warning systems include forecasting weather conditions associated with increased morbidity or mortality, predicting possible health outcomes, identifying triggers of effective and timely response plans that target vulnerable populations, communicating risks and prevention responses, and evaluating and revising the system to increase effectiveness in a changing climate (Lowe et al. 2011). Of eight studies of the effectiveness of heat wave early warning systems or heat prevention activities to reduce heat-related mortality, seven reported fewer deaths during heat waves after implementation of the system (Paleck, Changnon, and Kunkel 2001; Weisskopf et al. 2002; Ebi et al. 2004; Tan et al. 2007; Fouillet et al. 2008; Chau, Chan, and Woo 2009; Schifano et al. 2012); only Morabito et al. (2012) was inconclusive. For example, in summer 2006, France experienced high temperatures similar to those experienced during the 2003 heat wave, with about two thousand excess deaths. Far fewer deaths occurred than was anticipated on the basis of the experience in 2003. A national assessment attributed the lower death toll to greater public awareness of the health risks of heat, improved health care facilities, and the introduction in 2004 of a heat wave early warning system (Fouillet et al. 2008). A review of the heat wave early warning systems in the twelve European countries with such plans concluded that evaluations of the effectiveness of these systems are urgently needed to inform good practices, particularly understanding which actions increase resilience (Lowe et al. 2011).

Early warning systems also have been developed for vector-borne and food-borne infections using predictive models, although evidence of their effectiveness in reducing disease burdens is limited. In Botswana, interannual and seasonal variations in climate are associated with outbreaks of malaria (Thomson et al. 2006). These relationships were used to develop and operationalize an early warning system based on observed rainfall forecast malaria incidence up to four months in advance. Model outputs include probability distributions of disease risk and measures of the uncertainty associated with the forecasts.

E-Health

E-health and other emerging technologies offer opportunities to increase the effectiveness of early warning and response systems and to better target adaptation options to those most at risk (Holmner et al. 2012). E-health is not just telemedicine; it also includes activities such as home monitoring of vital parameters using mobile technology and electronic health surveillance systems. These applications can be broadly categorized into the use of distance-spanning technology for health care and the use of electronic documentation of health services (e.g., electronic health records, surveillance systems).

Possible examples of use of e-health in adaptation include telemedicine during disease outbreaks and extreme events, point-of-care diagnostic tools, strengthening of health system surveillance using mobile technologies, and promoting knowledge, awareness, and preparedness among the public, volunteers, and health workers.

CLINICAL CORRELATES 17.4 ELECTRONIC HEALTH RECORDS AND DISASTER MANAGEMENT

Clinicians working in areas susceptible to climate change are on the front lines of detecting and treating climate-sensitive health problems. The practice of medicine in vulnerable, low-resource settings is complicated by the fact that health records rarely exist to begin with and because paper records have the tendency to be destroyed and lost during disasters. Electronic health records have the potential to radically improve the way clinicians practice in disaster areas, as is being seen at the Hôpital universitaire de Mirebalais in Haiti. Here, Partners in Health has created an electronic health records system using open source software for their five-hundred-bed hospital. This technology has allowed for continuity in care and has greatly increased efficiency in the hospital and clinic system. In addition, these records are vital sources of real-time data that can allow clinicians and public health officials to develop early warning systems and have an evidence-based approach for handling community-level problems related to climate and disaster medicine. The medical community should continue to advocate for extension of electronic health records as a means of increasing adaptive management of climate related health issues.

Investing in medical information technology is a way to address issues related to continuity of care and disease surveillance in resource-poor environments.

Costs of Adaptation or Inaction

The UNFCCC states that all countries have a common but differentiated responsibility with respect to climate change (United Nations 1992). One consequence is that developed countries have a responsibility to help developing countries adapt to climate change within the context that developed countries are responsible for most of the cumulative greenhouse gases in the atmosphere. International negotiations on funding adaptation for low- and middle-income countries want to know the costs of inaction on climate change (e.g., the cost of impacts without adaptation or mitigation), the costs of impacts assuming various levels of adaptation (and mitigation for estimates later in the century), and the costs of residual impacts. Increasing research is focusing on providing estimates of these costs.

Global estimates of the costs of treating future cases of adverse health outcomes due to climate change are in the range of billions of dollars$ annually (Ebi 2008; Pandey 2010). Ebi (2008) estimated the worldwide costs in 2030 of additional cases of malnutrition, diarrheal disease, and malaria due to climate change, assuming no population or economic growth, emissions reductions resulting in stabilization at 750 parts per million CO_2 equivalent in 2210, and current costs of treatment in developing countries (e.g., cost of inaction). Estimated treatment costs in 2030 without adaptation could be $4 to $12 billion worldwide, depending on assumptions of the sensitivity of these health outcomes to climate change. Limitations of this estimate include that the costs for additional infrastructure and health care workers were not estimated, nor were the costs of additional health system services such as surveillance and monitoring, therefore suggesting this is an underestimate (Kovats 2009). The costs were unevenly distributed, with most of them borne by developing countries, particularly in South East Asia and Africa (Markandya and Chiabai 2009).

A second global estimate assumed UN population projections, strong economic growth, updated projections of the current health burden of diarrheal diseases and malaria, two climate scenarios, and updated estimates of the costs of malaria treatment (Pandey 2010). In 2010, the average annual costs for treating diarrheal disease and malaria due to climate change were estimated to be $3 to $5 billion, with the costs expected to decline over time with improvement in basic health services. Over the period 2010 to 2050, the average annual costs were estimated to be around $2 billion, with most of the costs related to treating diarrheal disease; the largest burden is expected to be in sub-Saharan Africa. The differences in costs from Ebi (2008) are primarily due to a reduction in the baseline burden of disease and lower costs for malaria treatment.

Watkiss and Hunt (2012) estimated the health impacts of climate change in Europe from 2071 to 2100 using physical and monetary metrics, taking socioeconomic change into consideration. Temperature-related mortality during winter and summer due to climate change included positive and negative effects, with welfare costs (and benefits) of up to 100 billion euro annually, with impacts unevenly distributed across countries. Assumptions about acclimatization influenced the size of the health impacts. The welfare costs for salmonellosis were estimated at potentially several hundred million euro annually, and those for the mental health impacts associated with coastal flooding due to climate change were up to 1.5 billion euro annually.

Assuming low- (high-)cost scenarios, the additional costs for the prevention and treatment of malaria in South Africa in 2025 were estimated to be approximately $280 million for the low-cost scenario and $3,764 million for the high-cost scenario (Van Rensburg and Blignaut 2002). Estimates for Botswana and Namibia were $9 million ($124 million) and $13 million ($177 million), respectively. The high-cost scenario for Namibia was about 4.6 percent of gross domestic product. The climate change-related malaria inpatient and outpatient treatments costs at the end of the century (2080–2100) in twenty-five African countries indicated that even marginal changes in temperature and precipitation could affect the number of malaria cases, with increases in most countries and decreases in a few (Egbendewe-Mondzozo et al. 2011). The end-of-century treatment costs as a proportion of annual year 2000 health expenditures per 1,000 people would increase in the vast majority of countries, with increases of more than 20 percent in inpatient treatment costs for Burundi, Côte d'Ivoire, Malawi, Rwanda, and Sudan.

The costs of cases of cholera in Tanzania due to climate change in 2030 were estimated to be in the range of 0.32 to 1.4 percent of GDP (Traerup, Ortiz, and Markandya 2011). The costs for treating additional cases of diarrhea and malaria in India in 2030 would depend on the emission scenario (Ramakrishnan 2011).

Estimates of how worker productivity could be affected by increasing heat stress due to climate change, assuming current work practices, indicate that productivity has already declined during the hottest and wettest seasons in parts of Africa and Asia, with more than half of afternoon hours projected to be lost to the need for rest breaks in 2050 in Southeast Asia and up to a 20 percent loss in global productivity in 2100 under a moderate scenario of greenhouse gas emissions (representative concentration pathway or RCP 4.5) (Kjellstrom, Kovats et al. 2009; Kjellstrom, Holmer, and Lemke 2009; Kjellstrom, Lemke, and Otto 2013; Dunne, Stouffer, and John 2013). Although not estimated, the costs associated with these decreases in productivity could be significant.

Cobenefits of Health Adaptation Strategies

Cheng and Berry (2013) reviewed public health policies to address the health risks of climate change to identify their associated health co-benefits and risks. Only 22 of 812 identified publications evaluated cobenefits, with most cobenefits related to improvements in health associated with building social capital (improved mental health) and urban design (reduced obesity, cardiovascular disease, and improved mental health) through increased physical activity, cooling spaces, and social connectivity. Risks included reinforcing existing misconceptions regarding health, pollen allergies with increased urban green space, and adverse health effects from heat waves through the use of air conditioning.

Conclusion

Avoiding, preparing for, responding to, coping with, and recovering from the health risks of climate change require urgent proactive adaptation if projected impacts over the next few decades are to be significantly reduced. Because many locations worldwide face similar risks or have experience relevant to other regions, there are significant opportunities to work across regions and countries to understand lessons learned and best practices for designing, implementing, monitoring, and evaluating adaptation options. Conducting an adaptation assessment is an important first step in understanding the sources of health risks of current and future climate variability and change and to identifying priority modifications of health system policies and programs to increase effective and efficient adaptation. Within and outside the health sector, a wide range of options is available that can facilitate building resilience. Research needs include developing new adaptation options to manage ever more complex and challenging risks and increasing understanding of how to implement iterative risk management approaches that explicitly incorporate climate change within the context of institutional structures in ministries of health. Failing to do so will leave populations ill prepared to manage what could be significant health risks, with increased morbidity and mortality, and their associated societal costs. The extent to which health impacts will occur depends on health system researchers and practitioners actively incorporating the risks of climate variability and change into all relevant activities.

DISCUSSION QUESTIONS

1. How has the framing of adaptation changed over time, and what difference does that framing make to when considering adaptation strategies, policies, and measures?

2. What factors together create risks of climate change?

3. What steps need to be considered in an adaptation assessment?

4. What are some adaptation options for managing the risks of extreme weather and climate events? The risks of communicable diseases?

5. What would you answer to the claim that adaptation will likely be inexpensive?

KEY TERMS

Adaptation: "In human systems, the process of adjustment to actual or expected climate and its effects, in order to moderate harm or exploit beneficial opportunities. In natural systems, the process of adjustment to actual climate and its effects; human intervention may facilitate adjustment to expected climate" (IPCC 2012).

Early warning systems: Systems designed specifically to monitor risk, warn the relevant population of that risk, and alert that population of how most effectively to prepare for and respond to that risk.

E-health: Health care supported by electronic processes and communication.

Mitigation: A human intervention to reduce the sources or enhance the sinks of greenhouse gases.

Transitional adaptation: Incorporates climate change into the design of adaptation programs and measures, accounting for both beneficial and deleterious effects that may be encountered.

Vulnerability mapping: The use of geospatial data and remote sensing technologies to understand where populations most susceptible to climate change are located.

References

Anderson, K., and A. Bows. 2011. "Beyond 'Dangerous' Climate Change: Emission Scenarios for a New World." *Philosophical Transactions of the Royal Society A* 369:20–44.

Bernard, S. M., and K. L. Ebi. 2001. "Comments on the Process and Product of the Health Impacts Assessment Component of the United States National Assessment of the Potential Consequences of Climate Variability and Change." *Environmental Health Perspectives* 109(Suppl. 2):177–84.

Black, R. E., S. Morris, and J. Bryce. 2003. "Where and Why Are 10 Million Children Dying Every Year?" *Lancet* 361:2226–34.

Bowen, K., and K. L. Ebi. 2015. "Governing the Health Risks of Climate Change: Towards Multi-Sector Responses." *Current Opinion in Environmental Sustainability* 12:80–85.

Bouzid, M., L. Hooper, and P. R. Hunter. 2013. "The Effectiveness of Public Health Interventions to Reduce The Health Impact of Climate Change: A Systematic Review Of Systematic Reviews." *PLoS ONE* 8(4):e62041.

Burton, I., A. Chandani, and T. Dickinson. 2011. "UNFCCC Article 2 Revisited." European Capacity Building Initiative Background Paper.

Carson, R. 1962. *Silent Spring.* New York: Houghton Mifflin.

Centers for Disease Control and Prevention. 2013. "Global Diarrhea Burden." http://www.cdc.gov/healthywater/global/diarrhea-burden.html

Chau, P. H., K. C. Chan, and J. Woo. 2009. "Hot Weather Warning Might Help to Reduce Elderly Mortality in Hong Kong." *International Journal of Biometeorology* 53:461–68.

Cheng, J., and P. Berry. 2013. "Health Co-Benefits and Risks of Public Health Adaptation Strategies to Climate Change: A Review of Current Literature." *International Journal of Public Health* 58:305–11.

Dunne, J., R. Stouffer, and J. John. 2013. "Reductions in Labour Capacity from Heat Stress under Climate Warming." *Nature Climate Change* 3(3):1–4.

Ebi, K. L. 2008. Adaptation Costs for Climate Change-Related Cases of Diarrhoeal Diseases, Malnutrition, and Malaria in 2030." *Globalization and Health* 4:9. doi:10.1186/1744–8603–4–9.

Ebi, K. L. 2009. "Public Health Responses to the Risks of Climate Variability and Change in the United States." *Journal of Occupational and Environmental Medicine* 51:4–12.

Ebi, K. 2011. "Climate Change and Health Risks: Assessing and Responding to Them through 'Adaptive Management.'" *Health Affairs (Millwood)* 30:924–30.

Ebi, K. L., E. Lindgren J. E. Suk, and J. C. Semenza. 2013. "Adaptation to the Infectious Disease Impacts of Climate Change." *Climatic Change* 118:355–65. doi:10.1007/s10584–012–0648–5

Ebi, K. L., and J. Semenza. 2008. "Community-Based Adaptation to the Health Impacts of Climate Change." *American Journal of Preventive Medicine* 35:501–507.

Ebi, K. L., T. J. Teisberg, L. S. Kalkstein, L. R. Robinson, and F. Weiher. 2004. "Heat Watch/Warning Systems Save Lives: Estimated Costs and Benefits for Philadelphia 1995–1998." *Bulletin of the American Meteorological Society* 85:1067–73.

Egbendewe-Mondzozo, A., M. Musumba, B. A. McCarl, and X. Wu. 2011. "Climate Change and Vector-Borne Diseases: An Economic Impact Analysis of Malaria in Africa." *International Journal of Environmental Research and Public Health* 8:913–30. doi:10.3390/ijerph8030913

Fouillet, A., G. Rey, V. Wagner, K. Laaidi, P. Empereur-Bissonnet, A. Le Tertre, P. Frayssinet, et al. 2008. "Has the Impact of Heat Waves on Mortality Changed in France since the European Heat Wave of Summer 2003? A Study of the 2006 Heat Wave." *International Journal of Epidemiology* 37:309–17.

Frumkin, H., J. Hess, G. Luber, J. Malilay, and M. McGeehin. 2008. "Climate Change: The Public Health Response." *American Journal of Public Health* 98:435–45.

Haines, A., K. L. Ebi, K. R. Smith, and A. Woodward. 2014. "Health Risks of Climate Change: Act Now or Pay Later." *Lancet* 384:1073–74.

Hess, J. J., J. Z. McDowell, and G. Luber. 2012. "Integrating Climate Change Adaptation into Public Health Practice: Using Adaptive Management to Increase Adaptive Capacity and Build Resilience." *Environmental Health Perspectives* 120:171–79.

Hirabayashi, Y., R. Mahendran, S. Koirala, L. Konoshima, D. Yamazaki, S. Watanabe, H. Kim, and S. Kanae. 2013. "Global Flood Risk under Climate Change." *Nature Climate Change* 3:816–21. doi:10.1038/NCLIMATE1911

Holmner, A., J. Rocklov, N. Ng, and M. Nilsson. 2012. "Climate Change and eHealth: A Promising Strategy for Health Sector Mitigation and Adaptation." *Global Health Action* 5:8428. http://dx.doi.org/10.3402/gha.v5i0.18428

Hutton, G., and B. Menne. 2014. "Economic Evidence on the Health Impacts of Climate Change in Europe." *Environmental Health Insights* 8:43–52.

Intergovernmental Panel on Climate Change (IPCC). 2012. "Summary for Policymakers." In *Managing the Risks of Extreme Events and Disasters to Advance Climate Change Adaptation: A Special Report of Working Groups I and II of the Intergovernmental Panel on Climate Change*, edited by C. B. Field, V. Barros, T. F. Stocker, D. Qin, D. J. Dokken, K. L. Ebi, M. Mastrandrea, et al., 3–21. Cambridge: Cambridge University Press.

Intergovernmental Panel on Climate Change (IPCC). 2014. *Climate Change 2014: Synthesis Report: Contribution of Working Groups I, II and III to the Fifth Assessment Report of the Intergovernmental Panel on Climate Change*, by R. K. Pachauri, L. Meyer, and the Core Writing Team. Geneva: IPCC.

Jackson, R., and K. N. Shields. 2008. "Preparing the U.S. Health Community for Climate Change." *Annual Reviews of Public Health* 29:57–73.

Kates, R. W., W. R. Travis, and T. J. Wilbanks. 2012. "Transformational Adaptation When Incremental Adaptations to Climate Change Are Insufficient." *Proceedings of the National Academies of Science* 109:7156–61.

Kjellstrom, T., I. Holmer, and B. Lemke. 2009. "Workplace Heat Stress, Health and Productivity: An Increasing Challenge for Low and Middle-Income Countries during Climate Change." *Global Health Action* 2.

Kjellstrom, T., R. S. Kovats, S. J. Lloyd, T. Holt, and R. S. Tol. 2009. "The Direct Impact of Climate Change on Regional Labor Productivity." *Archives of Environmental and Occupational Health* 64:217–27.

Kjellstrom, T., B. Lemke, and M. Otto. 2013. "Mapping Occupational Heat Exposure and Effects in South-East Asia: Ongoing Time Trends 1980–2009 and Future Estimates to 2050." *Industrial Health* 51:56–67.

Kovats, R. S. 2009. "Adaptation Costs for Human Health." In *Assessing the Costs of Adaptation to Climate Change: A Review of the UNFCCC and Other Recent Estimates*, edited by M. Parry, N. Arnell, P. Berry, D. Dodman, S. Fankhauser, C. Hope, S. Kovats, et al. London: Grantham Institute, Imperial College, IIED.

Kovats, R. S., S. Hajat, S. Edwards, K. L. Ebi, B. Menne, and the Collaborating Group. 2004. "The Effect of Temperature on Food Poisoning: A Time Series Analysis of Salmonellosis in 10 European Populations." *Epidemiology and Infection* 132:443–53.

Lackey, R. T., and R. L Blair. 1997. "Science, Policy, and Acid Rain: Lessons Learned." *Renewable Resources Journal* 15:9–13.

Last, J. M. 2001. *A Dictionary of Epidemiology*, 4th ed. New York: Oxford University Press.

Least Developed Countries Expert Group. 2012. *National Adaptation Plans: Technical Guidelines for the National Adaptation Plan Process.* Bonn: UNFCCC Secretariat. http://unfccc.int/NAP

Likens, G. E., and F. H. Bormann. 1974. "Acid Rain: A Serious Regional Environmental Problem." *Science* 184:1176–79.

Lim, B., E. Spanger-Siegfried, I. Burton, E. Malone, and S. Huq, eds. 2005. *Adaptation Policy Frameworks for Climate Change.* Cambridge: Cambridge University Press.

Lindgren, E., and R. Gustafson. 2001. "Tick-Borne Encephalitis in Sweden and Climate Change." *Lancet* 358(9275):16–18.

Lowe, D., K. L. Ebi, and B. Forsberg. 2011. "Heatwave Early Warning Systems and Adaptation Advice to Reduce Human Health Consequences of Heatwaves." *International Journal of Environmental Research and Public Health* 8:4623–48.

Marinucci, G. D., G. Luber, C. K. Uejio, S. Saha, and J. J. Hess. 2014. "Building Resilience against Climate Effects: A Novel Framework to Facilitate Climate Readiness in Public Health Agencies." *International Journal of Environmental Research and Public Health* 11:6433–58.

Markandya, A., and A. Chiabai. 2009. "Valuing Climate Change Impacts on Human Health: Empirical Evidence from the Literature." *International Journal of Environmental Research and Public Health* 6:759–86. doi:10.3390/ijerph6020759

McMichael, M., A. Githeko, R. Akhtar, R. Carcavallo, D. Gubler, A. Haines, R. S. Kovats, et al. 2001. "Human Health." In *Climate Change 2001: Impacts, Adaptation, and Vulnerability: Contribution of Working Group II to the Third Assessment Report of the Intergovernmental Panel on Climate Change*, edited by J. J. McCarthy, O. F. Canziani, N. A. Leary, D. J. Dokken, and K. S. White, 452–85. Cambridge: Cambridge University Press.

Morabito, M., F. Profili, A. Crisci, P. Francesconi, G. F. Gensini, and S. Orlandini. 2012. "Heat-Related Mortality in the Florence Area (Italy) before and after the Exceptional 2003 Heat Wave in Europe: An Improved Public Health Response?" *International Journal of Biometeorology* 56:801–10.

Morrow, G., and K. Bowen. 2014. "Accounting for Health in Climate Change Policies: A Case Study of Fiji." *Global Health Action* 7:23550. http://dx.doi.org/10.3402/gha.v7.23550

National Research Council. 2009. *America's Climate Choices: Panel on Adapting to the Impacts of Climate Change.* Washington, DC: National Academies Press.

Neira, M., D. Campbell-Lendrum, M. Maiero, C. Dora, and F. Bustreo. 2014. "Health and Climate Change: The End of the Beginning?" *Lancet* 384:2085–86.

Nurse, L., and R. Moore. 2005. "Adaptation to Global Climate Change: An Urgent Requirement for Small Island Developing States." *RECIEL* 14:100–107.

O'Brien, K., M. Pelling, A. Patwardhan, S. Hallegatte, A. Maskrey, T. Oki, U. Oswald-Spring, T. Wilbanks, and P. Z. Yanda. 2012. "Toward a Sustainable and Resilient Future." In *Managing the Risks of Extreme Events and Disasters to Advance Climate Change Adaptation: A Special Report of Working Groups I and II of the Intergovernmental Panel on Climate Change*, edited by C. B. Field, V. Barros, T. F. Stocker, D. Qin, D. J. Dokken, K. L. Ebi, M. Mastrandrea, et al., 437–86. Cambridge: Cambridge University Press.

Paleck, M. A., S. A. Changnon, and K. E. Kunkel. 2001. "Nature and Impacts of the July Heat Wave in the Midwestern United States: Learning from the lessons of 1995." *Bulletin of the American Meteorological Society* 82:1353–67.

Pandey, K. 2010. "Costs of Adapting to Climate Change for Human Health in Developing Countries." In *Development and Climate Change*, 1–19. Washington, DC: World Bank.

Parry, M. 2010. "Copenhagen Number Crunch." *Nature Climate Change* 4:18–19.

Partners in Health. 2013. "Open-Source EMR: A New Model for Evidence-Based Health Care in Haiti." http://www.pih.org/blog/university-hospitals-open-source-emr-a-model-for-evidence-based-health-care

Preston, B. L., E. J. Yuen, and R. M. Westaway. 2011. "Putting Vulnerability to Climate Change on the Map: A Review of Approaches, Benefits, and Risks." *Sustainability Science* 6:177–202. doi:10.1007/s11625–011–0129–1

Ramakrishnan, S. K. 2011. "Adaptation Cost of Diarrhea and Malaria in 2030 for India." *Indian Journal of Occupational and Environmental Medicine* 15(2):64–67.

Schifano, P., M., Leone De M. Sario, F. de'Donato, A. M. Bargagli, D. D'Ippoliti, C. Marino, and P. Michelozzi. 2012. "Changes in the Effects of Heat on Mortality among the Elderly from 1998–2010: Results from a Multicenter Time Series Study in Italy." *Environmental Health* 11:58. http://www.ehjournal.net/content/11/1/58

Schipper, E.L.F. 2006. "The History of Adaptation in the UNFCCC Process." *RECIEL* 15:82–92.

Semenza, J. C., and B. Menne. 2009. "Climate Change and Infectious Diseases in Europe." *Lancet Infectious Diseases* 9:365–75.

Semenza, J. C., B. Sudre, T. Oni, J. E. Suk, and J. Giesecke. 2013. "Linking Environmental Drivers to infectious Diseases: The European Environment and Epidemiology Network." *PLoS Neglected Tropical Diseases* 7(7):e2323. doi:10.1371/journal.pntd.0002323

Smith, J. B., S. H. Schneider, M. Oppenheimer, G. W. Yohe, W. Hare, M. D. Mastrandrea, A. Patwardhan, et al. 2009. "Assessing Dangerous Climate Change through an Update of the Intergovernmental Panel on Climate Change (IPCC) 'Reasons for Concern.'" *Proceedings of the National Academies of Science* 106:4133–37.

Smith, K. R., A. Woodward, M. D. Campbell-Lendru, D. D. Chadee, Y. Honda, Q. Liu, J. M. Olwoch, B. Revich, and R. Sauerborn. 2014. "Human Health: Impacts, Adaptation, and Co-Benefits." In *Climate Change 2014: Impacts, Adaptation, and Vulnerability. Part A: Global and Sectoral Aspects: Contribution of Working Group II to the Fifth Assessment Report of the Intergovernmental Panel on Climate Change*, edited by C. B. Field, V. Barros, D. J. Dokken, K. J. Mach, M. D. Mastrandrea, T. E. Bilir, et al., 709–54. Cambridge: Cambridge University Press.

Spickett, J. T., and D. Katscherian. 2014. "Health Impacts of Climate Change in the Solomon Islands: An Assessment and Adaptation Action Plan." *Global Journal of Health Science* 6:261–73.

Study of Critical Environmental Problems. 1970. *Man's Impact on the Global Environment: Assessment and Recommendations for Action.* Cambridge, MA: MIT Press. http://mitpress.mit.edu/books/mans-impact-global-environment

Sudre, B., M. Rossi, W. V. Bortel, K. Danis, A. Baka, N. Vakalis, and J. C. Semenza. 2013. "Mapping Environmental Suitability for Malaria Transmission, Greece." *Emerging Infectious Diseases* 19:784–86. doi:http://dx.doi.org/10.3201/eid1905.120811

Tan, J., Y. Zheng, G. Song, L. S. Kalkstein, A. J. Kalkstein, and X. Tang. 2007. "Heat Wave Impacts on Mortality in Shanghai, 1998 and 2003." *International Journal of Biometeorology* 51(3):193–200.

Thomson, M. C., F. J. Doblas-Reyes, S. J. Mason, R. Hagedorn, S. J. Connor, T. Phindela, A. P. Morse, and T. N. Palmer. 2006. "Malaria Early Warnings Based on Seasonal Climate Forecasts from Multi-Model Ensembles." *Nature* 439:576–79.

Tindyebwa, D. 2004. *Common Clinical Conditions Associated with HIV: Handbook on Paediatric AIDS in Africa.* Nairobi, Kenya: USAID.

Tindyebwa, D., J. Kayita, P. Musoke, B. Eley, R. Nduati,, H. Coovadia, R. Bobart, D. Mbori-Ngacha, and M. P. Kieffer. 2006. *Common Clinical Conditions Associated with HIV: Handbook on Paediatric AIDS in Africa.* Nairobi, Kenya: USAID.

Traerup, S.L.M., R. A. Ortiz, and A. Markandya. 2011. "The Costs of Climate Change: A Study of Cholera in Tanzania." *International Journal of Environmental Research and Public Health* 8:4386–4405.

UNICEF. 2013. "Mapping a City's Risks, Haiti Youth Learn about Health and Technology." http://www.unicef.org/infobycountry/haiti_70264.html

United Nations. 1992. *United Nations Framework Conventions on Climate Change.* Document FCCC/INFORMAL/84, GE.05–62220 (E) 200705. http://unfccc.int /essential_background/convention/items/2627.php

United Nations. 2009. *United Nations Framework Convention on Climate Change, Copenhagen Accord.* Document FCCC/CP/2009/L.7.

United Nations. 2010. *United Nations Framework Convention on Climate Change, Cancun Adaptation Framework.* Document FCCC/CP/2010/7/Decision 1 /CP.16.

United Nations. 2012. "Climate Change to Exacerbate Freshwater Problems of Pacific Islands." UN News Centre." April 23. http://www.un.org/apps/news /story.asp?NewsID=41845#.U-pMR1Za9uY

Van Rensburg, J.J.J., and J. N. Blignaut. 2002. "The Economic Impact of an Increasing Health Risk due to Global Warming." In *Forum for Economics and Environment: First Conference Proceedings.* Cape Town.

van Vuuren, D. P., J. A. Edmonds, M. Kainuma, K. Riahi, and J. Weyant. 2011. "A Special Issue on the RCPs." *Climatic Change* 109:1–4. doi:10.1007 /s10584–011–0157-y

Watkiss, P., and A. Hunt. 2012. "Projection of Economic Impacts of Climate Change in Sectors of Europe Based on Bottom Up Analysis: Human Health." *Climatic Change* 112:101–26. doi:10.1007/s10584–011–0342-z

Weisskopf, M. G., H. A. Anderson, S. Foldy, L. P. Hanrahan, K. Blair, and T. J. Török. 2002. "Heat Wave Morbidity and Mortality, Milwaukee, Wis, 1999 vs. 1995: An Improved Response?" *American Journal of Public Health* 29:830–33.

Wilson, M. L., and M. Anker. 2005. "Disease Surveillance in the Context of Climate Stressors: Needs and Opportunities." In *Integration of Public Health with Adaptation to Climate Change: Lessons Learned and New Directions,* edited by K. L. Ebi, J. Smith, and I. Burton, 191–214. London: Taylor & Francis.

World Bank. 2008. *Environmental Health and Child Survival: Epidemiology, Economics, Experiences.* Washington, DC: World Bank Economic and Health Sector, Environment Department.

World Health Organization. 2013. *Protecting Health from Climate Change: Vulnerability and Adaptation Assessment.* Geneva: WHO. http://www.who.int/globalchange/publications/vulnerability-adaptation/en/

World Health Organization. n.d. "Climate Change and Health." Fact sheet 266. http://www.who.int/mediacentre/factsheets/fs266/en/

CHAPTER 18

HEALTH COBENEFITS OF CLIMATE MITIGATION STRATEGIES

Linda Rudolph, Maxwell J. Richardson

Climate change mitigation refers to efforts to reduce the net amount of greenhouse gas emissions (GHGE) and increase carbon in order to slow climate change and reduce the long-term magnitude of climate change impacts on the environment and health (IPCC Working Group III 2001). Many climate change mitigation strategies directed at the reduction of greenhouse gas emissions also bring substantial public health cobenefits, particularly for the prevention of chronic illness and injury. Climate mitigation policies can also provide synergies with other strategies, such as local air pollution policies; for example, methane reduction also decreases background ground-level ozone concentrations (Shindell, Kuylenstierna, and Vignati 2012).

Climate mitigation cobenefits are the indirect public health (or other) benefits associated with GHGE reductions, independent of reductions to global warming (Parry et al. 2007; McMichael et al. 2003; Patz et al. 2005). Mitigation strategies with health cobenefits provide opportunities to simultaneously reduce the risk of catastrophic climate change and improve the public's health. Cobenefits are important for multiple reasons:

1. An increased awareness of health cobenefits may increase public and political support for policies that reduce GHGE (Krupnick, Burtraw, and Markandya 2000). Health cobenefits, such as increased physical activity and weight loss, are likely to accrue in the nearer term and be more direct and visible than the benefits of avoided climate-related health damage, which may occur over a much longer time horizon.

KEY CONCEPTS

-   **Cobenefits are the indirect public health (or other) benefits associated with greenhouse gas emissions reductions, independent of reductions to global warming.**

-   **Many climate mitigation strategies have significant health cobenefits; a few may have health co-harms.**

-   **Climate change mitigation strategies with health cobenefits present important opportunities for addressing key public health issues.**

-   **Cobenefits provide a framework for cross-sectoral partnerships and increased support for climate mitigation.**

These health cobenefits will also lower the net cost of implementing mitigation measures via a reduction in health care costs (Bollen et al. 2009).

2. Climate change mitigation strategies with health cobenefits present excellent opportunities for addressing key public health issues such as obesity and chronic illness, motor vehicle injuries, and health inequities/

3. Cobenefits provide a framework for strengthening cross-sectoral public health partnerships.

Quantitative analysis of health cobenefits requires the integration of multiple approaches/ including epidemiological, toxicological, and comparative risk assessment, and financial and economic analysis. Comprehensive and life cycle analysis of the health consequences of climate change mitigation strategies is important but remains rare and requires further methodological development, resources, and deployment (Smith and Haigler 2008).

This chapter provides an overview of the health cobenefits of climate change mitigation strategies in transportation, agriculture, energy production, buildings, **urban greening,** and population growth and includes a brief discussion of carbon capture and **geoengineering**.

Climate Change Impacts, Mitigation Strategies, and Cobenefits

Transportation and Land Use

Climate Impacts

In the United States, transportation is the second largest source of GHGE and contributed 31 percent of total US carbon dioxide (CO_2) emissions in 2010; passenger cars and light trucks accounted for 61 percent of total US transportation CO_2 emissions, or nearly 19 percent of total US CO_2 emissions (National Highway Traffic Safety Administration 2012). Newer sources of liquid fuels (used in transportation), such as shale oil and tar sands, may have even greater carbon footprints than conventional oil (Brandt 2008).

Transportation has been one of the fastest-growing sources of US GHGEs, accounting for nearly half of the increase in total US GHGEs since 1990. Total vehicle miles traveled (VMT) has increased due to population growth, offsetting gains in fuel efficiency and recent declines in VMT per capita (Ribeiro et al. 2007; Burbank, Wenger, and Sperling 2012). Freight transportation is now also a major driver of the sector's GHGE (Burbank, Wenger, and Sperling 2012).

Health Impacts

The adverse health impacts associated with the transportation sector are pervasive and well documented, including effects from fuel production, air pollution, motor vehicle injuries, sedentary behavior, noise, and stress (Woodcock et al. 2007; Dora and Phillips 2000; Douglas et al. 2011). Oil exploration, extraction, refining, and transport have been associated with a wide array of ecosystem, wildlife, economic, and health impacts (O'Rourke and Connolly 2003). Health risks associated with extraction of liquid fuels from oil shale and tar sands and from new oil and gas production methods such as hydraulic fracturing, remain controversial, but may include methane release and contamination of drinking water, earthquakes, and exposure to toxic chemicals in waste water (Jackson et al. 2011).

Motor vehicles contribute to air pollution through the combustion of petroleum-based fuels that release CO_2, ozone, particulate matter (PM), nitric oxide and nitrogen dioxide (NOx), sulfur dioxide (SO_2), and toxic air contaminants (California Air Resources Board 2004). Highway vehicles contribute nearly one-fourth of total nationwide emissions of volatile organic compounds (VOCs) and 31 percent of NOx, both of which are chemical precursors of ozone; NOx, SO_2, and VOCs also contribute to the formation of $PM_{2.5}$ (fine particulate matter) in the atmosphere (National Highway Traffic Safety Administration 2012). Ozone causes inflammation of the lining of the respiratory tract and is associated with increased hospitalizations for asthma and chronic obstructive pulmonary disease; particulate matter aggravates respiratory disease, causes premature deaths in those with lung and heart disease, and reduces lung function growth in children (California Air Resources Board 2004). In the Untied States, an estimated 21,000 premature deaths and 27,000 heart attacks each year result from exposure to particulate matter from mobile diesel sources alone (Hill 2005). The negative health impacts associated with air pollution are likely to be exacerbated by global warming as a result of increased ground-level ozone concentrations associated with increased temperature, synergistic interactions between high temperature and air pollution that aggravate the negative health impacts of pollution, and adaptive behaviors such as air-conditioner use that increase energy GHGE (Kinney 2008; Bernard et al. 2001).

Those who live or work near busy roads or spend more time in traffic experience higher exposure levels and health impacts; children living near major roads experience higher rates of asthma and impaired lung function (Bhatia and Rivard 2008; McConnell et al. 2006; Krzyzanowski, Kuna-Dibbert, and Schneider 2005; Giles-Corti et al. 2010). Low-income individuals and people of color often face more severe health effects associated with air pollution because of increased exposure due to residential proximity to roadways and stationary sources and greater susceptibility resulting from poorer overall health, increased psychosocial stress, and reduced access to health care (O'Neill et al. 2003; American Lung Association 2001).

Motor vehicle collisions result in approximately 1.2 million deaths and 50 million injuries worldwide each year and are one of the leading causes of disease burden globally (Richter et al. 2006). In 2010 there were over 37,000 US transportation-related deaths. Low-income individuals and children face a greater risk of death and injury due to motor vehicle collision (National Center for Health Statistics 2008).

Motorized transportation and supporting land use patterns (e.g., low-density neighborhoods with a poor mix of land uses) create disincentives for **active transport** and lead to reduced levels of physical activity (Woodcock 2007; Sallis et al. 2004). Motorized transportation is also a major source of noise pollution; excess noise has been associated with sleep disturbance, increased risk for cardiovascular disease, disrupted social behavior, stress, and disruptions at school and work (WHO Regional Office for Europe n.d.).

Active transport includes the use of nonmotorized forms of transportation, such as walking or cycling and public transit, as almost all trips include walking or cycling. The many health benefits of this relatively accessible form of exercise are well documented (Frank 2000; Maizlish et al. 2013).

Mitigation Strategies and Cobenefits

Mitigation options for reducing transportation GHGE fall into three categories: reducing vehicle miles traveled (VMT), increasing the fuel and operational efficiency of vehicles, and increasing the use of low-carbon fuels (Lutsey and Sperling 2008).)

A suite of tools exists to reduce VMT, including changes in land use patterns, carbon fees, VMT-based user fees, increased fuel pricing, congestion pricing, pay-as-you-drive auto insurance, parking pricing and parking supply management, carpooling and vanpooling, car sharing, telework programs, incentives for transit use, and optimizing freight use of rail and marine transportation (Burbank et al. 2012; Mackett and Brown 2011). Reverting to the walking patterns of 1975 would save nearly 6 percent of annual automobile CO_2 emissions in the United Kingdom; if all drivers walked as much as people who have no car, 11 megatonnes of CO_2 emissions (15.4 percent) could be avoided (Davis, Valsecchi, and Fergusson 2007).

VMT reduction is likely to yield the most significant public health benefits from transportation GHG mitigation strategies through decreased vehicle emissions and air pollution, reduced exposures to traffic collisions for motorists and pedestrians, and increased physical activity from active transport (Hosking, Mudu, and Dora 2011; Haines 2012). Any reduction in VMT will benefit health and reduce GHG, but strategies that also actively promote active transportation will have by far the most substantial health benefits.

Physical activity is associated with a decreased risk for cancer and diabetes; improved cardiovascular, musculoskeletal, and mental health; and reductions in all-cause mortality (Warburton, Nicol, and Bredin 2006; US Department of Health and Human Services 2002; Centers for Disease Control and Prevention 2011). Numerous recent studies project significant reductions in population disease burden with shifts from car travel to active transportation (Woodcock, Givoni, and Morgan 2013; Haines et al. 2009; Woodcock et al. 2009; Dhondt et al. 2013; Rojas-Rueda et al. 2012; Rabl and de Nazelle 2012; Lindsay, Macmillan, and Woodward 2011; Giles-Corti et al. 2010). A study in the San Francisco Bay Area found that increasing median daily walking and bicycling from four to twenty-two minutes reduces the burden of cardiovascular disease and diabetes by 14 percent and decreases GHGE by 14 percent, but without attention to pedestrian and bicycle infrastructure, increases in traffic injury burden by 39 percent are forecast (Maizlish et al. 2013). Researchers estimate that in the Upper Midwest, replacing half of short automobile trips with bicycle trips would yield net health benefits of nearly $5 billion per year (Grabow et al. 2012).

The health beneficial effects of increased physical activity associated with bicycling are substantially larger than the potential adverse impacts of increased air pollution exposure and injury (de Hartog et al. 2010). Increased pedestrian and bicycle injuries associated with increased active transportation can be reduced with investments in infrastructure (e.g., segregated cycle lanes and traffic calming measures), speed reduction, and cyclist training (Goodwin 2013; Bellefleur and Gagnon 2011). Increasing levels of bicycling and walking are associated with reduced injury rates (Swanson 2012).

Increased mode sharing for active transportation is associated with land use patterns that have increased street connectivity, improved bicycle and pedestrian infrastructure, and mixed-use and transit-oriented developments with higher residential densities within close proximity to a diversity of services and destinations (Saelens, Sallis, and Frank 2003; Frank 2000; Frank et al. 2010; Committee on Physical Activity, Health, Transportation, and Land Use, Transportation Research Board, and Institute of Medicine of the National Academies 2005). A Centers for Disease Control review of neighborhood design found that these "smart growth" characteristics may reduce the risk of obesity, heart disease, hypertension, asthma, and motor vehicle injuries; improve mental health; encourage healthier diets; and improve social connection and sense of community. However, higher property values and gentrification also associated with smart growth may lead to displacement of low-income residents without attention to equity issues (Centers for Disease Control and Prevention 2007; PolicyLink 2008). (See chapter 15 on environmental justice.) Neighborhood crime, poorly maintained pedestrian facilities, and time stress are likely to reduce use of active transport (Committee on Physical Activity, Health, Transportation, and Land Use 2005; Ferrell et al. 2012). Increasing heat may impede people's ability to be active outdoors, limiting active transport options (Tait 2011). Strategies to address urban heat islands would facilitate active transportation use.

Improved fuel efficiency and the use of low-carbon fuels have the potential to cut carbon emissions and reduce air pollution. The recently finalized 2025 US fuel economy standards are forecast to reduce GHGE from cars and light-duty trucks by almost half by 2025 and eliminate 6 billion metric tons of CO_2 over the life of the program (Vlasic 2012). US Environmental Protection Agency estimates up to 280 fewer premature deaths in 2030 due to the associated decrease in PM emissions, as well as health benefits associated with reductions in other pollutants (US Environmental Protection Agency Assessment and Standards Division 2012).

Operational efficiency can reduce fuel use and CO_2 emissions through such measures as speed enforcement and speed management, energy-efficient driving practices, synchronized traffic signals; anti-idling programs, traffic roundabouts,; and improved freight logistics (Burbank et al. 2012; Wilbers 2006; European Environmental Agency 2008). Raising motor vehicle speeds from 50 miles per hour to 70 miles per hour raises gasoline emissions of carbon monoxide (CO) and NO_x by factors of 3.5 and 1.7, respectively, and diesel emissions of PM (large particulates) over 200 percent; conversely, reducing the speed limit to 55 miles per hour would reduce vehicle GHGE by at least 10 percent (National Center for Health Statistics 2008; den Boer and Schroten 2007). Reduced vehicle speeds are also associated with lower motor vehicle injury and fatality rates, as well as noise reductions. The implementation of a 55 mile per hour speed limit in the 1970s resulted in nine thousand fewer US highway fatalities in the first year and up to five thousand fewer annual fatalities thereafter. Subsequent raising of state speed limits to at least 70 miles per hour resulted in between 35 percent and 38 percent more deaths (Richter, et al.

2006). The Netherlands lowered speed limits on various roadways near city dwellings in order to meet European Union air quality standards in 2006, with substantial improvements in air quality and noise (den Boer and Schroten 2007). Maintenance of proper tire pressure may also improve fuel efficiency and motor vehicle safety (Jones 2006; US Environmental Protection Agency 2010a).

Low-carbon fuel standards (LCFS), in place in California, Europe, and British Columbia, require fuel providers to reduce the average carbon intensity of the fuels that they provide through, for example, use of lower-carbon fuels such as biofuels, electricity, or natural gas (National Low Carbon Fuels Project 2013). California's LCFS was instituted in 2010 and is estimated to have prevented the emission of about 2.8 million metric tons of CO_2, equal to removing half a million vehicles (and their associated pollutant and toxic air contaminant emissions) from the road (Yeh, Witcover, and Kessler 2013). The US EPA (2010a) estimates that plug-in hybrid electric vehicles could achieve an 81 percent reduction in GHGE and associated tailpipe emissions. Converting all motor vehicles in California to zero emission could avoid an annual 110 million tons of GHGE, 300 premature deaths, and $2.2 billion in health costs from PM2.5 exposure (American Lung Association of California 2008). However, efforts to reduce transportation GHGE could backfire if coal-based electricity is increasingly used to fuel electric vehicles, with a possible net negative impact on air quality and GHGE (Frumkin, Hess, and Vindigni 2007). While diesel engines have lower CO_2 emissions, they increase PM and organic aerosol emissions (Ribeiro et al. 2007; Gentnera et al. 2012). Improved aerodynamics, low rolling resistance tires, advanced engines, and reduced truck idling may significantly decrease the GHGE and air pollution emissions of freight transport vehicles (US Environmental Protection Agency 2010a). (See table 18.1.)

Biofuels, produced from plant materials, have emerged as a popular strategy to reduce transportation GHGE and increase energy security (Paustian, Sheehan, and Paul 2006). The 2005 US Renewable Fuel Standard requires an increasing portion of fuels from renewable sources; California has a target of 20 percent biofuel use by 2020, as does the European Union, and many governments have 10 percent biofuel goals (MacDonald 2004; Boddiger 2007; Crane and Prusnek 2007; Howarth et al. 2009). The impact of ethanol use on GHGE is unclear, with estimates ranging from a 32 percent decrease to a 20 percent increase, the latter estimate due to increased emissions from converting lands to produce biofuels (Howarth et al. 2009). Large-scale expansion of biofuels plantations could also lead to biodiversity loss and plant disease emergence, eviction of subsistence farmers, pressure on freshwater resources, loss of indigenous residents' access to land and

Table 18.1 Cobenefits of Climate Change Mitigation Strategies in Land Use and Transportation

Mitigation Strategy	Intermediate Impacts	Health Impacts
Smart growth	Increase active transportation	Decrease premature mortality
Lower VMT	Increase physical activity	Decrease cardiovascular disease, diabetes, depression, osteoporosis, obesity, breast and colon cancer
		Increase social connection and well-being
		Possible increase bike and pedestrian injuries
	Decrease air pollution	Decrease respiratory disease, asthma, cardiovascular disease
Reduce speed	Decrease air pollution	Decrease respiratory disease, asthma, cardiovascular disease
	Lower vehicle speed	Reduce motor vehicle and pedestrian injuries, fatalities
	Decrease noise	Decrease CVD, increase well-being
Low carbon fuels	Unclear/mixed	Possible increase in food prices
	Possible land use changes	Possible population displacement
Fuel economy	Decrease PM and air pollution	Decrease premature mortality
		Decrease respiratory disease, asthma, cardiovascular disease

water resources through acquisition or diversion to large corporations or governments (also known as "grabbing"), and loss of grasslands with resultant erosion and "dust bowlification" (Patz et al. 2008; Rulli, Saviori, and D'Odorico 2013; Wright and Wimberly 2013; Stewart and Cromey 2012). Some analyses suggest that nitrous oxide (NO) emissions associated with corn ethanol production will significantly offset any CO_2 emissions benefits (Howarth et al. 2009). Cellulosic biofuels may have greater GHGE benefits, but debate as to net benefits of different fuels persists; moreover, there are not currently commercially viable biorefineries to convert cellulosic feedstock to biofuels (Committee on Economic and Environmental Impacts of Increasing Biofuels Production 2011). Full life-cycle assessment is critical to determine the GHGE of various biofuels, but is often lacking (Farrell 2008; Searchinger 2008; Burbank et al. 2012).

The health impacts of biofuel use remain inadequately researched and will depend on feedstock type, the net impact on climate change, air pollution, food security, and impacts on land use, water, and fertilizer use (Ridley et al. 2012; Howarth et al. 2009; Committee on Economic and Environmental Impacts 2011). Some biofuels blends (e.g., E85) are expected to increase emissions of formaldehyde and acetaldehyde, carcinogens that are important ozone precursors (Jacobson 2007). Ethanol from biomass may result in higher release of PM, ozone, and SO_2 than petroleum-based fuels (Committee on Economic and Environmental Impacts 2011), and some biofuel crops may significantly increase release of isoprene, another ozone precursor (Ashworth, Wild, and Hewitt 2013). Perennial biofuel crops such as miscanthus, switchgrass, or prairie produce significantly less nitrate leaching and N_2O emissions than corn or soybeans, and thus are preferred from both the GHG and water quality perspective (Smith et al. 2013).

Biofuels may also have an impact on food security as croplands shift to fuel production. Most current production of liquid biofuels uses food crops such as corn, sugarcane, and rapeseed (canola); in 2007, about one-quarter of the US corn harvest was used to produce ethanol contributing to just 1.3 percent of US liquid fuel use (Howarth et al. 2009). Food crop biofuels will likely exacerbate upward pressure on food prices that is already expected due to population growth and increases in meat consumption. In Mexico in 2007, tortilla prices rose between 40 and 100 percent, in part due to increased US ethanol demand (Burstein and Pérez Rocha 2007; Warner et al. 2013; Food and Agriculture Organization 2012). Bioenergy production that uses crop residues, excess agricultural products, or surplus land will better avoid negative effects on food production, but the impact of biofuels production on water use and water quality may still be significant (Smith et al. 2007). Research may identify commercially viable biofuels, such as made from waste biomass or from biomass grown on degraded and abandoned agricultural lands planted with perennials that will neither compete with food crops nor induce land use changes that negate GHGE reductions and impact biodiversity (Farrell 2008; Natural Resources Defense Council n.d.; Fargione et al. 2008; Tilman et al. 2009).

Agriculture Systems

Climate and Health Impacts

Agriculture accounts for an estimated 10 to 22 percent of total greenhouse gas emissions, but 52 percent and 84 percent of anthropogenic methane and nitrous oxide emissions, both of which have a considerably higher near term greenhouse warming potential than CO_2 (McMichael et al. 2007; Smith et al. 2008). (The lower estimates for agricultural GHG emissions do not count emissions from agricultural uses of electricity such as greenhouses and fuel for heavy machinery use and food transport, that are covered in the building and transport sectors, respectively, or emissions associated with the industrial production of agricultural inputs such as pesticides and fertilizer that are counted in the industrial sector; Smith et al. 2007.) Reduction of methane would lead to both a reduction in overall GHG concentration and a decrease in background tropospheric ozone concentrations, which also have detrimental impacts on human health and crops (Bollen et al. 2009). Application of nitrogen fertilizer accounts for nearly 80 percent of nitrous oxide (N_2O) emissions in the United States (Johnson et al. 2007). Nitrous oxide is a potent greenhouse gas, with three hundred times the warming impact of CO_2 (US Environmental Protection Agency 2013). When agricultural land use changes such as deforestation and soil depletion are taken into account, agriculture may account for as much as 35 percent of global GHGE. Livestock production alone contributes nearly 80 percent of global agricultural GHGE and is the largest source of nitrous oxide and methane, another highly potent greenhouse gas) emissions (Blashki, McMichael, and Karoly 2007). Livestock production also contributes significantly to the depletion of water resources, topsoil loss, and ecosystem damage (Food and Agriculture Organization of the United Nations 2006; Fiala 2006). Meat (especially red meat) and dairy production typically cause far greater GHGE than fruit and vegetable production, although recent studies suggest that GHGE emissions by the livestock sector could be cut by as much as 30 percent through the wider use of existing best practices (Saxe, Meinert Larsen, and Mogensen 2013; Gerber 2013).

Food production (growing, processing, and distribution) accounts for 17 percent of all US fossil fuel use. While it takes an average of 14 kcal of fuel energy to produce 1 calorie in food energy, energy input varies substantially, with lamb requiring about 57 calories of fossil energy to produce 1 kcal of animal protein (Garza 2013; Pimentel and Pimentel 2003). Vegetable and fruit shipments in the United States average sixteen hundred and twenty-four "food miles," respectively; food processing accounts for an estimated one-third of total food production energy use (Horrigan, Lawrence, and Walker 2002).

Agricultural systems affect public health by contributing to environmental risk factors that have a negative impact on health and by influencing dietary patterns. Industrialized animal production now accounts for 70 percent of all antibiotics produced in the United States, with negative implications for antibiotic resistance; organic pollutants used in animal feed may bioaccumulate in humans and increase the risk of poor health outcomes; and concentrated animal feeding operations may increase the risk of occupational respiratory diseases for farmworkers (Walker et al. 2005). The widespread use of pesticides and nitrogen fertilizers also contribute to GHGE, the degradation of potable water supplies, and the deterioration of fisheries, raising a variety of public health concerns (Tilman et al. 2001; Lewis et al. 2009). Nitrogen pollution in drinking water is associated with increased risks for cancer, miscarriages, and attention-deficit disorders (Howarth 2004). Pesticides are associated with cancer, reproductive defects, and impaired mental functioning; children and farmworkers are at particularly high risk of pesticide-related illness (Cohen 2007).

Dietary patterns have changed substantially over the past several decades, with increases in both total caloric intake and the consumption of energy-dense and high fat, high sugar foods (Farah and Buzby 2005). Large government subsidies for crops such as corn and soy have been implicated as key factors in the increased consumption of meat and high fructose corn syrup (Fields 2004). Such high-fat, high-sugar, and energy-dense foods are associated with obesity and increased risks for chronic diseases such as diabetes, heart disease, stroke, and certain types of cancer (McMichael et al. 2007). As developing countries increasingly adopt Western diets marked by high intakes of meat and processed foods, they face the same increased risks for chronic diseases (McMichael et al. 2007; Erlinger and Appel 2003; Friel 2010).

Parenthetically, efforts to address the global obesity epidemic may also reduce GHGE; food energy requirements rise with body mass index, as does energy required to transport a heavier population, with estimates that GHGE due to increases in adiposity in a population of 1 billion are between 0.4 and 1.0 gigatonnes of CO_2 annually (Edwards and Roberts 2009).

CLINICAL CORRELATES 18.1 ANTIBIOTIC RESISTANCE, CLIMATE CHANGE, AND FOOD CHOICES

The global increase in preference for animal-derived nutrition has many negative implications for human health and climate change. On the level of health, consumption of red meat is associated with ischemic heart disease, colorectal cancer, and obesity. On the larger scale, meat production accounts for 80 percent of agricultural greenhouse gas emissions and is an energy-inefficient way to derive nutrition, requiring more total inputs of water and energy per pound of food than plant sources. The meat industry also overutilizes human-grade antibiotics to increase yields. Prolonged and repeated administration of antibiotics, as is customary in industrialized meat production, is associated with the development of resistance among microorganisms. Drug-resistant bacteria are capable of transferring their resistance to other microorganisms, some of which infect humans (Okolo 1986). Based on a recent surveillance report, the World Health Organization states that worldwide antibiotic resistance is "a problem so serious that it threatens the achievements of modern medicine. A post-antibiotic era, in which common infections and minor injuries can kill, far from being an apocalyptic fantasy, is instead a very real possibility for the 21st century."

Increasing patterns of overconsumption of meat, particularly through industrialized animal production, risks higher chronic disease rates, increases greenhouse gas emissions, and contributes to rising rates of antibiotic resistance.

Mitigation Strategies and Cobenefits

Mitigation strategies to reduce agricultural GHGE include the promotion of sustainable land management practices, reductions in meat consumption, and the development of local food systems (table 18.2). Currently feasible and cost-effective best management agricultural practices could result in reductions of 5 to 14 percent of US agricultural GHGE and improve carbon storage, increase soil productivity and production efficiency, avoid soil erosion, and reduce runoff impacts on water quality. These practices include improved crop and land management, reduced fertilizer use, no-till, cover crops, restoration of soils, improved livestock and manure management including rotational grazing and use of methane digesters, restoration of degraded lands, and efficient irrigation (Glantz, Gommes, and Ramasamy 2009; Paustian, Sheehan, and Paul 2006; Smith et al. 2008; US Environmental Protection Agency 2010b; Johnson, et al. 2007). Livestock management practices such as pasture feeding also improve the fatty acid composition and the antioxidant content of beef (Daley et al. 2010). Reductions in the use of fossil fuels–based pesticides and pharmaceutical products could reduce pesticide-related illness and water contamination, and antibiotic resistance (Horrigan, Lawrence, and Walker 2002).

Reducing meat consumption could also decrease GHGE and yield substantial health benefits (Joyce et al. 2012). Estimates suggest that one

Table 18.2 Cobenefits of Climate Change Mitigation Strategies in Agriculture

Mitigation Strategy	Intermediate Impacts	Health Impacts
Sustainable local food systems	Increase school, community gardens Increase urban agriculture Increase healthy food access Increase nutritional awareness	Decrease obesity Decrease cardiovascular disease, diabetes Increase social capital
Improve land management and agricultural practices	Reduce fertilizer and pesticide use Reduce antibiotic use	Reduce pesticide illness Improve worker health Improve water quality Reduce antibiotic resistance
Equitable meat consumption	Reduce meat consumption Increase meat consumption	Decrease cardiovascular disease, cancers (developed nations) Reduce protein deficiency (poor nations)

kilogram of beef consumption is roughly equivalent to 160 highway miles in an average midsize car and that eating a plant-based versus meat-based diet is comparable to driving a Camry versus an SUV (Fiala 2006; Eshel and Martin 2006). A 30 percent reduction in consumption of animal source foods is estimated to produce about a 15 percent reduction in years of life lost from ischemic heart disease (Friel et al. 2009). Modeling studies also suggest significant reductions in diabetes and colorectal cancer risks with reduced meat consumption (Friel et al. 2009; Aston, Smith, and Powles 2012). Because a large proportion of cereal grains and wild fish catch goes for animal feed, decreased meat consumption could also increase food and water security globally (Scientific Committee on Problems of the Environment 2004). McMichaels et al. (2007) suggest an international "contraction and convergence strategy" to reduce the current tenfold variation in meat consumption between high-consuming and low-consuming populations, a policy that would reduce livestock emissions while addressing issues of global equity if people currently with inadequate protein consumption were to improve nutrition. Reducing consumption of foods low in nutritional value and reducing food waste could also decrease production-associated greenhouse gas emissions, have other positive environmental benefits, reduce nutrition-related chronic illness, and decrease food insecurity (Reddy, Lang, and Dibb 2009).

Current public health initiatives to promote local food systems may also yield numerous cobenefits by reducing the use of fossil fuels used to transport, process, package, and store agricultural products. An Iowa study found that a 10 percent increase in consumption of regional food would result in annual savings of 280,000 to 346,000 gallons of fuel and an annual reduction in CO_2 emissions of 6.7 to 7.9 million pounds (Pirog et al. 2001; Joyce et al. 2012). Local agricultural systems may simultaneously increase access to healthy fruits and vegetables, improve nutritional awareness, help build social capital and neighborhood support systems, and improve mental health (Hinrichs 2000; Bellows, Brown, and Smit 2003). It should be noted, however, that tens of millions of people, largely in the developing world, work in the global livestock and agricultural export sectors, and the impacts of a significant shift to local food systems on rural developing-nation workers and economies is unknown (Oliver 2008). The climate impacts of local food may not be universally positive and depend on the production method (Godfray et al. 2010; Edwards-Jones 2010); food product type (red versus white meat, meat versus vegetables) likely has a larger impact on GHGE than either method of production (organic versus conventional) or food transport (Saxe, Meinert Larsen, and Mogensen 2013).

Electricity and Energy Production

Climate and Health Impacts

Electricity production is a major source of greenhouse gas emissions. In 2011, 42 percent of US electricity was generated from coal combustion; other sources included natural gas (25 percent), nuclear (19 percent), hydropower (13 percent), and renewables such as biomass, wind, solar, and geothermal (5 percent) (US Energy Information Administration 2013a). Coal combustion is not only the greatest source of electricity but also produces the most CO_2 per kilowatt hour of electricity, contributing over 28 percent of total US GHGE in 2010 (US Energy Information Administration 2013b). Newer sources of energy such as shale oil and tar sands may have even greater carbon footprints (Brandt 2008). The use of coal in electricity production is declining in the United States in favor of cheaper natural gas and, to a lesser extent, renewables (Center for Climate and Energy Solutions 2013a). Natural gas energy production produces half as much carbon dioxide, and significantly fewer pollutants, than coal (USEPA Natural Gas n.d.; http://www.epa.gov/cleanenergy/energy-and-you/affect/natural-gas.html), but natural gas consists primarily of methane, with significantly higher global warming potential than CO_2, which can be emitted due to incomplete combustion, or during production, transmission, and distribution, thus offsetting some of the potential climate benefits of its expanded use (Center for Climate and Energy Solutions 2013b). Cradle to grave, solar, wind, and nuclear electricity release about one-twentieth the GHGEs per kilowatt-hour as coal (National Renewable Energy Laboratory 2013). The GHGE profile of energy from biomass (e.g., wood waste) is controversial and depends on source, production process, and transportation; life cycle assessment of climate impacts varies substantially by type of biomass and the energy source that bioenergy replaces (Kellerhals 2011).

Historically, electricity has had a profoundly positive impact on public health, enabling safer food, drug, and vaccine storage, enhanced educational opportunities, decreased indoor air pollution, and improved economic development and overall quality of life. Although electrification is now considered a basic standard for health, 1.3 billion people still lack electricity, primarily in rural areas in sub-Sarahan Africa and developing Asia (International Energy Agency 2013a).

The health risks associated with electricity production vary by source (Smith et al. 2013). Every phase of coal production and use has significant adverse impacts on health, including mining, transportation, washing, combustion, and disposal of postcombustion waste. Coal-burning power plants are the largest industrial source of air pollution, emitting NOx, SOx, mercury, selenium, and arsenic, and contributing to ozone and PM pollution (Smith et al. 2013). Coal combustion contributes to asthma, lung cancer, heart disease, stroke, adverse pregnancy outcomes, and impaired lung and neurodevelopment. Coal plant pollution is expected to cause over thirteen thousand deaths and more than twenty thousand heart attacks per year, at a total monetized value of more than $100 billion per year, with the greatest impacts on elderly, children, those with respiratory disease, the poor, minority groups, and people downwind of power plants (Schneider and Banks 2010). The Global Burden of Disease Study suggested more than 3 million premature deaths due to outdoor air pollution, much of that due to coal combustion (Smith et al. 2013). Coal miners face significant occupational risks including respiratory illnesses such as silicosis and coal workers' pneumoconiosis, lung cancer, noise-induced hearing loss, serious injury, and fatality (Markandya and Wilkinson 2007; Krewitt et al. 1998; Holmberg and Ahlborg 1983). Moreover, coal combustion accounts for a large fraction of PM pollution globally; PM resulted in over 3 million premature deaths in 2010 (Smith et al. 2013). Surface mining and mountaintop removal entail significant environmental risks including soil erosion with flooding, mudslide, and water contamination risks (Smith et al. 2013; Lockwood et al. 2009). The cumulative health costs of coal-based electricity in the United Stat4es have been estimated at $62 billion to $523 billion annually (Epstein et al. 2011; National Research Council 2010). Internationally, increasing coal consumption is associated with increased infant mortality and reduced life expectancy (Gohlke et al. 2011).

Natural gas extraction, production, and combustion may release methane, VOCs, and ultrafine PM, and may increase ambient ozone concentrations (Electric Power Research Institute 2012). Health risks associated with extraction from shale oil tar sands and growing oil and gas production methods such as hydraulic fracturing remain controversial, but may include methane release and contamination of drinking water, earthquakes, and exposure to toxic chemicals in wastewater (Jackson et al. 2011).

Nuclear power entails risks related to accidental releases of radiation and generates waste products containing highly radioactive substances with substantial health, environmental, and national security risks that persist over long periods of time. Uranium mining and milling is associated with high risks of lung cancer and other disease in miners, as well as environmental contamination with radioactive dust, radon gas, waterborne toxins, and increased levels of background radiation (Dewar, Harvey, and Vakil 2013; Holden and Smith 2000; Smith et al. 2013).

The known health impacts of hydroelectric power are related primarily to the occupational health risks, ecosystem and water access impacts, and large-scale community displacement due to construction of large dams, with concomitant sociocultural stress and health impacts of loss of livelihood (Holden and Smith 2000; Smith et al. 2013; Markandya and Wilkinson 2007).

The health impacts of wind and solar power appear to be relatively minimal; however, potential occupational and environmental hazards associated with exposure to silica and other toxic materials in the manufacture and disposal of solar panels, and health risks due to annoyance associated with noise and visual disturbance from wind turbines, merit further study as these power sources expand (Holden and Smith 2000; Markandya and Wilkinson 2007; Smith et al. 2013; Silicon Valley Toxics Coalition 2009; Michaud et al. 2012; Joshi et al. 2012; Expert Independent Panel on Wind Turbine Health Impacts 2012). Biomass health impacts remain controversial. Biomass combustion produces particulate matter; however, there is some suggestion that forest thinning or biomass clearance may reduce wildfire risk and the associated extremely high PM concentrations (Kellerhals 2011).

CLINICAL CORRELATES 18.2 GREENHOUSE GAS EMISSIONS OF THE US HEALTH CARE SECTOR

The health benefits of reducing GHG emissions have become abundantly clear. Paradoxically, the health care sector of the United States is a large contributor to GHG emissions. The sector encompasses hospital operation, home health care, nursing home care, prescription drugs, durable medical equipment, scientific research, and more. Based on estimates from 2007, health care activities contributed to 8 percent of the total US GHG emissions and 7 percent of the total carbon dioxide emissions. Health care institutions are increasingly aware of the need to reduce their GHG emissions. Many hospitals are now taking steps to increase procurement of renewable energy and reduce energy and water use and waste.

The health care sector is a major producer of greenhouse gas emissions.

Mitigation Strategies and Cobenefits

Strategies to reduce greenhouse gas emissions from electricity production include switching to low-carbon renewable and nuclear energy sources, use of new technologies such as carbon capture and sequestration, and energy efficiency (table 18.3). The health cobenefits of these strategies will be largely based on reductions achieved in exposures to the risks outlined above, balanced against any adverse health impacts associated with replacement power sources. Reducing US dependence on coal-generated electricity

Table 18.3   Cobenefits of Climate Change Mitigation Strategies in Electricity Production

Mitigation Strategy	Intermediate Impacts	Health Impacts
Decrease fossil fuel combustion	Decrease particulate matter	Decrease premature mortality
	Decrease air pollution	Decrease cardiovascular disease, respiratory disease, asthma
Increase renewable energy	Uncertain life cycle impacts	Possible worker health impacts

will clearly yield significant improvements in air quality with concomitant health benefits and mitigate global warming. Globally, GHGE reductions to 50 percent of 2005 levels by 2050 could lower premature deaths caused by air pollution by 20 to 40 percent (dependent on region) relative to business as usual (Bollen et al. 2009). A recent analysis of a plan to convert New York State's energy infrastructure to one derived entirely from renewables and hydrogen suggests a reduction of four thousand deaths per year due to air pollution, with an associated cost decline of $33 billion, enough to pay for the costs of conversion within seventeen years (Jacobson et al. 2013). Energy efficiency and conservation reduce energy demand and thus lower the need for energy production and any of its associated health impacts; energy efficiency may also alleviate energy poverty and free up income for spending on other critical needs (Ryan and Campbell 2012; International Energy Agency 2013a).

Increasing access to electricity in developing countries is an important public health goal. However, current strides in electrification in developing nations such as India and China may be accompanied by significant increases in global GHGE if electricity production relies on coal combustion. Solar energy offers a promising solution to provide electricity in areas without a grid and can provide basic electric service for critical needs such as cold storage of vaccines in health facilities without increasing GHG (PATH and World Health Organization 2012).

HOUSEHOLD ENERGY AND COOKSTOVES

Billions of poor people around the world continue to rely on solid fuels—charcoal, coal, dung, wood, and crop residues—for household energy needs such as cooking and heating. The common use of indoor fires or inefficient cookstoves in poorly ventilated spaces results in high levels of GHG production, including considerable amounts of short-lived climate-changed pollutants such as black carbon and methane, and indoor household air pollution with combustion products including particulates, carbon monoxide, SO_2, NO_2, and organic pollutants such as formaldehyde (World Health Organization 2012; Smith et al. 2013). It is estimated that universal adoption of advanced biomass cookstoves could have an impact equivalent to reducing CO_2 emissions by about 25 to 50 percent (Global Alliance of Clean Cookstoves 2013). Inefficient solid fuel cookstoves are also estimated to account for more than 15 percent of outdoor particulate air pollution worldwide, varying by region (Smith et al. 2013).

The health effects of household air pollution include pneumonia in young children, chronic obstructive pulmonary disease, lung cancer, cataracts, likely cardiovascular disease, low birth weight, tuberculosis, and impacts on child cognitive function. The 2010 Global Burden of Disease assessment estimated that household cooking with solid fuels resulted in about 3.5 million premature deaths in 2010, ranking as the second leading contributor to lost healthy life years for women and fourth for men (Smith et al. 2013).

Improved cookstove design potentially improves health, reduces GHG and air pollutant emissions, and preserves forests as fuel efficiency increases (Jeuland and Pattanayak 2012). An improved biomass cookstove may reduce CO_2 emissions by 161 kilograms annually (Panwar, Kurchania, and Rathore 2009). Projections of benefits from India's cookstove program suggest reduced childhood pneumonia, chronic obstructive pulmonary disease, and ischemic heart disease totaling 12,500 averted disability-adjusted life years (DALYs) and reduction of 0.1 to 0.2 megatonnes of CO_2 equivalent per year, mostly in short-lived GHGs (Wilkinson et al. 2009). However, to date, dissemination of improved cookstoves has been met with somewhat limited adoption due to multiple factors including user acceptability, education, availability of clean fuels, and household financial credit, among others (Lewis and Pattanayak 2012).

Buildings

Climate and Health Impacts

Buildings account for 41 percent of total US energy use, 65 percent of electricity consumption, and 30 percent of GHGE (US Green Building Council 2008; US Department of Energy 2011). housing consumes more than one-fifth of US energy (Wilson and Katz 2010; Laquatra et al. 2008). Buildings can have a dramatic impact on energy consumption and greenhouse gas emissions based on construction, design, and energy use over a building's life span; most emissions occur during their operational phase (United Nations Environmental Programme 2009). Because as much as 75 percent of the built environment is expected to be either constructed or renovated by 2035, the building sector may offer cost-effective potential for greenhouse gas emissions reductions (Levine et al. 2007; Architecture 2030 2011).

On average, people spend about 90 percent of their time indoors, and the indoor environment has a considerable impact on health (US Environmental

Protection Agency 2001). Certain building characteristics (e.g., closed windows, extensive air recirculation, fan versus window ventilation, moisture problems, dust mites, mold, and cockroach infestation) are associated with acute respiratory illness, asthma, allergies, sick building syndrome (SBS), decreased worker productivity, and lower student performance (Fisk 2000; Schneider 2002). Poor lighting has a negatively impact on performance in classrooms and workspaces (Fisk 2000; Schneider 2002; Levine et al. 2007).

Climate change could exacerbate negative health impacts from the indoor environment in a number of ways. First, changes in the outdoor environment—increases in pollution, severe weather and rainfall events, and excessive heat—will affect the indoor environment. Second, efforts to improve building efficiency and reduce building emissions could reduce ventilation rates, causing higher concentrations of and exposure to indoor pollutants or moisture. Finally, behavioral adaptations to changing climate, such as higher use of air-conditioning or portable generators, could lead to greater emissions and higher risk of carbon monoxide poisoning (Institute of Medicine 2011).

Mitigation Strategies and Cobenefits

Green buildings are those with a small carbon footprint, constructed with techniques and materials that minimize impacts on the natural environment and create healthy indoor environments (Laquatra et al. 2008). The greatest energy efficiency gains in the buildings sector can be produced using technologies that already exist (table 18.4 on page 554). Design and construction choices that can mitigate climate change while improving occupant health include (Levine et al. 2007; Kats et al. 2003):

- Low-impact indoor appliances and lighting, such as the EPA's Energy Star program
- Tightening the building envelope with improved insulation and modern heating, ventilation, and air-conditioning systems, coupled with proper ventilation and air filtering
- Green landscaping and cool roofs

Efficient building orientation and site selection A suite of existing practices is available to reduce building energy demand. Increased day lighting in a building can reduce lighting energy demands by 40 to 80 percent. Natural light also benefits building occupants by reducing stress, improving student performance, and increasing worker productivity (Boyce et al. 2003). Windows that let light in and provide a view of the outside environment may even improve postsurgery recovery times and improve an occupant's sense of well-being (Ulrich 1984; Kaplan 2001).

Improving building efficiency by tightening the building envelope will decrease energy consumption by reducing leakage. Adding insulation, installing modern high-efficiency heating, ventilation, and air-conditioning systems, and maintaining furnaces are easy ways to improve energy efficiency and lower utility bills. However, maintaining a balance between a tight building envelope and appropriate ventilation and air circulation is essential for capturing health cobenefits related to thermal stress, noise, moisture control, and indoor air quality (Institute of Medicine 2011).

Improving the building efficiency with sufficient ventilation to avoid overheating can reduce thermal stress in extreme temperatures (hot or cold), and most benefit populations susceptible to extreme temperatures, such as the elderly, those with preexisting health conditions, the poor, and children (Kovtas and Hajat 2008; Dengel and Swainson 2012; Medina-Ramon et al. 2006). This may be of particular importance in regions where populations are less physiologically and behaviorally adapted to deal with the effects of extreme heat (Knowlton et al. 2009).

Exposure to noise, even below levels needed to damage hearing, can harm health. Researchers have found that noise in the range of 60 to 70 decibels, roughly the equivalent of normal speech at three feet, can increase risks for hypertension and cardiovascular risk (Babisch 2008). Children who experience chronic noise at school or home have poorer school performance (Shield and Dockrell 2003). Building design and energy efficiency upgrades that can achieve emission reductions and dampen noise from outdoor sources include filtered mechanical ventilation to reduce the need to open windows, improving insulation, installing double-paned windows, and sealing openings that fit electrical, gas, or water conduits (Berendt, Corliss, and Ojalvo 1978).

Energy efficiency upgrades that do not consider ventilation, air exchange, and filtering systems could expose occupants to higher concentrations of indoor-emitted pollutants or indoor dampness, increasing occupant risks for asthma, allergies, and other respiratory ailments (Institute of Medicine 2011; Wilson and Katz 2010). Multiple federal and state programs incentivize home energy efficiency upgrades and, properly designed and executed, can improve the health of occupants compared to new homes using traditional practices. This can lead to less respiratory illness, fewer visits to primary care providers, and fewer days off from work or school.

The use of building orientation, shading, and site selection can reduce greenhouse gas emissions and have positive health effects for the building occupants (US Environmental Protection Agency 2012b). Before construction even begins on a new building, site selection and building orientation can have a tremendous impact on energy efficiency over the life span of the building. Selection of a site in a location that facilitates active transportation allows building occupants to substantially reduce transportation GHGE. Building orientation also influences the energy efficiency of a building and can decrease overall building emissions. Considerations of sun exposure, shading, window location, and ventilation can reduce energy costs, and promote natural ventilation (US Environmental Protection Agency 2012a). Building orientation is a cost-effective method to reduce thermal stress for building occupants and can be used to balance the need to make more energy-efficient buildings that also improve indoor air quality.

Addressing health effects caused by indoor environments would produce substantial economic benefits from reduced illness and increased productivity. Improving indoor air quality could result in savings of $6 billion to $14 billion from reduced respiratory disease, $1 billion to $4 billion from reduced allergies and asthmatic symptoms, $10 billion to $30 billion from reduced syndromes associated with discomfort and acute health effects from time spent inside buildings (broadly known as "sick building syndrome"), and improved worker productivity gains of $20 billion to $160 billion (Fisk 2000). Properly conducted energy retrofits and energy-efficient new home construction (compared to traditionally constructed homes) can improve occupant health, reduce fire risk, and save on utility bills, allowing expenditures on other essential needs; however, poorly executed energy-efficiency retrofits or construction can increase the risks of asthma, respiratory illness, and allergies associated with poor indoor air quality and mold. Furthermore, it can increase the risks of carbon monoxide poisoning and overheating in heat wave conditions unless measures are in place for adequate air exchange, venting of appliances and fans, and proper sealing of ductwork. Experts suggest that energy retrofits should also include smoke and CO_2 alarms, repair of water leaks, lead safety, radon testing, and (in hot climates) an air conditioner in at least one room (Howden-Chapman et al. 2011; Wilson and Katz 2010; Bone et al. 2010; Manuel 2011; Singh et al. 2010). A model projecting health impacts of improved household energy efficiency in England estimated 850 fewer disability-adjusted life years (DALYs), and a saving of 0.6 megatonnes of carbon dioxide per million population in one year (Wilkinson et al. 2009).

Air-conditioning is considered a key adaptation strategy to protect against extreme heat, but there are concerns that it is potentially maladaptive because its use during heat waves can cause blackouts. This in turn can lead to upgrading and adding energy production infrastructure to meet the added demand. Constructing additional infrastructure contributes to GHGE, and the associated costs have an adverse impact on households as electricity rates are raised to cover the expense (Farbotko and Waitt 2011).

Table 18.4   Cobenefits of Climate Change Mitigation Strategies in Buildings

Mitigation Strategy	Intermediate Impacts	Health Impacts
Green buildings and reduced toxics in building materials	Improve indoor air quality	Decrease sick building syndrome
Energy efficiency	Reduce pollutant emissions from electricity production	Decrease Cardiovascular disease, respiratory illness
	Reduce energy use	Reduce fuel poverty
Daylighting	Increase natural light, views of nature	Improve school and work performance

Urban Greening

Climate Impacts

Urban greening (parks, forests, trees, gardens, and agriculture) reduces greenhouse gas emissions through direct sequestration of CO_2 in trees and vegetation, and reduced demand for energy for heating and cooling due to lowering of surface and air temperatures (Wong 2008; McPherson et al. 2010). A tree sequesters several tons of CO_2 over its lifetime; urban trees in the United States sequestered an estimated 95.5 million metric tons (MMT) CO_2 in 2006 (McPherson 2007; McPherson et al. 2010; Groth et al. 2008).

Landscaping can directly sequester carbon and be used to increase building efficiency. Using deciduous trees to provide shade on south-facing facades can decrease air-conditioning costs by 20 percent. Conifer trees can be used to block northern winds to reduce heating costs in the winter (US Environmental Protection Agency 2012b). Green roofs have also been shown to decrease summer cooling costs, insulate buildings better during the winter, and lower concentrations of air pollution (Yang, Yu, and Gong 2008). En masse, creating green spaces around buildings and parking lots can reduce urban heat island effects and reduce energy use and thermal stress during extreme heat events (Institute of Medicine 2011).

Health Impacts and Cobenefits

Trees and vegetation remove pollutants such as ozone, NO_2, and to a lesser extent particulate matter through deposition on leaves and needles; however, biogenic hydrocarbons react with nitrogen oxides to form ozone, and trees and other plants are a source of pollens and other aeroallergens (California Air Resources Board 2012; McPherson et al. 2010; table 18.5). The careful selection of trees and vegetation to minimize biogenic emissions and aeroallergens can optimize the health cobenefits of greening (Lin and Zacharek 2012). Views of greenery have been associated with faster

Table 18.5   Cobenefits of Urban Greening

Mitigation Strategy	Intermediate Impacts	Health Impacts
Urban forestry	Decrease particulate matter	Decrease premature mortality
	Decrease air pollution	Decrease cardiovascular disease, respiratory disease, asthma
	Shading	
	Reduce energy use	Decrease heat risk
	Decrease flood risk	Reduce fuel poverty
	Increase groundwater recharge	Increase drought and flood resilience
	Filter water	
School and community gardens	Increase healthy food access	Decrease obesity
Urban agriculture	Increase nutritional awareness	Decrease cardiovascular disease, diabetes
		Increase social capital
Parks and open space	Space for activity	Increase physical activity
	Venues for social engagement	Increase social capital

recovery times in hospital patients, reduced stress, and lowered annoyance from noise (Lottrup, Grahn, and Sigsdotter 2013; Li, Chau, and Tang 2010).

Urban greening provides spaces for recreation, relaxation, and social engagement. It can increase physical activity and, if green spaces are well placed, reduce motor vehicle trips for recreation. Tree shade can slow deterioration of sidewalk pavement, making walking safer for pedestrians; however, consideration must be given to minimizing root damage to sidewalks. Green infrastructure increases stormwater retention and groundwater recharge, with reduced risk of stormwater runoff, flooding, and water shortages. Tree planting—in combination with water management tools such as permeable pavements and rain barrels—is estimated to be three to six times more effective in managing stormwater per one thousand dollars invested than conventional gray water infrastructure (Groth et al. 2008; Foster, Lowe, and Winkelman 2011). Tree selection mindful of regional drought potential may limit urban forest damage in prolonged drought conditions. Green roofs also significantly reduce stormwater runoff and energy consumption (Foster, Lowe, and Winkelman 2011). Finally, urban greening brings social, economic, and cultural benefits, improving the quality of life and increasing property values and the aesthetic quality of neighborhoods (Haq 2011). As with smart growth, these positive improvements may be associated with displacement of lower- income neighborhood residents, without explicit attention to social equity (Wolcha, Bynreb, and Newell 2014). (See chapter 15 on environmental justice.)

Urban greening is also an important public health climate adaptation strategy, as reducing temperatures in urban heat islands can significantly decrease the risk of heat illness. Australian researchers found that a 0.5°C reduction in the maximum and minimum temperature resulted in a 50 percent reduction in heat-related mortality in two cities, and that green infrastructure could reduce temperatures by 0.3°C to 0.7°C (Chen 2012). Heat morbidity may increase when low-income people fail to use air-conditioning due to concerns about energy costs (English et al. 2008). Reduced energy demand can lessen the burden of high energy costs. The increased temperature in urban heat islands is responsible for 5 to 10 percent of urban peak electric demand for air conditioning (Akbari 2003). Shaded surfaces may be 20°F to 45°F (11°C to 25°C) cooler than unshaded surfaces, and together shading and evapotranspiration can reduce peak summer ambient temperatures by 2°C to 9°F (1°C to 5°C), yielding significant reductions in energy demand and emissions (Wong 2008).

Market Mechanisms

Market mechanisms for climate change mitigation, such as a carbon tax, northeast US states, and cap and trade, increase the price of carbon and create a financial incentive to reduce the use of fossil fuels by consumers, or of CO_2 and other GHGE by commercial and industrial processes.

Under cap and trade, which has been instituted by the European Union, northeast US states, and the State of California, a ceiling for CO_2 emissions is established and then reduced over time. Carbon "credits" are allocated or auctioned that can be used to purchase the right to emit CO_2 up to the value of the credits or can be traded among companies with different CO_2 emissions needs. The purchase of offsets that reduce or sequester CO_2 emissions (e.g., tree planting, methane digesters) provides another mechanism for emitting industries to attain their CO_2 emissions allocations (California Air Resources Board 2015).

Supporters of cap and trade maintain that the establishment of a defined cap on emissions leads to a certain reduction in emissions over time, with associated reductions in harmful air pollutants. However, the trading and offset mechanism in cap-and-trade schemes allows continued high levels of emissions in communities already highly affected by air pollution from refineries and other carbon-intensive industries. Thus, many environmental justice advocates have opposed cap and trade because of concerns that it may perpetuate existing pollution inequities (California Environmental Justice Movement 2008). Offset projects, such as methane digesters or tree planting, could have health benefits in the communities in which they are implemented (Richardson, English, and Rudolph 2012).

All market mechanisms intentionally increase the price of carbon. Economists estimate, for example, that a 10 percent rise in prices will reduce gas consumption by 7 percent, through consumers shifting to cars with better mileage and driving less (Krugman 2008). The overall health effects of rising carbon prices will depend on the impacts on copollutants and, potentially more significant, how tax or auction revenues are allocated (Dinan 2013). Price increases will have the greatest impact on people with low-incomes, potentially increasing fuel poverty or limiting available dollars for food (Richardson, English, and Rudolph 2012). A study by the Organization of Economic Cooperation and Development suggests that a carbon tax that reduces carbon emissions by 5 percent annually in China would reduce local health losses by 0.2 percent of GDPH annually (Garbaccio, Ho, and Jorgenson 2000).

CLINICAL CORRELATES 18.3 BEHAVIOR CHANGES TO COMBAT CHILDHOOD OBESITY AND CLIMATE CHANGE

Childhood obesity is a rising problem in United States and in developed countries worldwide. In 2012, more than one-third of children and adolescents in the United States were obese (http://www.cdc.gov/healthyyouth/obesity/facts.htm), which raises the concern that these children will early in their adult lives develop the negative comorbidities associated with obesity, such as heart disease and diabetes. On a basic level, weight gain occurs when energy expenditure is less than energy consumption. Recent studies have shown that physical activity, or the lack thereof, plays a major role in determining weight gain among children (Anderson and Butcher 2006). Modeling and practicing healthy living choices, such as physical activity, are essential during childhood development, when strong behavioral habits are formed. In addition, modeling physical activity as an alternative means of transportation has benefits in terms of preparing the future generation to become energy conscious. Pediatric practitioners can help by educating and encouraging parents to model exercise as a form of enjoyment and a means of alternative transportation.

Teaching the next generation to understand that our health and the environment are linked and that we all have a role in taking care of the environment should be part of pediatric well-child care.

Women's Rights, Population Growth, and Consumption

The relationship between environment, climate change, and population is complex, mediated by development practices, institutions and social organization (United Nations Population Fund 2012).

Several recent papers present evidence that stabilization of population growth is simultaneously a significant climate mitigation strategy, a core element in climate adaptation, and one of the most effective strategies to advance global health equity, gender equality, and human development (Howat and Stoneham 2011; Stott 2010; Stephenson, Newman, and Mayhew 2010; Mutunga and Hardee 2010). Empowering women, improving their social conditions, and ensuring reliable access to safe reproductive health services would serve to reduce poverty, hasten population stabilization, and curb overall population pressure on environmental resources (United Nations Population Fund 2012).

Climate Impacts

The UN projects world population will grow from today's nearly 7 billion to 8 to 10.5 billion by 2050 (Food and Agriculture Organization of the United Nations n.d.). Population control will have only limited impact on short- to medium-term GHGE, because population growth now is due to previous high-fertility cohorts, but it can contribute significantly to long-term GHGE reduction (Kippen, McCalman, and Wiseman 2010). It has been suggested that slowing population growth could provide 16 to 29 percent of the emissions reductions suggested to be necessary by 2050 to avoid dangerous climate change and that stabilizing the climate may be impossible without slowing population growth (O'Neill et al. 2012; Martin 2011). Voluntary family planning, a natural outgrowth of women's empowerment and education, mitigates 100 percent of GHGE for each person whose unwanted conception is averted, as well as that of their nonexistent descendants. It is less costly than many technologically driven mitigations such as low carbon fuel or carbon capture strategies and is cost-competitive with forest conservation and improvements in agricultural practices (Martin 2011; Wheeler 2010). More important, it provides a human-based dimension to climate solutions that can also address fundamental issues of gender, social, and income inequality.

While no person is carbon neutral, economic consumption drives GHGE more than population growth in and of itself. Historically, CO_2 emissions from energy use have grown proportionately to changes in population size, but with industrialization, developed nations with low or negative fertility rates have been responsible for the bulk of GHGE. Cumulative GHGE to date are largely the responsibility of wealthy nations; per capita GHGE in the United States remains about four times that of China, ten times that of India, and more than twenty times that of sub-Saharan Africa. The future interplay between population, development, economic growth, and consumption will drive future GHGE. Interventions to promote education, alleviate poverty, and stabilize population are essential. There is also a need to reduce per capita emissions as economies grow; but it is critically important that the issues of global equity be addressed, potentially through the "contraction and convergence" mechanism that would lead toward a declining but equitable global per capita share of GHGE (Rao and Samarth 2010; Stott 2010; Stephenson, Newman, and Mayhew 2010; Global Commons Institute 1996).

Health Impacts

Projected population growth is concentrated in poor, urban, and coastal populations that are highly vulnerable to climate change, with women being most susceptible to the negative impacts. Rapid population growth will stunt development and perpetuates poverty, increasing climate vulnerability. Slowed population growth will reduce the number of future victims of climate change and reduce the scale of many other environmental problems that adversely impact health, including deforestation, freshwater shortage, food shortages and fisheries loss, land scarcity, waste production, traffic congestion, lack of affordable housing, unemployment, and related mass migration, urbanization, and unemployment (Martin 2011). Policies that slow population, such as educational and economic opportunities for women and access to reproductive health and family planning, can simultaneously reduce poverty, empower women, improve maternal and child health outcomes, and reduce climate vulnerability (Stephenson, Newman, and Mayhew 2010; Blomstrom, Cunningham, Johnson, and Owen 2009).

Dramatic reductions in GHGE in industrialized nations, coupled with increases to an agreed level consistent with poverty reduction, provide a route to sustainable, equitable human development (Stephenson, Newman, and Mayhew 2010; Stott 2010; Rao and Samarth 2010). Substantial declines in consumption in the industrialized world are unlikely to have a significant impact on well-being and could lead to reduced long-term carbon intensity in developing nations (Cohen and Vandenbergh 2008).

Carbon Capture and Geoengineering

Carbon capture and storage (CCS) refers to emerging technologies that capture CO_2 from coal- or gas-burning power plants and other large industrial sources before it reaches the atmosphere, and then transporting it for injection into deep underground geological formation for storage, presumably forever. The US EPA has proposed GHGE standards for new electric generating–units that coal-fired plants could not meet without CCS, but the feasibility of commercial CCS has not been fully demonstrated (Fogarty and McCally 2010; Haszelidine 2009; McCarthy 2013; World Resources Institute n.d.; International Energy Agency 2013c).

There are few studies on the health risks or environmental consequences of CCS. The ability to store large quantities of CO_2 permanently without leakage or unintentional release remains unclear. such release could lead to concentrations of CO_2 capable of causing asphyxiation; lower levels of leakage could offset GHGE benefits of CCS. CO_2 could also increase drinking water contamination through increased leaching of contaminants due to acidification (Fogarty and McCally 2010). CCS impacts on air pollutant emissions are likely to depend on specific technologies employed and the magnitude of the "energy penalty" of CCS; increases in NO_x, NH_3, and PM are likely, while SO_2 emissions will decrease. Life cycle assessment of CCS suggests significant additional indirect emissions from increases in fuel extraction, production, and transportation; if CO_2 is stored in the ocean, acidification could affect marine ecosystems (Tzanidakis et al 2013; van Harmelen et al. 2011; Metz et al. 2005).

Geoengineering has been proposed in the face of little progress in reducing GHGE. There is wide range of proposed geoengineering techniques, large-scale interventions to counteract climate through solar radiation management (SRM), which aims to reflect some of the sun's energy back into space, and carbon dioxide removal. SRM approaches include the use of space reflectors (e.g., large mirrors) or stratospheric aerosols (e.g., sulfur dioxide) to enhance earth's albedo. CDR techniques remove CO_2 from the atmosphere, including global-scale tree planting, biochar, use of large machines to suck CO_2 from the air, ocean fertilization to increase plankton production (e.g., using iron filings), or ocean alkalinity enhancement through addition of crushed rocks (e.g., limestone) (Oxford Geoengineering Program 2015).

The risks of geoengineering are unknown, and their deployment is controversial, but as GHGE continue apace, the push for more research and trial deployment of geoengineering strategies increases. Injecting SO_2 into the atmosphere would lower global temperatures (similar to cooling after volcanic eruptions such as Mt. Pinatubo), but it would not halt ocean acidification, would threaten the ozone layer, could alter monsoon cycles and global rainfall patterns, and, if such a program were to be disrupted, could lead to catastrophic rapid warming. Ocean iron fertilization would interfere with marine ecosystems and affect cloud formation. Some fear that discussion of geoengineering solutions may diminish efforts to achieve serious GHGE reductions. The costs and risks are high, but no mechanism is yet in place for regulating geoengineering (Bellamy et al. 2012; Specter 2012; "Hidden Dangers of Geoengineering" 2008; Hamilton 2013; Irfan 2013; Cressey 2013; Oxford Geoengineering Program 2015).

Conclusion

Urgent implementation of robust climate change mitigation strategies is required to avert climate scenarios with devastating global health impacts that would overwhelm our adaptation and response capacities. Many climate change mitigation strategies offer remarkable opportunities to simultaneously improve population health. Some climate mitigation strategies may have adverse health impacts. Judicious use of health impact assessment and life cycle analysis may identify health cobenefits and potential adverse impacts of various mitigation strategies, thus optimizing opportunities for climate mitigation actions to improve health and reduce health inequities.

Public health professionals have compelling reason and responsibility to lend their full support to efforts at all levels to reduce GHGE, with an emphasis on mitigation strategies with public health cobenefits. These strategies include:

- Land use patterns and transportation infrastructure changes that increase active transportation and reduce vehicle miles traveled

- Local sustainable food systems and agricultural practices and reduced meat consumption in developed countries

- Increased energy efficiency in appliances, buildings, and motorized vehicles

- Decarbonization of energy sources to diminish reliance on coal and other solid and fossil fuel–based household energy and electricity, through increased use of renewable energy and low carbon fuels

- Family planning and women's education and economic development to stabilize and slow population growth

- Consumption contraction and convergence to reduce per capita consumption that contributes to GHGE in wealthy nations while permitting those in poor nations to increase consumption to an established maximum, thus promoting global equity while addressing climate change.

DISCUSSION QUESTIONS

1. Discuss some of the potential trade-offs in the use of biofuels as a strategy for greenhouse gas emissions reduction.

2. What are some of the tools and strategies that might be implemented to incorporate consideration of health cobenefits in climate policy and program planning?

3. Discuss some of the equity issues associated with climate change mitigation strategies such as "smart growth" and urban greening, and how these might be addressed.

KEY TERMS

Active transport: Includes the use of nonmotorized forms of transportation, such as walking, cycling, and public transit, as almost all trips include walking or cycling.

Biofuels: Fuels produced by plant materials.

Carbon capture and storage (CCS): Refers to emerging technologies that capture carbon dioxide from coal or gas burning power plants and other large industrial sources before it reaches the atmosphere. The carbon dioxide is then injected into deep underground geological formation for storage, presumably forever.

Climate mitigation cobenefits: The indirect public health (or other) benefits associated with greenhouse gas emission reductions, independent of reductions to global warming.

Geoengineering: Deliberate, large-scale intervention in the Earth's natural systems to counteract climate change,

Urban greening: The installation of parks, forests, trees, gardens, and agriculture in urban environments.

References

Akbari, H. 2003. "Energy Saving Potentials and Air Quality Benefits of Urban Heat Island Mitigation." Berkeley, CA: Heat Island Group, Lawrence Berkeley National Laboratory.

American Lung Association. 2001. "Urban Air Pollution and Health Inequities: A Workshop Report." *Environmental Health Perspectives* 109:357–74.

American Lung Association of California. 2008. *The Road to a Cleaner Future.* Sacramento.

Anderson, P.M., and K.F. Butcher. 2006. "Childhood Obesity: Trends and Potential Cause." *The Future of Children* 16(1):19–45.

"Architecture 2030. A Historic Opportunity." 2011. http://architecture2030.org/the_solution/buildings_solution_how

Ashworth, K., O. Wild, and C. Hewitt. 2013. "Impacts of Biofuel Cultivation on Mortality and Crop Yields." *Nature Climate Change* 3:492–96.

Aston, L. M., J. N. Smith, and J. W. Powles. 2012. "Impact of a Reduced Red and Processed Meat Dietary Pattern on Disease Risks and Greenhouse Gas Emissions in the UK: A Modelling Study." *BMJ Open* 2:e001072.

Babisch, W. 2008. "Road Traffic Noise and Cardiovascular Risk." *Noise and Health* 10(38):27–33.

Bellamy, R., J. Chilvers, N. Vaughan, and T. Lenton. 2012. "A Review of Climate Geoengineering Appraisals." *Wiley Interdisciplinary Reviews: Climate Change* 3(6):597–615.

Bellefleur, O., and F. Gagnon. 2011. *Urban Traffic Calming and Health: A Literature Review.* Quebec: National Collaborating Centre for Healthy Public Policy.

Bellows, A. C., K. Brown, and J. Smit. 2003. "Health Benefits of Urban Agriculture: Public Health and Food Security." Community Food Security Coalition. http://www.foodsecurity.org/UAHealthFactsheet.pdf

Berendt, R., E. Corliss, and M. Ojalvo. 1978. "Quieting in the Home." Washington, DC: US Environmental Protection Agency, Office of Noise Abatement and Control.

Bernard, S. M., J. M. Samet, A. Grambsch, K. L. Ebi, and I. Romieu. 2001. "The Potential Impacts of Climate Variability and Change on Air Pollution-Related Health Effects in the United States." *Environmental Health Perspectives* 109(Suppl.):199–209.

Bhatia, R., and T. Rivard. 2008. *Assessment and Mitigation of Air Pollutant Health Effects from Intra-Urban Roadways: Guidance for Land Use Planning and Enviornmental Review.* San Francisco: San Francisco Department of Public Health.

Blashki, G., T. McMichael, and D. J. Karoly. 2007. "Climate Change and Primary Health C." *Australian Family Physician* 36:986–89.

Blomstrom, E., S. Cunningham, N. Johnson, and C. Owen. 2009. "Climate Change Connections: A Resource Kit on Climate, Population and Gender." United Nations Population Fund.

Boddiger, D. 2007. "Boosting Biofuel Crops Could Threaten Food Security." *Lancet* 370:923–24.

Bollen, J., B. Guay, S. Jamet, and J. Corfee-Morlot. 2009. "Cobenefits of Climate Change Mitigation Policies: Literature Review and New Results Economics Department." Working paper 693. Paris: OECD.

Bone, A., V. Murray, I. Myers, A. Dengel, and D. Crump. 2010. "Will Drivers for Home Energy Efficiency Harm Occupant Health?" *Perspectives in Public Health* 130(5):233–38.

Boyce, P., C. Hunter, and O. Howlet. 2003. *The Benefits of Daylight through Windows.* Troy, NY: Rensselaer Polytechnic University, Lighting Research Center.

Brandt, A. R. 2008. "Converting Oil Shale to Liquid Fuels: Energy Inputs and Greenhouse Gas Emissions of the Shell in Situ Conversion Process." *Environmental Science and Technology* 42:7489–95.

Burbank, C. J., J. A. Wenger, and D. Sperling. 2012. "Climate Change and Transportation: Summary of Key Information." Washington, DC: Transportation Research Board.

Burstein, J., and M. Pérez Rocha. 2007. "Mexico Pays Heavy Price for Imported Corn." *Foreign Policy in Focus.*

California Air Resources Board. 2012. "Trees and Air Quality." Sacramento: California Air Resources Board. http://www.arb.ca.gov/research/ecosys/tree-aq/tree-aq.htm

California Air Resources Board. 2015. "Cap-and-Trade Program." Sacramento: Calfornia Air Resources Board, California Environmental Protection Agency. http://www.arb.ca.gov/cc/capandtrade/capandtrade.htm

California Air Resources Board. 2004. "Recent Research Findings: Health Effects of Particulate Matter and Ozone Air Pollution." California Air Resources Board, American Lung Association of California. January.

"California Environmental Justice Movement's Declaration Against the Use of Carbon Trading Schemes to Address Climate Change." 2008. Environmental Justice Matters. http://www.ejmatters.org/declaration.html

Center for Climate and Energy Solutions. 2013a. "Coal." Arlington, VA: Center for Climate and Energy Solutions.

Center for Climate and Energy Solutions. 2013b. "Leveraging Natural Gas to Reduce Greenhouse Gas Emissions." Arlington, VA: Center for Climate and Energy Solutions.

Centers for Disease Control and Prevention. 2007. *LEED-ND and Healthy Neighborhoods: An Expert Panel Review.* Atlanta: Centers for Disease Control.

Centers for Disease Control and Prevention. 2011. *Physical Activity and Health.* http://www.cdc.gov/physicalactivity/everyone/health/

Chen, D. 2012. "Green Infrastructure in Mitigating Extreme Summer Heat." Climate Adaptation Flagship. https://wiki.csiro.au/confluence/download /attachments/442597561/Thursday+Chen_1140Th.pdf

Cohen, M. 2007. "Environmental Toxins and Health: The Health Impact of Pesticides." *Australian Family Medicine* 36(12):1002–1004.

Cohen, M. A., and M. P. Vandenbergh. 2008. *Consumption, Happiness, and Climate Change.* Washington, DC: Resources for the Future.

Committee on Economic and Environmental Impacts of Increasing Biofuels Production. 2011. *Renewable Fuel Standard: Potential Economic and Environmental Effects of U.S. Biofuel Policy.* Washington, DC: National Academy of Sciences.

Committee on Physical Activity, Health, Transportation, and Land Use, Transportation Research Board, and Institute of Medicine of the National Academies. 2005. *Does the Built Environment Influence Physical Activity?* Washington DC: Institute of Medicine, Transportation Research Board

Crane, D., and B. Prusnek. 2007. *The Role of a Low Carbon Fuel Standard in Reducing Greenhouse Gas Emissions and Protecting Our Economy.* Sacramento: Office of the Governor.

Cressey, D. 2013. "Climate Report Puts Geoengineering in the Spotlight: IPCC Statement Suggests Tinkering with the atmosphere Could Be Necessary to Meet Climate Goals." *Nature,* October 2. http://www.nature.com/news /climate-report-puts-geoengineering-in-the-spotlight-1.13871

Daley, C. A., A. Abbott, P. S. Doyle, G. A. Nader, and S. A. Larson. 2010. "A Review of Fatty Acid Profiles and Antioxidant Content in Grass-Fed and Grain-Fed Beef." *Nutrition Journal* 9:10.

Davis, A., C. Valsecchi, and M. Fergusson. 2007. *Unfit for Purpose: How Car Use Fuels Climate Change and Obesity.* London: Institute for European Environmental Policy.

de Hartog, J. J., H. Boogaard, H. Nijland, and G. Hoek. 2010. "Do the Health Benefits of Cycling Outweigh the Risks?" *Environmental Health Perspectives* 118(8):1109–16.

den Boer, L. C., and A. Schroten. 2007. *Traffic Noise Reduction in Europe: Health Effects, Social Costs and Technical and Policy Options to Reduce Road and Rail Traffic Noise.* European Federation for Transport and Environment.

Dengel, A., and M. Swainson. 2012. "Overheating in New Homes: A Review of the Evidence." NHBC Foundation.

Dewar, D., L. Harvey, and C. Vakil. 2013 . "Uranium Mining and Health." *Canadian Family Physicians* 59:469–71.

Dhondt, S., B. Kochan, C. Beckx, W. Lefebvre, A. Pirdavani, B. Degraeuwe, T. Bellemans, L. Int Panis, C. Macharis, and K. Putman. 2013. "Integrated Health Impact Assessment of Travel Behaviour: Model Exploration and Application to a Fuel Price Increase." *Environment International* 5:45–58.

Dinan, T. 2013. "Effects of a Carbon Tax on the Economy and the Environment." Washington, DC: Congressional Budget Office.

Dora, C., and M. Phillips, eds. 2000. *Transport, Environment, and Health.* World Health Organization. Regional Office for Europe.

Douglas, M. J., S. J. Watkins, D. R. Gorman, and M. Higgins. 2011. "Are Cars the New Tobacco?" *Journal of Public Health* 33:160–69.

Edwards, P., and I. Roberts. 2009. "Population Adiposity and Climate Change." *International Journal of Epidemiology* 38:1137–40.

Edwards-Jones, G. 2010. "Does Eating Local Food Reduce the Environmental Impact of Food Production and Enhance Consumer Health?" *Proceedings of the Nutrition Society* 69:582–91.

Electric Power Research Institute. 2012. "Air Quality Impacts from Natural Gas Extraction and Combustion."

English, P. K. Fitzsimmons, S. Hoshiko, T. Kim, H. G. Margolis, T. E. McKone, M. Rotkin-Ellman, G. Solomon, R. Trent, Z. Ross. 2008. "Public Health Impacts of Climate Change in California: Community Vulnerability Assessments and Adaptation Strategies." California Department of Public Health.

Epstein, P. R., J. J. Buonocore, K. Eckerle, M. Hendryx, B. M. Stout III, R. Heinberg R. W. Clapp, et al. 2011. "Full Cost Accounting for the Life Cycle of Coal." *Annals of the New York Academy of Sciences* 1219:73–98.

Erlinger, T. P., and L. J. Appel. 2003. *The Relationship between Meat Intake and Cardiovascular Disease.* Baltimore, MD: Johns Hopkins Center for a Livable Future.

Eshel, G., and P. A. Martin. 2006. "Diet, Energy, and Global Warming." *Earth Interactions* 10:1–17.

European Environmental Agency. 2008. *Success Stories within the Road Transport Sector on Reducing Greenhouse Gas Emission and Producing Ancillary Benefits.* Copenhagen: European Environmental Agency.

Expert Independent Panel on Wind Turbine Health Impacts. 2012. *Wind Turbine Health Impact Study: Report of Independent Expert Panel:* Boston: Massachusetts Departments of Health and Environmental Protection.

Farah, H., and J. Buzby. 2005. "U.S. Food Consumption Up 16 Percent since 1970." Washington, DC: Economic Research Service, US Department of Agriculture.

Farbotko, C., and W. Waitt. 2011 "Residential Air-Conditioning and Climate Change: Voices of the Vulnerable." *Health Promotion Journal of Australia* (22):S13–16.

Fargione, J., J. Hill, D. Tilman, S. Polasky, and P. Hawthorne. 2008. "Land Clearing and the Biofuel Carbon Debt." *Science* 319(5867):1235–38.

Farrell, A. 2008. "Better Biofuels before More Biofuels." *San Francisco Chronicle,* February 13.

Ferrell, C., S. Mathur, J. Meek, and M. Piven. 2012. N*eighborhood Crime and Travel Behavior: An Investigation of the Influence of Neighborhood Crime Rates on Mode Choice—Phase II.* San Jose, CA: Mineta Transportation Institute, San Jose State University.

Fiala, N. 2006. *Economic and Environmental Impact of Meat Consumption.* University of Caliornia, Irvine. http://www.imbs.uci.edu/files/docs/2006/grad_conf/06-Fiala-Pa0er.pdf

Fields, S. 2004. "The Fat of the Land: Do Agricultural Subsidies Foster Poor Health?" *Environmental Health Perspectives* 112(14):A820–30.

Fisk, W. 2000. "Better Indoor Environments and Their Relationship with Building Energy Efficiency." *Annual Review of Energy and the Environment* 25:537–66.

Fogarty, J., and M. McCally. 2010. "Health and Safety Risks of Carbon Capture and Storage." *JAMA* 303(1):67–68.

Food and Agriculture Organization. n.d. http://www.un.org/en/development/desa/publications/world-population-prospects-the-2012-revision.html

Food and Agriculture Organization. 2006. *Livestock's Long Shadow: Environmental Issues and Options.* Rome: UN Food and Agriculture Organization.

Food and Agriculture Organization. 2012. *The State of Food and Agriculture.* Rome: UN Food and Agriculture Organization.

Foster, J., A. Lowe, and S. Winkelman. 2011. "The Value of Green Infrastructure for Urban Climate Adaptation." Washington, DC: Center for Clean Air Policy.

Frank, L. 2000. " Land Use and Transportation Interaction: Implications on Public Health and Quality of Life." *Journal of Planning Education and Research* 20:6–22.

Frank, L. D., M. J. Greenwald, S. Winkelman, J. Chapman, and S. Kavage. 2010. " Carbonless Footprints: Promoting Health and Climate Stabilization through Active Transportation." *Preventive Medicine* 50(Suppl. 1):S99–105.

Friel, S. 2010. "Climate Change, Food Insecurity and Chronic Diseases: Sustainable and Healthy Policy Opportunities for Australia." *NSW Public Health Bulletin* 21:129–33.

Friel., S., A. D. Dangour, T. Garnett, K. Lock, Z. Chalabi, I. Roberts, A. Butler, C. D. Butler, et al. 2009. "Public Health Benefits of Strategies to Reduce Greenhouse-Gas Emissions: Food and Agriculture." *Lancet* 374(9706):2016–25.

Frumkin, H., J. Hess, and S. Vindigni. 2007. "Peak Petroleum and Public Health." *JAMA* 298:1688–90.

Garbaccio, R., M. S. Ho, and D. W. Jorgenson. 2000. "The Health Benefits of Controlling Carbon Emissions in China." Organisation for Economic Co-operation and Development. http://www.oecd.org/environment/cc/2053233.pdf

Garza, E. 2013. "Counting Calories: The Energy Cost of Food." Burlington: University of Vermont, Sustainable Food Systems.

Gentnera, D., G. Isaacman, D. Worton, A.W.H. Chan, T. R. Dallman, L. Davis, S. Liu, et al. 2012. "Elucidating Secondary Organic Aerosol from Diesel and Gasoline Vehicles through Detailed Characterization of Organic Carbon Emissions." *PNAS* 109(45):18318–323.

Gerber, P. J., H. Steinfeld, B. Henderson, A. Mottet, C. Opio, J. Dijkman, A. Falcucci, and G. Tempio. 2013. "Tackling Climate Change through Livestock: A Global Assessment of Emissions and Mitigation Opportunities." Rome: UN Food and Agriculture Organization. http://www.fao.org/docrep/018/i3437e/i3437e.pdf

Giles-Corti, B., S. Foster, T. Shilton, and R. Falconer. 2010. "The Cobenefits for Health of Investing in Active Transportation." *NSW Public Health Bulletin* 21(5–6):122–27.

Glantz, M. H., R. Gommes, and S. Ramasamy. 2009. *Coping with a Changing Climate: Considerations for Adaptation and Mitigation in Agriculture.* Rome: UN Food and Agriculture Organization.

Global Alliance of Clean Cookstoves. 2013. "Clean Cookstoves and Climate Change." Global Alliance of Clean Cookstoves.

Global Commons Institute. 1996. "Contraction and Convergence: Climate Justice without Vengeance." *www.gci.org.uk/Documents/ECOSOCIALIST.pdf.*

Godfray, H. C., I. R. Crute, L. Haddad, D. Lawrence, J. F. Muir, N. Nisbett, J. Petty, S. Robinson, C. Toulmin, and R. Whitely. 2010. " The Future of the Global Food System." *Philosophical Transactions of the Royal Society B* 365(1554):2769–77.

Gohlke, J. M., T. R. Woodward, D. Campbell-Lendrum, A. Prüss-üstün, S. Hales, and C. J. Portier. 2011. "Estimating the Global Public Health Implications of Electricity and Coal Consumption." *Environmental Health Perspectives* 119:821–86.

Goodwin, P. 2013. *Get Britain Cycling.* London: All Party Parliamentary Cycling Group, House of Commons.

Grabow, M.L., S. N. Spak, T. Holloway, B. Stone, A. C. Mednick, and J. A. Patz. 2012. "Air Quality and Exercise-Related Health Benefits from Reduced Car Travel in the Midwestern United States." *Environmental Health Perspectives* 120(1):66–76.

Groth, P., R. Miller, N. Nadkarni, M. Riley, and L. Shoup. 2008. "Quantifying the Greenhouse Gas Benefits of Urban Parks." San Francisco: Trust for Public Lands.

Haines, A. 2012. " Health Benefits of a Low Carbon Economy." *Public Health* 126(Suppl. 1):S33–39.

Haines, A., A. J. McMichael, K. R. Smith, I. Roberts, J. Woodcock, A. Markandya, B. G. Armstrong, et al. 2009. "Public Health Benefits of Strategies to Reduce Greenhouse-Gas Emissions: Overview and Implications for Policy Makers." *Lancet* 374:2104–14.

Hamilton, O. 2013. "Geoengineering: Our Last Hope, or a False Promise?" *New York Times*, May 26.

Haq, S. 2011. "Urban Green Spaces and an Integrative Approach to Sustainable Environment." *Journal of Environmental Protection* 2:601–608.

Haszelidine, R. S. 2009. "Carbon Capture and Storage: How Green Can Black Be?" *Science* 325(5948):1647–52.

"The Hidden Dangers of Geoengineering." 2008. *Scientific American* (November). http://www.scientificamerican.com/article/the-hidden-dangers-of-geoengineering/

Hill, L. B. 2005. *An Analysis of Diesel Air Pollution and Public Health in America.* Boston: Clean Air Task Force.

Hinrichs C. 2000. "Embeddedness and Local Food Systems: Notes on Two Types of Direct Agricultural Markets." *Journal of Rural Studies* 16(3):295–303.

Holden, J. P., and K. R. Smith. 2000. "Energy, the Environment, and Health." *Energy and the Challenge of Sustainability.* New York: United Nations Development Programme. http://belfercenter.ksg.harvard.edu/publication/2429/energy_the_environment_and_health.html

Holmberg, B., and U. Ahlborg. 1983. "Consensus Report: Mutagenicity and Carcinogenicity of Car Exhausts and Coal Combustion Emissions." *Environmental Health Perspectives* 47:1–30.

Horrigan, L., R. S. Lawrence, and P. Walker. 2002. "How Sustainable Agriculture Can Address the Environmental and Human Health Harms of Industrial Agriculture." *Environmental Health Perspectives* 110:445–56.

Hosking, J., P. Mudu, and C. Dora. 2011. *Health Cobenefits of Climate Change Mitigation—Transport Sector.* Geneva: World Health Organization.

Howarth, R. W. 2004. "Human Acceleration of the Nitrogen Cycle: Drivers, Consequences, and Steps toward Solutions." *Water Science and Technology* 49(5–6):7–13.

Howarth, R. W., S. Bringezu, M. Bekunda, L. de Fraiture, L. Maene, L. A. Martinelli, and O. E. Sala. 2009. "Executive Summary: Rapid Assessment on Biofuels and the Environment: Overview and Key Findings. In *Biofuels: Environmental Consequences and Interactions with Changing Land Use. Proceedings of the Scientific Committee on Problems of the Environment (SCOPE) International Biofuels Project Rapid Assessment*, edited by R. W. Howarth and S. Bringezu, 1–13. Gummersbach, Germany.

Howat, P., and M. Stoneham. 2011. "Why Sustainable Population Growth Is a Key to Climate Change and Public Health Equity." *Health Promotion Journal of Australia* 2:S34–38.

Howden-Chapman, P., J. Crane, R. Chapman, and G. Fougere. 2011. "Improving Health and Energy Efficiency through Community-Based Housing Interventions." *International Journal of Public Health* 56(6):583–88.

Institute of Medicine. 2011. *Climate Change, the Indoor Environment, and Health* Washington, DC: Institute of Medicine.

Intergovernmental Panel on Climate Change Working Group III. 2001. "Summary for Policymakers. Climate Change 2001: Mitigation Intergovernmental Panel on Climate Change." Geneva: IPCC.

International Energy Agency. 2013a. "Energy Poverty." International Energy Agency.

International Energy Agency. 2013b. *Energy Efficiency Market Report.* International Energy Agency.

International Energy Agency. 2013c. "Topics: Carbon Capture and Storage." International Energy Agency.

Irfan, U. 2013. "Has the Time Come to Consider Geoengineering?" *Scientific American,* July 18. https://www.scientificamerican.com/article/has-the-time-come-to-consider-geoengineering/

Jackson, R. B., B. R. Pearson, S. G. Osborn, N. R. Warner, and A. Vengosh. 2011. *Research and Policy Recommendations for Hydraulic Fracturing and Shale-Gas Extraction.* Durham, NC: Center on Global Change, Duke University.

Jacobson, M. 2007. "Effects of Ethanol (E85) versus Gasoline Vehicles on Cancer and Mortality in the United States." *Environmental Science and Technology* 41(11):4150–57.

Jacobson, M. T., W. Howarth, M. Delucchi, S. R. Scobie, J. M. Barth, M. J. Dvorak, M. Klevze, et al. 2013. "Examining the Feasibility of Converting New York State's All-Purpose Energy Infrastructure to One Using Wind, Water, and Sunlight." *Energy Policy* 57:585–601.

Jeuland, M. A., and S. K. Pattanayak. 2012. "Benefits and Costs of Improved Cookstoves: Assessing the Implications of Variability in Health, Forest and Climate Impacts." *PLoS One* 7(2):e30338.

Johnson, J.M.F., A. J. Franzluebbers, S. L. Weyers, and D. C. Reicosky. 2007. "Agricultural Opportunities to Mitigate Greenhouse Gas Emissions." *Environmental Pollution* 150:107–24.

Jones, R. 2006. "Tire Upkeep Can Boost Safety, Fuel Economy." MSNBC. May 3.

Joshi, S., J. Douglas, A. Hamberg, S. Teshale, D. Cain, and J. Early-Alberts. 2012. *Strategic Health Impact Assessment on Wind Energy Development in Oregon.* Health Impact Assessment Program, Public Health Division, Oregon Health Authority.

Joyce, A., S. Dixon, J. Comfort, and J. Hallett. 2012. "Reducing the Environmental Impact of Dietary Choice: Perspectives from a Behavioural and Social Change Approach." *Journal of Environmental and Public Health,* article 978672. doi:10.1155/2012/978672

Kaplan, R. 2001. "The Nature of the View from Home: Psychological Benefits." *Environment and Behavior* 33(4):507–42.

Kats, G., L. Alevantis, A. Berman, E., Mills and J. Perlman. 2003. *The Costs and Financial Benefits of Green Buildings.* Sacramento: California Integrated Waste Management Board, California Sustainable Building Task Force.

Kellerhals, M. 2011. "Biomass, Climate, and Health: British Columbia Government Perspective." Paper presented at the Eighth Annual Air Quality and Health Workshop. Vancouver.

Kinney, P. L. 2008. "Climate Change, Air Quality, and Human Health." *American Journal of Preventive Medicine* 35:459–67.

Kippen, R., J. McCalman, and J. Wiseman. 2010. "Climate Change and Population Policy: Towards a Just and Transformational Approach." *Journal of Public Health* 32(2):161–62.

Knowlton, K., M. Rotkin-Ellman, G. King, H. G. Margolis, D. Smith, G. Solomon, R. Trent, and P. English. 2009. "The 2006 California Heat Wave: Impacts on Hospitalizations and Emergency Department Visits." *Environmental Health Perspectives* 117(1):61–67.

Kovtas, S. R., and S. Hajat. 2008. "Heat Stress and Public Health: A Critical Review." *Annual Review of Public Health* 29:41–55.

Krewitt, W., F. Hurley, A. Trukenmuller, and R. Friedrich. 1998. "Health Risks of Energy Systems." *Risk Analysis* 18:377–83.

Krugman, P. 2008. "Price and Gasoline Demand." *New York Times*, May 9.

Krupnick, A., D. Burtraw, and A. Markandya. 2000. "The Ancillary Benefits and Costs of Climate Change Mitigation: A Conceptual Framework." In *Ancillary Benefits and Costs of Greenhouse Gas Mitigation: Proceedings of an Expert Workshop*. Paris: OECD.

Krzyzanowski, M., B. Kuna-Dibbert, and J. Schneider. 2005. *Health Effects of Transport-Related Air Pollution*. Geneva: World Health Organization.

Laquatra, J., G. Pillai, A. Singh, and G. Syal. 2008. "Green and Healthy Housing." *Journal of Architectural Engineering* 14(4):94–97

Levine, M., D. Ürge-Vorsatz, K. Blok, L. Geng, D. Harvey, S. Lang, G. Levermore, et al. 2007. "Residential and Commercial Buildings." In *Climate Change Mitigation. Contribution of Working Group III to the Fourth Assessment Report of the Intergovernmental Panel on Climate Change*, edited by B. Metz, O. R. Davidson, P. R. Bosch, R. Dave, and L. A. Meyer, 389–427. Cambridge: Cambridge University Press.

Lewis, J. M., and S. K. Pattanayak. 2012. "Who Adopts Improved Fuels and Cookstoves? A Systematic Review." *Environmental Health Perspectives* 120(5):637–45.

Lewis, S. E., J. E. Brodie, Z. T. Bainbridge, K. W. Rohde, A. M. Davis, B. L. Masters, M. Maughan, M. J. Devlin, J. F. Mueller, and B. Schaffelke. 2009. "Herbicides: A New Threat to the Great Barrier Reef." *Environmental Pollution* 157(8–9):2470–84.

Li, H.N.C., K. Chau, and S. K. Tang. 2010. "Can Surrounding Greenery Reduce Noise Annoyance at Home?" *Science of the Total Environment* 408(20):4376–84.

Lin, G. C., and M. A. Zacharek. 2012. "Climate Change and Its Impact on Allergic Rhinitis and Other Allergic Respiratory Diseases." *Current Opinion in Otolaryngology & Head and Neck Surgery* 20(3):188–93.

Lindsay, G., A. Macmillan, and A. Woodward. 2011. "Moving Urban Trips from Cars to Bicycles: Impact on Health and Emissions." *Australian and New Zealand Journal of Public Health* 35(1):54–60.

Lockwood, A. H., K. Walker-Hood, M. Rauch, and B. Gottlieb. 2009. "Coal's Assault on Human Health: A Report from Physicians for Social Responsibility." Washington, DC: Physicians for Social Responsibility.

Lottrup, L., P. Grahn, and U. K. Sigsdotter. 2013. "Workplace Greenery and Perceived Level of Stress: Benefits of Access to a Green Outdoor Environment at the Workplace." *Landscape and Urban Planning* 110:5–11.

Lutsey, N., and D. Sperling. 2008. Transportation and Greenhouse Gas Mitigation." In *Climate Action*, 191–94. United Nations Environmental Program.

MacDonald, P. 2004. *Ethanol Fuel Incentives Applied in the U.S.* Sacramento: California Energy Commission.

Mackett, R., and B. Brown. 2011. *Transport, Physical Activity and Health: Present Knowledge and the Way Ahead.* London: Centre for Transport Stuides, University College London.

Maizlish, M., M. Woodcock, S. Co, B. Ostro, A. Fanai, and D. Fairley. 2013. "Health Cobenefits and Transportation-Related Reductions in Greenhouse Gas Emissions in the San Francisco Bay Area." *American Journal of Public Health* 104(4):703–709.

Manuel, J. 2011. "Avoiding Health Pitfalls of Home Energy-Efficiency Retrofits." *Environmental Health Perspectives* 119(2):A76–9.

Markandya, A., and P. Wilkinson. 2007. "Electricity Generation and Health." *Lancet* 370(9591):979–90.

Martin, R. M. 2011. "Population and Adaptation to Climate Change: A Complementary Analysis for the UNFCCC." Ouagadougou, Burkina Faso: Conference of the Union of African Scientists.

McCarthy, J. E. 2013. "EPA Standards for Greenhouse Gas Emissions from Power Plants: Many Questions, Some Answers." Washington, DC: Congressional Research Service.

McConnell, R., K. Berhane, L. Yao, M. Jettett, F. Lurmann, F. Gilliland, N. Künzli, et al. 2006. "Traffic, Susceptibility, and Childhood Asthma." *Environmental Health Perspectives* 114:766–72.

McMichael, A. J., D. Campbell-Lendrum, C. F. Corvalän, K. L. Ebi, A. Githeko, J. D. Scheraga, and A. Woodward, eds. 2003. *Climate Change and Human Health: Risks and Responses.* Geneva: World Health Organization.

McMichael, A. J., J. W. Powles, C. D. Butler, and R. Uauy. 2007. "Food, Livestock Production, Energy, Climate Change, and Health." *Lancet* 370(9594):1253–63.

McPherson, G. 2007. "Urban Tree Planting and Greenhouse Gas Reductions." USDA Forest Service.

McPherson, E. G., J. R. Simpson, P. J. Peper, A. Crowell, and Q. Xiao. 2010. "Northern California Coast Community Tree Guide: Benefits, Costs, and Strategic Planting." General Technical Report PSW-GTR-228. Albany, CA.

Medina-Ramon, M., A. Zanobetti, D. P. Cavanagh, and J. Schwartz. 2006. "Extreme Temperatures and Mortality: Assessing Effect Modification by Personal Characteristics and Specific Cause of Death in a Multi-City Case-Only Analysis." *Environmental Health Perspectives* 114(9):1331–36.

Metz, B., O. Davidson, H. C. de Coninck, M. Loos, and L. A Meyer, eds. 2005. *Working Group III of the Intergovernmental Panel on Climate Change: Special Report on Carbon Dioxide Capture and Storage.* Cambridge: IPCC.

Michaud, D., S. Keith, K. Feder, and T. Bower. 2012. *Health Impacts and Exposure to Wind Turbine Noise: Research Design and Noise Exposure Assessment.* Health Canada.

Mutunga, C., and K. Hardee. 2010. "Population and Reproductive Health in National Adaptation Programmes of Action (NAPAs) for Climate Change in Africa." *African Journal of Reproductive Health* 14(4):127–39.

National Center for Health Statistics. 2008. " Fastats: Accidents/Unintentional Injuries." Atlanta: Centers for Disease Control and Prevention.

National Highway Traffic Safety Administration. 2012. "Corporate Average Fuel Economy Standards Passenger Cars and Light Trucks Model Years 2017–2025: Final Environmental Impact Statement Summary." http://www.nhtsa.gov/staticfiles/rulemaking/pdf/cafe/FRIA_2017–2025.pdf

National Low Carbon Fuels Project. 2013. *The Basics of Low Carbon Fuel Standards.* Davis: University of California Davis.

National Renewable Energy Laboratory. 2013. "Life Cycle Greenhouse Gas Emissions from Electricity Generation." US Department of Energy, Office of Energy Efficiency and Renewable Energy.

National Research Council. 2010. *The Hidden Cost of Energy: Unpriced Consequences of Energy Production and Use.* Washington, DC: National Academies Press.

Natural Resources Defense Council. n.d. "Biomass Energy and Cellulosic Ethanol." In *Renewable Energy for America: Harvesting the Benefits of Homegrown Renewable Energy.* Washington, DC: Natural Resources Defense Council.

O'Neill, B. C., L. Jiang, K. R. Smith, S. Pachauri, M. Dalton, and R. Fuchs. 2012. "Demographic Change and Carbon Dioxide Emissions." *Lancet* 380(9837):157–64.

O'Neill, M. S., M. Jerrett, I. Kawachi, J. I. Levy, A. J. Cohen, N. Gouveia, P. Wilkinson, T. Fletcher, L. Cifuentes, and J. Schwartz. 2003. "Health, Wealth, and Air Pollution: Advancing Theory and Methods." *Environmental Health Perspectives* 111:1861–70.

O'Rourke, D., and S. Connolly. 2003. "Just Oil? The Distribution of Environmental and Social Impacts of Oil Production and Consumption." *Annual Review of Environment and Resources* 36:193–222.

Okolo, M.I. 1986. "Bacterial Drug Resistance in Meat Animals: A Review." *International Journal of Zoonoses* 13(3):143–52.

Oliver, R. 2008. "Food and Fossil Fuels." CNN.com.

Oxford Geoengineering Program. 2015. *What Is Geoengineering?* University of Oxford. http://www.geoengineering.ox.ac.uk/what-is-geoengineering/what-is-geoengineering/

Panwar, M., A. Kurchania, and N. Rathore. 2009. "Mitigation of Greenhouse Gases by Adoption of Improved Biomass Cookstoves." *Mitigation and Adaptation Strategies for Global Change* 14(6):569–78.

Parry, M. L., J. P. Palutikof, P. J. van der Linden, C. E. Hanson, eds. 2007. "IPCC, 2007: Climate Change 2007: Impacts, Adaptation, and Vulnerability." *Contribution of Working Group II to the Third Assessment Report of the Intergovernmental Panel on Climate Change.* Cambridge: Cambridge University Press.

PATH and World Health Organization. 2012. *Harnessing Solar Energy for Health Needs: World Health Organization.* Program for Appropriate Technology in Health.

Patz, J., D. Campbell-Lendrum, H. Gibbs, and R. Woodruff. 2008. "Health Impact Assessment of Global Climate Change: Expanding on Comparative Risk Assessment Approaches for Policy Making." *Annual Review of Public Health* 29:27–39.

Patz, J., D. Campbell-Lendrum, T. Holloway, and J. Foley. 2005. "Impact of Regional Climate Change on Human Health." *Nature* 438:310–18.

Paustian, K.A.J., J. Sheehan, and E. Paul. 2006. *Agriculture's Role in Greenhouse Gas Mitigation.* Arlington, VA: Pew Center on Global Climate Change.

Pimentel, D., and M. Pimentel. 2003. "Sustainability of Meat-Based and Plant-Based Diets and the Environment." *American Journal of Clinical Nutrition* 78:6605–35.

Pirog, R., T. Van Pelt, K. Enshayan, and E. Cook. 2001. "Food, Fuel, and Freeways: An Iowa Perspective on How Far Food Travels, Fuel Usage, and Greenhouse Gas Emissions." Ames, IA: Leopold Center for Sustainable Agriculture.

PolicyLink. 2008. *Equitable Development Toolkit: Transit-Oriented Development.* Oakland, CA: PolicyLink.

Rabl, A., and A. Nazelle. 2012. "Benefits of Shift from Car to Active Transport." *Transportation Policy* 19:121–31.

Rao, M., and A. Samarth. 2010. "Population Dynamics and Climate Change: Links and Issues for Development." *Journal of Public Health* 32(2):163–64.

Reddy, S., T. Lang, and S. Dibb, S. 2009. "Setting the Table: Advice to Government on Priority Elements of Sustainable Diets." UK Sustainable Development Commission. http://www.scp-knowledge.eu/knowledge/setting-table-advice-government-priority-elements-sustainable-diets

Ribeiro, K. S., S. Kobayashi, M. Beuthe, J. Gasca, D. Greene, D. S. Lee, Y. Muromachi, et al. 2007. "Transport and Its Infrastructure." In *Climate Change 2007: Mitigation. Contribution of Working Group III to the Fourth Assessment Report of the Intergovernmental Panel on Climate Change*, edited by B. Metz, O. R. Davidson, P. R. Bosch, R. Dave, and L. A. Meyer. Cambridge: Cambridge University Press, 2007.

Richardson, M. J., P. English, and L. A. Rudolph. 2012. "Health Impact Assessment of California's Proposed Cap-and-Trade Regulations." *American Journal of Public Health* 102(9):e52–58.

Richter, E. D., T. Berman, L. Friedman, and G. Ben-David 2006. "Speed, Road Injury, and Public Health." *Annual Review of Public Health* 27:125–52.

Ridley, C. E., C. M. Clark, S. D. LeDuc,, B. G. Bierwagen, B. B. Lin, A. Mehl, and D. A. Tobias. 2012. "Biofuels: Network Analysis of the Literature Reveals Key Environmental and Economic Unknowns." *Environmental Science and Technology* 46:1309–15.

Rojas-Rueda, D., A. de Nazelle, O. Teixido, and M. J. Niewenhuijsen. 2012. "Replacing Car Trips by Increasing Bike and Public Transport in the Greater Barcelona Metropolitan Area: A Health Impact Assessment Study." *Environment International* 49:100–109.

Rulli, M. C., A. Saviori, and P. D'Odorico. 2013. "Global Land and Water Grabbing." *PNAS* 110:892–97.

Ryan, L., and N. Campbell. 2012. *Spreading the Net: The Multiple Benefits Of Energy Efficiency Improvements.* Paris: International Energy Agency/OECD.

Saelens, B. E., J. F. Sallis, and L. D. Frank 2003. "Environmental Correlates of Walking and Cycling: Findings from the Transportation, Urban Design, and Planning Literatures." *Annals of Behavioral Medicine* 25(2):80–91.

Sallis, J. F., L. D. Frank, B. E. Saelens, and M. K. Kraft. 2004. " Active Transportation and Physical Activity: Opportunities for Collaboration on Transportation and Public Health Research." *Transportation Research Part A* 38:249–68.

Saxe, H., T. Meinert Larsen, and L. Mogensen. 2013. " The Global Warming Potential of Two Healthy Nordic Diets Compared with the Average Danish Diet." *Climatic Change* 116:249–62.

Schneider, C., and J. Banks. 2010. "The Toll from Coal." Boston: Clean Air Task Force.

Schneider, M. 2002. "Do School Facilities Affect Academic Outcomes?" Washington, DC: National Clearinghouse for Educational Facilities.

Scientific Committee on Problems of the Environment. 2004. *Consequences of Industrialized Animal Production Systems.* Paris: Scientific Committee on Problems of the Environment.

Searchinger, T. 2008. "Use of U.S. Croplands for Biofuels Increases Greenhouse Gases through Emissions from Land-Use Change." *Science* 319:1238–40.

Shield, B. M., and J. E. Dockrell. 2003. "The Effects of Noise on Children at School: A Review." *Journal of Building Acoustics* 203:97–106.

Shindell, D., J. Kuylenstierna, and E. Vignati. 2012. "Simultaneously Mitigating Near-Term Climate Change and Improving Human Health and Food Security." *Science* 335:183–89.

Silicon Valley Toxics Coalition. 2009. *Toward a Just and Sustainable Solar Energy Industry.* San Jose, CA. http://svtc.org/wp-content/uploads/Silicon_Valley _Toxics_Coalition_-_Toward_a_Just_and_Sust.pdf

Singh, A., M. Syal, S. Grady, and S. Korkmaz. 2010. "Effects of Green Buildings on Employee Health and Productivity." *American Journal of Public Health* 100(9):1665–68.

Smith, K. 2013. "Smoked Out: The Health Hazards of Burning Coal." *Lancet* 381(9882):1979.

Smith, K. R., H. Frumkin, K. Balakrishnan, C. D. Butler, Z. A. Chafe, I. Fairlie, P. Kinney, et al. 2013. "Energy and Human Health." *Annual Review of Public Health* 34:159–88.

Smith, C., M. David, C. Mitchellab, M. D. Masters, K. J. Anderson-Teixeira, C. J. Bernacchi, and E. H. DeLucia. 2013. "Reduced Nitrogen Losses after Conversion of Row Crop Agriculture to Perennial Biofuel Crops." *Journal of Environmental Quality* 42(1):219–28.

Smith, K., and E. Haigler. 2008. "Cobenefits of Climate Mitigation and Health Protection in Energy Systems: Scoping Methods." *Annual Review of Public Health* 29:11–25.

Smith, P., D. Martino, Z. Cai, D. Gwary, H. Janzen, P. Kumar, B. McCarl, et al. 2008. "Greenhouse Gas Mitigation in Agriculture." *Philosophical Transactions of the Royal Society B* 363:789–813.

Smith, P., D. Martino, Z. Cai, D. Gwary, H. Janzen, P. Kumar, B. McCarl, et al. 2007. "Agriculture." In *Climate Change 2007: Mitigation. Contribution of Working Group III to the Fourth Assessment Report of the, Intergovernmental Panel on Climate Change*, edited by B. Metz, O. R. Davidson, P. R. Bosch, R. Dave, and L. A. Meyer, 499–532. Cambridge: Cambridge University Press.

Specter, M. 2012. "The Climate Fixers." *New Yorker*, May 14.

Stephenson, J., K. Newman, and S. Mayhew. 2010. "Population Dynamics and Climate Change: What Are the Links?" *Journal of Public Health* 32(2):150–56.

Stewart, A., and M. Cromey. 2012. "Biofuels: The Need for Disease Risk Management." *Biofuels* 3(1):1–3.

Stott, R. 2010. "Population and Climate Change: Moving toward Gender Equality Is the Key." *Journal of Public Health* 32(2):159–60.

Swanson, K. 2012. *Bicycling and Walking in the United States: 2012 Benchmarking Report*. Washington, DC: Alliance for Biking and Walking.

Tait, P. W. 2011. "Active Transport and Heat." *Asia Pacific Journal of Public Health* 23:634–35.

Tilman, D., J. Fargione, B. Wolff, C. D'Antonio, A. Dobson, R. Howarth, D. Schindler, W. H. Schlesinger, D. Simberloff, and D. Swackhamer. 2001. "Forecasting Agriculturally Driven Global Environmental Change." *Science* 292:281–84.

Tilman, D., R. Socolow, J. Foley, J. Hill, E. Larson, L. Lynd, S. Pacala, et al. 2009. "Beneficial Biofuels: The Food, Energy, and Environment Trilemma." *Science* 325:270–71.

Tzanidakis, K., T. Oxley, T. Cockerill, and H. ApSimon. 2013. "Illustrative National Scale Scenarios of Environmental and Human Health Impacts of Carbon Capture and Storage." *Environment International* 56:48–64.

UN Environmental Programme. 2009. "Buildings and Climate Change: Summary for Decision-Makers."

UN Population Fund. 2012. UNFPA Population matters for Sustainable Development. http://www.unfpa.org

US Department of Energy. 2011. *Buildings Energy Data Book: Buildings Share of U.S. Primary Energy Consumption*. Washington, DC: US Department of Energy.

US Department of Health and Human Services. 2002. *Physical Activity Fundamental to Preventing Disease*. Washngton, DC: US Department of Health and Human Services.

US Energy Information Administration. 2013a. "Electricity Explained: Electricity in the United States." Washington, DC: US Energy Information Administration.

US Energy Information Administration. 2013b. "Frequently Asked Questions: How Much CO2 Is Produced per Kilowatt Hour When Generating Electricity with Fossil Fuels?" Washingon, DC: US Energy Information Administration.

USEPA Natural Gas. n.d. http://www.epa.gov/cleanenergy/energy-and-you/affect /natural-gas.html

US Environmental Protection Agency. 2001. *Healthy Buildings, Healthy People: A Vision for the 21st Century.* Washington, DC: US EPA.

US Environmental Protection Agency. 2010a. *EPA Analysis of the Transportation Sector.* Washington, DC: US EPA.

US Environmental Protection Agency. 2010b. "Methane and Nitrous Oxide Emissions from Natural Sources." Washington, DC: US EPA.

US Environmental Protection Agency. 2012a. "Green Building: Home Selection/ Site Selection." Washington, DC: US EPA.

US Environmental Protection Agency. 2012b. "IAQ Tools for Schools." Washington, DC: US EPA.

US Environmental Protection Agency. 2013. "Overview of Greenhouse Gases: Nitrous Oxide Emissions." Washington DC: US EPA. http://epa.gov/climate -change/ghgemissions/gases/n2o.html.

US Environmental Protection Agency Assessment and Standards Division Office of Transportation and Air Quality. 2012. *2017 and Later Model Year Light-Duty Vehicle Greenhouse Gas Emissions and Corporate Average Fuel Economy Standards: EPA Response to Comments.* Washington, DC: US Environmental Protection Agency.

US Green Building Council. 2008. "Why Build Green?" US Green Building Council.

Ulrich, R. S. 1984. "View Through a Window May Influence Recovery from Surgery." *Science* 224(4647):420–21.

van Harmelen, T., A. van Horssen, M . Jozwicka, T. Pulles, and N. Odeh. 2011. "Air Pollution Impacts from Carbon Capture and Storage (CCS)." Copenhagen: European Environment Agency.

Vlasic, B. 2012. "U.S. Sets Higher Fuel Efficiency Standards." *New York Times,* August 28.

Walker, P., P. Rhubart-Berg, S. McKenzie, K. Kelling, and R. S. Lawrence. 2005. "Public Health Implications of Meat Production and Consumption." *Public Health Nutrition* 8:348–56.

Warburton, D.E.R., C. W. Nicol, and S. D. Bredin. 2006. "Health Benefits of Physical Activity: The Evidence." *Canadian Medical Association Journal 174*:801–809.

Warner, E., D. Inman, B. Kunstman, B. Bush, L. Vimmerstedt, S. Peterson, J. Macknick, and Y. Zhang. 2013. "Modeling Biofuel Expansion Effects on Land Use Change Dynamics." *Environmental Research Letters* 8:015003. http:// iopscience.iop.org/1748–9326/8/1/015003/pdf/1748–9326_8_1_015003.pdf

Wheeler, D. 2010. *The Economics of Population Policy for Carbon Emissions Reduction in Developing Countries.* Washington, DC: Center for Global Development.

Wilbers, P. 2006. "What Is Ecodriving?" http://www.ecodrive.org/What-is-ecodriving.228.0.html

Wilkinson, P., K. R. Smith, M. Davies, H. Adair, B. G. Armstrong, M. Barrett, N. Bruce, et al. 2009. "Public Health Benefits of Strategies to Reduce Greenhouse-Gas Emissions: Household Energy." *Lancet* 374(9705):1917–29.

Wilson, J., and A. Katz. 2010. "Integrating Energy Efficiency and Healthy Housing." Briefing paper for the National Healthy Housing Policy Summit. Washington, DC: National Safe and Healthy Housing Coalition.

Wolcha, J. R., J. Bynreb, and J. P. Newell. 2014. "Urban Green Space, Public Health, and Environmental Justice: The Challenge of Making Cities 'Just Green Enough.'" *Landscape and Urban Planning* 125:234–44.

Wong, E. 2008. "Trees and Vegetation." In *Reducing Urban Heat Islands: Compendium of Strategies.* Washington, DC: US Environmental Protection Agency, Climate Protection Partnership Division, Office of Atmospheric Programs.

Woodcock, J., D. B. Banister, P. Edwards, A. M. Prentice, and I. Roberts. 2007. "Energy and Transport." *Lancet* 370:1078–88.

Woodcock, J. 2007. " Energy and Transport: Londoners' Physical Activity." *Lancet,* September 13. http://www.thelancet.com/cms/attachment/2000990379/2003649828/mmc3.pdf

Woodcock, J., P. Edwards, C. Tonne, B. G. Armstrong, O. Ashiru, D. Banister, S. Beevers, et al. 2009. "Public Health Benefits of Strategies to Reduce Greenhouse-Gas Emissions: Urban Land Transport." *Lancet* 374:1930–43.

Woodcock, J., M. Givoni, and A. S. Morgan. 2013. "Health Impact Modelling of Active Travel Visions for England and Wales Using an Integrated Transport and Health Impact Modelling Tool (ITHIM)." *PLoS One* 8(1).

World Health Organization. 2012. *Health Indicators of Sustainable Energy.*

World Health Organization Regional Office for Europe. n.d. *Noise and Health.* http://www.euro.who.int/Noise

World Resources Institute. n.d. "Carbon Dioxide Capture and Storage." World Resources Institute. http://www.wri.org/our-work/project/carbon-dioxide-capture-and-storage-ccs.

Wright, C. K., and M. C. Wimberly. 2013. "Recent Land Use Change in the Western Corn Belt Threatens Grasslands and Wetlands." *PNAS* 110(10):4134–39.

Yang, J., Q. Yu, and P. Gong. 2008. "Quantifying Air Pollution Removal by Green Roofs in Chicago." *Atmospheric Environment* 42(31):7266–73.

Yeh, S., J. Witcover, and J. Kessler. 2013. *Status Review of California's Low Carbon Fuel Standard—Spring,* Rev. ed. Davis: Institute of Transportation Studies, University of California, Davis.

CHAPTER 19

MITIGATION

International Institutions and Global Governance

Farah Faisal, Perry Sheffield

Acknowledgment of the severe public health impacts from climate change is gaining traction in the US government, governments worldwide, and in international institutions. Growing interaction between public health and environmental officials, scholars, and experts will help to expand our knowledge of this interaction, and reframe the issue for a more robust global response.

Climate change is an urgent threat to human health and well-being. Climate experts estimate a rise in temperature of as high as 4°degrees Celsius by 2100 if the global response to climate change remains at current levels (World Bank Group 2015). The consequences for global public health range from a rise in infectious disease and respiratory illness to reduced food and water security to large-scale migration and civil unrest ("Health and Climate Change" 2015), factors that can lead to exponential increases in human morbidity and premature fatality. But who has the authority to control the climate? And why have public health concerns not factored into major policy debates? These questions require significant international cooperation to even begin to answer.

The various efforts by countries, intergovernmental institutions, and nongovernmental actors contribute to the global regime for climate change. This chapter introduces some of the important players in these efforts and describe some of their actions. In broad strokes, the global governance architecture for climate change aims to reduce greenhouse gas emissions to a level that would prevent excessive disruption of the world's climate—referred to as *mitigation*—and to reduce the impact of climate variability

KEY CONCEPTS

- **Climate change is an urgent threat to human health. Global health gains achieved over the past decades could be reversed as a result of the direct and indirect impacts of climate change.**

- **Climate change governance is the combined efforts of countries, intergovernmental groups, and nongovernmental actors to prevent human contribution to climate change and reduce the impact of climate variability on humans and the environment.**

- **The global governance architecture for climate change and public health is stovepiped and fragmented. The climate change regime has focused on economic consequences, with insufficient attention to multifaceted social, environmental, and development implications, including those on human health.**

on livelihoods, the environment, and human health—known as *adaptation.* In terms of health, there are two main ways that climate change governance is important. The first is through the mitigation efforts, where reducing greenhouse gas emissions can have both immediate health benefits and long-term health benefits from reduced climate variability and exposure to pollutants. The second is through adaptation efforts where, through better preparedness, human health can be protected from the dire effects of climate change.

This chapter gives an overview of the predominant climate change governance institutions and instruments while highlighting the nexus with global public health governance (WHO 2012a).

The Climate Threat for Human Health

Human development and public health have benefited from resounding gains over the past decades as a result of increased funding and a proliferation of actors and programs dedicated to reduce the levels of poverty and disease worldwide. Alarmingly, however, many of these gains could be reversed because of the potentially catastrophic effects of climate change (UNDP 2013). In particular, the existing and potential effects are most stark in developing countries, coastal regions, and drylands, where either the climate is already harsh or countries do not have the financial or technical means to protect their populations from an altering climate. Increasingly, however, industrialized countries are also wrestling with a weak response to climate change, as can be witnessed by the effects of recent hurricanes, floods, heat waves, and droughts.

The implications on human health are indeed severe and wide ranging, as described in earlier chapters of this text. A hugely complicating ethical element in global climate change governance is that many states that have contributed the most to rising greenhouse gas emissions are not expected to experience the greatest human health impacts.

CLINICAL CORRELATES 19.1 CALL TO ACTION ON GLOBAL WARMING

The response to climate change among the US health care community has been as fragmented as the international response. One physician action group, Physicians for Social Responsibility, has taken a strong stance to address and meaningfully mitigate the situation. They call for dramatic reductions in greenhouse gas emissions and place responsibility on the United States, which, they recognize as a major contributor to global warming (Physicians for Social Responsibility 2014). More concerted efforts are needed on behalf of health care providers, who are likely to serve on the front lines to care for those patients affected by climate change.

Fragmented approaches to climate change also occur among the US health care community. Stronger organization is needed to multiply efforts to educate the profession and to mount mitigation and adaptation efforts.

Climate Change Governance

Efforts to build a meaningful regime to tackle climate change began in 1992 with the eventual adoption of the **United Nations Framework Convention on Climate Change (UNFCCC)** and the **Kyoto Protocol**. These two agreements are the centerpiece of today's climate change regime, but they are woefully inadequate in both reducing greenhouse gas emissions and addressing the multifaceted impacts of climate change, including those on human health.

The objective of the UNFCCC is to limit man-made (or "anthropogenic") greenhouse gas emissions to levels that "would prevent dangerous anthropogenic interference with the climate system." To achieve this objective, the UNFCCC encourages industrialized countries to take measures to stabilize emissions, and introduces the concept of common but differentiated responsibilities (CBDR) as the guiding principle to attain emission-reduction goals. In essence, CBDR places responsibility of emissions reduction on industrialized countries based on historical levels of industrial activity, in theory applying concepts of distributive justice to climate action. Since its introduction, CBDR has become a divisive and politically contentious topic between industrialized countries and the Global South. Rich industrialized countries say the concept is outdated and call for more rigorous measures for developing countries, particularly major emitters such as China and India; at the same time, developing countries continue to place the responsibility for emission reduction on the industrialized North based on past levels of activity that have enabled the conditions for present-day climate change.

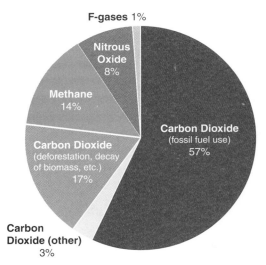

Figure 19.1   Greenhouse Emissions by Gas

Note: F-gases = fluorinated gases.

In 1997, the international community came together for a second time to establish a new climate treaty with stronger enforcement stipulations. The new treaty, known as the Kyoto Protocol, again prioritized a CBDR approach, and this time placed mandatory obligations that "commits" industrialized countries to stabilize seven greenhouse gases: carbon dioxide (CO_2), methane (CH_4), nitrous oxide (N_2O), hydrofluorocarbons (HFC), perfluorocarbons (PFC), sulphur hexafluoride, and nitrogen triflouride (NF_3)(UNFCCC 2012). Carbon dioxide is the predominant gas in terms of proportion of emissions (see figure 19.1) but other gases play important roles based on their potency and other human and environmental health impacts.

The target reduction set by the Kyoto Protocol was a global reduction of 5 percent of greenhouse gas emissions, measured against 1990 levels, for the first commitment period, 2008–2012. (The protocol came into force in 2005 when the requisite number of countries ratified it.) The second commitment period (2013–2020), commits parties to reduce emissions by at least 18 percent below 1990 levels (UNFCCC 2014a).

As it exists, the Kyoto Protocol relies on countries to pursue domestic policies to reach their emissions goals based on internationally agreed-on targets (a top-down approach). In addition, it offers three market mechanisms: emissions trading, clean development mechanism (CDM), and joint implementation (JI), to help achieve emission reduction goals.

*   *Emissions trading (carbon markets):* A central authority assigns caps on emissions across industries. The same authority awards emission

permits (or carbon units), which are distributed to firms. These firms can sell unused permits in an open market to firms that are over their emissions cap. The European Union's Emission Trading Scheme (EU ETS) is the largest carbon trading model. In this case, the EU sets a cap for specific industries and awards permits accordingly.

- *Clean development mechanism (CDM):* Industrialized countries with emission reduction targets under the Kyoto Protocol can invest in an emission-reduction project in a developing country. This in turn, generates a credit (a certified emission reduction or CER) that can be applied to meeting the industrialized country's own emission reduction targets.

- *Joint implementation:* Industrialized countries with emission reduction targets under the Kyoto Protocol can assist other industrialized countries with emission reduction projects. Similar to the CDM scheme, countries leading the project can earn credits (emission reduction units, ERU) that are counted towards their own targets.

At the time of writing this chapter, the UNFCCC has 194 (plus the European Union) state parties and the Kyoto Protocol has 191 state parties (plus the European Union) (UNFCCC 2014b, 2014c). The second period, however, has seen dwindling support from key member states, with Canada withdrawing all together from the protocol, and Russia, New Zealand, and Japan not taking part in this commitment. For its part, the United States never ratified the Kyoto Protocol. The main issues for the United States are the lack of demands on developing countries to reduce their greenhouse gas emissions and the potential harm to the US economy from an international agreement restricting GHG emissions (US Senate Committee on Foreign Relations 1997).

Today, one of the main objectives of international climate negotiations is to create a new framework to replace the Kyoto Protocol once it expires in 2020 with one that would include all major emitters, including the United States and emerging economies.

UNFCCC and Health

Overall, the UNFCCC pays insufficient attention to health. The UNFCC mentions public health indirectly by calling on parties to "take climate change considerations into account . . . with a view to minimizing adverse effects . . . on public health and on the quality of the environment, of projects or measures undertaken by them to mitigate or adapt to climate change" (UNFCCC 1992). However, this vague reference to adverse health impacts does not provide a foundation for policy formulation at the domestic level

(Onzivu 2010). For its part, the Kyoto Protocol makes no mention of public health impacts.

On an operational level, the UNFCCC process—through conferences, funding instruments, and publications—has recognized the interlinkage between health and climate change, albeit the attention is still tangential. For instance, public health has increasingly gained a platform at UNFCCC annual conferences. Twelve health-related side events were organized for the UNFCCC conference in Doha, including a high-level meeting on health adaptation framework in Africa featuring Lord Nicholas Stern, adviser to the UK government on the economics of climate change and author of major report on the economic impact of climate change (Stern 2011; figure 19.2). The Adaptation Fund, a financing vehicle established by the UNFCCC (2014d), invests in flood management and agricultural sector resilience projects (Adaptation Fund 2014a)—elements indirectly related to human health. However, available funding as of August 2012 was approximately $115 million, far short of what is needed globally (Adaptation Fund 2014). The UNFCCC also requires parties to share scientific and technological knowledge that can positively affect human health conditions. Yet even here, the sharing of best practices is on an ad hoc basis, and does not necessarily involve public health solutions.

Figure 19.2   The 2012 UNFCCC Gathering in Doha

Source: http://www.theguardian.com/environment/2012/nov/26/doha-2012-us-carbon-emissions.

At the heart of the problem are the mismatched goals of an international climate regime focused on mitigation and the public health impacts, which are largely related to adaptation. Developing countries—those bearing the brunt of the ills from climate change—are poorly equipped with adaptive response capacities and have limited influence on emission reduction policies of the industrialized North. Helping to raise the concerns of poor nations requires a more concerted integration of the public health domain in climate circles. While this is slowly occurring, it remains an uphill challenge as global health activism and climate activism are two very distinct disciplines with tailored governance solutions, specific lexicons, and unique histories. This divide is evident in the UNFCCC process, a framework centered on environmental policymakers with little space for public health officials to influence or reframe the climate challenge as a public health concern that would allow them to raise awareness of the immediate health benefits from reduced emissions (Inter Academy Medical Panel 2010), as well as the urgency for action for vulnerable populations.

Beyond the UNFCCC Process

In addition to the UNFCCC and Kyoto Protocol, a fragmented but engaged climate regime that includes international institutions, countries, and civil society have rallied to form a range of initiatives at the multilateral, regional, and local levels to either extend and improve the existing instruments, or to test new approaches for effective cooperation. Below is a discussion of several other institutions and coalitions.

The IPCC

The **Intergovernmental Panel on Climate Change (IPCC)** predates the UNFCCC by four years. Established in 1988 by the World Meteorological Organization (WMO) and the United Nations Environment Program (UNEP), the IPCC consists of a group of over twenty-five hundred international voluntary scientists who assemble periodic "Assessment Reports" that summarize the state of the science on climate change, impacts, and policy response strategies. These reports are reviewed by representatives of the member states of the UN who ultimately accept or reject them. The first assessment produced in 1990 played a pivotal role in the establishment of the UNFCCC two years later and, in 2007, the fourth assessment report was jointly awarded the Nobel Peace Prize with Al Gore.

In addition to the assessment reports, the IPCC has produced several special reports on various topics. Human health has taken an increasingly prominent role in the assessment reports, starting as a portion of a chapter on human impacts, and as of the third assessment report representing a stand-alone chapter with over three hundred references. The fourth assessment report also included a stand-alone chapter with over five hundred references (Parry et al. 2007). This change is likely reflective of both an increasing international awareness and a concomitant growth in the body of publications focusing on climate and health impacts. Overall, the IPCC contends that the impact of climate change will be particularly dire in developing countries, especially in the tropics and subtropics. However, the extent of global impact more generally is difficult to quantify as it is interrelated with other factors, including "migration, provision of clean urban environments, improved nutrition, increased availability of potable water, improvements in sanitation, the extent of disease vector-control measures, changes in resistance of vector organisms to insecticides, and more widespread availability of health care" (Watson, Zinyowera, and Moss 1997).

Other UN Bodies

A number of UN agencies are involved directly or indirectly in climate change work. This section offers two diverse examples: the Food and Agriculture Organization (FAO) and the World Meteorological Organization (WMO). The United Nations Environment Programme (UNEP) and the United Nations Development Programme (UNDP) are two other significant players.

Food and Agriculture Organization

The Food and Agriculture Organization is a specialized agency of the United Nations that works to achieve food security for all. This organization focuses not only on agriculture but also forestry and fishery practices. While not explicitly framing their work in terms of health, the FAO's central mission around ending hunger globally is implicitly a public health mandate. Its climate change initiative, Climate-Smart Agriculture, has a two-prong approach: reducing global greenhouse gas emissions from agriculture, a contribution to mitigation efforts, and improving food practice productivity and resilience in the face of climate change, an adaptation effort.

The FAO's role with the UNFCCC is one of advocacy and support around both mitigation and adaptation actions. The specific activities have included workshops, written submissions, and action pledges (Food and Agriculture Organization 2010, 2015a, 2015b).

World Meteorological Organization

The World Meteorological Organization is also a specialized agency of the United Nations but with a focus on meteorology which includes climate change (World Meteorological Organization n.d.; Matthies et al. 2008). The WMO in collaboration with the United Nations Environment Program created the Intergovernmental Panel on Climate Change, which through its periodic assessment reports, summarizes the state of the art research on climate science and impacts, including health. The fifth such assessment report was completed in 2014. Other efforts to date related specifically to health have been copublication with the World Health Organization of the *Atlas on Health and Climate* (World Health Organization 2012b), collaborations on the development of climate forecasts for use in early warning systems such as those used to predict malaria outbreaks, and issuing guidance on the development of heat-health action plans for municipalities to use during extreme heat events.

Regional and Plurilateral Organizations

In addition to the UN bodies, there are numerous important groups at the regional and plurilateral level. Brief descriptions of the European Union, Arctic Council, the Group of Eight, the Group of Twenty, and the Major Economies Forum are included here.

Other groups, like Asia-Pacific Economic Cooperation (APEC) (Asia-Pacific Economic Cooperation n.d.), Organization for Economic Cooperation and Development (OECD) (Organisation for Economic Co-operation and Development n.d.) and Brazil, Russia, India, China bloc (BRIC) (Birdsall and MacDonald 2014; Huifang et al. 2009) also play a role.

European Union

The EU, a twenty-eight–member state union as of July 2013 with the addition of Croatia, originated as a six-country union in the 1950s. The EU is a legislative entity that can create regulations that override national law of the individual member states. The European Union has the most developed emissions trading of multinational organizations but even this framework is still in its relative infancy and threatened by political forces (Council on Foreign Relations 2013). The European Climate Change Program was created in 2000 to address climate mitigation by responding to the Kyoto Protocol but a more broadly focused entity, the Directorate-General for Climate Action, was created in 2010 with the objective of mitigation and adaptation following the development of an adaptation framework in 2009 (European Commission—Climate 2012; European Commission 2009). Health, specifically, however, plays only a small part in the overall adaptation planning efforts though a number of the initiatives such as changes to building codes and flood defenses that will likely also be health protective (European Commission—Climate Action 2015). Overall, the EU has embraced its role in leading international climate policy negotiations and will likely play an increasingly pivotal role in helping to broker both mitigation and adaptation treaties moving forward.

Arctic Council

The Arctic Council is an intergovernmental membership group consisting of the eight arctic states and six organizations representing Arctic Indigenous Peoples established in 1996 to promote better cooperation on issues that are common to arctic nations. To date the council has sponsored a study of climate impacts in the arctic that emphasizes the joint need for both mitigation and adaptation efforts with a particular focus on protecting sensitive and vulnerable natural and human systems ("Arctic Council" 2004). Chapin et al. (2006) propose that the Arctic Council is well-positioned to "co-manage" marine areas to "sustain resources and meet community needs." They also highlight that unlike other countries in marginal environments, the member nations of the council have sufficient resources to appropriately invest in and guide necessary development. Borgerson (2008) argues that while it exists to manage pan-arctic environmental concerns, the council does have the authority to manage the necessary security concerns around economic development in the region and a new treaty is needed to establish a clearer picture of overall governance in the region and also to further empower the council for action.

Group of Eight and the Group of Twenty

Originally formed by six countries in the 1970s, the Group of Eight (G8) to which it grew over the next decades was intended to convene the leaders of the world's largest economies for improved international cooperation. As early as 1997, the leaders in this group acknowledged that climate change would have negative effects on health and would require immediate action, yet little action resulted (Kirton and Guebert 2010). The G8 is now largely replaced as an economic decision-making forum by the Group of Twenty (G20). While the G8 and G20 focus primarily on finance, climate change has been recurred as an agenda item with variable attention devoted to this issue (Council on Foreign Relations 2013). John Kirton, codirector and founder of the G20 Research Group at the Munk School of Global Affairs at the University of Toronto, argues that the core directive of the G20, that of economic sustainability, is achievable only if obtained with ecologic sustainability and that climate change control, including "adaptation, mitigation and resilience," is the linchpin without which there will be no progress (G20, 2012).

Major Economies Forum on Energy and Climate Change

Similar to the G20, the Major Economies Forum on Energy and Climate Change (MEF) is described by the Council on Foreign Relations as part of the increasingly popular "à la carte multilateralism" that is being used as an attempt to find a more flexible approach, outside the UNFCCC mechanism, for climate change initiatives. The MEF, established in 2009, consists of seventeen members from both developed and developing countries that produce, collectively, approximately 80 percent of global emissions. These economies are Australia, Brazil, Canada, China, the European Union, France, Germany, India, Indonesia, Italy, Japan, Korea, Mexico, Russia, South Africa, the United Kingdom, and the United States. The forum's focus is primarily to tackle strategies to reduce emissions without any specific stated adaptation or health initiative (Council on Foreign Relations 2013). Revisiting the initial questions of this chapter about who has the authority and the ethical responsibility around controlling climate change, we see from this survey of UN, regional, and plurilateral mechanisms that the intention to take action is coupled with complex layers of negotiation that can slow or stall action. Global governance itself is a challenge to conceptualize, and taken in light of one of the largest transboundary issues that the world has ever faced, that of climate change, it becomes even more complex.

Climate and Clean Air Coalition to Reduce Short-Lived Climate Pollutants

In 2012, a coalition of six countries and the UN Environment Program established a partnership to tackle emissions from pollutants that remain in the atmosphere only for a limited time; they are known as short-lived pollutants: hydrofluorocarbons, black carbon, and methane. These greenhouse gases are responsible for up to one-third of global emissions (US Department of State 2012). Short-lived pollutants have a particularly strong linkage to poor public health in developing countries because of the high number of fatalities from the use of indoor cooking stoves and dirty fuel in the transportation sector.

The objective of this minilateral forum is to establish policies in developing countries to reduce short-lived gases and mobilize funding, among other broader goals. The coalition has been successfully ramping up its partners, which now include thirty-two countries and a host of international partners. By coemphasizing the immediate benefits to health, such as reduced childhood mortality from lower respiratory tract infections, that result from improved air quality, such an effort can better harness the public health community's resources while simultaneously working toward the longer-term goal of climate change mitigation.

The last section of this chapter provides more concrete examples of some specific actions that are taking place at the nexus of climate and health.

CLINICAL CORRELATES 19.2 DUAL BENEFITS OF ADDRESSING SHORT-LIVED CLIMATE POLLUTANTS

Experts estimate that short-lived climate pollutants (black carbon, hydrofluorocarbons, methane, and ozone) account for 40 to 45 percent of anthropogenic climate warming chemicals. Therefore, reduction in the production of these chemicals is essential to slow global climate change and protect human health. Black carbon and ozone are major air pollutants that contribute to more than 6 million deaths annually. Household burning of solid fuels accounts for more than half of mortality (Lim et al. 2012). In South Asia, indoor air pollution is the leading risk factor for early mortality and years lived at less than optimal health (WHO 2013). Efforts to control release of black carbon in indoor environments include replacing traditional cooking stoves with clean-burning biomass stoves, modern brick kilns, and modern coke ovens. Clinicians working in these environments can encourage communities to adopt these technologies that improve health, decrease strain on local environment carbon sources, improve ambient air quality, and reduce global warming (Barnes et al. 1994).

Reducing short-lived climate pollutants and improving indoor ambient air is essential for respiratory health and for the environment.

Public Health Governance

The first part of this chapter provided an overview of how entities charged with governing climate change address health. This section explores briefly how the World Health Organization, the leading international institution on global health, addresses climate change. In most cases, this involves adaptation efforts—ones which have the goal of reducing the negative impacts of climate change—rather than mitigation efforts to reduce greenhouse gas production.

The World Health Organization (WHO) is one of the oldest UN agencies whose current mandate includes collecting data, conducting research, establishing norms and standards, providing input to policy processes, and supporting countries with technical assistance (CFR 2013). Over the past seventy years, the WHO has improved global human health conditions, including spearheading a program that eradicated smallpox.

Yet while the organization remains the central body on global public health, it faces considerable challenges in addressing the scope of public health challenges. The organization suffers from a shortfall in funding, an expansive and long list of priority areas—with the recent inclusion of new public health threats such as climate change—and competition from new actors in the public health space. In an effort to address these challenges, the WHO has initiated a comprehensive reform agenda that looks to update its administrative, financial, and managerial directives. This process, alongside all agenda setting, is spearheaded by the WHO's internal committee of member states, known as the World Health Assembly (WHA). At the time of writing this chapter, the WHA comprises 193 countries.

The WHO has underscored the risks of climate change on human health since the early 1990s, but it has increased its focus on the subject in the past five years. In 2008, members passed a pioneering resolution calling on the WHO "to strengthen its work in raising awareness about the health implications of climate change, support capacity building and research in health protection from climate change in countries, and urge action by the health sector" (WHO n.d.). As a follow-up to the resolution, the WHO instituted a five-pronged research agenda to evaluate the climate-health nexus (WHO 2008), and evaluate possible policy responses (Campbell-Lendrum, Corvalan, and Neira 2007).

Moreover, in 2009, the WHO executive board approved a plan to launch programs on the climate-health nexus to address four priority areas: advocacy and raising awareness, strengthening partnerships across the UN family, enhancing scientific evidence on the linkage between climate and health, and helping states build climate-resilient health systems (Chan 2009). On all four counts, the WHO has made significant progress. Foremost, the WHO has been more active in advocating for public health interests in the UNFCCC process with side sessions and panels on health-related issues. At the UNFCCC conference in Durban in 2011, the WHO organized a side event on the social dimensions of climate change in collaboration with the International Labor Organization. At the UNFCCC conference in Doha in 2012, the WHO also hosted side events and distributed promotional material outlining top-line messages on climate-health interlinkage (IFMSA/WHO 2012).

WHO has also ramped up its research on health impacts. In 2012 it launched a new publication, *Health in the Green Economy*, examining the health benefits of lower-emissions transportation systems, improved rapid-transit systems, and more walking and cycling routes. The report finds that a transition to a low carbon-infrastructure "can help reduce risks from urban air pollution, traffic injuries and the growing burden of noncommunicable diseases associated with physical inactivity."

At the same time, WHO has continued to provide scientific evidence to the IPCC and monitor the impact of factors prone to climatic reconditioning, such as water scarcity and air pollution.

Finally, the WHO has instituted regional frameworks to act on the 2008 WHA resolution and provided assessments and technical guidance on adaptation. To date, the WHO, alongside other international and regional partners, helped establish five regional frameworks that provide guidance on strengthening the public health sector's resilience to climate change (WHO 2015). In particular, the Framework for Public Health Adaptation to Climate Change in the African Region (WHO-Africa 2011) has been endorsed by the ministers of health and ministers of environment of Africa. As of 2012, the WHO had seventeen major projects on health adaptation to climate change in fourteen countries (Public Health and Environment Department 2012). It has also supported climate change assessments in over thirty countries (http://www.who.int/globalchange/health_policy /WHO_submission_on_NAPs_13_Feb2012.pdf).

Clinical Correlations

Although the topic of this chapter does not lend itself specifically to cases that a clinician would observe in a one-on-one patient interaction, this section provides an opportunity to explore national, regional, and even local public health entities' role in climate change adaptation. The case studies that follow describe some specific preparedness activities.

Recent US Government Activities on Climate and Health

Despite never ratifying the Kyoto Protocol, the United States has made some specific efforts around climate change over the last decade. Two angles pertain to health. First of all, the Obama administration acknowledges that there will be harmful effects to health from "heat stress, air pollutants, extreme weather events, and diseases carried by food, water, and insects" (White House 2013). Second, certain adaptation efforts include public health preparedness. Many of the advances have been spearheaded by the Interagency Climate Change Adaptation Task Force, a task force convened by the Obama administration in 2009 as a result of Executive Order 13514 (White House, Council on Environmental Quality n.d.). This order also required executive branch agencies to develop adaptation plans.

The Centers for Disease Control and Prevention has developed the Building Resilience Against Climate Effects (BRACE) framework for use by jurisdictions to develop strategies and programs to reduce climate-related health impacts. Through its Climate and Health Program, this federal entity has dedicated resources toward participation with both the IPCC and Interagency Workgroups of the US Global Change Research Program (Centers for Disease Control and Prevention 2015).

At the predominant US governmental health research organization, the activities of the National Institutes of Health (NIH) around climate change and health have been spearheaded by the National Institute of Environmental Health Science under its Climate Change and Human Health program, as well as the Fogarty International Center (NIEHS 2015). In comparison to the overall portfolio of the combined institutes, specific climate change activities represent a small but arguably growing portion. As of 2008, climate and health research made up only 0.17 percent of the National Institutes of Health's over fifty thousand awards (NIEHS 2015). A more recent analysis is not available. However, in 2010 the first climate change and health-specific request for proposals was issued by multiple institutes within the NIH and, over the subsequent several years, resulted in the launch of more than a dozen climate and health-focused projects.

As a third federal locus of activity, mandated by Congress in the Global Change Research Act of 1990, the US Global Change Research Program (USGCRP) has continued to produce periodic National Climate Assessments (NCA), which directly inform the IPCC process. The USGCRP efforts are led by representatives from thirteen federal agencies, including the Department of Health and Human Services. Work is underway on the latest NCA, which will potentially include a new web-based interface and a platform for an ongoing assessment process that will further contribute to the climate and health platform. Additionally, an interagency group of the USGCRP has recently launched a new tool, the Metadata Access Tool for Climate and Health (MATCH) (USGCRP n.d.) Regional Greenhouse Gas Initiative, a searchable database of publicly available federal metadata to facilitate research and cross-communication around climate and health issues.

Finally, there has been considerable state-led activity primarily concentrated in the Northeast Untied States. This extensive US. regional initiative, the Regional Greenhouse Gas Initiative (RGGI), is a market-based cap-and-trade program now involving nine states. While the primary focus is mitigation, a peripheral motivator for RGGI and other state-led initiatives is the short-term public health benefits that will come from reduced regional air pollution (RGGI Benefits n.d.; Shonkoff et al. 2009).

Disaster Relief/Migration: UN Office for the Coordination of Humanitarian Affairs

The UN Office for the Coordination of Humanitarian Affairs (OCHA; n.d.) asserts that the overarching humanitarian challenge of climate change is how to bring about "effective disaster response." The office cites the response to the 2007 floods in Mozambique as an example of exemplary national preparedness and international cooperation.

The assertion is that disasters, over 70 percent of which are now considered climate related, are not altogether unpredictable and the charge is thus to "act sooner and act smarter."

In Mozambique, the 2007 disaster included a Category 4 cyclone that compounded flooding that was already present in two major rivers and affected up to 500,000 people. The high baseline rate of poverty in Mozambique (54 percent) meant the floods exacerbated existing vulnerabilities. However, prior to the 2007, disaster a number of efforts occurred that contributed to a notable absence of both widespread suffering and avoidable deaths. These efforts included both national and international measures:

*   Strong national leadership and political commitment to preparedness. Clear political support and direction led to the creation of the national disaster management institute (INGC) in 2000. The INGC looked to countries such as Honduras and Guatemala for preparedness solutions, rather than developed countries, and subsequently implemented preparedness measures including building a new national emergency operation center, and carrying out simulation exercises

*   Increased availability of resources, technical support, and funds for preparedness. In addition to national resources, international donor investment and support to the INGC and related preparedness action was instrumental. Funding supported staff employment and training with the Germany agency, GTZ, playing an instrumental role.

*   Active involvement of communities, civil society and agencies in the implementation of disaster preparedness measures in advance. Local civil society networks helped reach larger population centers in rural areas through radio broadcasts, field trips, and mobile telephones. Many village committees were trained to organize and carry out evacuations.

*   Rapid availability of sufficient funds during the response provided almost a third of the international funds committed to the flood response and helped to ensure a rapid response. The availability of such funds meant UN agencies were able to spend their own resources and deploy their stockpiles because of preexisting agreements that the resources would be replenished.

CLINICAL CORRELATES 19.3 BUILDING RESILIENCE AGAINST CLIMATE EFFECTS (BRACE)

The Centers for Disease Control and Prevention have created the following five-step model for local health departments to organize their adaptation planning:

Step 1: Forecasting Climate Impacts and Assessing Vulnerabilities. A health department identifies the scope of the most likely climate impacts, the potential health outcomes associated with those climatic changes, and the locations of vulnerable populations within a jurisdiction.

Step 2: Projecting the disease burden. A health department estimates or quantifies the additional burden of health outcomes due to climate change to support prioritization and decision making.

Step 3: Assessing public health interventions. A health department seeks to identify the most suitable health interventions for the health impacts of greatest concern.

Step 4: Developing and implementing a climate and health adaptation plan. A health department develops and implements a health adaptation plan for climate change that addresses health impacts, gaps in critical public health functions and services, and a plan for enhancing adaptive capacity in the jurisdiction.

Step 5: Evaluating impact and improving quality of activities step for the framework. A health department evaluates the processes it has used, determines the value of using the framework, and the value of climate and health activities undertaken.

Stepwise and organized efforts are required at local levels to identify and anticipate the burden of climate related health issues in vulnerable populations.

Way Forward

Moving forward, public health experts, climate scientists, policymakers, scholars, and advocacy groups need to reframe the issue to improve public understanding and awareness of the massive human health threats posed by catastrophic climate change. Measures to consider include:

- Increasing climate- and health-impact and adaptation research, particularly in developing countries with weak public health systems as underscored by the IPCC (World Health Organization 2012a).

- Raising awareness of climate change effects on human well-being to increase preparedness to major climatic events and raising funding for adaptive capacity.

- Using rating efforts such as the Council on Foreign Relations's Global Governance Report Card (CFR 2014) to critically assess and improve governance activities and organizational structures.

- Incorporating a "health in all policies" approach on the part of multinational agencies, and thereby including projected health impacts of climate change in planning and policymaking. Entities like the World Trade Organization, for example, could "give greater priority to averting the adverse health and environmental effects of international free trade." (McMichael 2013).

Conclusion

This chapter underscores the fractured and largely ineffective global response to the increasing influence of climatic factors on the emergence and spread of disease and public health emergencies. The existing global institutional architecture for climate change does not provide immediate solutions to tackling the health risks, which are often considered tangential to the actual problem of reducing carbon emissions. Driven primarily by climate activists who are all too often operating separately from public health activists, various multilateral groups are spearheading their own initiatives outside of the cumbersome UNFCCC mechanism. Without a more unified approach and specific prioritization of public health, countless unnecessary deaths and additional cases of disease are impending. New minilateral movements that emphasize short-term cobenefits to health and development are gaining traction and represent a bright spot in this unprecedented transboundary global issue.

DISCUSSION QUESTIONS

1. How do you define climate change governance? What entities should be responsible for legislating on and creating regulations regarding climate change?

2. The main GHG contributor states are not the same as those where the most health impacts are being experienced and expected to worsen the most. How is this discrepancy a North-South equity issue? How is this being addressed by the international community?

3. Why has the UNFCCC framework failed to deliver significant reductions in greenhouse gas emissions?

4. Is climate governance more effective at the minilateral level (note the climate and clean air coalition)? Can we expect to achieve significant gains without a universal agreement on climate change?

5. How can the adaptive capacity of public health systems to climate change be enhanced, particularly in developing countries?

6. Which climate change impacts should the global public health regime prioritize (e.g., air pollution, water and sanitation, effects of heat)?

KEY TERMS

Intergovernmental Panel on Climate Change (IPCC): Established in 1988 by the World Meteorological Organization and the United Nations Environment Program, the IPCC consists of a group of over twenty-five hundred international voluntary scientists who assemble periodic Assessment Reports that summarize the state of the science on climate change, impacts, and policy response strategies.

Kyoto Protocol: An international agreement that is independent of but linked to the United Nations Framework Convention on Climate Change. It sets binding targets for the reduction of greenhouse gas emissions by industrialized nations.

United Nations Framework Convention on Climate change (UNFCCC): An international environmental treaty negotiated at the United Nations Conference on Environment and Development in 1992. Its goal is to stabilize greenhouse gas emissions so as to prevent detrimental climate change.

References

Adaptation Fund. 2014. "Endorsed Concepts." https://www.adaptation-fund.org/projects-programmes/endorsed_concepts

"Arctic Council." 2004. http://www.arctic-council.org/index.php/en/

Asia-Pacific Economic Cooperation. n.d. "Climate Change—Fact Sheet." http://www.apec.org/About-Us/About-APEC/Fact-Sheets/Climate-Change.aspx

Barnes, D. F., K. Openshaw, K. R. Smith, and P. van der Plas. 1994. "What makes People Cook with Improved Biomass Stoves?" World Bank Technical Paper 242—Energy Series.

Borgerson, S. G. 2008. "Arctic Meltdown: The Economic and Security Implications of Global Warming." *Foreign Affairs* 87:63–77.

Birdsall, N., and L. MacDonald. 2014. "Could China and Its Fellow BRICs Nations Lead the Way on Climate Change?" *Guardian*, January 28. http://www.guardian.co.uk/global-development/poverty-matters/2013/jan/28/china-brics-lead-climate-change

Campbell-Lendrum, D., C. Corvalan, and M. Neira. 2007. "Global Climate Change: Implications for International Public Health Policy." *Bulletin of the World Health Organization* 85(3):161–244.

Centers for Disease Control and Prevention. 2015. "Climate and Health Program." http://www.cdc.gov/climateandhealth/default.htm

CFR (Council on Foreign Relations). 2014. "Global Governance Report Card." http://www.cfr.org/thinktank//iigg/reportcard/

Chan, M. 2009. "The Impact of Global Crises on Health: Money, Weather and Microbes." World Health Organization. http://www.who.int/dg/speeches/2009/financial_crisis_20090318/en/

Chapin F. S. III, M. Hoe, S. R. Carpenter, J. Lubchenco, B. Walker, T. V. Callaghan, C. Folke, et al. 2006. "Building Resilience and Adaptation to Manage Arctic Change." *Ambio* 35:198–202.

"Climate Change." United Nations Development Programme. http://www.undp.org/content/undp/en/home/ourwork/environmentandenergy/strategic_themes/climate_change.html

Council on Foreign Relations. 2013. "The Global Climate Change Regime—Issue Brief." April 23. http://www.cfr.org/climate-change/lobal-climate-change-regime/p21831

European Commission. 2009. "Adapting to Climate Change: A Framework for EU Action." http://ec.europa.eu/clima/summary/docs/adapting_en.pdf

European Commission—Climate. 2012. "European Climate Change Programme." September 7. http://ec.europa.eu/clima/policies/eccp/index_en.htm

European Commission—Climate Action. 2015. "What Is the EU Doing About Climate Change?" http://ec.europa.eu/clima/policies/brief/eu/index_en.htm

Food and Agriculture Organization. 2010. "UNFCCC Process: The Nairobi Work Programme on Impacts, Vulnerability, and Adaptation to Climate Change." http://www.fao.org/climatechange/unfccc-process/63662/en/

Food and Agriculture Organization. 2015a. "Climate Change." http://www.fao.org/climatechange/en/

Food and Agriculture Organization. 2015b. "UNFCCC Process: Key Submissions by FAO and Partners." Food and Agriculture Organization of the United Nations. 2015b. http://www.fao.org/climatechange/unfccc-process/63661/en/

G20. December 19, 2012. "John Kirton: We Have to Unleash the Power of Young Entrepreneurship. We Need More Steve Jobs." http://en.g20russia.ru/news/20121219/781086187.html

"Health and Climate Change: Policy Responses to Protect Public Health." 2015. *Lancet*, June 23. http://www.thelancet.com/commissions/climate-change-2015

Huifang, T., J. Whalley, and C. Yuezhou. 2009. "Trade Sanctions, Financial Transfers, and BRIC's Participation in Global Climate Change Negotiations." http://www.econstor.eu/bitstream/10419/30642/1/604952872.pdf

IFMSA/WHO. 2012. "Health Coverage at the 18th Conference of the Parties to the UN Framework Convention on Climate Change." http://www.who.int/globalchange/mediacentre/events/cop18reports.pdf

Inter Academy Medical Panel. 2010. "IAMP Statement on the Health Co-Benefits of Policies to Tackle Climate Change." http://www.iamp-online.org/sites/iamp-online.org/files/IAMP%20Climate%20STATEMENT%20eng.pdf

Kirton, J., and J. Guebert. 2010. "The Climate Change-Health Connection: Compounding Challenges for Scholars and Practitioners." www.g8.utoronto.ca/scholar/kirton-guebert-isa-100217.pdf

Lim, S., et al. 2012. "A Comparative Risk Assessment of Burden of Disease and Injury Attributable to 67 Risk Factors and Risk Factor Clusters in 21 Regions, 1990–2010: A Systematic Analysis for the Global Burden of Disease Study 2010." *The Lancet* 380(9859):2224–60.

Matthies, F., G. Bickler, N. C. Marín, and S. Hales, eds. 2008. "Heat-Health Action Plans." World Health Organization Europe. http://www.euro.who.int/__data/assets/pdf_file/0006/95919/E91347.pdf

McMichael, A. J. 2013. "Globalization, Climate Change, and Human Health." *New England Journal of Medicine* 369(1):96. doi:10.1056/NEJMc1305749

NIEHS (National Institute of Environmental Health Services). 2015. "Climate Change and Human Health." http://www.niehs.nih.gov/research/programs /geh/climatechange/

Onzivu, W. 2010. "Health in Global Climate Change Law: The Long Road to an Effective Legal Regime Protecting Both Public Health and the Climate." *Carbon and Climate Law Review* 4:364.

Organisation for Economic Co-operation and Development. n.d. "Climate Change." http://www.oecd.org/env/cc/

Parry, M. L., O. F. Canziani, J. P. Palutikof, P. J. van der Linden, and C. E. Hanson. 2007. *Climate Change 2007: Impacts, Adaptation and Vulnerability.* Cambridge: Cambridge University Press. http://www.ipcc.ch/pdf/assessment -report/ar4/wg2/ar4_wg2_full_report.pdf

Physicians for Social Responsibility. 2014. "Climate Change Is a Threat to Human Health." http://www.psr.org/environment-and-health/climate-change/

Public Health and Environment Department. 2012. "WHO Information Session on Health in the UN Framework Convention on Climate Change." http://www .who.int/globalchange/mediacentre/events/key_messages_cop18.pdf

Regional Greenhouse Gas Initiative. n.d. "RGGI Benefits." http://www.rggi.org /rggi_benefits

Shonkoff, S. B., R. Morello-Frosch, M. Pastor, and J. Sadd. 2009. "Minding the Climate Gap: Environmental Health and Equity Implications of Climate Change Mitigation Policies in California." December 15. http://online.liebertpub.com /doi/pdf/10.1089/env.2009.0030

Stern, N. 2011. "Climate and Health in a Post-Kyoto World." *Lancet* 378:1825.

United Nations Development Program. 2013. "The Rise of the South: Human Progress in a Diverse World." http://www.undp.org/content/dam/undp/library /corporate/HDR/2013GlobalHDR/English/HDR2013%20Report%20English.pdf

United Nations Framework Convention on Climate Change. 1992. http://unfccc .int/resource/docs/convkp/conveng.pdf

United Nations Framework Convention on Climate Change. 2012. Conference of the Parties serving as the Meeting of the Parties to the Kyoto Protocol (CMP). Outcome of the Work of the Ad Hoc Working Group on Further Commitments for Annex I Parties Under the Kyoto Protocol. December 8. http://unfccc.int /resource/docs/2012/cmp8/eng/109.pdf

United Nations Framework Convention on Climate Change. 2014a. "Kyoto Protocol." http://unfccc.int/kyoto_protocol/items/2830.php

United Nations Framework Convention on Climate Change. 2014b. "Parties to the Convention and Observer States." http://unfccc.int/parties_and_observers /parties/items/2352.php

United Nations Framework Convention on Climate Change. 2014c. "Status of Ratification of the Kyoto Protocol." http://unfccc.int/kyoto_protocol/status_of _ratification/items/2613.php

United Nations Framework Convention on Climate Change. 2014d. "Developments at Past COP and SB Sessions: Marrakesh Accords and COP7." http://unfccc.int/methods_and_science/lulucf/items/3063.php.

United Nations Office for the Coordination of Humanitarian Affairs. n.d. "Climate Change—Case Study." http://www.unocha.org/what-we-do/advocacy/thematic-campaigns/climate-change/case-study

US Department of State. 2012. "The Climate and Clean Air Coalition to Reduce Short-Lived Climate Pollutants." http://www.state.gov/r/pa/prs/ps/2012/02/184055.htm

USGCRP (United States Global Change Research Program) n.d. "Metadata Access Tool for Climate and Health (MATCH)." http://match.globalchange.gov

US Senate Committee on Foreign Relations. 1997. Senate Resolution 98: Conditions Regarding U.N. Framework Convention on Climate Change. S.Rept. 105–54, July 21.

Watson, R. T., M. C. Zinyowera, and R. H. Moss, eds. 1997. *The Regional Impacts of Climate Change: An Assessment of Vulnerability.* Cambridge: Cambridge University Press. http://www.ipcc.ch/pdf/special-reports/spm/region-en.pdf

White House. 2013. "President Obama's Plan to Fight Climate Change." http://www.whitehouse.gov/share/climate-action-plan

White House, Council on Environmental Quality. n.d. "Climate Change Adaptation Task Force." http://www.whitehouse.gov/administration/eop/ceq/initiatives/adaptation

World Bank Group. 2015. "Climate Change." http://climatechange.worldbank.org/sites/default/files/Turn_Down_the_heat_Why_a_4_degree_centrigrade_warmer_world_must_be_avoided.pdf

World Health Organization. 2008. "WHO Agreed on a Research Agenda on Climate Change and Public Health." World Health Organization, October 8. http://www.who.int/mediacentre/news/releases/2008/pr36/en/

World Health Organization. 2012a. "Building Sustainable Health Systems: Focus on Climate Resilience." December 3. http://www.who.int/globalchange/mediacentre/events/cop18_concept_note.pdf

World Health Organization. 2012b. *Atlas of Health and Climate.* World Meteorological Organization. http://www.wmo.int/ebooks/WHO/Atlas_EN_web.pdf

World Health Organization. 2013. "About the Global Burden of Disease (GBD) Projects." http"//who.int/healthinfo/global_burden_disease/about/en/

World Health Organization. 2015. "Health Policy and Climate Change." http://www.who.int/globalchange/health_policy/en/

World Health Organization. n.d. "Climate Change and Health—World Health Organization." http://unfccc.int/files/adaptation/sbi_agenda_item_adaptation/application/pdf/who.pdf

World Health Organization—Africa. 2011. "Framework for Public Health Adaptation to Climate Change in the African Region." http://www.unep.org/roa/amcen/Amcen_Events/4th_ss/Docs/AMCEN-SS4-INF-4.pdf

World Meteorological Organization. n.d. "Climate Applications in Health Sector." http://www.wmo.int/pages/themes/climate/applications_health.php

CHAPTER 20

CLIMATE CHANGE AND THE RIGHT TO HEALTH

Carmel Williams

Human rights are the entitlements everybody has, by virtue of being born, to live a life of equality and dignity. These rights are inherent in all people, everywhere in the world, regardless of their nationality, place of residence, sex, ethnicity, disability, or any other status. International human rights law includes the fundamental commitments of states to treat all people equally and without discrimination, to enable them to enjoy all their human rights, including the right to health. Health rights entitlements are not just to health services but also to information about health and to the underlying determinants of health, such as potable water, sanitation, an adequate supply of nutrition, safe housing, and clean air (UN Committee on Economic, Social and Cultural Rights 2000).

Because climate change threatens people's health, as well as people's access to these determinants of health, it has enormous human rights implications. Fortunately, key human rights principles offer processes to guide climate change mitigation and adaptation proposals so that those whose health is most threatened are made central to remedial and other actions and are actively involved in all climate change decisions.

What Is the Right to Health?

The right to health is included in the Universal Declaration of Human Rights (1948), where it is stated in Article 25 that everyone has the right to a standard of living adequate for the health and well-being of self and family, including food, clothing, housing, and medical care and necessary social services, and the right to security in the event of unemployment, sickness, disability, widowhood, old age, or other lack of livelihood in circumstances beyond one's

KEY CONCEPTS

- **The right to health is not just aspirational; rather, it is a legal entitlement that carries state obligations and has significant and legal bearing on how states must engage with other states when there are consequences on health in these engagements.**

- **Climate change will have an impact on people's right to health.**

- **Those whose health rights are not realized are most vulnerable to climate change.**

- **Human rights principles guide an equitable response to climate change health impacts.**

control. In addition, mothers and children are entitled to special care and assistance.

The right to the highest attainable standard of physical and mental health (abbreviated to the **right to health**) more specifically arises from the International Convention on Economic, Social and Cultural Rights, Article 12, and is thus part of the International Bill of Rights, which is legally binding on state members of the UN through international human rights law. (The conventions can be viewed online at www.ohchr.org.) Of importance in the context of climate change, Article 12 includes entitlements to health care as well as "all aspects of environmental and industrial hygiene" as part of the right to health.

In 2000, the meaning of health rights entitlements was further clarified by the UN Committee on Economic Social and Cultural Rights in **General Comment 14**, which was UN state members adopted. State obligations include the provision of primary health services such as maternal and child health and essential medicines, among many others. The General Comment is not unrealistic, and accordingly it allows for the impossibility of all states being able to meet the same standards of health care immediately. But it does specify that over time, there must be a gradual improvement in the provision of health care and in access to the underlying determinants of health, which is called **progressive realization of the right to health**. This means that when states report every four years to the committee on their right to health achievements, they must demonstrate that health entitlements have improved—that there is greater realization of people's health rights.

There are also rights to health obligations that the state must implement immediately. These include the fundamental human rights principle that all people must be treated equally and without discrimination. In practice, this means that no one can be denied access to health care on the basis of discrimination and all people have an equal right to participate in decisions about their own health. Principles of equality and nondiscrimination also mean that people living remotely, or indigenous people, people in poverty, and women and children are entitled to the same access to health care and the same quality of water, sanitation, nutrition, clean air, and other public goods as everyone else. In order to achieve equality, the most disadvantaged people are entitled to have their rights to health addressed soonest.

The right to health is a legal entitlement. In the past ten years, there has been an exponential increase in the number of health-related rights cases being taken to court. This "has begun to have a substantial impact in countries across the world affecting tens of thousands of individual entitlements to medications and treatments a year in some countries, but also rewriting intellectual property rules, ensuring regulation of laws, causing changes in policies of various kinds, and influencing health priority-setting processes and budgetary allocations" (Yamin 2014). Although access to legal redress varies within and between countries, it is now evident in principle and practice that the right to health is not just aspirational; rather, it is a legal entitlement that carries state obligations and also has significant and legal bearing on how states must engage with other states when there are consequences on health in these engagements.

General Comment 14 enabled the development of a framework through which the right to health could be operationalized. Illustrated by the first special rapporteur on the right to health, the ten-point framework provides a guide to the various elements and processes required when wanting to formulate a plan to meet or examine the right to health:

The Right-to-Health Analytical Framework

1. Identification of the relevant national and international human rights laws, norms, and standards.

2. The right to health is subject to resource availability, but states are obliged to progressively realize the right over time and must identify indicators and benchmarks to measure progress.

3. States have obligations of immediate effect.

4. The right to health includes freedoms and entitlements.

5. All health services, goods, and facilities shall be available, accessible, acceptable, and of good quality (AAAQ).

6. States have duties to respect, protect, and fulfill the right to health.

7. Because of their crucial importance, the analytical framework demands that special attention is given to issues of nondiscrimination, equality, and vulnerability.

8. The right to health requires that there is an opportunity for the active and informed participation of individuals and communities in decision making that affects their health.

9. Developing countries have a responsibility to seek international assistance and cooperation, while resource-rich states have responsibilities toward the realization of the right to health in developing countries.

10. Monitoring and accountability mechanisms that are transparent, effective, and accessible and include redress, are crucial.

Climate Change and Its Impact on the Right to Health

As illustrated in the other chapters of this book, there are numerous ways in which climate change has an effect on health. These include the increase in vector-borne and waterborne diseases, rising temperatures that will likely increase respiratory diseases, and physical and mental stresses that arise from decreased water supply as well as its impact on nutrition (Smith et al. 2014).

These impacts are felt most acutely by poor and marginalized people who are most vulnerable to ill health and usually have the least access to quality health care or quality underlying determinants of health, such as water and sanitation, nutritious food, and secure housing. Mary Robinson, former president of Ireland and UN high commissioner for human rights from 1997 to 2002, describes the impact of extreme weather events, as well as sea level rise and glacial melt, as destroying the homes of vulnerable and poor people who "face increasing struggles to feed themselves and their families, and are more susceptible to diseases while having their access to health care diminished" (Robinson 2014).

The World Health Organization calculates that weather-related natural disasters have more than tripled since the 1960s, resulting in over 60,000 deaths each year, mainly in developing countries. It further estimates that between 2030 and 2050, climate change will cause approximately 250,000 additional deaths per year from malnutrition, malaria, diarrhea, and heat stress (World Health Organization 2014). The UN Human Rights Council adopted a resolution in 2009 that identified direct and nondirect implications of climate change on the right to life, the right to adequate food, the right to the highest attainable standard of health, the right to adequate housing, the right to self-determination, and human rights obligations related to access to safe drinking water and sanitation (Human Rights Council 2009). It also acknowledged that "while these implications affect individuals and communities around the world, the effects of climate change will be felt most acutely by those segments of the population who are already in vulnerable situations owing to factors such as geography, poverty, gender, age, indigenous or minority status and disability" (Human Rights Council 2009).

Furthermore, people who are in vulnerable situations are often not likely to have access to good health services, especially in developing countries where health systems are struggling to provide appropriate and good-quality care (World Health Organization 2007; Williams, Ashton, and Bullen 2014; Freedman 2005). These health systems will be facing even greater demands arising from increased levels of waterborne and vector-borne diseases and the other climate-related illnesses arising from heat stress, poor nutrition, and poor air quality. For example, as more people experience malaria or dengue fever, the understaffed and frequently distant health clinics that have irregular supplies of appropriate medicines will be under more strain to cope with additional patients. In these ways, the health rights of the people who are already suffering the consequences of human rights failings, such as poor health, poor education, and inaccessible health services, are most at risk of further deterioration.

The governments of the states in which people are vulnerable to the impact of climate change have human rights obligations to mitigate these impacts and to provide health care and nutrition, clean air, sanitation, and potable water systems for all their citizens—and especially for those most vulnerable and unable to pay for these services and facilities. But these governments commonly have financial and other resource deficits that leave them unable to make an adequate response that would protect and fulfill their citizens' right to health.

Fortunately, General Comment 14 has made the duties of international states and partners clear: subject to adequate resourcing, states are expected to offer financial and technical assistance to less-well-resourced states to realize human rights. This has a direct bearing on climate change response because states must ensure that their actions in their own countries and elsewhere respect and protect human rights, including the right to health. Therefore, the right to health can be the basis on which developing countries ask for international assistance to support climate change mitigation and adaptation plans.

It isn't possible to clearly attribute causation of climate change impacts to specific countries, despite universal agreement that developed countries have contributed a vastly disproportionate volume of the greenhouse gases to the environment. Even so, human rights provide mechanisms and processes through which the most vulnerable can be protected and human rights violators held to account. "Such procedures include information-sharing, grievance redress mechanisms and the active participation of various participants including rights-holders in decision making. These procedures can help guide iterative, participatory and accountable solutions, offering an avenue for equitable decision making, including over rights conflicts" (Hall 2014). Use of these procedures constitutes a **human rights–based approach** (HRBA) to climate change. These are explored more fully in the next section.

Human Rights–Based Approaches to Climate Change

HRBA to policies, programs, and agreements are a means and an end: they use human rights principles as the means to guide processes toward achieving the end goal, which is the realization of human rights. An HRBA explicitly assists governments to meet their internationally and nationally binding human rights obligations. But it is more than just this: this approach also empowers people to know and claim their rights. It provides them with knowledge and tools to challenge power imbalances or discriminatory practices. In this way, the state is held accountable for its human rights obligations.

Key human rights principles and concepts are consistent across all human rights conventions. The principles are equality and nondiscrimination, participation, transparency, and accountability. The principles as applied to the right to health, arising from General Comment 14, and the work of many human rights experts, including the first special rapporteur on the right to health, are quite specific.

The following ten sections examine these right-to-health principles in a climate change context and draw on the work of various authors, many of whom published their work in a special climate justice edition of the *Health and Human Rights Journal* (www.hhrjournal.org) in June 2014.

1. *Identification of the relevant national and international human rights laws, norms, and standards.* An HRBA places emphasis on ensuring an enabling legal and policy framework and environment. It requires an understanding of how laws and social or institutional practices affect the enjoyment of human rights (Yamin and Cantor 2014). In the context of climate change and its impact on health, this involves examining domestic and international law, conventions, and climate change negotiations to determine whether enjoyment of the right to health is protected or, if not, whether there is a remedy for violations to rights. As with all other elements of this framework, such examination requires participation from diverse sectors to ensure protection is afforded to all people. For example, inadequate regulation and legislation has failed to protect people living alongside fossil fuel railway corridors in Canada and the United States. In Canada's worst rail catastrophe, forty-seven people died, and many lost their homes in the destruction of downtown Lac Mégantic (Burton and Stretesky 2014). Burton argues that the US and Canadian governments must implement regulations and specific rail reform to honor their obligations to citizens who are paying a high human cost for the material benefits associated with increased energy production.

2. *The right to health is subject to resource availability, but states are obliged to progressively realize the right over time and must identify indicators and benchmarks to measure progress.* In climate change practice, this means that states must make national plans, after meaningful engagement with communities, health professionals, and indigenous people, among many others, to address climate change and its health impacts and agree on appropriate indicators of progress. These plans must include the increased

provision of health care and underlying determinants over time and ensure that those most vulnerable to climate change impacts will have their rights entitlements addressed first.

3. *States have obligations of immediate effect.* Obligations of equality and nondiscrimination are immediate. This requires that states plan for access to health-related services and facilities on a nondiscriminatory basis, especially for disadvantaged individuals, communities, and populations. "This means, for example, that a state has a core obligation to establish effective outreach programs for those living in poverty" (Hunt and Backman 2008). People living in malarial areas, for example, have the right to at least the same level of access to health services as those living in urban areas. This often requires plans to address an urgent scale-up of health services to poorer and more remote regions.

4. *The right to health includes freedoms and entitlements.* Generally human rights guarantee people freedom to control the decisions about their health and confer the right to be free from nonconsensual medical treatment and experimentation. Entitlements include the right to a system of health protection. In the case of climate change, freedom means choosing whether to participate in decisions regarding, for example, the relocation of communities threatened by rising oceans. Entitlements also mean participating in decisions on how the state is obligated to ensure survival in the face of imminent threats to life, health, and livelihoods.

5. *All health services, goods, and facilities shall be available, accessible, acceptable, and of good quality (AAAQ).* The services needed to address the health impacts of climate change must become progressively available and accessible, as well as culturally appropriate and of good quality, especially in the face of the increasing need for vulnerable people. Health service development must ensure these rights are achieved for those likely to be hardest hit by climate change, which cannot be achieved without their active participation in the process. Health systems have six component parts: human resources, facilities, medical supplies, financing, health information systems, and management (World Health Organization 2007). Quality health services cannot become increasingly available and accessible without addressing all of these components of the health system; for example, planning for an increase in human resources can take up to ten years to achieve. Therefore, planning health system responses to climate change has to begin immediately to be effective when needed, and in the countries that are most vulnerable, planning is urgent.

6. *States have duties to respect, protect, and fulfill the right to health.* *Respecting* the right to health involves ensuring that state action or inaction does not undermine health rights. States must take action to mitigate

increased risk to climate change health impacts and also ensure that infrastructure or industrial development does not increase risks to weather events. For example, when Hurricane Katrina hit the city of New Orleans in 2005, over one thousand people drowned, and many more lost their homes. Jean Carmalt (2014) claims the US government "violated the obligation to respect health by building a shipping canal that substantially increased the threat of flooding in New Orleans."

Protecting the right to health places an obligation on the state to ensure that third parties do not interfere with attainment of this right. States have a human rights responsibility to ensure that other parties, in their own countries and internationally, honor their climate agreements, especially regarding emissions. As an example of protecting the right to health, in the small Pacific island country of the Marshall Islands, there is increasing dependence on food aid as a result of war, nuclear testing, and, most recently, climate change (Ahlgren, Yamada, and Wong 2014). Ahlgren and colleagues argue that the government of the Marshall Islands must protect the health of the islanders by ensuring food aid is adequately nutritious. Currently it is not. "Accordingly," they write, "donors and the government should reexamine the content of food aid and ensure it is of sufficient quality to meet the right to health obligations."

Fulfilling the right to health requires the delivery of services and facilities, including those pertaining to the underlying determinants of health, to meet people's increased climate change–related health demands. The state has an obligation to plan for these climate impacts in a way that is nondiscriminatory and results in equitable outcomes, with disadvantaged communities receiving the same quality of health services, air, water, and nutrition as others. Fulfilling the right to health also requires robust health systems that function adequately. However, the generally weak and underresourced health systems in developing countries are not equipped to tackle the increased demands arising from climate change (Hunt and Khosla 2010). This places human rights responsibilities on underresourced states to strengthen health systems and to seek international assistance when necessary to do so.

7. *Because of their crucial importance, the right to health analytical frameworks demands that special attention is given to issues of nondiscrimination, equality, and vulnerability.* In the aftermath of Hurricane Katrina, New Orleans residents were able to evacuate the devastated city only if they had access to private transport. In effect, this was an entirely discriminatory evacuation plan, which resulted in the poor and marginalized communities being stranded without adequate access to food or clean water, despite the fact that the authorities had several days' warning that the hurricane would

hit the city (Carmalt 2014). The discriminatory suffering of these residents is a human rights violation that could have been avoided if people in these communities had played an active role in the design of evacuation plans.

Principles of equality and nondiscrimination require responses to climate change impacts to be considered in terms of impacts on all citizens. The most vulnerable people to climate change—the elderly, the young, the poor, indigenous peoples, and people living in coastal, atoll, or low-lying islands (Robinson 2014; Lemery, Williams, and Farmer 2014)—must be part of climate change adaptation and mitigation plans. But equality does not just mean people have equal opportunity to participate in planning; it also means ensuring an equality of achievement of human rights, so that all people will have the same degree of access to health care or the same quality of water and sanitation, and nutrition. This frequently requires a greater level of resource commitment to communities that are now disadvantaged to achieve an equality of outcome. Health care services, information, and education for people at greater risk of climate-related diseases must increase proportionately to their risk.

Similarly, health benefits from some climate change responses should be equitable. Climate change campaigns to increase active transport and reduce animal fat consumption are beneficial to health. But the benefits might not be available to everyone unless policies and interventions are designed to promote the benefits specifically to those who are most disadvantaged (Jones et al. 2014). This might require use of different languages or media in the distribution of messages. Another mitigation measure is taxation on the cost of carbon, intended to reduce emissions; but this usually increases the costs of goods and services, which in turn imposes a disproportionate financial burden on poor people. New technologies that reduce emissions can also have negative impacts on people living in poverty. Electric car batteries and solar energy units contain heavy metals and toxic substances that create health hazards associated with their disposal. Currently between 50 and 80 percent of this e-waste is shipped to China or India for disposal, predominantly by poor women and children (McAllister, Magee, and Hale 2014). So while these technological solutions may help reduce emissions, they violate the right to health in the impoverished and marginalized communities that eke out a living from working in disposal areas. Special attention must be given to all climate change responses to check for equitable impacts.

8. *The right to health requires that there is an opportunity for the active and informed participation of individuals and communities in decision making that affects their health.* Participation is crucial to the achievement of human rights. It is central to human rights-based approaches because

meaningful participation converts passive targets of policies and programs into active agents who demand their rights with respect to their own well-being (Yamin and Cantor 2014). Meaningful participation is not achieved simply by inviting representatives to state- or donor-funded climate change meetings, where the powerful and privileged set the agenda and control decision-making processes and outcomes. This has particular and urgent relevance to indigenous people and those who are losing their land to climate change in small island states. In New Zealand, meaningful participation and respect for Maori rights to self-determination require recognizing Maori concepts of health. Not only does this enable relevant and appropriate climate change strategies to protect Maori health, but their traditional ecological knowledge and expertise mean they have much to contribute to developing and implementing effective, sustainable mitigation and adaptation strategies (Jones et al. 2014). Meaningful participation can thus be a win-win for all parties.

The Committee on the Rights of the Child, in its recent General Comment on the right to health, described climate change as one of the biggest threats to child health and one that exacerbates inequalities (UN Committee on the Rights of the Child 2013). Accordingly, child rights advocates have called for children's participation in global forums on climate change and lament children's absent voices and influence in declarations, while noting also the absence of other vulnerable and minority groups, including women, indigenous people, and people with disabilities (Gibbons 2014).

Meaningful participation takes place when people who are at risk of rights violations actively pursue solutions to overcome their disadvantages and have their rights respected, protected, and fulfilled. In so doing, they hold the powerful to account. "In reality, effective participation (like access to information) is power" (Hunt 2008).

True participation in climate change is not limited to just one phase of developing climate change plans; rather, participation extends through whole cycles from planning, to implementing adaptation or mitigation plans, determining indicators, monitoring and adjusting the project in accordance with indicator feedback and other data, and holding those responsible for action (nationally and internationally) to account.

9. *Developing countries have a responsibility to seek international assistance and cooperation, while resource-rich states have responsibilities to the realization of the right to health in developing countries.* General Comment 14 is clear and explicit regarding the duties of states toward each other in matters impinging on the right to health. In the first instance, human rights duties to protect health rights place an obligation on states to

take measures to prevent third parties from interfering with health rights. Thus, states must take whatever measures are possible to reduce emissions and hold other states to account for their global warming activities in order to protect their citizens' rights. In addition, there are specific international obligations: "Depending on the availability of resources, States should facilitate access to essential health facilities, goods and services in other countries, wherever possible and provide the necessary aid when required" (UN Committee on Economic, Social and Cultural Rights 2000). Of further relevance is the responsibility of states to cooperate in providing disaster relief and humanitarian assistance in times of emergency, including assistance to refugees and internally displaced persons. "Priority in the provision of international medical aid, distribution and management of resources, such as safe and potable water, food and medical supplies, and financial aid should be given to the most vulnerable or marginalized groups of the population" (UN Committee on Economic, Social and Cultural Rights 2000). So although it is not possible to draw direct causal links between climate change events, gradual or otherwise, and specific countries and take legal action against any one country, international human rights obligations pertaining to the right to health show that developed countries, which have contributed far more to the climate change crisis, have obligations to at least support health systems in countries that will bear the brunt of climate change health damage.

10. *Monitoring and accountability mechanisms that are transparent, effective, and accessible and include redress, are crucial.* Employing the key human rights principles of participation, equality, and nondiscrimination brings a deeper meaning to accountability. Currently there is little in the way of accountability for climate change action or redress, which has led human rights experts to call for mechanisms to hold states accountable for their damaging impacts on climate, as well as for their duties to protect citizens' rights. Suggestions include public forums for debate, citizens' charters, and grievance redress mechanisms, including litigation (Hall 2014). The first special rapporteur on the right to health, Paul Hunt, has also sought strong international accountability mechanisms for climate change that would give adequate attention to the impact of a developed country's policies on climate change and the right to health. He emphasizes the importance of effective, transparent, and accessible accountability mechanisms, including for international assistance and cooperation in health. He describes the need for these accountability mechanisms as urgent and suggests they must allow for the differentiated responsibilities of states, reflecting their differentiated contribution to climate change in the first place (Hunt and Khosla 2010).

CLINICAL CORRELATES 20.1 PROTECTING THE VULNERABLE AGAINST CLIMATE CHANGE

Understanding that the most vulnerable among us will bear the brunt of climate change health impacts is a recurring theme throughout this book. It is predicted that heat-related illness, food insecurity, and waterborne and vector-borne infectious disease will increase this century, especially among vulnerable populations living in developing countries. Climate change will act as a threat multiplier, worsening human security through population displacement, violent conflict, and poverty entrenchment.

Clinicians will bear witness to this in both primary events (heat waves, extreme weather events such as floods or hurricanes, infectious disease outbreaks) and secondary events (disruption in health care services subsequent to extreme weather or forced migrations).

Adopting a rights-based approach to climate change begins by recognizing the obligations of states to respect, protect, and fulfill all human rights threatened by climate change. It then requires states to begin a transparent and participatory process with their own people, and international partners, to determine a plan of mitigation and adaptation, addressing the rights of the most vulnerable first. Clinicians hold a powerful fulcrum to affect change in this regard— over both policymakers and patients—and they have the unique perspective to keep the climate change conversation relevant to individuals worldwide.

The Universal Declaration of Human Rights was created in response to global outrage at the human suffering and atrocities of World War II. The world united to ensure that humankind would never again experience such loss of dignity and freedom. Unabated climate change poses exactly this threat. A rights-based approach will provide the imperative to guide the process and actions to mitigate such disaster (Lemery, Williams, and Farmer 2014).

Conclusion

All people have a right to health regardless of their nationality, sex, or socioeconomic status. The impact of climate change on health will be significant to all people, but people whose health is already compromised and who have little access to appropriate and good-quality health care will suffer the most. Their right to health, which includes the right to health care and to the underlying determinants of health, will be further eroded unless positive action is taken expeditiously. Strengthening health systems in countries most vulnerable to climate change is a crucial element in the protection and fulfillment of health rights. So too is the empowerment of people living in at-risk situations, so that they have the knowledge and confidence to engage meaningfully in the domestic and international forums where decisions affecting their lives, livelihoods, and health, and those of their children, are being made. In this chapter, we have used a right-to-health framework to explore what a human rights–based approach to climate change would incorporate. The key human rights principles of equality and nondiscrimination, participation, and accountability apply to each element of the framework to ensure all voices are heard and states are held to their human rights obligations as the world addresses its health-threatening warmer future.

DISCUSSION QUESTIONS

1. Why are people living in poverty considered most vulnerable to the impacts of climate change on their health?

2. Why does a human rights–based approach focus on getting health care to the most disadvantaged people even if this is more costly than treating greater numbers of people?

3. Why are already weak health systems going to be disproportionately burdened by climate change?

KEY TERMS

General Comment 14: Drafted by the Committee on Economic, Social and Cultural Rights to explain the meaning of the right to health; adopted by UN members in 2000.

Human rights: The entitlements everybody has, by virtue of being born, to live a life of equality and dignity.

Human rights–based approach (HRBA): An approach that explicitly assists governments to meet their internationally and nationally binding human rights obligations and empower people to know and claim their rights.

Progressive realization of the right to health: A specific and continuing state obligation to move as expeditiously and effectively as possible toward the full realization of the right to health. Retrogressive measures are not permissible (health rights must not deteriorate), and states must prove any such measures were introduced only after the most careful consideration of all alternatives.

Right to health: Arising from the International Covenant on Economic, Social and Cultural Rights (Article 12) and spelled out most clearly in UN General Comment 14 that all people are entitled to the highest attainable standard of mental and physical health. This extends to timely and appropriate health care, as well as access to the underlying determinants of health, such as access to safe and potable water and adequate sanitation, safe food, nutrition and housing, healthy occupational, and environmental conditions and health information.

References

Ahlgren, I., S. Yamada, and A. Wong. 2014. "Rising Oceans, Climate Change, Food Aid, and Human Rights in the Marshall Islands." *Health and Human Rights Journal* 16(1):69–81.

Burton, L., and P. Stretesky. 2014. "Wrong Side of the Tracks: The Neglected Human Costs of Transporting Oil and Gas." *Health and Human Rights Journal* 16(1):82–92.

Carmalt, J. 2014. "Prioritizing Health: A Human Rights Analysis of Disaster, Vulnerability, and Urbanization in New Orleans and Port-au-Prince." *Health and Human Rights Journal* 16(1):41.

Freedman, L. P. 2005. "Achieving the MDGs: Health Systems as Core Social Institutions." *Development* 48(1):19–24.

Gibbons, E. 2014. "Climate Change, Children's Rights, and the Pursuit of Intergenerational Climate Justice." *Health and Human Rights Journal* 16(1):19–31.

Hall, M. 2014. "Advancing Climate Justice and the Right to Health through Procedural Rights." *Health and Human Rights Journal* 16(1):8–18.

Human Rights Council. 2009. "Human Rights and Climate Change." UN Resolution 10/4. A_HRC_RES_10_4. 10th sess. http://ap.ohchr.org/documents/E/HRC/resolutions/A_HRC_RES_10_4.pdf

Hunt, P. 2008. Foreword to H. Potts, *Participation and the Right to the Highest Attainable Standard of Health.* Colchester: Human Rights Centre, Essex University.

Hunt, P., and G. Backman. 2008. "Health Systems and the Right to the Highest Attainable Standard of Health." *Health and Human Rights* 10(1):81–92.

Hunt, P., and R. Khosla. 2010. "Climate Change and the Right to the Highest Attainable Standard of Health." In *Human Rights and Climate Change*, edited by S. Humphreys, 238–57. Cambridge: Cambridge University Press.

Jones, R., H. Bennett, G. Keating, and A. Blaiklock. 2014. "Climate Change and the Right to Health for Māori in Aotearoa/New Zealand." *Health and Human Rights Journal* 16(1): 54–68.

Lemery, J., C. Williams, and P. Farmer. 2014. "Editorial: The Great Procrastination." *Health and Human Rights Journal* 16(1):1–3.

McAllister, L., A. Magee, and B. Hale. 2014. "Women, E-Waste, and Technological Solutions to Climate Change." *Health and Human Rights Journal* 16(1):166–78.

Robinson, M. 2014. Foreword to *Health and Human Rights Journal* 16(1):4–7.

Smith, K. R., A. Woodward, D. Campbell-Lendrum, D. D. Chadee, Y. Honda, Q. Liu, J. M. Olwoch, B. Revich, and R. Sauerborn. 2014. "Human Health: Impacts, Adaptation, and Co-Benefits." In *Climate Change 2014: Impacts, Adaptation, and Vulnerability. Part A: Global and Sectoral Aspects. Contribution of Working Group II to the Fifth Assessment Report of the Intergovernmental Panel of Climate Change*, edited by C. B. Field, V. R. Barros, D. J. Dokken, K. J. Mach, M. D. Mastrandrea, T. E. Bilir, M. Chatterjee, et al., 709–54. Cambridge: Cambridge University Press.

UN Committee on Economic, Social and Cultural Rights. 2000. "General Comment No. 14: The Right to the Highest Attainable Standard of Health." E/C.12/2000/4. United Nations.

UN Committee on the Rights of the Child. 2013. "General Comment No. 15." CRC/C/GC/15. United Nations.

UN General Assembly. 1948. "Universal Declaration of Human Rights." 217A(111). http://www.refword.org/docid/3ae6b3712c.html

Williams, C., T. Ashton, and C. Bullen. 2014. "Using Health Rights to Design Aid-Funded Health Programs So They First Do No Harm." *Human Rights Quarterly* 36:428–46.

World Health Organization. 2007. *Everybody's Business: Strengthening Health Systems to Improve Health Outcomes. WHO's Framework for Action.* Geneva: World Health Organization.

World Health Organization. 2014. "Climate Change and Health." Fact sheet 266. Geneva: WHO.

Yamin, A. E. 2014. "Editorial: Promoting Equity in Health: What Role for Courts?" *Health and Human Rights Journal* 16(2):1–9.

Yamin, A. E., and R. Cantor. 2014. "Between Insurrectional Discourse and Operational Guidance: Challenges and Dilemmas in Implementing Human Rights-Based Approaches to Health." *Journal of Human Rights Practice* 6:451–85.

1